GETTING TO ZERO ALCOHOL-IMPAIRED DRIVING FATALITIES

A Comprehensive Approach to a Persistent Problem

Steven M. Teutsch, Amy Geller, and Yamrot Negussie, *Editors*

Committee on Accelerating Progress to Reduce Alcohol-Impaired Driving Fatalities

Board on Population Health and Public Health Practice

Health and Medicine Division

A Consensus Study Report of

The National Academies of
SCIENCES • ENGINEERING • MEDICINE

THE NATIONAL ACADEMIES PRESS
Washington, DC
www.nap.edu

THE NATIONAL ACADEMIES PRESS 500 Fifth Street, NW Washington, DC 20001

This project was supported by the National Highway Traffic Safety Administration (Contract No. 10002951). Any opinions, findings, conclusions, or recommendations expressed in this publication do not necessarily reflect the views of any organization or agency that provided support for the project.

International Standard Book Number-13: 978-0-309-46826-8
International Standard Book Number-10: 0-309-46826-4
Digital Object Identifier: https://doi.org/10.17226/24951
Library of Congress Control Number: 2018932638

Additional copies of this publication are available for sale from the National Academies Press, 500 Fifth Street, NW, Keck 360, Washington, DC 20001; (800) 624-6242 or (202) 334-3313; http://www.nap.edu.

Printed in the United States of America

Suggested citation: National Academies of Sciences, Engineering, and Medicine. 2018. *Getting to zero alcohol-impaired driving fatalities: A comprehensive approach to a persistent problem*. Washington, DC: The National Academies Press. doi: https://doi.org/10.17226/24951.

The National Academies of
SCIENCES • ENGINEERING • MEDICINE

The **National Academy of Sciences** was established in 1863 by an Act of Congress, signed by President Lincoln, as a private, nongovernmental institution to advise the nation on issues related to science and technology. Members are elected by their peers for outstanding contributions to research. Dr. Marcia McNutt is president.

The **National Academy of Engineering** was established in 1964 under the charter of the National Academy of Sciences to bring the practices of engineering to advising the nation. Members are elected by their peers for extraordinary contributions to engineering. Dr. C. D. Mote, Jr., is president.

The **National Academy of Medicine** (formerly the Institute of Medicine) was established in 1970 under the charter of the National Academy of Sciences to advise the nation on medical and health issues. Members are elected by their peers for distinguished contributions to medicine and health. Dr. Victor J. Dzau is president.

The three Academies work together as the **National Academies of Sciences, Engineering, and Medicine** to provide independent, objective analysis and advice to the nation and conduct other activities to solve complex problems and inform public policy decisions. The National Academies also encourage education and research, recognize outstanding contributions to knowledge, and increase public understanding in matters of science, engineering, and medicine.

Learn more about the National Academies of Sciences, Engineering, and Medicine at **www.nationalacademies.org.**

The National Academies of
SCIENCES • ENGINEERING • MEDICINE

Consensus Study Reports published by the National Academies of Sciences, Engineering, and Medicine document the evidence-based consensus on the study's statement of task by an authoring committee of experts. Reports typically include findings, conclusions, and recommendations based on information gathered by the committee and the committee's deliberations. Each report has been subjected to a rigorous and independent peer-review process and it represents the position of the National Academies on the statement of task.

Proceedings published by the National Academies of Sciences, Engineering, and Medicine chronicle the presentations and discussions at a workshop, symposium, or other event convened by the National Academies. The statements and opinions contained in proceedings are those of the participants and are not endorsed by other participants, the planning committee, or the National Academies.

For information about other products and activities of the National Academies, please visit www.nationalacademies.org/about/whatwedo.

COMMITTEE ON ACCELERATING PROGRESS TO REDUCE ALCOHOL-IMPAIRED DRIVING FATALITIES

STEVEN M. TEUTSCH (*Chair*), Adjunct Professor, University of California, Los Angeles, Fielding School of Public Health; Senior Fellow, Public Health Institute; Senior Fellow, Leonard D. Schaeffer Center for Health Policy and Economics, University of Southern California

JULIE A. BALDWIN, Professor, Department of Health Sciences, Director, Center for Health Equity Research, Northern Arizona University

LINDA C. DEGUTIS, Executive Director, Defense Health Horizons, Henry M. Jackson Foundation; Adjunct Professor, Rollins School of Public Health, Emory University

MUCIO KIT DELGADO, Assistant Professor of Emergency Medicine and Epidemiology, Perelman School of Medicine, University of Pennsylvania

DAVID H. JERNIGAN, Associate Professor, Department of Health, Behavior and Society, Bloomberg School of Public Health, Johns Hopkins University

KATHERINE KEYES, Associate Professor of Epidemiology, Mailman School of Public Health, Columbia University

RICARDO MARTINEZ, Chief Medical Officer, Adeptus Health; Assistant Professor of Emergency Medicine, School of Medicine, Emory University

TIMOTHY S. NAIMI, Associate Professor of Medicine, School of Medicine, School of Public Health, Boston University; Clinician-Investigator, Section of General Internal Medicine, Boston Medical Center

JEFF NIEDERDEPPE, Associate Professor, Department of Communication, Cornell University

CHARLES P. O'BRIEN, Kenneth Appel Professor and Founding Director, Center for Studies of Addiction, University of Pennsylvania

JODY L. SINDELAR, Professor, Public Health (Policy) and Economics, School of Public Health, Yale University

JOANNE E. THOMKA, Program Counsel, National Association of Attorneys General

DOUGLAS WIEBE, Associate Professor of Epidemiology, Department of Biostatistics, Epidemiology, and Informatics, University of Pennsylvania

Study Staff

AMY GELLER, Study Director
YAMROT NEGUSSIE, Research Associate
AIMEE MEAD, Research Associate (from June 2017)
SOPHIE YANG, Research Assistant (from June 2017)
MARJORIE PICHON, Senior Program Assistant (until September 2017)
JENNIFER COHEN, Program Officer (July 2017–January 2018)
HOPE HARE, Administrative Assistant
MISRAK DABI, Financial Associate
BERNARDO KLEINER, Associate Division Director, Transportation Research Board
ROSE MARIE MARTINEZ, Senior Board Director, Board on Population Health and Public Health Practice

Reviewers

This Consensus Study Report was reviewed in draft form by individuals chosen for their diverse perspectives and technical expertise. The purpose of this independent review is to provide candid and critical comments that will assist the National Academies of Sciences, Engineering, and Medicine in making each published report as sound as possible and to ensure that it meets the institutional standards for quality, objectivity, evidence, and responsiveness to the study charge. The review comments and draft manuscript remain confidential to protect the integrity of the deliberative process.

We thank the following individuals for their review of this report:

KRISTINE M. GEBBIE, Torrens Resilience Institute, Flinders University
NORMAN GIESBRECHT, Institute for Mental Health Policy Research, Centre for Addiction and Mental Health
RALPH HINGSON, National Institute on Alcohol Abuse and Alcoholism, National Institutes of Health
ANNE McCARTT, formerly with Insurance Institute for Highway Safety
SCOTT C. RATZAN, AB InBev Foundation
EDUARDO ROMANO, Pacific Institute for Research and Evaluation
RUTH SHULTS, Centers for Disease Control and Prevention
MICHAEL D. SLATER, The Ohio State University

FRANK A. SLOAN, Duke University
GORDON SMITH, West Virginia University
SRINIVASAN SUNDARARAJAN, Ford Motor Company
STEPHEN K. TALPINS, Rumberger Kirk & Caldwell and National Partnership on Alcohol Misuse and Crime
LAWRENCE WALLACK, Portland State University

Although the reviewers listed above provided many constructive comments and suggestions, they were not asked to endorse the conclusions or recommendations of this report nor did they see the final draft before its release. The review of this report was overseen by **ROBERT B. WALLACE,** The University of Iowa, and **RICHARD J. BONNIE,** University of Virginia. They were responsible for making certain that an independent examination of this report was carried out in accordance with the standards of the National Academies and that all review comments were carefully considered. Responsibility for the final content rests entirely with the authoring committee and the National Academies.

Acknowledgments

The Committee on Accelerating Progress to Reduce Alcohol-Impaired Driving Fatalities wishes to acknowledge the many people whose contributions and support made this report possible. The committee benefited from presentations made by a number of experts. The following individuals shared their research, experience, and perspectives with the committee: Nadia Anderson, Douglas Beirness, Nancy Bill, Jessica Cicchino, Phillip Cook, James C. Fell, Debra Furr-Holden, Jacqueline Gillan, Thomas Greenfield, J. T. Griffin, Frank Harris, Ralph Hingson, Tara Kelley-Baker, Bill Kerr, Russ Martin, Jim McDonnell, Jeff Michael, Keith Nothacker, M. J. Paschall, Francesca Polletta, Rebecca Ramirez, Craig Reinarman, Lawrence Robertson, Steve Schmidt, Clint Shrum, Brooke Stringer, Steve Taylor, Anne Teigen, Nick Van Dyke, Robert Voas, Diane Wigle, and Thomas Woodward.

The following individuals were important sources of information, generously giving their time and knowledge to further the committee's efforts: Thomas F. Babor, Charles DiMaggio, Lori Dorfman, Deborah Fisher, Adnan Hyder, Jonathan Noel, Jamie Oliver, Katherine Robaina, Robert Strassburger, Andres Vecino-Ortiz, and Katherine Wheeler-Martin.

The committee is thankful to the study staff for their support of this study: Amy Geller, Yamrot Negussie, Aimee Mead, Sophie Yang, Marjorie Pichon, Jennifer Cohen, Bernardo Kleiner, and Rose Marie Martinez. The committee also acknowledges the support of other National Academies of Sciences, Engineering, and Medicine staff, especially Daniel Bearss, Clyde Behney, Misrak Dabi, Iliana Espinal, Chelsea Frakes, Greta Gorman,

Hope Hare, Nicole Joy, Sarah Kelley, Ellen Kimmel, Dana Korsen, Rebecca Morgan, Tina Ritter, Doris Romero, Barbara Schlein, Lauren Shern, Elizabeth Tyson, and Taryn Young.

The committee also benefited from past National Academies studies relevant to this report, particularly the 2004 report *Reducing Underage Drinking: A Collective Responsibility*.

Finally, funding for this project was provided by the National Highway Traffic Safety Administration. The committee extends special thanks for that support.

Contents

Acronyms and Abbreviations

AASHTO	American Association of State Highway and Transportation Officials
ABI	American Beverage Institute
ABV	alcohol by volume
ACEP	American College of Emergency Physicians
ACTS	Automotive Coalition for Traffic Safety
AHA	American Hospital Association
AI/AN	American Indian/Alaska Native
AIS	Abbreviated Injury Scale
ALR	administrative license revocation
ALS	administrative license suspension
AMERSA	Association for Medical Education and Research in Substance Abuse
APIS	Alcohol Policy Information System
ASSIST	American Stop Smoking Intervention Study
AUD	alcohol use disorder
BAC	blood alcohol concentration/content
BrAC	breath alcohol concentration
BRFSS	Behavioral Risk Factor Surveillance System
CADCA	Community Anti-Drug Coalitions of America
CBA	cost-benefit analysis
CBT	cognitive behavioral therapy

CDC	Centers for Disease Control and Prevention
CEA	cost-effectiveness analysis
CI	confidence interval
CIREN	Crash Injury Research and Engineering Network
CODES	Crash Outcome Data Evaluation System
CPSTF	Community Preventive Services Task Force
CVD	cardiovascular disease
DADSS	Driver Alcohol Detection System for Safety
DMV	Department of Motor Vehicles
DOT	Department of Transportation
DUI	driving under the influence
DWI	driving while impaired
ED	emergency department
EMS	emergency medical services
ESV	Enhanced Safety of Vehicles
FARS	Fatality Analysis Reporting System
FAST	Fixing America's Surface Transportation
FBI	Federal Bureau of Investigation
FDA	Food and Drug Administration
FHWA	Federal Highway Administration
FMCSA	Federal Motor Carrier Safety Administration
FY	fiscal year
GHSA	Governors Highway Safety Association
GIS	geographic information system
HVMT	highway vehicle miles traveled
IIHS	Insurance Institute for Highway Safety
ITE	Institute of Transportation Engineers
MADD	Mothers Against Drunk Driving
MAP-21	Moving Ahead for Progress in the 21st Century Act
MLDA	minimum legal drinking age
NCSA	National Center for Statistics and Analysis
NCSL	National Conference of State Legislators
NEISS	National Electronic Injury Surveillance System
NESARC	National Epidemiologic Survey on Alcohol-Related Conditions

NHTS	National Household Travel Survey
NHTSA	National Highway Traffic Safety Administration
NIAAA	National Institute on Alcohol Abuse and Alcoholism
NIBRS	National Incident-Based Reporting System
NRS	National Roadside Survey of Alcohol and Drug Use by Drivers
NSC	National Safety Council
NSDUH	National Survey on Drug Use and Health
NTDB	National Trauma Data Bank
NTSB	National Transportation Safety Board
NTX	Naltrexone
OECD	Organisation for Economic Co-operation and Development
OR	odds ratio
PAHO	Pan American Health Organization
PAR	police accident report
PAS	passive alcohol sensor
PBT	preliminary breath test
POLD	place of last drink
RBS	responsible beverage service
RID	Remove Intoxicated Drivers
ROADS SAFE	Research of Alcohol Detection Systems for Stopping Alcohol-Related Fatalities Everywhere
RR	relative risk
SAMHSA	Substance Abuse and Mental Health Services Administration
SBIRT	screening, brief intervention, and referral to treatment
SCC	Safe Communities Coalition
SDLP	standard deviation of lane position
SDOH	social determinants of health
SDS	State Data System
SDSP	standard deviation of speed
SES	socioeconomic status
SFST	standardized field sobriety test
SHS	secondhand smoke
SIP	sales to intoxicated persons
STRADA	Swedish Traffic Accident Data Acquisition

TAC	transdermal alcohol content
UCR	Uniform Crime Reporting System
UPPL	Uniform Accident and Sickness Policy Provision Law
V2I	vehicle to infrastructure
V2V	vehicle to vehicle
VMT	vehicle miles traveled
WHO	World Health Organization
WISQARS	Web-based Injury Statistics Query and Reporting System
YRBSS	Youth Risk Behavior Surveillance System

Glossary

Alcohol-impaired driving crash/fatality—In all U.S. states[1] drivers are considered legally impaired to drive when their blood alcohol concentration (BAC) is greater than or equal to 0.08 grams per deciliter (g/dL, often expressed as %, as in 0.08%).[2] Thus, in the United States, any crash involving one or more drivers with a BAC of 0.08% or higher is typically referred to by the National Highway Traffic Safety Administration (NHTSA) as an alcohol-impaired driving crash, and fatalities stemming from those crashes are defined as being alcohol-impaired driving crash fatalities. Of note, however, is that impairment begins below 0.08%, so this is an underestimate relative to all crash fatalities in which impairment from alcohol may have contributed.[3]

Alcohol-related crash/fatality—A crash or a fatality from a crash that involves one or more drivers of a motor vehicle with any alcohol in their system (i.e., a BAC greater than 0.00%). This term also subsumes alcohol-impaired driving crashes. It is a useful umbrella term for all motor vehicle

[1] Utah recently passed legislation to lower the BAC law to 0.05% beginning in December 2018.

[2] States may have lower BAC laws for individuals under the minimum legal drinking age of 21 and for commercial drivers.

[3] Of note, a crash involving a nonimpaired motor vehicle driver and an impaired pedestrian or cyclist is not counted as an alcohol-impaired motor vehicle crash by NHTSA's Fatality Analysis Reporting System, which collects information about all motor vehicle crash fatalities occurring on U.S. public roadways.

crashes that involve any alcohol. Some have also used the term *alcohol-involved* to convey the same idea.

Alcohol use disorder (AUD)—The current *Diagnostic and Statistical Manual of Mental Disorders* (DSM-5) combines previously separate disorders (alcohol abuse and alcohol dependence) into one alcohol use disorder with a continuum of mild, moderate, and severe subclassifications. A patient is diagnosed with AUD if he or she displays 2 of the 11 symptoms during a 12-month period; the subclassifications are based on the number of symptoms the patient has (mild AUD = 2 or 3 of the symptoms, moderate AUD = 4 or 5 symptoms, and severe AUD = 6 or more symptoms).

Binge drinking—Used to connote drinking at or above levels during a drinking occasion/episode that typically results in impairment-level BAC (i.e., ≥0.08%) for most men and women drinking at typical drinking rates. This corresponds to drinking five or more drinks for men and four or more drinks for women in about 2 hours. Most public health and epidemiologic studies use five/four thresholds, and members of the general public interpret the term *binge drinking* to mean drinking to the point of impairment or intoxication.

Blood alcohol concentration/content (BAC)—The percentage (%) of ethanol in the blood, based on the mass of alcohol per mass of blood. For instance, a BAC of 0.10 (0.10%, or one-tenth of 1 percent) means that there are 0.10 grams of alcohol for every deciliter (100 ml) of blood. Blood alcohol concentrations can also be derived from breath tests or transcutaneous monitors. This is sometimes expressed in milligrams per deciliter, in which case a BAC of 0.1% is expressed as 100 mg/dL.

Driver—Refers to the operator of any motor vehicle, including a motorcycle or motorboat. For surveillance purposes (e.g., NHTSA), this is usually restricted to motor vehicles operating on land, meaning motor vehicles, including motorcycles and related vehicles, operating on public roadways.

Driving under the influence (DUI), driving while impaired (DWI)—These are legal terms that refer to operating a motor vehicle while one's blood alcohol concentration is above the limit set by state law, or on the basis of field sobriety tests or observed behavior. Colloquial terms for DUI and DWI include

> **Drink-driving**—Refers to driving or operating a motor vehicle while impaired or while one's blood alcohol concentration is above the limit set by law (more commonly used in the United Kingdom).

Drunk driving crash/fatality—Widely used and recognized, and generally refers to driving or crashes or fatalities that are related to alcohol impairment (in most U.S. states based on BAC levels ≥ 0.08%; see footnote 1).

Impairment—Refers to the deterioration of an individual's judgment and/or physical ability. Physiological and cognitive impairment begin at BAC levels below those that are associated with intoxication. As a legal standard, impairment and DWI laws are based on a person's physical or mental impairment as judged on the basis of BAC level, performance in standardized field sobriety tests, or observed behavior. Although this report is focused on impairment from alcohol, impairment can result from other substance use, distracted driving, and other reasons.

Intoxication—Refers to the condition of having physical or mental control markedly diminished by the effects of alcohol or drugs. This is usually based on a subjective determination (one feels the sensation, or observes a behavior in another person). Physiological impairment begins at BAC levels below those that are associated with intoxication. Intoxication is not a legal standard.

Motor vehicle crash fatality—NHTSA defines a motor vehicle crash fatality as one that (1) involves at least one motor vehicle (e.g., car, motorcycle); (2) results in the death of a driver, passenger, cyclist, pedestrian, or occupant of a vehicle in transit within 30 days of the crash; and (3) occurs on a public U.S. roadway.

Per se laws—Per se laws in DUI or DWI cases generally establish that once an individual is shown to have a BAC at or above a certain limit (e.g., 0.08%) that person will be considered impaired by law. In such circumstances, no further evidence of intoxication or impairment need be demonstrated for the purpose of a DUI case. Currently, all states have per se DUI laws.

U.S. standard drink—In the United States, a standard drink is 14 grams or 0.6 ounces of pure ethanol (a weight-based measure). This is the amount of ethanol in 12 ounces of 5 percent alcohol-by-volume (ABV) beer, 5 ounces of 12 percent ABV wine, or 1.5 ounces of 40 percent ABV distilled spirits (40 percent ABV, or 80 proof, is the concentration in most brands of whiskey, vodka, rum, gin, etc.).

Preface

More than 10,000 people are killed in the United States each year from alcohol-impaired driving, and that number is on the rise. After decades of progress, the number of alcohol-impaired driving deaths first stagnated and is now actually increasing. Alcohol-impaired driving remains the greatest single cause of motor vehicle fatalities, significantly exceeding the number of deaths from distracted driving and drugged driving. Passengers, pedestrians, cyclists, and occupants of other vehicles—who make up almost 40 percent of alcohol-impaired driving fatalities[1]—are secondhand victims, and their fatalities are just as intolerable as those of the victims of cigarette secondhand smoke. For each death, hundreds more are injured or disabled.

Our apathy toward 29 alcohol-impaired driving deaths per day is unacceptable, particularly because these tragic events can be prevented. This report describes how this can be accomplished with the tools already at our disposal and on the near-term horizon. By marshalling real-time, comprehensive data and the collective action of all the relevant stakeholders, we can make step-by-step progress toward eliminating these needless deaths and injuries. Vision Zero—the framework for eliminating motor vehicle deaths—provides the road map. Policy makers can enact and implement evidence-based policies, the clinical care system can identify and manage those at risk, the enforcement and legal systems can

[1] NCSA (National Center for Statistics and Analysis). 2016. Alcohol-impaired driving: 2015 data. DOT HS 812 350. Washington, DC: National Highway Traffic Safety Administration.

identify and manage offenders, the alcohol beverage industry can support and implement effective actions grounded in evidence and take steps to reduce harmful drinking, engineers and the private sector can partner to develop and incorporate effective technologies into vehicles and devices, government agencies can provide the leadership and research to enact and enforce policies to reinvigorate progress, and the public can advocate for effective actions. These collaborations can establish processes for the actions that need to be taken, determine the entities primarily responsible, assess progress toward implementation, and develop mechanisms to identify problems, investigate them, and take effective action. As some Organisation for Economic Co-operation and Development nations have demonstrated, alcohol-impaired driving deaths can be virtually eliminated. This report provides the science base to do so.

I want to extend my gratitude to the National Highway Traffic Safety Administration for stimulating and sponsoring this report. It is another step in its continued leadership in making our roadways safer. Thanks, too, to the committee, staff, and consultants for their creativity and energy in bringing this report to fruition.

Steven M. Teutsch, *Chair*
Committee on Accelerating Progress to Reduce
Alcohol-Impaired Driving Fatalities

Summary

ABSTRACT

Despite widespread public attention to distracted and drug-impaired driving in recent years, alcohol-impaired driving remains the deadliest and costliest danger on U.S. roads today. One person dies in an alcohol-impaired driving crash every 49 minutes. The causes of alcohol-impaired driving are complex and multifaceted, but these deaths are entirely preventable. This report offers a blueprint for solving the problem by identifying numerous evidence-based and promising policies, programs, and systems changes to accelerate national progress in reducing alcohol-impaired driving fatalities. The committee embraces a vision in which no alcohol-impaired driving deaths are acceptable—Vision Zero. Each alcohol-impaired driving crash represents a failure of the system—whether that is excessive alcohol service, poor road design, or lack of effective policies or enforcement—and is preventable with a coordinated, systematic approach across multiple sectors. This report offers interventions and actions to accelerate progress to reduce alcohol-impaired driving fatalities and offers concrete recommendations to galvanize stakeholder action.

The committee's recommendations include increasing alcohol excise taxes, lowering state per se laws for alcohol-impaired driving to 0.05% blood alcohol concentration (BAC), preventing illegal alcohol sales to underage persons and to already-intoxicated adults, strengthening regulation of alcohol marketing, and implementing policies to reduce the physical availability of alcohol. The report also emphasizes the need for enhanced enforcement, including sobriety checkpoints and the use of DWI courts. It describes the need for engineering solutions, such as ignition interlocks and the Driver Alcohol Detection System for Safety

(DADSS). This report underscores the value of comprehensive clinical interventions such as screening, brief intervention, and referral to treatment (SBIRT), as well as effective treatment for alcohol use disorders (AUDs) with medications and other evidence-based treatments.

The report also offers conclusions about what should be done to improve important existing interventions such as administrative license suspension/revocation laws; professional education for the judiciary, law enforcement, and health professionals; limits on diversion programs and plea agreements; and universal primary seatbelt laws. The committee suggests ways to ensure that these policies will have maximum impact—for instance, that the National Conference of State Legislatures update and develop model legislation for the effective policies identified in this report to give states benchmarks for progress.

The report also provides an overview of available data and surveillance systems and gaps and offers recommendations to provide a more comprehensive understanding of the problem of alcohol-impaired driving, identify the critical intervention points, and monitor the progress of interventions.

Taken together, the committee's recommendations have the potential to reinvigorate commitment and accelerate progress to eliminate deaths from alcohol-impaired driving. Many of these strategies are not new. However, systematically implementing these policies, programs, and systems changes would renew progress and save lives. The critical need is to revive public and policy-maker attention and resolve, and the report concludes by offering a variety of strategies to turn public concern into decisive action to address this tragic and preventable problem.

Alcohol-impaired driving remains the most deadly yet entirely preventable danger on U.S. roads today.[1] Alcohol-impaired driving fatalities have remained a fairly constant proportion of all traffic deaths since 2000. Each day 29 people in the United States die in an alcohol-impaired driving crash; that is one person every 49 minutes. Despite years of success, traffic deaths from all causes are on the rise in the United States for the third straight year, and crashes remain a leading killer and cause of disabling injuries. In 2016, 37,461 people died from traffic crashes, an increase of 5.6 percent from 2015. In 2016, alcohol-impaired driving fatalities accounted for 28 percent of traffic deaths—the largest percentage of all traffic fatalities—with a total of 10,497 lives lost, a 1.7 percent increase from 2015. In comparison, distracted driving accounted for 9 percent of traffic deaths, with a total of 3,450 deaths in 2016. These data create a growing sense of urgency to reverse the current trend and improve the safety of communities, decrease associated health care costs, and save lives. (See Box S-1 for key alcohol-impaired driving facts and Figure S-1 for trends in alcohol-impaired driving fatalities over time.)

[1] All references and sources can be found in the report chapters.

BOX S-1
Key Facts About Alcohol-Impaired Driving

- Each day 29 people in the United States die in an alcohol-impaired driving crash; that is one person every 49 minutes.
- On average since 1982, one-third of all traffic fatalities were alcohol-impaired driving fatalities with more than 10,400 people killed in 2016.
- Almost 40 percent of alcohol-impaired driving fatalities are victims other than the drinking driver.
- 214 children aged 14 years or younger were killed in alcohol-impaired driving crashes in 2016.
- Rural areas are disproportionally affected by alcohol-impaired driving crashes and fatalities.
- The total economic cost of alcohol-impaired driving crashes was $121.5 billion in 2010 (including medical costs, earnings losses, productivity losses, legal costs, and vehicle damage).

Alcohol-impaired driving is a growing public health problem that transcends the transportation, law enforcement, and clinical care systems. Despite its persistent nature, the problem is not intractable. There are many existing evidence-based and promising strategies to address alcohol-impaired driving; however, a coordinated, multilevel approach across multiple sectors will be required to accelerate change. This report presents these interventions and opportunities.

To accelerate progress to reduce alcohol-impaired driving fatalities, the National Highway Traffic Safety Administration (NHTSA) asked the Health and Medicine Division of the National Academies of Sciences, Engineering, and Medicine to help identify promising interventions to reduce the fatalities caused by alcohol-impaired driving in the United States to be implemented over the next 30 to 40 years (the full charge to the committee is provided in Box S-2).

Successful past efforts to reduce alcohol-impaired driving are well recognized. In the early 1980s alcohol-impaired driving rose to the forefront of the public's attention. Attitudes toward drinking and driving shifted as groups such as Mothers Against Drunk Driving (MADD) began opening chapters across the country and sharing victims' experiences with policy makers. From the 1980s through the early 2000s alcohol-related fatalities steadily decreased as numerous new laws were passed that helped decrease alcohol-impaired driving, including laws making it illegal to purchase alcohol under the age of 21, or to drive with a BAC of 0.10% or greater. Other alcohol-impaired driving laws increased the

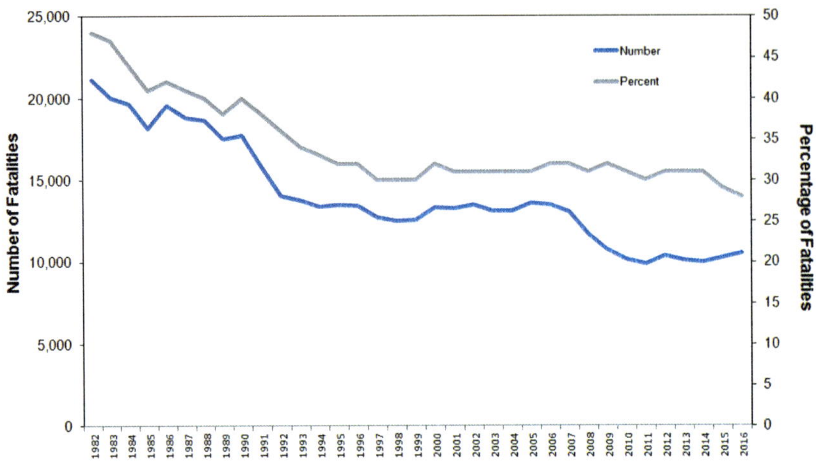

FIGURE S-1 Number of alcohol-impaired driving fatalities and percentage of all traffic fatalities in the United States, 1982–2016.

authority of law enforcement, allowing them to conduct sobriety checkpoints and to revoke a driver's license. Fell and Voas estimated that from 1982 to 2001 these actions saved more than 300,000 lives.

Although much progress has been made as states passed and implemented policies, these heterogeneous policies lacked benchmarks and

---

BOX S-2
Statement of Task for the Committee on Accelerating Progress to Reduce Alcohol-Impaired Driving Fatalities

The National Highway Traffic Safety Administration requests that the Health and Medicine Division of the National Academies of Sciences, Engineering, and Medicine convene a committee to examine

- which interventions (programs, systems, and policies) are most promising to prevent injuries and deaths from alcohol-impaired driving;
- the barriers to action and approaches to overcome them; and
- which interventions need to be changed or adopted.

In conducting its work, the committee may consider interventions implemented by other countries. The committee's recommendations will be broad reaching and serve as a blueprint for the nation to accelerate the progress in reducing alcohol-impaired driving fatalities.

---

have been enforced with varying intensity. Progress has stagnated and even reversed. The plateauing fatality rates indicate that what has been done to decrease deaths from alcohol-impaired driving has been working but is no longer sufficient. Changes that call on contributions from the transportation, law enforcement, clinical care systems, and others are needed to accelerate progress and save more lives.

Conclusion 1-1: Alcohol-impaired driving is a complex preventable public health problem that requires a comprehensive and collaborative multisector approach.

ABOUT THIS REPORT

The Committee's Approach

While recognizing that alcohol-impaired driving is a crime, and enforcement and criminal justice approaches are critically important, the committee took a holistic public health approach. The committee's approach is focused on population-level strategies aimed at providing the maximum benefit at the population level. This includes understanding the problem based on available data and surveillance, identifying risk and protective factors, reviewing the evidence for interventions, implementing interventions that will likely have the largest public health impact, and monitoring progress. A public health approach allows for exploration of the complex intersections of social, cultural, political, economic, legal, and systems-level influences on health and safety. There are often inherent tensions that exist between control measures to protect the public's health and civil/personal liberties. Reducing alcohol-impaired driving injuries and fatalities is difficult to separate from the broader public health rationale for reducing excessive alcohol consumption since drinking is the precursor for alcohol-impaired driving. In particular, while recognizing that many people enjoy alcohol responsibly, the committee believes that the evidence shows that placing some limits on the alcohol environment is warranted by the public health and safety benefits of decreasing alcohol-related driving deaths.

Conceptual Framework for Preventing Alcohol-Impaired Driving Fatalities

Traditional approaches to preventive countermeasures for motor vehicle crashes are categorized as being implemented before the event, during the event, or after the event—each point represents opportunities to intervene.[2] There are many upstream or causal factors that may affect alcohol use and subsequent driving, but for the purpose of this report the committee primarily covers interventions directly related to the prevention of alcohol-impaired driving fatalities. This includes precrash interventions, such as alcohol policies that affect price, the physical availability of alcohol, and alcohol consumption, as well as alternative transportation and ridesharing options that may affect whether an impaired person chooses to drive. Figure S-2 illustrates the sequence of behaviors leading to an alcohol-impaired driving fatality, the potential intervention opportunities, and the important factors that shape the outcomes.

In each phase of the framework, the additional layer around the perimeter of the shapes (e.g., one layer around "drink to impairment," two around "drive impaired") signifies increased likelihood or risk of a negative outcome among the behaviors (squares) and increased severity in the outcomes (diamond shape). An individual can exit this sequence at any point; for example, a person may consume alcohol, but not to the level of impairment. Furthermore, there are individual risk factors that affect the likelihood of drinking to impairment (e.g., being a binge drinker or meeting the criteria for AUD) and driving while impaired (e.g., prior DWI, availability of a vehicle, or possession of a driver's license). In addition, driving while impaired does not always lead to a collision and an alcohol-impaired collision does not always result in an injury or fatality. These are *potential* outcomes of impaired driving, as indicated by the dashed lines leading up to them. The intervention opportunities interact with one another and target multiple levels (e.g., individual, interpersonal, institutional, community, and societal). The strategies, programs, policies, and systems within these intervention opportunities need to take into account the varied environmental contexts within which they will be implemented. There are several effective and important interventions that can prevent fatalities that are not reflected in the conceptual framework or this report (for example, the automobile manufacturing process and highway and road design).

Methodology

The literature on the effectiveness and applicability of interventions provides important information for assessing which interventions are

[2] One such approach is the use of the Haddon Matrix, which is commonly used in the injury field and looks at human, environmental, and vehicle factors before, during, and after a crash. The Haddon Matrix paradigm provides an important organization to the many inputs to address alcohol-impaired driving crashes, and the committee's conceptual framework grows from that approach.

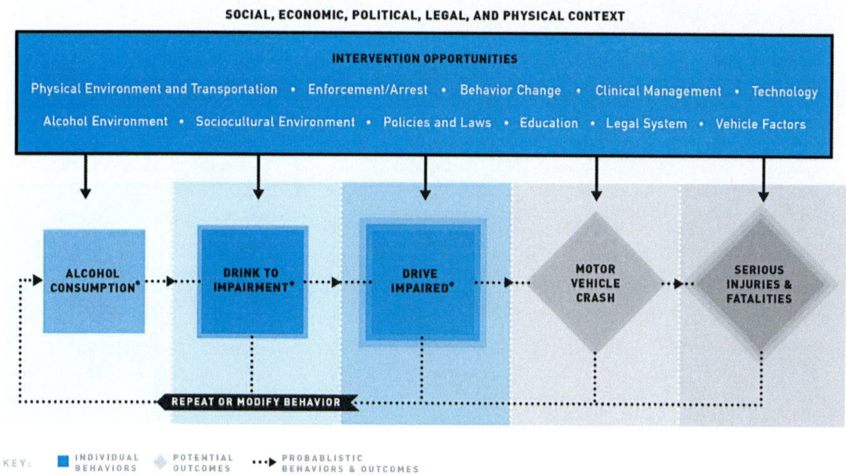

FIGURE S-2 Preventing alcohol-impaired driving fatalities conceptual framework.
NOTES: Each of the phases in this figure represents an opportunity to intervene and prevent alcohol-impaired driving fatalities. A square denotes a behavior, a diamond denotes an outcome, and dotted lines denote potential progression to an outcome. Extra layers around a square or a diamond denote increased likelihood or increased severity, respectively. The asterisks signify that there are alternative behaviors not represented in the first three phases that would preclude an alcohol-impaired driving fatality (e.g., not drinking or not drinking to the level of impairment).

most effective, cost-effective, and suitable for either a general or more specific population. Selection of interventions ought to be based on the extant literature; however, many interventions have not been adequately evaluated for general or specific effectiveness, or evaluated for effectiveness when brought to scale. In addition, comparisons of interventions are often incomplete and difficult to conduct because studies vary in dimensions such as the appropriateness of the study design and setting, outcomes measured, failure to consider other consequences, quality of execution, interactions with other interventions, and inclusion of economic consequences. With this in mind, the committee examined the available literature on alcohol-impaired driving interventions that target alcohol consumption, drinking to impairment, driving while impaired, and the postcrash and/or postarrest phase. The committee was not charged with undertaking a systematic review of the evidence, but rather to identify which interventions are most promising to prevent alcohol-impaired driving injuries and fatalities given the current state of knowledge and environment.

A Comprehensive Approach to Address Alcohol-Impaired Driving

There is no one-size-fits-all approach that will solve the problem of alcohol-impaired driving. For a problem this large and widespread a systematic population approach is needed. Therefore, the committee does not prioritize among its recommendations; while each state needs to take a comprehensive approach to addressing alcohol-impaired driving, the exact combination of interventions for particular states will vary. When identifying conclusions and recommendations, the committee focused on interventions that are evidence based, promising, and relevant in the current environment, or where improvements are needed to increase effectiveness. While many of the strategies outlined in this report are not new, systematically implementing these policies, programs, and systems changes would renew progress and save lives.

THE ROAD AHEAD

Vision Zero

NHTSA (the sponsor of this report), the Federal Motor Carrier Safety Administration, the Federal Highway Administration, and the National Safety Council launched the Road to Zero coalition in 2016 with the bold goal to end all traffic fatalities within 30 years. The Road to Zero is consistent with the goals of Vision Zero—a philosophical approach to road safety that was crafted in the 1990s and adopted in Sweden in 1997. Vision Zero, as a unifying philosophy, has expanded to other countries and can be expanded to address alcohol-impaired driving. Its principal aim is to eliminate all serious road traffic injuries and fatalities. This innovative approach transformed the traditional approach of transportation design in which the roadbuilders simply expected road users to use the road as designed. Vision Zero was a drastic change in approach and places the responsibility for traffic safety problems on the infrastructure system designers instead of only on the drivers. The framework centers on the idea that the design and structure of roads and cars should account and accommodate for individual mistakes and choices. Each alcohol-impaired fatality represents a system failure. This approach brings in new stakeholders and creates innovative partnerships where everyone has a role and an opportunity to contribute to the shared goals.

Achieving Vision Zero in the United States

Although still in its infancy in the United States, the Vision Zero concept continues to expand as it has been adopted by over two dozen American cities. However, there are many other variations of Vision Zero that exist in the United States (for example, the Vision Zero Network, Toward Zero Deaths, and Vision Zero Task Force). The Vision Zero philosophy is spreading across the country but in a disjointed and fragmented fashion, rather than as a coordinated approach.

Implementing Vision Zero as a U.S. policy to reduce alcohol-impaired driving injuries and fatalities would be a bold step, but it is important that partners beyond the transportation and transportation system design sector recognize that traffic safety deaths are preventable and acknowledge the need for a spectrum of partners to join efforts to implement systems change to address this public health crisis. These partners include government agencies, car manufacturers, auto insurers, advocacy organizations, state and local public health agencies, technology companies, health care systems, clinicians, employers, alcohol retailers, wholesale distributors, alcohol producers, the hospitality industry, and law enforcement. Importantly, the public itself can also directly participate in preventing alcohol-impaired driving through participation in Vision Zero.

Bold goals are important and can be used to galvanize action, change social norms, and bring stakeholders together around a common vision and goal. The committee recognizes that in an economic sense, eliminating all roadway fatalities would require investments that have diminishing returns and that there are important alternate uses of those resources; however, Vision Zero is not primarily an economic goal. It is about establishing an aspirational goal that can rally stakeholders, provide focus, and make substantial progress toward achieving that goal.

Key Terms

Box S-3 highlights key terms related to impairment used throughout the report. For the purpose of this report the term *alcohol-impaired driving* will be used, as will *DWI* (instead of *DUI* or similar). See the report glossary for definitions of other terms in this report. Discussion of what it means to be alcohol impaired follows.

What Is Alcohol Impairment?

The current legal definition of alcohol impairment in all 50 states is a BAC of 0.08% or higher.[3] Although this is the limit set by state law, impairment begins at lower levels; even small amounts of alcohol affect the brain. Biologically, alcohol impairment occurs before reaching a BAC of 0.08%, and impairment affects driving-related skills and behaviors.

---

[3] Utah recently passed legislation to lower the BAC law to 0.05% beginning in December 2018.

BOX S-3
Key Impairment Terms from the Glossary

Alcohol-impaired driving crash/fatality—In all U.S. states[a] drivers are considered legally impaired to drive when their BAC is greater than or equal to 0.08 grams per deciliter (g/dL, often expressed as %, as in 0.08%).[b] Thus, in the United States, any crash involving one or more drivers with a BAC of 0.08% or higher is typically referred to by NHTSA as an alcohol-impaired driving crash, and fatalities stemming from those crashes are defined as alcohol-impaired driving crash fatalities. Of note, however, is that impairment begins below 0.08%, so this is an underestimate relative to all crash fatalities in which impairment from alcohol may have contributed.[c]

Alcohol-related crash/fatality—A crash or a fatality from a crash that involves one or more drivers of a motor vehicle with any alcohol in their system (i.e., a BAC greater than 0.00%). This term also subsumes alcohol-impaired driving crashes. It is a useful umbrella term for all motor vehicle crashes that involve any alcohol. Some have also used the *alcohol-involved* term to convey the same idea.

Impairment—Refers to the deterioration of an individual's judgment and/or physical ability. Physiological and cognitive impairment begin at BAC levels below those that are associated with intoxication. As a legal standard, impairment and DWI laws are based on a person's physical or mental impairment as judged on the basis of BAC level, performance in standardized field sobriety tests, or observed behavior. Although this report is focused on impairment from alcohol, impairment can result from other substance use, distracted driving, and other reasons.

---

[a] Utah recently passed legislation to lower the BAC law to 0.05% beginning in December 2018.

[b] States may have lower BAC laws for individuals under the minimum legal drinking age of 21 and commercial drivers.

[c] Of note, a crash involving a nonimpaired motor vehicle driver and an impaired pedestrian or cyclist is not counted as an alcohol-impaired motor vehicle crash fatality by NHTSA's Fatality Analysis Reporting System, which collects information about all motor vehicle crash fatalities occurring on U.S. public roadways.

The effects of alcohol include psychomotor impairment, decreased inhibition, diminished alertness and sleepiness, confusion and problems with concentration, reduced visual focus, and slurred speech. Driving requires several complex skills, and alcohol affects the capacity to drive safely by impairing information processing and reaction time and compromising judgment and coordination.

Understanding Impairment

It can be difficult for individuals to understand what it means to be impaired. Individuals differ in their degree of impairment at a given BAC.

Several individual-level factors affect alcohol's physiological influence, including weight, age, sex, race, and ability to metabolize alcohol. In addition, alcohol content varies across beverage types and serving sizes differ among environments. Therefore a "drink" commonly contains more (or less) than 14 grams of pure alcohol. Alcoholic beverages themselves have changed significantly in the past 25 years. They are more affordable, of far greater variety, and more widely advertised and promoted than in earlier periods. In addition, inconsistent serving sizes and the combination of alcohol with caffeine and energy drinks, among other factors, undermine individuals' ability to estimate their level of impairment.

THE CURRENT ENVIRONMENT

It is important to understand the context in which alcohol-related fatalities occur, as noted in the committee's conceptual framework. There are two contexts that are especially salient and worth examining: the alcohol environment (e.g., social and cultural drinking norms, availability, pricing, and regulation) and the driving environment (e.g., road safety infrastructure, public transportation, and driving patterns). Especially noteworthy is the proximal relationship between binge drinking and alcohol-impaired driving.[4] There is a substantial body of evidence that indicates that binge drinking is strongly associated with alcohol-impaired driving.

> *Conclusion 2-2: Policies to reduce binge drinking are also protective against alcohol-impaired driving, and the adoption of a comprehensive set of effective interventions and population-based strategies that take advantage of synergies across interventions would further help to reduce binge drinking and related harms.*

The lack of a comprehensive population-based strategy may partly explain why the proportion of crash fatalities that are alcohol related has not declined in the last decade and has begun to increase.

---

[4] *Binge drinking* refers to drinking at or above levels during a drinking occasion/episode that typically results in impairment-level BAC (i.e., ≥0.08%) for most men and women drinking at typical drinking rates. This corresponds to drinking five or more drinks for men and four or more drinks for women in about 2 hours. Most public health and epidemiological studies use five/four thresholds, and members of the general public often interpret the term *binge drinking* to mean drinking to the point of impairment or intoxication.

ALCOHOL-IMPAIRED DRIVING INTERVENTIONS

The committee provides a suite of recommendations that when implemented together have the potential to save lives. Below and in the report, the recommendations are organized by the first four phases in the conceptual framework (alcohol consumption, drinking to impairment, driving while impaired, and postarrest and/or postcrash); they are then followed by recommendations on data and surveillance systems and for generating action. Because rural areas are disproportionately affected by alcohol-impaired driving crashes and fatalities, the report notes opportunities for this population throughout.

Interventions to Reduce Drinking to Impairment

Most interventions to reduce alcohol-impaired driving have focused on decreasing the likelihood that someone will drive after they are already impaired by alcohol. Conversely, less policy attention has been focused on reducing drinking to impairment before driving. However, there are a number of effective interventions to reduce drinking to the point of impairment (i.e., binge drinking), and some of these interventions have an independent effect on reducing impaired driving and alcohol-impaired crashes. Therefore, increasing adoption of interventions that have been proven to reduce excessive drinking is an important and underused strategy to reduce morbidity and mortality from alcohol-impaired driving.

Raising Alcohol Taxes

Alcohol taxes have perhaps the strongest and most consistent evidence base of any U.S. policy for reducing binge drinking, and strong direct evidence shows that higher alcohol taxes reduce alcohol-impaired driving and motor vehicle crash fatalities. For example, there is research suggesting that a doubling of alcohol taxes would lead to an 11 percent reduction in traffic crash deaths. Another study indicates that a 10 percent increase in alcohol price is associated with a 6 percent reduction in consumption. Despite this evidence, alcohol taxes have declined in inflation-adjusted terms at both federal and state levels. At present, alcohol taxes are considerably less than alcohol-related costs (such as health care, lost productivity, or criminal justice costs). Current federal plus state taxes do not cover alcohol-related costs, which are approximately \$2.00 per U.S. standard drink. Among states, the average excise tax is only \$0.03 per standard drink of beer, \$0.03 per standard drink of wine, and \$0.05 per standard drink of distilled spirits. Federal taxes are currently \$0.05 for a standard drink of beer, \$0.04 for a standard drink of wine, and $0.13 for a standard drink of distilled spirits. Given the efficacy of increased prices and taxes for reducing binge drinking and alcohol-related motor vehicle crash fatalities in particular, the committee recommends:

Recommendation 3-1: Federal and state governments should increase alcohol taxes significantly.

By "significantly," the committee means that alcohol taxes should be increased enough to have a meaningful impact on price and therefore on reducing alcohol-related crash fatalities. The increases should comprise a meaningful percent of the net-of-tax price (e.g., 30 percent or more) of alcohol products, and cover the marginal, external (i.e., secondhand) costs incurred by the sale of alcohol. Specific excise taxes may be preferred because it is the volume of ethanol that leads to impaired driving. However, volume-based excise taxes erode with inflation and therefore should be indexed to inflation. Ideally, taxes should be based on ethanol content rather than beverage type. Taxes can be earmarked to support alcohol-related activities (e.g., funding sobriety checkpoints or alcohol prevention and treatment programs), which may enhance public support.

Policies to Address Physical Availability of Alcohol

Addressing the physical availability of alcohol has strong evidence for reducing excessive drinking and related harms. Among these alcohol-related harms are alcohol-impaired driving and crashes, which have a strong link to excessive consumption.

Recommendation 3-2: State and local governments should take appropriate steps to limit or reduce alcohol availability, including restrictions on the number of on- and off-premises alcohol outlets, and the days and hours of alcohol sales.

In addition, states could consider reducing or eliminating alcohol sales concurrent with driving, such as sales at drive-through retailers or gas stations, as a common sense measure.

Policies to Reduce Illegal Sales of Alcohol and Strengthen Enforcement

To reduce excessive alcohol consumption prior to driving, at the population level, there is a need for a comprehensive set of policies that minimize the illegal sale of alcohol to underage persons and already intoxicated persons beyond the laws currently in place.[5]

Recommendation 3-3: Federal, state, and local governments should adopt and/or strengthen laws and dedicate enforcement resources to stop illegal alcohol sales (i.e., sales to already-intoxicated adults and sales to underage persons).

This includes having strong penalties for licensed retailers or purveyors who engage in illegal alcohol sales to already-intoxicated adults; having dram shop liability laws without caps;[6] high-quality, mandatory training in responsible beverage service for managers and sellers; having strong social host laws and other laws to limit adults from providing alcohol to underage persons; improving enforcement of minimum legal drinking age laws including passing laws to permit compliance checks using underage decoys and conducting those compliance checks; collection of data regarding place of last drink; and adequate enforcement personnel to enforce existing laws in this area.

Alcohol Advertising and Marketing

Given that young people are at higher risk of alcohol-impaired driving, that the evidence is substantial that they are influenced by alcohol marketing, and that numerous studies have found the alcohol industry's self-regulation of its marketing ineffective and insufficient because the voluntary standards are permissive and vague, not consistently followed, and without penalties for violations, the committee recommends:

Recommendation 3-4: Federal, state, and local governments should use their existing regulatory powers to strengthen and implement standards for permissible alcohol marketing content and placement across all media, establish consequences for violations, and promote and fund countermarketing campaigns.

Mass Media Campaigns

There is strong evidence based on findings from a variety of high-quality systematic reviews, across numerous health behavior domains, that large-scale media campaigns can promote meaningful changes in

[5] Underage persons are defined as individuals who are under 21 years old, the minimum legal age to purchase and possess alcohol in the United States.

[6] Dram shops are commercial establishments where alcoholic beverages are sold.

health behavior at the population level when implemented alongside broader, community-level interventions. The evidence is strongest for campaigns implemented alongside other community initiatives such as increased enforcement or community mobilization.

Conclusion 3-2: There is sufficient evidence to conclude that well-funded media campaigns are an important component of alcohol-impaired driving enforcement policy interventions to ensure their successful adoption and impact. Campaigns are more likely to be effective when rigorous formative research and behavioral change theories inform their design and dissemination.

Interventions to Reduce Driving While Impaired

There are several intervention opportunities for reducing alcohol-impaired driving, including changes in policies, laws, and enforcement; technological advances and vehicle features that could offer protections to drivers, occupants, and others; and programs or policies that could impact the sociocultural environment.

BAC Laws

BAC laws have been, and continue to be, a key intervention for reducing alcohol-impaired driving and reducing injuries and fatalities. Currently, in each state in the United States, drivers 21 years of age and older are prohibited from driving with a BAC greater than or equal to 0.08% (younger drivers have lower BAC requirements), which is the limit proscribed in state per se laws for alcohol-impaired drivers.[7] In December 2018, however, Utah will be the first state to lower the BAC per se law to 0.05%. Based on the available evidence from laboratory and epidemiological studies, the committee concludes that an individual's ability to operate a motor vehicle (including a motorcycle) begins to deteriorate at BAC levels well below 0.05%, increasing a driver's risk of being in a crash. Data from countries that have decreased their legal BAC to 0.05% suggest that this is an effective policy for reducing alcohol-impaired driving injuries and fatalities. The benefits of lowering BAC are on a continuum, but they are enhanced when introduced alongside high-visibility enforcement, sobriety checkpoints, and publicity. The committee concludes that reducing the BAC law to 0.05% is an effective strategy and has the greatest potential impact on those at the highest risk of alcohol-impaired traffic fatalities.

[7] A per se law means that the act in question is illegal in and of itself.

Recommendation 4-1: State governments should enact per se laws for alcohol-impaired driving at 0.05% blood alcohol concentration (BAC). The federal government should incentivize this change, and other stakeholders should assist in this process. The enactment of 0.05% per se laws should be accompanied by media campaigns and robust and visible enforcement efforts.

The effectiveness of this policy will be enabled by legislation that currently applies to 0.08% per se laws, including, but not limited to, use of sobriety checkpoints, administrative license revocation, and penalties for refusing preliminary breath tests or blood tests that are equal to or greater than penalties for alcohol-impaired driving offenses. This means that the same laws and sanctions that currently apply to 0.08% per se laws could remain in place but enforceable at the 0.05% BAC limit. Effectiveness will also be enhanced by efforts to publicize 0.05% per se laws through mass media campaigns, by strong and sustained enforcement efforts, and through the implementation and enforcement of laws and policies to prevent illegal alcohol sales to underage or intoxicated persons (e.g., underage compliance checks with alcohol licensees and dram shop liability laws).

Sobriety Checkpoints

Sobriety checkpoints are a high-visibility enforcement strategy that aims to identify and arrest alcohol-impaired drivers as well as increase the perceived risk of arrest to deter alcohol-impaired driving. There is strong evidence supporting the effectiveness of publicized sobriety checkpoint programs to reduce alcohol-impaired driving fatalities in both urban and rural areas. The ideal frequency of sobriety checkpoints needs further research. Low-staff checkpoints have been shown to be effective and are useful in rural areas, when resources for full-scale checkpoints are not available, and other circumstances.

Recommendation 4-2: States and localities should conduct frequent sobriety checkpoints in conjunction with widespread publicity to promote awareness of these enforcement initiatives.

Driver Alcohol Detection System for Safety

The DADSS program is a cooperative research partnership between NHTSA and the Automotive Coalition for Traffic Safety to develop non-invasive, in-vehicle technology that prevents drivers from operating vehicles when their BAC exceeds the limit set by state law. Given strong public support and endorsement from various sectors, as well as having significant potential impact for reducing alcohol-impaired driving fatalities, and to leverage advancements in technology for primary prevention of alcohol-impaired driving fatalities, the committee recommends:

Recommendation 4-3: When the Driver Alcohol Detection System for Safety (DADSS) is accurate and available for public use, auto insurers should provide policy discounts to stimulate the adoption of DADSS. Once the cost is on par with other existing automobile safety features and the technology is demonstrated to be accurate and effective, the National Highway Traffic Safety Administration should make DADSS mandatory in all new vehicles.

Alternative Transportation

Alternative transportation includes smartphone-enabled ridesharing, safe ride programs, and public transportation. These services provide intoxicated people with additional ways to avoid driving while impaired. Although the evidence is mixed or emerging for the various alternative transportation options, it is an area with great promise to reduce alcohol-impaired driving fatalities.

Recommendation 4-4: Municipalities should support policies and programs that increase the availability, convenience, affordability, and safety of transportation alternatives for drinkers who might otherwise drive. This includes permitting transportation network company ridesharing, enhancing public transportation options (especially during nighttime and weekend hours), and boosting or incentivizing transportation alternatives in rural areas.

Postarrest and Postcrash Interventions

While the two previous sets of recommendations are aimed at influencing behaviors such as drinking to impairment and driving while impaired, the following recommendations focus on reducing the potential negative outcomes of these behaviors: motor vehicle crashes and serious injuries and fatalities. There were more than 1 million arrests for driving under the influence in 2015. About 20 to 28 percent of first-time DWI offenders will repeat the offense, and recidivists are 62 percent more likely to be involved in a fatal crash.

Treatment Related to the Alcohol-Impaired Driving Adjudication Process

DWI courts are specialized courts aimed at changing DWI offenders' behavior through comprehensive monitoring and substance abuse treatment. As a part of the DWI control system, these postconviction courts are a systematic mechanism for holding offenders accountable for their actions while treating the underlying causes of their impaired driving. To ensure effective oversight for high-rate recidivists and/or high BAC offenders, the committee recommends:

Recommendation 5-1: Every state should implement DWI courts, guided by the evidence-based standards set by the National Center for DWI Courts, and all DWI courts should include available consultation or referral for evaluation by an addiction-trained clinician.

An arrest for DWI or admission to the hospital for an alcohol-impaired driving injury represents an opportunity to screen and treat individuals who engage in hazardous drinking. The offender should be evaluated by a clinician with addiction training and, if medically indicated, placed in a program that includes relapse prevention medication and requires an extended period of attendance in cognitive behavioral therapy.

Recommendation 5-2: All health care systems and health insurers should cover and facilitate effective evaluation, prevention, and treatment strategies for binge drinking and alcohol use disorders including screening, brief intervention, and referral to treatment (SBIRT), cognitive behavioral therapy, and medication-assisted therapy.

Ignition Interlock Devices

Strong evidence from the United States and other countries shows that individuals convicted of alcohol-impaired driving who have an ignition interlock installed on their vehicles are less likely than others to be rearrested for alcohol-impaired driving or to crash while the device is installed. This technology is affordable for many individuals, and it is made affordable for others through funds for low-income offenders. States that have introduced all-offender ignition interlock laws appear to have experienced reductions in alcohol-related motor vehicle crash deaths.

Recommendation 5-3: All states should enact all-offender ignition interlock laws to reduce alcohol-impaired driving fatalities. An ignition interlock should be required for all offenders with a blood alcohol concentration (BAC) above the limit set by state law. To increase effectiveness, states should consider increased monitoring periods based on the offender's BAC or past recidivism.

Evidence shows that a minimum monitoring period for interlock devices of 2 years is effective for a first offense, and 4 years is effective for a second offense.

Other promising interventions in the postcrash or postarrest phase include limits on diversion programs and plea agreements; education of professionals in law enforcement to improve identification of alcohol-impaired individuals; training for prosecutors and for judges on what constitutes impairment and the proper protocols for screening for AUD; more widely and systematically used administrative license suspension or revocation laws; systems alcohol monitoring programs; and a coordinated and continuous learning trauma care system.

Data and Surveillance Needs and Opportunities

There are a variety of datasets and surveillance systems that provide information on alcohol-impaired driving in the United States. These data systems each have their respective strengths and limitations, but examining them together allows a picture of the state of alcohol-impaired driving in the United States to emerge. Having a comprehensive understanding of alcohol-impaired driving, both in regard to the rates of occurrence, traffic crashes, injuries, fatalities, arrests, and convictions as well as qualitative data on when and why people drive impaired, is vital to create specific and targeted interventions. There are data gaps (such as lack of data on place of last drink), methodological issues (such as inconsistent data collection), and a lack of integration of datasets (e.g., how many people are arrested, outcomes of arrest, and long-term outcomes in terms of recidivism).

Conclusion 6-1: Data collection and reporting of high-risk intersections, outlets, drinking behaviors before driving, risk factors, and demographic trends are needed to measure, evaluate, and accelerate progress in reducing risk of fatalities. This evaluation would be facilitated by regular, systematic data collection on geocoded crash locations linked to data systems that monitor injury and fatality information, as well as criminal justice outcomes.

Recommendation 6-1: The National Highway Traffic Safety Administration should ensure that timely standardized data on alcohol-impaired driving, crashes, serious injuries, and fatalities are collected and accessible for evaluation, research, and strategic public dissemination; ensure that data from other government agencies and private organizations are included as needed; and explore the usefulness of big data for inclusion in alcohol-impaired driving information strategies.

Reducing alcohol-impaired driving requires diligent and accurate collection of surveillance data. Examples of improvements necessary for advancing the science include standardized data definitions, harmonization of reported data, and increased capacity for data linkages.

Recommendation 6-2: To facilitate surveillance of alcohol-impaired driving that is timely, ongoing, concise, and actionable, the National Highway Traffic Safety Administration should convene a diverse group of stakeholders that includes academic researchers, law enforcement, city and state public health, transportation sector, and other federal agency representation to create and maintain a metrics dashboard, and publish brief, visually appealing quarterly and annual national and state-by-state reports that analyze and interpret progress in reducing alcohol-impaired driving.

This recommendation entails identifying the data elements and data sources that are needed to monitor changes in rates of alcohol-impaired driving risk factors (including place of last drink), arrests, crashes, injuries, and fatalities, as well as data elements needed to inform quarterly metrics and reports designed to effectively communicate such findings to the public, various public and private stakeholders, and local, state, and national policy makers. In addition, this recommendation involves ensuring that data for research on the effectiveness of interventions to reduce alcohol-impaired driving are accessible and available using techniques that reflect contemporary standards for data acquisition and downloading. The dashboard, a user-friendly interface, should contain analyzed data, including longitudinal data linking crash data with licensing data, hospital data that include costs for care, arrest data, and the results of arrest. To be most effective, and to raise awareness of alcohol-impaired driving, the data should be strategically released to inculcate action.

GENERATING ACTION

To initiate and sustain action that will bolster progress to reduce alcohol-impaired driving fatalities, a strategic and comprehensive effort needs to be put forth nationwide. Such an effort requires the engagement of stakeholders across multiple sectors such as transportation, law enforcement, public health, the private sector, and philanthropy. Table S-1 (see page 24) summarizes the stakeholders who are needed to ensure implementation of the evidence-based and promising tools discussed throughout this report. Furthermore, initiating sustainable action will require garnering public will to address alcohol-impaired driving and allocating the resources needed to do so by creating and sustaining public discourse to underscore the magnitude of the problem and strategies to move these efforts forward. Chapter 7 highlights the key elements, approaches, innovations, and partnerships that could generate such action and overcome barriers.

The Role of Social Movements

The report examines the history of the alcohol-impaired driving social movement that took place in the 1980s, including the groundbreaking work of MADD. For an organization or movement to lift up the cause of alcohol-impaired driving as a social issue, it will likely need to be able to capture media attention. The role of funding from NHTSA in getting MADD off the ground, and the lessons it has for the ability of well-aimed seed funding to "sprout" results, provides a successful example of funding community-level demonstration projects to identify innovative solutions and tactics. Based on extensive evidence and experience in the use of community coalitions both in the alcohol field and in other areas of public health, the committee recommends:

Recommendation 7-3: The National Highway Traffic Safety Administration, other federal partners, and private funding sources free of conflicts of interest should support training, technical assistance, and demonstration projects in the implementation of effective strategies, including policy changes, for reducing alcohol-impaired driving.

Interagency Coordination

To ensure a comprehensive approach, input and collaboration from multiple sectors are needed. Specifically, coordination and cooperation across federal agencies will be an important element in making the best use of limited resources.

Recommendation 7-2: The National Highway Traffic Safety Administration should create a federal interagency coordinating committee to develop and oversee an integrated strategy for reducing alcohol-impaired driving, ensure collaboration, maintain accountability, and share information among organizations committed to reducing alcohol-impaired driving.

The coordinating body could include the U.S. Department of Health and Human Services (Centers for Disease Control and Prevention, Substance Abuse and Mental Health Services Administration, Indian Health Service, the National Institutes of Health), the Alcohol and Tobacco Tax and Trade Bureau, the U.S. Department of Transportation (National Highway Traffic Safety Administration, Federal Highway Administration), U.S. Homeland Security (emergency services sector), U.S. Department of Justice, U.S. Department of Defense, and U.S. Department of Veterans Affairs. The interagency group could convene other stakeholders such as private philanthropy, schools, hospitals, public health, health care, hospitality and the restaurant industry, payers, medical insurers, and trial lawyers to further maintain accountability and share information. At a minimum, such an approach would combine one or more coordinating centers providing training, technical assistance, and ongoing coaching with demonstration project sites in a diverse array of states and settings.

The Role of Alcohol Industry

Alcohol companies have taken on an active role in traffic safety and alcohol-impaired driving. However, they generally promote ineffective or non-evidence-based policies, and generally oppose effective population-based strategies to reduce binge drinking and impaired driving.

Conclusion 7-2: Alcohol companies and alcohol-related businesses could assist efforts to reduce alcohol-impaired driving fatalities by reducing the alcohol content of existing products, refraining from marketing including sponsorships that are likely to influence excessive alcohol use, and supporting or at least not opposing effective alcohol-impaired driving countermeasures.

Actions by the alcohol industry to support efforts to reduce alcohol-impaired driving could also include, at a minimum, adhering to and strengthening self-regulatory standards, sharing needed data on alcohol sales and consumption, and subjecting industry activities to reduce harmful use of alcohol to rigorous independent evaluations, free of conflicts of interest (i.e., employing evaluation design methods as robust as those of public health interventions).

Model Legislation

States implement different alcohol-impaired driving laws and policies, and when the same policies are in place in multiple states, there is considerable variation in how they are implemented. Given the lack of progress over the last decade in reducing alcohol-impaired fatalities, a more uniform approach is needed to move toward best practices. While each state could design and implement the policies and laws that are tailored to its respective population, benchmarks for the states could provide guidance on which evidence-based strategies to adopt.

Recommendation 7-1: The National Conference of State Legislatures should draft model legislation to provide benchmarks for states that seek to reduce alcohol-impaired driving fatalities.

This recommendation is intended to improve uniformity across states and move toward best practices—it is not meant to be a coercive measure. The model legislation would also inform community coalitions and policy makers who do not have technical expertise in this area on the composition of various legal actions. A good starting point would be for the National Conference of State Legislatures to develop model legislation on lowering the BAC limit to 0.05% (see Recommendation 4-1).

ACHIEVING ZERO DEATHS

To achieve zero alcohol-impaired driving fatalities—where every alcohol-impaired driving death could be thought of as a failure of the system—a systematic, multipronged approach with clear roles and accountabilities across sectors (including public health, transportation, law enforcement, and clinical care) is needed. Victims are dying each day, and fatality rates are rising—substantial progress has been made in the past, and that progress needs to be jump-started again. Applying a Vision Zero approach where every stakeholder has an opportunity and responsibility to take action and hold others accountable will help sustain solutions for alcohol-impaired driving. This report lays out a comprehensive set of evidence-based and promising interventions and system improvements (see Table S-1) to eliminate these preventable deaths.

TABLE S-1 Tools and Stakeholders to Accelerate Progress to Reduce Alcohol-Impaired Driving Fatalities

	Alcohol Consumption and Drinking to Impairment	
Evidence-based	Increase alcohol taxes	**Stakeholders:** *State and federal governments; alcohol producers; consumers; community coalitions **Time frame:** short term
	Implement policies to address physical availability of alcohol	**Stakeholders:** *Local and state governments; alcohol producers; hospitality and retail sectors; community coalitions **Time frame:** short term
	Implement policies to reduce illegal sales of alcohol	**Stakeholders:** *Local, state, and federal governments; alcohol producers; hospitality and retail sectors; community coalitions **Time frame:** short term
	Regulate alcohol marketing	**Stakeholders:** *Local, state, and federal governments; alcohol producers; hospitality and retail sectors; media (television, radio, print, social media); community coalitions **Time frame:** short term
	Driving While Impaired	
Evidence-based	Lower BAC per se laws to 0.05%	**Stakeholders:** *State and federal governments; law enforcement; news media/advertising (television, radio, print, social media); alcohol producers; hospitality and retail sectors; public/consumers; community coalitions **Time frame:** short term
	Conduct frequent, publicized sobriety checkpoints	**Stakeholders:** *Local and state governments; law enforcement, news media/advertising (television, radio, print, social media) **Time frame:** short term
	Universal primary seat belt laws	**Stakeholders:** *Local and state governments; law enforcement; public/consumers **Time frame:** short term

TABLE S-1 Continued

Promising	Future use of DADSS	**Stakeholders:** *NHTSA; automobile industry; automobile insurance industry; Congress; health insurers **Time frame:** long term
	Increase availability of transportation alternatives	**Stakeholders:** *Local government; transportation sector; hospitality and retail sectors; news media/advertising (television, radio, print, social media); public/consumers; private sector **Time frame:** short term
	Postcrash and/or Arrest	
Evidence-based	Evaluation and treatment of binge drinking and AUD (e.g., SBIRT, CBT, medication-assisted therapy)	**Stakeholders:** *Health care sector; *health insurers; *state government; law enforcement; legal sector **Time frame:** short term to midterm
	Implement DWI courts using standards set by National Center for DWI Courts	**Stakeholders:** *Legal sector; law enforcement; National Center for DWI Courts; victims' rights organizations (e.g., MADD) **Time frame:** short term to midterm
	Increased use of ignition interlocks and extended monitoring periods	**Stakeholders:** *State governments; legal sector; law enforcement **Time frame:** short term
	Improving administrative license suspension/revocation laws	**Stakeholders:** *Local, state, and federal governments; law enforcement; legal sector **Time frame:** short term
	Coordinated and continuous learning trauma care system	**Stakeholders:** *Health care sector; law enforcement **Time frame:** short term to midterm
Promising	Professional education and training (judiciary, law enforcement, health professionals)	**Stakeholders:** *Law enforcement; *legal sector; *health care sector; state and local public health **Time frame:** short term to midterm
	Limits on diversion programs and plea agreements	**Stakeholders:** *Research sector; legal sector; law enforcement **Time frame:** short term
	Use of systems alcohol monitoring programs	**Stakeholders:** *Law enforcement; legal sector; local and state government **Time frame:** short term to midterm

continued

TABLE S-1 Continued

Tools for Addressing the Social, Economic, Political, Legal, and Physical Context		
System-level interventions	Systematic approach to alcohol law enforcement	**Stakeholders:** *Law enforcement; health care sector, local and state government **Time frame:** short term
	Ensure timely, standardized, and accessible data on alcohol-impaired driving with strategic dissemination to the public, and explore big data opportunities	**Stakeholders:** *NHTSA **Time frame:** short term
	Convening of diverse stakeholders to create and maintain a metrics dashboard for alcohol-impaired driving	**Stakeholders:** *NHTSA; academia/research; law enforcement; state and local public health; transportation sector; other federal agencies as needed **Time frame:** short term
	Publish brief, visually appealing quarterly and annual reports that analyze and interpret progress in reducing alcohol-impaired driving	**Stakeholders:** *NHTSA; academia/research; law enforcement; state and local public health; transportation sector; other federal agencies as needed; news media/advertising (television, radio, print, social media) **Time frame:** short term
	Funding and support for community-level demonstration projects	**Stakeholders:** *NHTSA; other federal agencies as needed; private funders **Time frame:** short term
	Create interagency coordinating committee on alcohol-impaired driving	**Stakeholders:** *NHTSA; other DOT agencies as needed; HHS; TTB; DHS; DOJ; NIH; IHS; other federal agencies as needed; state and local governments **Time frame:** short term
	Development of model legislation from NCSL	**Stakeholders:** *National Conference of State Legislatures; NHTSA; state governments **Time frame:** short term to midterm
	Update Healthy People 2030 objectives for alcohol-impaired driving fatalities	**Stakeholders:** *HHS; other federal agencies as needed **Time frame:** short term

TABLE S-1 Continued

NOTES: Stakeholders marked with an asterisk are the primary actor(s) responsible for initiating action for the intervention. The rows shaded in gray are report conclusions and those in white are recommendations. The committee applied the Healthy People 2020 typology to inform the classification of evidence-based, promising, and emerging tools in this table. Time frame (approximations of when these interventions could be in place): short term is 0–2 years, midterm is 3–10 years; long term is 10 years or more. In some cases, the time horizon may be longer depending on the length of time it takes for a bill to be passed and signed into law. AUD = alcohol use disorder; CBT = cognitive behavioral therapy; DADSS = Driver Alcohol Detection System for Safety; DHS = U.S. Department of Homeland Security; DOJ = U.S. Department of Justice; DOT = U.S. Department of Transportation; DWI = driving while impaired; HHS = U.S. Department of Health and Human Services; IHS = Indian Health Service; NCSL = National Conference of State Legislators; NHTSA = National Highway Traffic Safety Administration; NIH = National Institutes of Health; SBIRT = screening, brief intervention, and referral to treatment; TTB = Alcohol and Tobacco Tax and Trade Bureau.

1

Introduction and Context

INTRODUCTION

Traffic deaths remain a leading killer of Americans of all ages in the United States today. Injury and violence cause more deaths than noncommunicable and infectious diseases among people ages 1–44 (see Figure 1-1). Unintentional injury, including traffic fatalities (which make up 26 percent of unintentional injury deaths), is the fourth leading cause of death for all Americans (CDC, 2017d,e). Despite years of success, traffic deaths from all causes are on the rise in the United States for the third straight year. In 2016, 37,461 people died from traffic crashes, an increase in deaths of 5.6 percent from 2015 (NCSA, 2017a). For each death, there are many more injuries. The estimated number of people injured from traffic crashes increased in 2015[1] from 2.34 to 2.44 million (NCSA, 2016a).

Since 1982, alcohol-impaired driving has accounted for approximately one-third of all traffic deaths on average (34 percent from 1982 to 2016 and 31 percent in the last 10 years—2006 to 2016 [Michael, 2017; NCSA, 2016b, 2017a]). Furthermore, 29 people in the United States die each day from an alcohol-impaired driving crash—that is one person every 49 minutes (NCSA, 2017a). Alcohol-impaired driving is a growing public health and safety problem that transcends the transportation, law enforcement, and clinical systems. Despite this trend, the problem is not intractable. There

[1] The 2016 fatal traffic crash data became available late in the study process (October 2017); however, in-depth analyses had not yet been completed during the writing of this report. When 2016 analyses were not available, 2015 (or most recent) data were used.

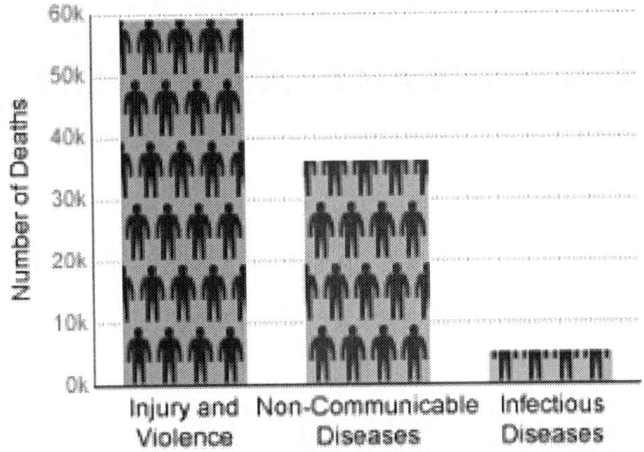

FIGURE 1-1 Deaths from injury and violence, noncommunicable diseases, and infectious diseases for Americans ages 1–44, 2013.
NOTES: Traffic fatalities are the leading cause of death for people ages 1–44. Ages <1, 45–54, 55–64, and 65+ have leading causes of death other than unintentional injury.
SOURCE: CDC, 2016a.

are many existing evidence-based and promising strategies to address alcohol-impaired driving; however, a coordinated, multilevel approach across multiple sectors will be required to accelerate change. This report presents these interventions and opportunities.

To accelerate progress to reduce alcohol-impaired driving fatalities, the National Highway Traffic Safety Administration (NHTSA) asked the Health and Medicine Division of the National Academies of Sciences, Engineering, and Medicine to identify promising interventions to reduce the fatalities caused by alcohol-impaired driving in the United States (the full charge to the committee is provided in Box 1-1). To respond to the charge, the Committee on Accelerating Progress to Reduce Alcohol-Impaired Driving Fatalities was formed.

At the first committee meeting, Jeff Michael, Associate Administrator for Research and Program Development at NHTSA, described the mission of the committee as twofold. First, the committee was tasked with identifying promising interventions that could be used to decrease alcohol-impaired driving fatalities in the United States, including interventions to be applied in the short and long term. NHTSA has been striving to reduce alcohol-impaired driving fatalities since it was founded in 1970 (*Federal Register*, n.d.). The committee's task was to build on that work, identifying which interventions have been effective and which interventions need to be modified and how, and proposing new interventions that may emerge,

BOX 1-1
Statement of Task for the Committee on Accelerating Progress to Reduce Alcohol-Impaired Driving Fatalities

The National Highway Traffic Safety Administration requests that the Health and Medicine Division of the National Academies of Sciences, Engineering, and Medicine convene a committee to examine

- which interventions (programs, systems, and policies) are most promising to prevent injuries and deaths from alcohol-impaired driving;
- the barriers to action and approaches to overcome them; and
- which interventions need to be changed or adopted.

In conducting its work, the committee may consider interventions implemented by other countries. The committee's recommendations will be broad reaching and serve as a blueprint for the nation to accelerate the progress in reducing alcohol-impaired driving fatalities.

such as advances in technology. The committee was given discretion on whether to consider interventions implemented by other countries to inform their conclusions and recommendations. Second, Michael expressed the need to increase public and policy maker attention to the issue of alcohol-impaired driving. He explained that recently distracted driving and cannabis use and driving have overshadowed alcohol-impaired driving in the public and political spheres despite alcohol-impaired driving having higher fatality rates. There is a wide breadth of literature on the efficacy of different interventions to reduce alcohol-impaired driving fatalities. The challenge presented to the committee was not only to review that literature, but also to conceptualize new ways of approaching the problem and to revitalize old ones.

The data outlined above on alcohol-impaired driving present a growing sense of urgency to reverse the current trend and improve the safety of communities, decrease associated health care costs, and save lives. Alcohol-impaired driving is entirely preventable and accounts for the largest percentage of traffic deaths. Between 2009 and 2015 the number of alcohol-impaired driving traffic deaths plateaued at about 10,000 deaths per year (NCSA, 2016b) (see Figure 1-2). Now the number of deaths from alcohol-impaired driving fatalities is beginning to rise again (although as a proportion of all traffic fatalities, the percentage has stayed about the same for alcohol-impaired driving) (NCSA, 2016a, 2017a). In 2016, alcohol-impaired driving fatalities accounted for 28 percent of traffic deaths with

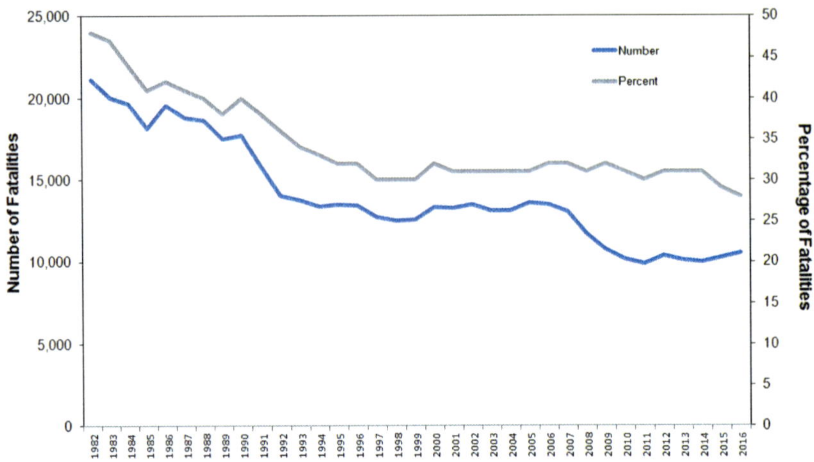

FIGURE 1-2 Number of alcohol-impaired driving fatalities and percentage of all traffic fatalities in the United States, 1982–2016.
SOURCE: Adapted from Michael, 2017.

a total of 10,497 lives lost, a 1.7 percent increase from 2015 (NCSA, 2017a). In comparison, distracted driving accounted for 9 percent of traffic deaths in 2016, with a total of 3,450 deaths (NCSA, 2017a) (see Figure 1-3). In 2015, 48 percent of alcohol-impaired driving fatalities occurred in rural areas (NCSA, 2017b). Similar to smoking, there are secondhand effects of alcohol-impaired driving; in 2015, almost 40 percent of alcohol-impaired driving fatalities were victims other than the drinking driver (NCSA, 2016b). Comparatively, victim deaths from secondhand smoke exposure were responsible for about 8.5 percent of all smoking deaths in the same year (HHS, 2014). These consequences justify interventions to protect the public. Box 1-2 contains key statistics about alcohol-impaired driving.

Alcohol-impaired driving remains the most deadly yet preventable danger on U.S. roads. The United States has the highest number of alcohol-impaired traffic deaths per capita among 10 Organisation for Economic Co-operation and Development countries based on 2015 data (see Figure 1-4).[2] In 2013, the United States had the second highest percentage of traffic fatalities attributed to alcohol-impaired driving (31 percent) when compared to 18 other high-income countries; other countries'

[2] The Redelmeier and Detsky (2017) paper does not discuss vehicle miles traveled; this can affect alcohol-impaired traffic death comparisons among countries.

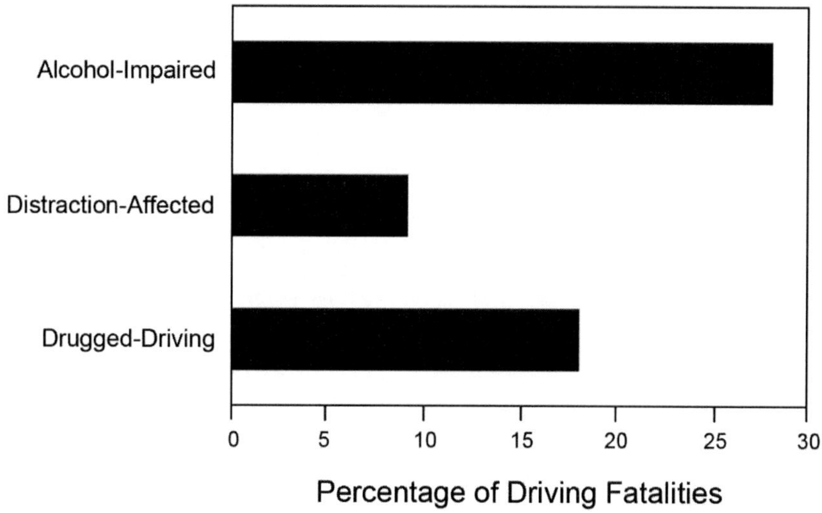

FIGURE 1-3 Comparison of traffic fatalities by select human choice categories, 2016.
NOTES: The percentage of traffic fatalities caused by drugged drivers comes from a 2009 study, the most recent year analysis is available. However, drug test results of fatally injured drivers are not always available, in part because the practice varies by state (Berning and Smither, 2014). Furthermore, it is important to note that drugged-driving data in the Fatality Analysis Reporting System (FARS) have many limitations (see Chapter 6 for information on calculating drug-impaired driving fatalities). Cell phones caused 14 percent of distracted driving fatalities in 2015.
SOURCES: NCSA, 2017a; NHTSA, 2010.

proportion of crash fatalities involving alcohol ranged from 3.2 (Israel) to 33.6 percent (Canada) (Sauber-Schatz et al., 2016). It is important to note that these studies did not use vehicle miles traveled in their analysis—doing so would likely make the U.S. less of an outlier.

Alcohol-impaired driving is an important health and social issue as it remains a major risk to Americans' health today, surpassing deaths per year of certain cancers,[3] HIV/AIDS,[4] and drownings,[5] among others (CDC, 2016b, 2017b,c,f), and contributing to long-term disabilities from head and spinal injuries from those injured in alcohol-impaired crashes.

---

[3] For example, in 2014, there were 9,324 melanoma fatalities and 4,115 cervical cancer fatalities (CDC, 2017b,f).

[4] In 2014, there were 6,721 fatalities from HIV/AIDS (CDC, 2017c).

[5] There was an average of 3,536 drownings per year from 2005 to 2014 (CDC, 2016b).

BOX 1-2
Key Facts and Statistics About Alcohol-Impaired Driving

- Each day, 29 people in the United States die in an alcohol-impaired driving crash; that is 1 person every 49 minutes.
- On average since 1982, one-third of all traffic fatalities were from alcohol-impaired driving fatalities (meaning a driver's blood alcohol concentration, or BAC, was at least 0.08%); more than 10,400 people were killed in alcohol-impaired driving crashes in 2016.
- 214 children aged 14 years or younger were killed in alcohol-impaired driving crashes in 2016.
- Rural areas are disproportionately affected by alcohol-impaired driving crashes and fatalities.
- Like smoking, there are secondhand effects of alcohol-impaired driving in which the injured have no voice in the harmful decision. Almost 40 percent of alcohol-impaired driving fatalities in 2015 were victims other than the drinking driver; for comparison, about 8.5 percent of smoking-related deaths were due to secondhand smoke in 2015.
- The economic cost, including medical costs, legal expenses, and property damages, of alcohol-impaired driving crashes was $121.5 billion in 2010, the most recent year for which data are available.

SOURCES: HHS, 2014; Michael, 2017; NCSA, 2016b, 2017a,b; Zaloshnja et al., 2013.

Progress has been made over the past three decades, but that advancement has been incremental and has stagnated more recently. Importantly, social interest has lagged over time (Hedlund and McCartt, 2002; IIHS, n.d.; Redelmeier and Detsky, 2017; Williams, 2006), leading to missed opportunities for implementing effective countermeasures throughout society (e.g., a missed opportunity is the lack of changes to some policies based on the best available evidence). Without a concerted effort, the number of alcohol-impaired driving injuries and deaths could continue to increase.

Successful past efforts are well recognized. In the early 1980s alcohol-impaired driving rose to the forefront of the public's attention (Fell and Voas, 2006). Attitudes toward drinking and driving shifted as groups like Mothers Against Drunk Driving (MADD), which was founded by a mother whose 13-year-old daughter was killed by an alcohol-impaired driver, began opening chapters across the country and sharing victims' experiences with policy makers (Fell and Voas, 2006). Alcohol-impaired driving penetrated the media through campaigns such as the U.S. Department of Transportation and the Ad Council's "Friends don't let friends

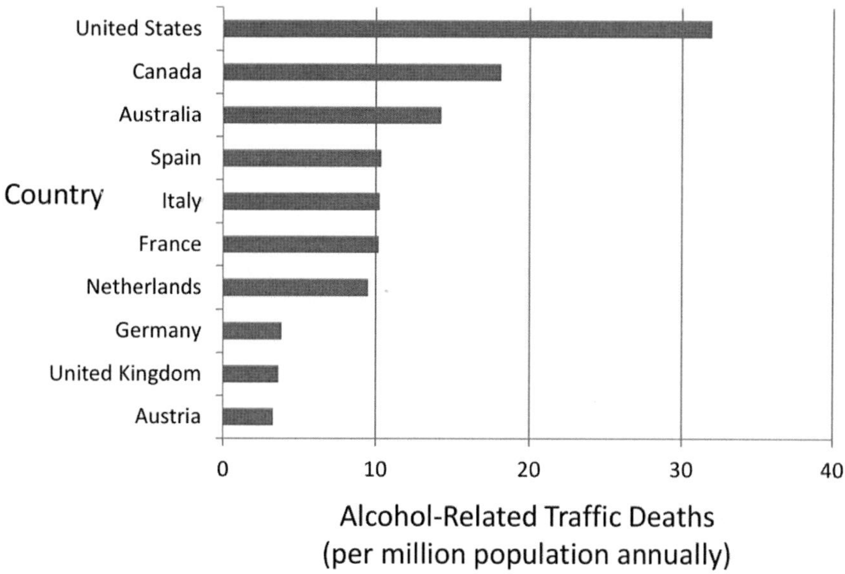

FIGURE 1-4 Annual alcohol-impaired driving traffic deaths per million.
SOURCE: Redelmeier and Detsky, 2017.

drive drunk" public service announcements. Although this national campaign has not been rigorously evaluated, it is often credited with contributing to the shift in social norms around drinking and driving (Ad Council, n.d.; Glascoff et al., 2013). According to Voas and Lacey (2011) and Subramanian (2002), in 1982, which was the first year that alcohol-impaired driving was included in the current system for estimating the number of traffic fatalities in the United States, alcohol-impaired driving caused 26,173 deaths—the highest number recorded to date (Voas and Lacey, 2011). From the 1980s through the early 2000s, alcohol-impaired driving fatalities steadily decreased (Voas and Lacey, 2011). Numerous new laws were passed that helped decrease alcohol-impaired driving, including laws making it illegal to purchase alcohol under the age of 21 (minimum legal drinking age), or to drive with a blood alcohol concentration (BAC) of 0.10% or greater (Fell and Voas, 2006). Other laws increased law enforcement authority, allowing them to conduct sobriety checkpoints and to confiscate the licenses of driving while impaired (DWI) offenders (Fell and Voas, 2006). Fell and Voas (2006) and Voas and Lacey (2011) estimated that these actions saved more than 300,000 lives from 1982 to 2001.

Although much progress has been made as states passed and implemented policies, these heterogeneous policies lacked benchmarks and have been enforced with varying intensity. Progress has stagnated and even reversed. It will likely worsen without renewed and innovative efforts, which are now possible. The plateauing fatality rates indicate that what has been done to decrease deaths from alcohol-impaired driving has been working but is no longer enough. Changes are needed to accelerate progress and save additional lives (see additional alcohol-impaired driving trends in Chapter 2 and Appendix A).

Why Now?

Social, technological, financial, and clinical changes provide a timely opportunity to reinvigorate successful efforts to reduce alcohol-impaired driving injuries and deaths. These changes present greater opportunities for individuals and community movements, greater insights into underlying causes, improved targeting of effective interventions, and enhanced data systems that offer a greater understanding of causes and contributing factors as well as more effective targeting of solutions and tracking progress. Every individual and stakeholder now has the opportunity to better recognize the problem, identify ways risks can be addressed, and work together to minimize or eliminate them.

At the societal level there is a greater understanding of how individual and population actions and the environment affect health. Clinical changes include hospital-based interventions that have transitioned to population- and community-based interventions, with a greater focus on early intervention, and with that framework there is a better understanding of how various segments of society can work together in innovative ways toward a common goal.

The transformation of technology includes interconnectivity of information; the growth of "big data" analytics provides new insights that help delineate cause and effect and better identify problem areas and target interventions (see Chapter 6 for additional discussion). Together, these trends provide the substrate for a dramatic shift in addressing alcohol-impaired driving and making significant gains. Technologically, the emergence of big data has provided organizations, policy makers, and stakeholders tremendous insight that allows them to have a data-driven approach for targeting high-risk individuals, geographic zones, and roadway hotspots for specific interventions, as well as more rapidly seeing the effects of directed countermeasures and the return-on-share investments (see Chapter 6 for additional discussion). In addition, technology has allowed new interventions like ignition interlock devices and ridesharing opportunities using smartphone technology that provide new potential countermeasures in ways never available before.

Given these advances and the current focus on reducing traffic fatalities, there are many opportunities to involve traditional and novel stakeholders in innovative ways and to leverage newly available societal and technological infrastructure to break through the stagnation and accelerate progress on the path toward a new, comprehensive approach to confronting alcohol-impaired driving (see Chapters 7 and 8 for more on the roles of various stakeholders).

ABOUT THIS REPORT

The Committee's Approach

Though recognizing that alcohol-impaired driving is a crime, and that enforcement and criminal justice approaches are critically important, the committee takes a holistic public health approach. The committee's approach is focused on population-level strategies aimed at providing the maximum benefit at the population level. This includes understanding the problem based on available data and surveillance, identifying risk and protective factors, reviewing the evidence for interventions, implementing interventions that will likely have the largest public health impact, and monitoring progress. A public health approach also uses a social determinants of health[6] lens. The social determinants of health allow for exploration of the complex intersections of social, cultural, political, economic, legal, and systems-level influences on health and well-being. The social determinants of health framework considers access to health care, economic stability, education, neighborhood and built environment, and social and cultural contexts as influential on health and wellness outcomes. Such an approach enables key health issues to be considered in the context of the social and physical environments in which people live, enriching opportunities for cross-sector data analytics and collaborative solution development. Individual behaviors, physical and social environments, and access to services and information all play a role in facilitating or mitigating risky behavior and risky situations and the negative health outcomes associated with them (Stockwell et al., 2015). Social determinants of health can play a large role in advancing health equity as well. Health equity means that everyone has full and equal access to opportunities that allow them to lead healthy lives. To achieve health equity, people's health and wellness ought not be compromised or disadvantaged because of race/ethnicity, sex, income, sexual orientation, education, neighborhood, rural residence, or any other social condition.

---

[6] The World Health Organization describes the social determinants of health as "the conditions in which people are born, grow, live, work, and age . . . circumstances shaped by the distribution of money, power, and resources at global, national, and local levels" (WHO, n.d.).

These concepts are discussed in more detail in Chapter 2 as they relate to alcohol-impaired driving.

Conceptual Framework for Preventing Alcohol-Impaired Driving Fatalities

Traditional approaches to preventive countermeasures are categorized as being implemented before the event, during the event, or after the event—each point represents opportunities to intervene. One such approach is the use of the Haddon Matrix, which is commonly used in the injury field and looks at human, environmental, and vehicle factors before, during, and after a crash (Haddon, 1980). The Haddon Matrix paradigm provides an important organization to the many inputs that address alcohol-impaired driving crashes, and the committee's conceptual model grows from that approach. There are many contextual factors that may affect alcohol use and driving, but for the purpose of this report the committee primarily discusses interventions directly related to the prevention of alcohol-impaired driving crash fatalities. This includes pre-crash interventions, such as alcohol policies that affect price and physical availability of alcohol and alcohol consumption, alternative transportation and ridesharing options that may affect whether an impaired person chooses to drive, and enforcement policies such as ignition interlocks for repeat offenders that may affect whether an impaired person drives once in his or her vehicle. Figure 1-5 (the committee's conceptual framework) illustrates the sequence of behaviors leading to an alcohol-impaired driving fatality, the potential intervention opportunities, and the important factors that shape the outcomes.

The sequence of events in the framework begins with drinking alcohol, which can lead to drinking to the level of impairment, driving while impaired, being involved in an alcohol-impaired motor vehicle crash, and finally to crashes that result in serious injuries and fatalities. The injuries and fatalities can include the driver, occupants, pedestrians, bicyclists, or drivers and occupants of other vehicles. Within the phases, the additional layer around the perimeter of the shapes (e.g., one layer around "drink to impairment," two around "drive impaired") signifies increased likelihood or risk of a negative outcome among the behaviors (squares), and increased severity among the outcomes (diamonds). An individual can drop off of this sequence at any point; for example, a person may consume alcohol, but not to the level of impairment, or may plan an alternative mode of transportation. Furthermore, there are individual risk factors that affect the likelihood of drinking to impairment (e.g., being a binge drinker or having an alcohol use disorder) and driving while impaired (e.g., prior DWI, availability of a vehicle, or possession of a driver's license). While

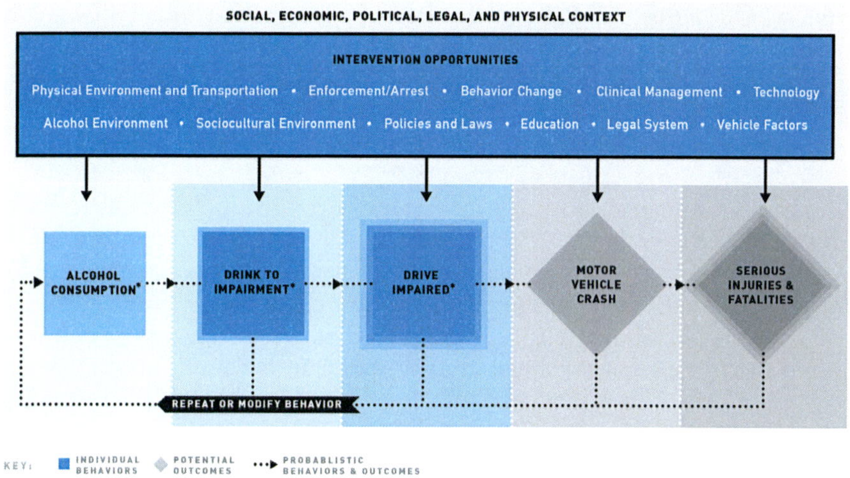

FIGURE 1-5 Preventing alcohol-impaired driving crash fatalities conceptual framework.
NOTES: Each of the phases in this figure represents an opportunity to intervene and prevent alcohol-impaired driving fatalities. A square denotes a behavior, a diamond denotes an outcome, and dotted lines denote potential progression to an outcome. Extra layers around a square or a diamond denote increased likelihood or increased severity, respectively. The asterisks signify that there are alternative behaviors not represented in the first three phases that would preclude an alcohol-impaired driving fatality (e.g., not drinking or not drinking to the level of impairment).

these are not reflected in the framework, they are important individual-level considerations and will be discussed in the report as they relate to alcohol-impaired driving and effective interventions.

In addition, driving while impaired does not always lead to a collision and an alcohol-impaired driving collision does not always result in an injury or fatality. These are potential outcomes of impaired driving, as indicated by the dashed lines leading up to them. However, the extensive literature on alcohol-impaired driving demonstrates a causal effect between impaired driving and increased risk for motor vehicle crashes and fatalities (Blomberg et al., 2005; Compton and Berning, 2015; Voas and Lacey, 2011). Thus, while the committee's ultimate goal is to accelerate progress to reduce alcohol-impaired driving fatalities, the major task is to reduce alcohol-impaired driving.

Above the sequence of events, the figure highlights intervention opportunities that consist of effective or promising solutions to reduce alcohol-impaired driving. These opportunities include the sociocultural environment; the alcohol environment; clinical treatment; behavior change; education; policies and laws; enforcement and arrest; the legal system; the physical environment and transportation; vehicle factors; and technologies. These areas of intervention opportunity interact with one another and target multiple levels (e.g., individual, interpersonal, institutional, community, and societal). The strategies, programs, policies, and systems within these intervention opportunities need to take into account the varied environmental contexts within which they will be implemented. These are the social, economic, political, legal, and physical contexts. The socioecological model (see Figure 1-6) is also a useful framework for understanding alcohol-impaired driving and how to prevent it, as the model reflects the interactions among individual, interpersonal, community, institutional, and societal levels, and it presents opportunities for potential interventions in each level.

Interventions for alcohol-impaired driving can target various points along the sequence at the bottom of the conceptual framework, and many

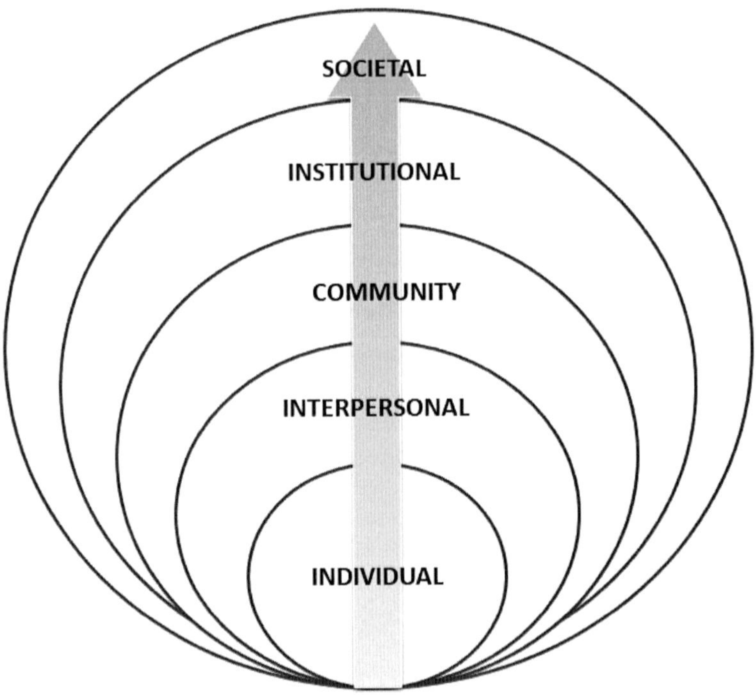

FIGURE 1-6 The socioecological model.
SOURCE: Concept from McLeroy et al., 1988.

affect outcomes through complex pathways (see, for example, Figure 11 in Voas and Lacey, 2011). For instance, the legal consequences of driving while impaired can have a deterrent effect, preventing someone from drinking to the level of impairment (Voas and Lacey, 2011), and they can also deter someone who has been arrested for involvement in an alcohol-impaired driving crash from reoffending (Sloan et al., 2011).

For the purpose of this report, the committee applied a socioecological viewpoint while evaluating interventions and making recommendations (see Figure 1-6). Alcohol-impaired driving is a complex, multicomponent problem requiring a multifaceted set of synergistic interventions. The individual level consists of knowledge, attitudes, behavior, self-concept, and skills related to alcohol-impaired driving (such as drinking behavior or perceived risk of being pulled over and arrested by law enforcement for driving while impaired). These beliefs and attitudes could be linked to policies and interventions that are shown to affect them (e.g., minimum legal drinking age laws or mass media campaigns). The interpersonal level includes interpersonal processes and primary groups, such as formal and informal social networks, family, friends, treating physicians, and work groups. These groups could include bystanders who may or may not intervene when a person is making the decision to drive while impaired. At the institutional level (also sometimes called "organizational"), there are social institutions with organizational characteristics and rules for operation that affect alcohol-impaired driving (e.g., MADD, the alcohol industry, and law enforcement). The community level describes the relationships among organizations, institutions, and informal networks with specific boundaries (e.g., the alcohol environment and transportation alternatives). At the public policy and societal level, there are local, state, and national laws and policies that influence alcohol-impaired driving and the associated risk factors such as excessive drinking. This model illustrates the multiple levels at which a comprehensive approach to reducing alcohol-impaired driving could intervene, as well as the actors involved. There is substantial overlap across the levels of the model, and the interventions and actors within each level interact with one another. Interventions presented in this report range from the individual level to population-level approaches to reduce alcohol-impaired driving.

There are several effective and important interventions that can prevent fatalities that are not reflected in the conceptual framework or this report (e.g., the automobile manufacturing process and highway and road design). For example, the committee focused on postcrash interventions directly related to reducing DWI recidivism (e.g., legal consequences, brief interventions in emergency rooms, and continuing education) or those that are important for specific populations (e.g., rural communities).

In an effort to produce a report that focuses on what actions need to be taken over the next 30 to 40 years, the committee does not fully address many issues less directly related to alcohol-impaired driving crashes and fatalities, including postcrash survival interventions, highway and road design, and vehicle safety crash tests. Though each of these is important in its own right, they are not the focus of this report.

Methodology

As noted in the committee's statement of task, an intervention could be a program, system, or policy. The literature on the effectiveness and applicability of alternative interventions provides important information for assessing which interventions are most effective, cost-effective, and suitable for either a general or more specific population. Selection of interventions ought to be based on the extant literature; however, many interventions have not been adequately evaluated for general or specific effectiveness, or evaluated for effectiveness when brought to scale. In addition, comparisons of interventions are often incomplete and difficult to conduct because studies vary in dimensions such as the appropriateness of the study design and setting, outcomes measured, failure to consider other consequences (that is, externalities), quality of execution, interactions with other interventions, and inclusion of economic consequences. Furthermore, a lack of studies on an intervention does not equate to lack of effectiveness. Conversely, the presence of methodologically flawed studies that conclude an intervention is effective are of limited value.

With the above in mind, the committee examined the available literature on alcohol-impaired driving interventions that target alcohol consumption, drinking to impairment, driving while impaired, and the postcrash and/or postarrest phase. The committee was not charged with undertaking a systematic review of the evidence, but rather to identify which interventions are most promising to prevent alcohol-impaired driving injuries and fatalities given the current state of knowledge and environment. The committee did, however, conduct a comprehensive literature review to gather information on interventions and barriers to action from the peer-reviewed and grey literature. This entailed a systematic search of academic and governmental databases and websites for studies that evaluated or assessed the effects of interventions on any one of the following outcomes: alcohol consumption, binge drinking, alcohol-impaired driving, arrests, recidivism, and alcohol-impaired driving crashes, injuries, and fatalities.[7] The sources of evidence spanned across

---

[7] Search terms included alcohol terms (such as alcohol-impaired fatalities, alcohol-impaired driving, alcohol-related deaths, binge drinking, blood alcohol concentration/

multiple sectors, including transportation, the criminal justice system (e.g., law enforcement and courts), and public health (e.g., injury prevention and substance use). Each field has its own scientific methods and standards. In general, the committee's assessment of individual studies and an overall body of literature followed the methodologic approach of the Community Preventive Services Task Force (Task Force on Community Preventive Services, 2000).[8] For example, the Task Force evaluates the body of evidence around a specific intervention by factoring in the number of available studies, the strength of the study design and execution, and the size and consistency of observed effects. In assessing the evidence, the committee relied on existing systematic reviews and meta-analyses with strong methodologies from credible organizations with clear and established evidentiary standards and review processes such as the Centers for Disease Control and Prevention and the Cochrane Collaboration.[9] In addition, the committee drew from existing, comprehensive reviews of the evidence, such as NHTSA's *Countermeasures That Work* to inform its work. The following section describes some of the factors that the committee took into consideration when assessing the impact of interventions.

Considerations for Assessing Alcohol-Impaired Driving Interventions

When assessing specific interventions, the committee considered total population impact (how much alcohol-impaired driving would be reduced), cost-effectiveness, feasibility, and values and public acceptance. The committee considered the following factors when examining and comparing studies.

Suitability of study design and quality of execution Quality and sophistication vary across studies. Randomized controlled studies and randomized field studies can assess the causal effect, but they are often unsuitable for evaluation of population-based interventions. Other approaches use observational data and can capitalize on, for instance,

---

content, drunk driving) paired with traffic terms (such as accidents, traffic fatalities, traffic safety, crashes) and intervention terms, among others.

[8] The Community Preventive Services Task Force was formerly known as the Task Force on Community Preventive Services. Task Force publications prior to 2012 are cited as the latter, and those published after 2012 are cited as the former.

[9] Cochrane defines a systematic review as "a review of a clearly formulated question that uses systematic and explicit methods to identify, select, and critically appraise relevant research, and to collect and analyze data from the studies that are included in the review." Relatedly, a meta-analysis involves "the use of statistical techniques in a systematic review to integrate the results of included studies" (http://community.cochrane.org/glossary [accessed November 29, 2017]).

variations in policies over time and across jurisdictions to assess the effect. The design and statistical approach, such as controlling for confounding factors, can affect the results and the confidence a decision maker has that the intervention is effective.

Real-world effect The applicability of the findings to the real world (effectiveness, studies with high external validity) often differs from the findings in a more controlled experiment (efficacy, studies with high internal validity). Similarly, the results of a project implemented on a small scale may differ from the results when the project is implemented nationally. In general, real-world implementation falls short of the results of studies conducted in ideal settings. The committee was most concerned about findings in real-world situations.

Examined outcomes and measurement of spillover effects Importantly, the outcomes measured (i.e., only considering alcohol-impaired driving crashes or fatalities, including only those in a car, not pedestrians) and how they are measured are critical, yet commonly differ from study to study. The extent to which benefits and harms (positive and negative spillovers) are measured matters because the total population effect (net benefit) is important in selecting interventions.

Heterogeneity in effect across populations The effectiveness of interventions can also vary among different populations. For example, some interventions may be more effective for young people and less effective for adults, and others, such as ignition interlock devices, will be effective only for drivers of vehicles that have them equipped. Among the numerous factors that lead to heterogeneity are location (e.g., rural versus urban), demographics (e.g., age, gender, and race/ethnicity), and drinking habits (e.g., heavy, light, or binge drinkers). Understanding these differences is important for comparing study results and for selecting interventions most suitable for target populations.

Scale, intensity, or focus of interventions The estimated effectiveness of interventions may depend on the scale or intensity with which they are implemented. For example, if a sobriety checkpoint is implemented only occasionally, it could have a small effect and a high cost per death averted. But, if it is scaled up, the marginal cost could decline and the marginal effect could increase.

Optimal set of interventions Alcohol-impaired driving results from a complex set of factors. Consequently, reducing alcohol-impaired driving requires a *set* of interventions. Because some interventions are already in place, the key question to address is which additional approaches, or scaled-up approaches of current tactics, will reduce alcohol-impaired driving the most. Unfortunately, few studies assess the synergies among interventions.

Sets of interventions and synergies (positive or negative externalities) Adopting a set of interventions can modify the effectiveness of individual approaches, as interventions can have positive or negative synergies. For example, sobriety checkpoints may be enhanced by a media campaign and vice versa. By the same token, an intervention that reduces alcohol-impaired driving crashes might affect other alcohol-related outcomes in similar or different ways (such as consequences of alcohol on families) as well. If only alcohol-impaired driving fatalities are considered as the outcome, an intervention might not seem very effective, but if all the benefits (harms and costs) are included, then the intervention may be sufficiently effective to be worth implementing. This comprehensive approach of including negative and positive spillovers is the gold standard for analyses but demands more information than is generally available to inform published studies.

Match of intervention to population Some approaches might be most effective when they are aimed at high-risk groups. For example, alcohol treatment combined with ignition interlock devices may be most effective in reducing alcohol-impaired driving fatalities if they are aimed at repeat offenders or young drivers.

In sum, comparisons across studies are needed to better assess intervention opportunities; however, such comparisons are often not available or are difficult to interpret. The committee used the available evidence and balanced the concepts above in considering effective and promising interventions to reduce alcohol-impaired driving fatalities.

Cost-Effectiveness and Cost-Benefit

Interventions will also likely vary in the degree to which the costs of the intervention are a good use of governments', or more broadly, society's resources. In the literature the committee reviewed, value for use of resources is typically analyzed as being "cost-effective" or "cost-beneficial." A cost-effectiveness analysis compares the effect (e.g., alcohol-impaired driving fatalities) of an intervention to the costs of implementing the intervention; other costs can be included as well, depending on the perspective of the study. In contrast, a complete cost-benefit analysis values all effects in dollar terms and sums them, and then compares this value to the dollar costs of implementing the intervention. If the monetary benefits outweigh the dollar costs, the intervention is considered to be cost-beneficial. However, there are relatively few studies that provide consistent, empirical estimates of either of these measures for the interventions that the committee reviewed. Furthermore, not all interventions have been evaluated by a cost-effectiveness or cost-benefit study. Although the committee was not specifically asked to review cost-effectiveness of the interventions, where analyses were available that were robust enough to provide some insight, the committee included an overview.

International Comparisons

In its statement of task the committee was asked to look at international examples addressing alcohol-impaired driving as appropriate. While looking at examples outside of the United States can be informative, certain caveats on applicability are important. For example, some differences in fatality rates or other measures of progress in the United States compared to other countries may be explained by differences in population density, availability of mass transit, and other factors. O'Neill and Kyrychenko (2006) note that comparisons of the United States and other countries can mask the vast differences across U.S. states, largely explained by population density and other non-highway safety factors, and fail to address the underlying differences that do not relate to highway safety policy. This is not to say that comparisons are not helpful, but these potential differences are important to consider. In terms of the acceptance and success of various interventions, differences in culture, laws, and implementation need to be considered as well. In this report the committee points to international examples and lessons learned when appropriate and notes what does (or does not) make these examples relevant to the U.S. context.

Tension Between Civil Liberties and Needed Interventions

There are often inherent ethical tensions that exist between control measures to protect the public's health and civil/personal liberties—the tension between the good of the collective and rights of the individual. This tension has existed since the fight against infectious disease in the nineteenth and twentieth centuries and continues today in efforts to address chronic conditions (Bayer, 2007) and more recently with tobacco use, fluoridation, food regulations, and traffic safety laws. These trade-offs can be difficult to address but are important to consider. In relation to alcohol-impaired driving, for example, impairment can be measured in several ways by a law enforcement officer (and all 50 states and the District of Columbia have *implied consent* laws),[10] although drivers may refuse BAC testing (states vary on whether refusal is a criminal offense) and this can hinder the prosecution process. Another example is sobriety checkpoints—some states do not allow checkpoints as they believe they impinge on personal liberties. While mandatory BAC testing would be beneficial to arresting officers and prosecutors and the allowance of sobriety checkpoints is critically important, the committee did not make recommendations on whether these laws should be changed at the state level. The committee does recommend, for example, the use of sobriety checkpoints, but it will be up to the states which have laws against their use to weigh the potential benefits of using them for the health of their population against the need to uphold personal liberties in that instance. A balance inevitably needs to be struck based on the values of the community. Furthermore, reducing alcohol-impaired driving injuries and fatalities is difficult to separate from the broader public health rationale for reducing excessive alcohol consumption since drinking is the precursor for alcohol-impaired driving.

A Comprehensive Approach to Address Alcohol-Impaired Driving

There is no one-size-fits-all approach that will solve the problem of alcohol-impaired driving. For a problem this large and widespread, a systematic population approach is needed. In addition, each state is unique in terms of laws in place, population needs, transportation options, roadway conditions, and many other factors, so an intervention that is appropriate in one state or locality might not be as impactful in another (e.g., in an urban population versus a rural one). Therefore, the committee does not prioritize among its recommendations; while each state needs to take a comprehensive approach to addressing alcohol-impaired driving (see Figure 1-5), the exact combination of interventions for particular states will vary. While targeted interventions for important subpopulations would be beneficial, more data are needed to accurately implement these (see Chapter 6). Generally, alcohol-impaired driving studies do not focus on subpopulations.

When identifying conclusions and recommendations the committee focused on interventions that are evidence based, promising, and relevant in the current environment, or where improvements are needed to increase effectiveness. When the committee identified the need for a specific action and a specific actor, a recommendation was provided.

[10] Meaning that drivers using state roads (or federally owned park roads) have "consented" to comply with sobriety testing if there is indication that they are driving while impaired. More detail is provided in Chapter 5.

Where the available evidence and the committee's expertise led the committee to reach a conclusion about the state of the evidence or the need for a particular action, a conclusion was provided. While many of the strategies outlined in this report are not new, systematically implementing these policies, programs, and systems changes would renew progress and save lives.

Behavioral Insights

Conventional behavior change models assume individuals consistently act in their own interest and form behavioral change intentions based on a rational assessment of the costs and benefits. Behavioral economics, for example, applies psychological insights to understand the many natural decisions people make that routinely deviate from their best interests. Along with several other fields, the behavioral economics literature demonstrates cases where rationality is limited by impulsiveness, social norms, and the context in which choices are made (Cohen et al., 2000; Matjasko et al., 2016; Rice, 2013; Thorgeirsson and Kawachi, 2013; Zimmerman, 2009). These insights help explain why many traditional health promotion efforts have limited success, such as simply increasing awareness of the risks of drinking and driving. Policies and interventions to improve public health can therefore be made more effective if designed with insights from behavioral economics. For example, individuals show status quo bias and tend not to deviate or opt out from default options (the events that will occur if no alternatives are selected). For example, many people do not deviate from default options for retirement savings, generic medications, and health insurance plans (Halpern et al., 2007, 2013). Therefore, changing environments to make the healthy or less risky option the default is highly likely to be successful (Frieden, 2010).

Research shows that those who repeatedly drink and drive compared to those who do not engage in such behavior actually know DWI laws better, but are poorer planners (i.e., in planning a transportation alternative), lack self-control, and are more impulsive with much higher temporal discounting rates,[11] preferring short-term rewards over bigger, long-term rewards (Sloan et al., 2014). Because those who drive while impaired by alcohol have difficulty improving their behavior, a productive approach would be to implement policies and interventions that make the transportation and drinking environments safer. Furthermore, these insights suggest that stringent policies are needed to counter the impulsivity and lack of self-control especially among DWI offenders. Finally, the high personal discount rates among those who drive while impaired by alcohol

[11] The rate at which individuals discount future costs and benefits.

suggest swiftness of punishment and increasing the perceived chances of getting caught are critical to deterrence. Accelerating progress to reduce alcohol-impaired driving fatalities thus will require a system designed to accommodate the shortfalls in decision making by those who drive while impaired by alcohol.

With these ideas and the conceptual model in mind, the committee recognizes the need for an overarching philosophy and process for improvement, tailored to local environments and involving a range of stakeholders motivated by a common goal to reduce alcohol-impaired driving fatalities.

THE ROAD AHEAD

Vision Zero

NHTSA (the sponsor of this report), the Federal Motor Carrier Safety Administration (FMCSA), the Federal Highway Administration (FHWA), and the National Safety Council launched the Road to Zero coalition in 2016 with the bold goal to end all traffic fatalities within 30 years (NHTSA, 2016). With more than 360 partners nationwide, the coalition has pledged to focus on evidence-based strategies to reduce traffic fatalities, such as the use of seat belts, rumble strips, behavior change campaigns, and data-driven enforcement (NHTSA, 2016; NSC, 2017). The Road to Zero expands the discussion to include not only representatives of roadway, behavioral, and vehicle safety, but also nonprofit groups, public health officials, and technology companies—dozens of organizations working together to develop a coordinated approach (NSC, 2017). While the Road to Zero effort acknowledges that zero deaths is a "lofty" goal, it notes that it is attainable because traffic fatalities are preventable and no traffic fatality is acceptable; a future with zero traffic deaths is more certain than ever with the emergence of self-driving cars and the Safe Systems transportation approach; and a coordinated effort that brings together multiple stakeholders with the same goal can achieve more than individual organizations working independently.

The Road to Zero is consistent with Vision Zero—a philosophical approach to road safety that was crafted in the 1990s and adopted in Sweden in 1997 (see Box 1-3). Vision Zero, as a unifying philosophy, has expanded to the United States and other countries. While originally focused on road builders and design, Vision Zero continues to have an increasing breadth of participants. Its principal aim is to eliminate all serious traffic injuries and fatalities (Rosencrantz et al., 2007). Described as "audacious," "bold" (Aboelata et al., 2017), and "radical" (Belin et al., 2012), this innovative approach transformed the traditional approach of

BOX 1-3
The Swedish Experience with Vision Zero

Since the implementation of Vision Zero, the Swedish government has made changes in four areas: road and infrastructure, vehicle technology, services and education, and control and surveillance. The Swedish Traffic Accident Data Acquisition (STRADA) information system collects data on crashes and injuries occurring nationwide from police crash reports and hospital medical reports (Swedish Transport Administration, 2015). By combining these two sources of information, STRADA is able to give a robust account of traffic crashes and their consequences while identifying cases often not reported to the traffic police (usually involving pedestrians, cyclists, or mopeds) (Swedish Transport Administration, 2015). The Swedish government has also partnered with the automotive industry to develop new technologies such as antiskid systems and antilock brakes, and there is a push toward automated driving and the digitalization of roads, which would include automated sobriety checkpoints (Government Offices of Sweden, 2016).

Although Vision Zero places ultimate responsibility for traffic fatalities on system designers, a higher demand is also placed on road users to comply with traffic regulations (Belin et al., 2012; Tingvall and Haworth, 2000). A large component of the Swedish success story has been in creating a social norm in which impaired driving is not only rare, but seriously frowned upon (Tingvall and Haworth, 2000).

Vision Zero has succeeded at reducing traffic fatalities, even as the traffic volume in Sweden has increased (Swedish Transport Administration, n.d.). When Vision Zero was launched, traffic deaths exceeded 500 people per year (Swedish Transport Administration, 2017). By 2015 this number had been reduced almost by half (Swedish Transport Administration, 2017).

transportation design, in which the road builders simply expected road users to use the road as designed, and instead shifts responsibility to the transportation system and road designers to prevent injury and death. This brings in new stakeholders and creates innovative partnerships. Everyone has a role and an opportunity to contribute to the shared goals. Vision Zero is a starting point that can be expanded to address alcohol-impaired driving. Therefore, each alcohol-impaired driving fatality could be thought of as a system failure and understanding the reason for that failure facilitates interventions to prevent recurrence. Vision Zero continues to expand and has been adopted by more than two dozen U.S. cities.

Achieving Vision Zero in the United States

Other initiatives or programs aimed at achieving zero deaths from traffic fatalities in the United States include the Vision Zero Network, which is composed of U.S. cities that have made the pledge to pursue continuous elimination of traffic fatalities and serious injuries within a designated time period (Vision Zero Network, 2017). Toward Zero Deaths: A National Strategy on Highway Safety is an initiative that was created in 2009 by a steering committee cooperative with the aim of eliminating traffic injuries and fatalities nationwide. It receives technical support from FHWA, FMCSA, and NHTSA and is promoted by many groups including the American Association of State Highway and Transportation Officials, the Governors Highway Safety Association, and numerous state departments of transportation (AASHTO, 2015; TZD, 2015). The Institute of Transportation Engineers also launched a Vision Zero Task Force in 2016 that supports Vision Zero efforts in U.S. cities through public–private partnerships, volunteerism, and raising awareness (ITE, 2017, n.d.).

The Vision Zero philosophy is spreading throughout the country but in a disjointed and fragmented fashion. Instead of working together, invested partners are creating their own, slightly different Vision Zero programs. Implementing a unified Vision Zero as a U.S. policy to reduce alcohol-impaired driving injuries and fatalities is an important step. To fulfill Vision Zero successfully, shared goals and continued progress toward reducing alcohol-impaired driving fatalities is essential. Vision Zero will need to include interventions to modify drinking as well as alcohol-impaired driving (see Chapter 2 for information on the relationship between drinking and impaired driving), in addition to more traditional engineering solutions. More data at the community level are also needed, as is the integration of data systems to better target where alcohol-impaired traffic fatalities occur and to make the appropriate changes (see Chapter 6 for more information on data system needs). To address this growing public health and safety problem, an integrated systems change requires many varied partners to join the transportation and transportation system design sector in recognizing that alcohol-impaired driving fatalities are preventable. These partners include government agencies, state and local public health departments, clinicians, health care systems, law enforcement, car manufacturers, auto insurers, advocacy organizations, technology companies, employers, alcohol retailers, wholesale distributors, alcohol producers, and the hospitality industry, among others (see Chapters 7 and 8 for further explanation of stakeholder accountability).

Vision Zero aspires to reach zero traffic fatalities. Reducing alcohol-impaired driving is, in part, a means to that end. A public health approach to injury prevention that encompasses the full array of contributing variables or causes for the target harm is needed. From this perspective, reducing excessive alcohol consumption and reducing alcohol-impaired driving are two of the logically available means. As discussed throughout the report, altering the alcohol and driving environments often entails trade-offs, as described above. Vision Zero is an aspirational goal, not a policy prescription.

Bold goals are important and can be used to galvanize action, change social norms, and bring stakeholders together around a common vision and goal. The committee recognizes that in an economic sense, eliminating all roadway fatalities would require investments that have diminishing returns and that there are important alternate uses of those resources; however, Vision Zero is not primarily an economic goal. It is about establishing an aspirational goal that can rally stakeholders, provide focus, and make substantial progress toward achieving that goal.

If Vision Zero is further expanded to specifically address the largest killer on the road—alcohol-impaired driving—and the wide range of stakeholders were to unite behind one comprehensive, overarching approach to Vision Zero with clearly defined roles and responsibilities, they would be able to provide a stronger message, provide more targeted and effective interventions, and tackle alcohol-impaired driving more cohesively. Table 8-1 outlines the stakeholders who are needed to ensure implementation of the evidence-based and promising interventions discussed throughout this report.

Importantly, the public itself can also directly participate in preventing alcohol-impaired driving through Vision Zero. Introducing a goal of zero alcohol-impaired driving injuries or fatalities requires the country to adopt a new, multisector approach and system for improvement, driven by stakeholders motivated by a common goal. Throughout this report the Vision Zero philosophy is applied to alcohol-impaired driving with the aim of developing a comprehensive approach that involves stakeholders across sectors.

Conclusion 1-1: Alcohol-impaired driving is a complex preventable public health problem that requires a comprehensive and collaborative multisector approach.

WHAT IS ALCOHOL IMPAIRMENT?

Terms

Box 1-4 highlights key terms related to impairment used throughout the report. For the purpose of this report, the term *alcohol-impaired driving* is used. While impairment can be caused by other substances or conditions, and although it begins before reaching the BAC limit set by state law, this report generally uses the term to mean driving with a BAC of 0.08% or higher. The term applies to drivers of all vehicle types and does not include pedestrians or cyclists.

BOX 1-4
Key Impairment Terms from the Glossary

Alcohol-impaired driving crash/fatality—In all U.S. states[a] drivers are considered legally impaired to drive when their blood alcohol concentration (BAC) is greater than or equal to 0.08 grams per deciliter (g/dL, often expressed as %, as in 0.08%).[b] Thus, in the United States, any crash involving one or more drivers with a BAC of 0.08% or higher is typically referred to by the National Highway Traffic Safety Administration (NHTSA) as an alcohol-impaired driving crash, and fatalities stemming from those crashes are defined as being alcohol-impaired driving crash fatalities. Of note, however, is that impairment begins below 0.08%, so this is an underestimate relative to all crash fatalities in which impairment from alcohol may have contributed.[c]

Alcohol-related crash/fatality—A crash or a fatality from a crash that involves one or more drivers of a motor vehicle with any alcohol in their system (i.e., a BAC greater than 0.00%). This term also subsumes alcohol-impaired driving crashes. It is a useful umbrella term for all motor vehicle crashes that involve any alcohol. Some have also used the *alcohol-involved* term to convey the same idea.

Driving under the influence (DUI), driving while impaired (DWI)—These are legal phrases that refer to handling a motor vehicle while one's BAC is above the limit set by state statute, or on the basis of field sobriety tests or observed behavior.

Drunk driving crash/fatality—A colloquial term, widely used and recognized, and generally refers to driving or crashes or fatalities that are related to alcohol impairment (in most U.S. states based on a BAC ≥0.08%).

Impairment—Refers to the deterioration of an individual's judgment and/or physical ability. Physiological and cognitive impairment begin at BAC levels below those that are associated with intoxication. As a legal standard, impairment and driving under the influence laws are based on a person's physical or mental impairment as judged on the basis of BAC level, performance in standardized field sobriety tests, or observed behavior. Although this report is focused on impairment from alcohol, impairment can result from other substance use and distracted driving, among others.

---

[a] Utah recently passed legislation to lower the BAC law to 0.05% beginning in December 2018.

[b] States may have lower BAC laws for individuals under the minimum legal drinking age of 21 and commercial drivers.

[c] Of note, a crash involving a nonimpaired motor vehicle driver and an impaired pedestrian or cyclist is not counted as an alcohol-impaired motor vehicle crash fatality by NHTSA's FARS, which collects information about all motor vehicle crash fatalities occurring on U.S. public roadways.

This report also uses *DWI* (instead of *DUI* or a similar state-specific phrase). DWI is a legal term; states vary in how they designate the violation of driving while impaired by alcohol. See the report glossary for definitions of other terms in this report. Discussion of what it means to be impaired follows.

Alcohol's Physiological Effects and Influence on Driving

As noted in Box 1-4, the current legal definition of alcohol impairment in almost all 50 states is a BAC of 0.08%. Although this is the limit set by state law, impairment begins at lower levels; even small amounts of alcohol affect the brain.

Biologically, alcohol impairment occurs before reaching BAC of 0.08%, and impairment affects driving-related skills and behaviors. A standard drink in the United States has 14 grams of pure alcohol, which is the amount of alcohol in approximately 12 ounces of beer of 5 percent alcohol by volume (ABV), 5 ounces of wine of 12 percent ABV, or 1.5 ounces of distilled spirits of 40 percent ABV (NIAAA, n.d.-b) (see Figure 1-7). However, alcohol content varies by beverage type and serving size and therefore a "drink" may contain either more (or less) than the standard 14 grams of pure alcohol (Kerr et al., 2005, 2008, 2009).

Once consumed, alcohol is absorbed from the stomach and small intestine into the bloodstream. Most alcohol metabolism takes place in the liver, but the gastrointestinal tract, pancreas, and brain also metabolize alcohol. Most alcohol is chemically broken down by a process with two enzymes into acetaldehyde and acetate,[12] which is further metabolized and eliminated as water and carbon dioxide (CDC, 2017a; NIAAA, 2007). Alcohol circulates in the bloodstream until the body can metabolize it.

Individuals differ in their degree of impairment at a given BAC. Several factors affect alcohol's physiological influence, including weight, age, sex, race, and ability to metabolize alcohol. Women are often more sensitive to the effects of alcohol and have a higher BAC than men after drinking the same amount of alcohol, in part because women usually have a higher percentage of body fat than men (Cederbaum, 2012; Frezza et al., 1990). Additionally, genetic variations in enzymes affect the clearance of one of the by-products of alcohol metabolism, resulting in an intensified physiological reaction and altering the risk of developing alcohol dependence. Genetic differences interact with other individual

[12] Alcohol dehydrogenase and aldehyde dehydrogenase. Other enzymes have similar roles but may only be active after consumption of large amounts of alcohol.

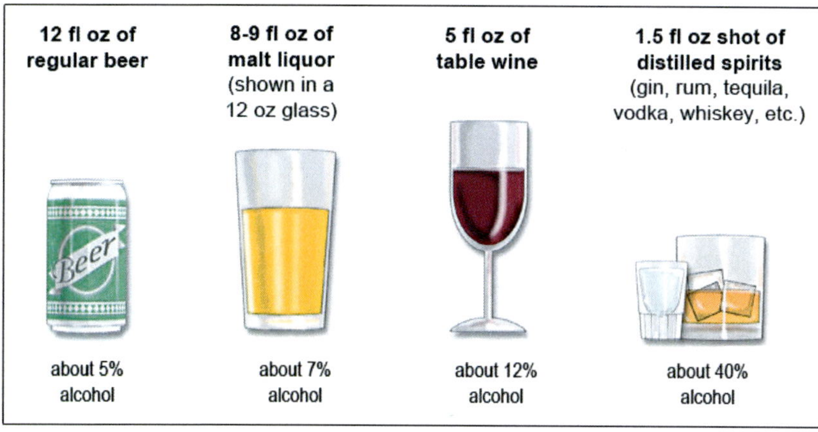

FIGURE 1-7 Standard drinks in the United States.
NOTES: Each beverage portrayed above represents one standard drink of "pure" alcohol, defined in the United States as 0.6 fl oz or 14 grams. The percent of pure alcohol, expressed here as alcohol by volume (ABV), varies within and across beverage types. Although the standard drink amounts are helpful for following health guidelines, they may not reflect customary serving sizes.
SOURCE: NIAAA, n.d.-b.

and environmental elements in determining an individual's response to alcohol (Ehlers and Gizer, 2013; Wall et al., 2016).

The amount and rate of alcohol an individual consumes, along with how often one drinks, and the use of drugs or prescription medications can also affect the body's response to alcohol (CDC, 2017a; NIAAA, n.d.-a). For example, alcohol interacts with a variety of medications such as antibiotics, antidepressants, and opioids and other pain medicines, and can either heighten or hinder the medication's effect (Weathermon and Crabb, 1999). Over-the-counter medications, herbal supplements, and cannabis also alter alcohol metabolism (Ronen et al., 2010; Weathermon and Crabb, 1999).

Alcohol is a central nervous system depressant (Dry et al., 2012). The effects of alcohol include psychomotor impairment, decreased inhibition, diminished alertness and sleepiness, confusion and problems with concentration, reduced visual focus, and slurred speech. At higher BAC levels, alcohol can induce vomiting, blackouts, disrupted breathing, seizures, coma, and death (NHTSA, n.d.; NIAAA, n.d.-a).

Driving requires several complex skills. A driver must maintain the correct speed and keep their vehicle within the appropriate lane while observing and processing their surroundings for safety information (such as traffic signs, other vehicles, and pedestrians). Alcohol affects the capacity to drive safely by impairing information processing and reaction time and compromising judgment and coordination (CDC, 2017a), and the risk of crash increases with higher BAC levels (Hingson et al., 2000; Martin et al., 2013; Starkey and Charlton, 2014). Chapter 4 describes the effects of escalating BAC levels on driving abilities in more detail.

OVERVIEW OF THE STUDY PROCESS

To address its charge, the committee gathered information through a variety of means. It held three information-gathering meetings that were webcast live. The first, held in February 2017, focused on obtaining information on the history of alcohol-impaired driving and interventions currently being used in the United States. The second meeting, held in March 2017, focused on obtaining information on the current alcohol environment, stakeholder activities, relevant surveillance systems, and social movements. The third meeting was held in May 2017; presentation topics included pertinent technological innovations, alcohol policy (such as taxes and warning labels), DWI arrests in tribal communities, and automobile and insurance industry perspectives (committee meeting agendas are listed in Appendix E). The committee also met in deliberative meetings throughout the study process. The committee received public submissions of materials for its consideration throughout the course of the study.[13] The committee's online activity page provided information to the public about the committee's work and facilitated communication with the public.[14]

Throughout this report the committee provides conclusions and recommendations for short-, mid-, and long-term interventions. Chapter 2 provides an overview of the current alcohol and transportation environments. Chapters 3 through 5 target intervention points identified in the conceptual framework: Chapter 3 describes interventions to reduce drinking to impairment, Chapter 4 discusses interventions that affect an individual's likelihood to drive once impaired, and Chapter 5 describes postcrash and postarrest interventions. Chapter 6 identifies data and surveillance needs and opportunities. Chapter 7 considers the importance of social movements and other approaches to generate stakeholder action, and Chapter 8 ties together the previous chapters' recommendations and conclusions. The committee also commissioned four papers

---

[13] Public access materials can be requested from http://www8.nationalacademies.org/cp/projectview.aspx?key=49848 (accessed April 26, 2017).

[14] See http://nationalacademies.org/hmd/Activities/PublicHealth/ReduceAlcoholImpairedDrivingFatalities.aspx (accessed April 26, 2017).

to offer additional context and perspective on alcohol-impaired driving. These papers helped to fill gaps in the literature and were considered in conjunction with other literature on these topics. Appendix A describes data and surveillance systems that could better inform alcohol-impaired driving interventions in the United States. Appendix B presents a content analysis of how alcohol-impaired driving is framed in the news. Appendix C provides an overview of the role of the alcohol industry in alcohol-impaired driving interventions. Finally, Appendix D gives insight into international alcohol-impaired driving countermeasures.

CONCLUSION

To achieve zero alcohol-impaired crash fatalities—where every alcohol-impaired driving death could be thought of as a failure of the system—a systematic, multipronged approach with clear roles and accountabilities across sectors (including public health, transportation, law enforcement, and clinical care) is needed. Victims are dying each day, and fatality rates are rising—substantial progress has been made in the past, and that progress needs to be jump-started again. As a philosophy, Vision Zero offers a system for improvement and a way to rally stakeholders from many arenas around a common goal. No one intervention will solve the preventable deaths resulting from alcohol-impaired driving. This report lays out a comprehensive set of evidence-based and promising interventions and system improvements that when implemented together have the potential to eliminate these preventable deaths.

REFERENCES

AASHTO (American Association of State Highway and Transportation Officials). 2015. *AASHTO introduces Toward Zero Deaths plan to reduce roadway fatalities*. https://news.transportation.org/Pages/NewsReleaseDetail.aspx?NewsReleaseID=1440 (accessed August 17, 2017).

Aboelata, M., E. Yanez, and R. Kharrazi. 2017. *Vision Zero: A health equity road map for getting to zero in every community*. Los Angeles, CA: Prevention Institute.

Ad Council. n.d. *Drunk driving prevention*. https://www.adcouncil.org/Our-Campaigns/The-Classics/Drunk-Driving-Prevention (accessed November 27, 2017).

Bayer, R. 2007. The continuing tensions between individual rights and public health. Talking point on public health versus civil liberties. *EMBO Reports* 8(12):1099–1103.

Belin, M.-Å., P. Tillgren, and E. Vedung. 2012. Vision Zero—A road safety policy innovation. *International Journal of Injury Control and Safety Promotion* 19(2):171–179.

Berning, A., and D. D. Smither. 2014. *Understanding the limitations of drug test information, reporting, and testing practices in fatal crashes*. Traffic Safety Facts Research Note. Report no. DOT HS 812 072. Washington, DC: National Highway Traffic Safety Administration.

Blomberg, R. D., R. C. Peck, H. Moskowitz, M. Burns, and D. Fiorentino. 2005. *Crash risk of alcohol involved driving: A case-control study*. Stamford, CT: Dunlap and Associates, Inc.

CDC (Centers for Disease Control and Prevention). 2016a. *Injury prevention and control: Key injury and violence data.* https://www.cdc.gov/injury/wisqars/overview/key_data.html (accessed September 20, 2017).

CDC. 2016b. *Unintentional drowning: Get the facts.* https://www.cdc.gov/homeandrecreationalsafety/water-safety/waterinjuries-factsheet.html (accessed September 26, 2017).

CDC. 2017a. *Alcohol and public health: Frequently asked questions.* https://www.cdc.gov/alcohol/faqs.htm (accessed May 16, 2017).

CDC. 2017b. *Cervical cancer statistics.* https://www.cdc.gov/cancer/cervical/statistics/index.htm (accessed October 2, 2017).

CDC. 2017c. *HIV/AIDS: Basic statistics.* https://www.cdc.gov/hiv/basics/statistics.html (accessed September 26, 2017).

CDC. 2017d. *Injury prevention and control: Ten leading causes of death and injury.* https://www.cdc.gov/injury/images/lc-charts/leading_causes_of_death_age_group_2015_1050w740h.gif (accessed September 20, 2017).

CDC. 2017e. *Leading causes of death.* https://www.cdc.gov/nchs/fastats/leading-causes-of-death.htm (accessed September 20, 2017).

CDC. 2017f. *Skin cancer statistics.* https://www.cdc.gov/cancer/skin/statistics/index.htm (accessed October 2, 2017).

Cederbaum, A. I. 2012. Alcohol metabolism. *Clinical Liver Disease* 16(4):667–685.

Cohen, D. A., R. A. Scribner, and T. A. Farley. 2000. A structural model of health behavior: A pragmatic approach to explain and influence health behaviors at the population level. *Preventive Medicine* 30(2):146–154.

Compton, R. P., and A. Berning. 2015. *Drug and alcohol crash risk.* Washington, DC: National Highway Traffic Safety Administration.

Dry, M. J., N. R. Burns, T. Nettelbeck, A. L. Farquharson, and J. M. White. 2012. Dose-related effects of alcohol on cognitive functioning. *PLoS ONE* 7(11):e50977.

Ehlers, C. L., and I. R. Gizer. 2013. Evidence for a genetic component for substance dependence in Native Americans. *American Journal of Psychiatry* 170(2):154–164.

Federal Register. n.d. *National Highway Traffic Safety Administration.* https://www.federalregister.gov/agencies/national-highway-traffic-safety-administration (accessed April 26, 2017).

Fell, J. C., and R. B. Voas. 2006. Mothers Against Drunk Driving (MADD): The first 25 years. *Traffic Injury Prevention* 7(3):195–212.

Frezza, M., C. di Padova, G. Pozzato, M. Terpin, E. Baraona, and C. S. Lieber. 1990. High blood alcohol levels in women. The role of decreased gastric alcohol dehydrogenase activity and first-pass metabolism. *New England Journal of Medicine* 322(2):95–99.

Frieden, T. R. 2010. A framework for public health action: The health impact pyramid. *American Journal of Public Health* 100(4):590–595.

Glascoff, M. A., J. S. Shrader, and R. K. Haddock. 2013. Friends don't let friends drive drunk, but do they let friends drive high. *Journal of Alcohol and Drug Education* 57(1):66–84.

Government Offices of Sweden. 2016. *Renewed commitment to Vision Zero: Intensified efforts for transport safety in Sweden.* Stockholm: Government Offices of Sweden.

Haddon, Jr., W. 1980. Advances in the epidemiology of injuries as a basis for public policy. *Public Health Reports* 95(5):411–421.

Halpern, S. D., P. A. Ubel, and D. A. Asch. 2007. Harnessing the power of default options to improve health care. *New England Journal of Medicine* 357(13):1340–1344.

Halpern, S. D., G. Loewenstein, K. G. Volpp, E. Cooney, K. Vranas, C. M. Quill, M. S. McKenzie, M. O. Harhay, N. B. Gabler, T. Silva, R. Arnold, D. C. Angus, and C. Bryce. 2013. Default options in advance directives influence how patients set goals for end-of-life care. *Health Affairs (Millwood)* 32(2):408–417.

Hedlund, J., and A. T. McCartt. 2002. *Drunk driving: Seeking additional solutions.* Washington, DC: AAA Foundation for Traffic Safety.

HHS (U.S. Department of Health and Human Services). 2014. *The health consequences of smoking: 50 years of progress. A report of the Surgeon General.* Atlanta, GA: Office on Smoking and Health.

Hingson, R., T. Heeren, and M. Winter. 2000. Effects of recent 0.08% legal blood alcohol limits on fatal crash involvement. *Injury Prevention* 6(2):109–114.

IIHS (Insurance Institute for Highway Safety). n.d. *Impaired driving.* http://www.iihs.org/iihs/topics/t/impaired-driving/topicoverview (accessed December 4, 2017).

ITE (Institute of Transportation Engineers). 2017. *ITE Vision Zero.* http://www.ite.org/visionzero/default.asp (accessed August 17, 2017).

ITE. n.d. *ITE Vision Zero task force: Statement of intent.* library.ite.org/pub/ed59a040-caf4-5300-8ffc-35deb33ce03d (accessed October 15, 2017).

Kerr, W. C., T. K. Greenfield, J. Tujague, and S. E. Brown. 2005. A drink is a drink? Variation in the amount of alcohol contained in beer, wine and spirits drinks in a US methodological sample. *Alcoholism: Clinical and Experimental Research* 29(11):2015–2021.

Kerr, W. C., D. Patterson, M. A. Koenen, and T. K. Greenfield. 2008. Alcohol content variation of bar and restaurant drinks in northern California. *Alcoholism: Clinical and Experimental Research* 32(9):1623–1629.

Kerr, W. C., D. Patterson, M. A. Koenen, and T. K. Greenfield. 2009. Large drinks are no mistake: Glass size, not shape, affects alcoholic beverage drink pours. *Drug and Alcohol Review* 28(4):360–365.

Martin, T. L., P. A. Solbeck, D. J. Mayers, R. M. Langille, Y. Buczek, and M. R. Pelletier. 2013. A review of alcohol-impaired driving: The role of blood alcohol concentration and complexity of the driving task. *Journal of Forensic Sciences* 58(5):1238–1250.

Matjasko, J. L., J. H. Cawley, M. M. Baker-Goering, and D. V. Yokum. 2016. Applying behavioral economics to public health policy: Illustrative examples and promising directions. *American Journal of Preventive Medicine* 50(5 Suppl 1):S13–S19.

McLeroy, K. R., D. Bibeau, A. Steckler, and K. Glanz. 1988. An ecological perspective on health promotion programs. *Health Education & Behavior* 15(4):351–377.

Michael, J. 2017. PowerPoint presentation to the Committee on Accelerating Progress to Reduce Alcohol-Impaired Driving Fatalities in Washington, DC, February 16, 2017. http://www.nationalacademies.org/hmd/~/media/Files/Activity%20Files/AcceleratingProgresstoReduceAlcoholImpairedDrivingFatalities/16%20FEB%202017/1%20Michael.pdf (accessed September 26, 2017).

NCSA (National Center for Statistics and Analysis). 2016a. *Alcohol-impaired driving: 2015 data.* Traffic Safety Facts. Report no. DOT HS 812 350. Washington, DC: National Highway Traffic Safety Administration.

NCSA. 2016b. *Traffic safety facts 2015: A compliation of motor vehcile crash data from the Fatality Analysis Reporting System and General Estimates System.* Report no. DOT HS 812 384. Washington, DC: National Highway Traffic Safety Administration.

NCSA. 2017a. *2016 fatal motor vehicle crashes: Overview.* Traffic Safety Facts. Report no. DOT HS 812 456. Washington, DC: National Highway Traffic Safety Administration.

NCSA. 2017b. *Rural/urban comparison of traffic fatalities: 2015 data.* Traffic Safety Facts. Report no. DOT HS 812 393. Washington, DC: National Highway Traffic Safety Administration.

NHTSA (National Highway Traffic Safety Administration). 2010. *Drug involvement of fatally injured drivers.* Traffic Safety Facts. Report no. DOT HS 811 415. Washington, DC: National Highway Traffic Safety Administration.

NHTSA. 2016. *U.S. DOT, National Safety Council launch "Road to Zero" Coalition to end roadway fatalities.* https://www.nhtsa.gov/press-releases/us-dot-national-safety-council-launch-road-zero-coalition-end-roadway-fatalities (accessed July 20, 2017).

NHTSA. n.d. *Drunk driving*. https://www.nhtsa.gov/risky-driving/drunk-driving (accessed May 16, 2017).

NIAAA (National Institute on Alcohol Abuse and Alcoholism). 2007. Alcohol metabolism: An update. *Alcohol Alert* 72.

NIAAA. n.d.-a. *Overview of alcohol consumption*. https://www.niaaa.nih.gov/alcohol-health/overview-alcohol-consumption (accessed May 16, 2017).

NIAAA. n.d.-b. *What is a standard drink?* https://www.niaaa.nih.gov/alcohol-health/overview-alcohol-consumption/what-standard-drink (accessed March 30, 2017).

NSC (National Safety Council). 2017. *Road to Zero coalition marks first anniversary in October 2017*. http://www.nsc.org/learn/NSC-Initiatives/Pages/The-Road-to-Zero.aspx (accessed October 13, 2017).

O'Neill, B., and S. Y. Kyrychenko. 2006. Use and misuse of motor-vehicle crash death rates in assessing highway-safety performance. *Traffic Injury Prevention* 7(4):307–318.

Redelmeier, D. A., and A. S. Detsky. 2017. Clinical action against drunk driving. *PLoS Medicine* 14(2):e1002231.

Rice, T. 2013. The behavioral economics of health and health care. *Annual Review of Public Health* 34:431–447.

Ronen, A., H. S. Chassidim, P. Gershon, Y. Parmet, A. Rabinovich, R. Bar-Hamburger, Y. Cassuto, and D. Shinar. 2010. The effect of alcohol, THC and their combination on perceived effects, willingness to drive and performance of driving and non-driving tasks. *Accident Analysis & Prevention* 42(6):1855–1865.

Rosencrantz, H., K. Edvardsson, and S. O. Hansson. 2007. Vision Zero—Is it irrational? *Transportation Research Part A: Policy and Practice* 41(6):559–567.

Sauber-Schatz, E. K., D. J. Ederer, A. M. Dellinger, and G. T. Baldwin. 2016. Vital signs: Motor vehicle injury prevention—United States and 19 comparison countries. *Morbidity and Mortality Weekly Report* 65(26):672–677.

Sloan, F., L. Eldred, and A. Platt. 2011. Deterring rearrests for drinking and driving. *Duke University Department of Economics*. https://thew.web.unc.edu/files/2013/09/sloan2.pdf (accessed May 8, 2017).

Sloan, F. A., L. M. Eldred, and Y. Xu. 2014. The behavioral economics of drunk driving. *Journal of Health Economics* 35:64–81.

Starkey, N. J., and S. G. Charlton. 2014. The effects of moderate alcohol concentrations on driving and cognitive performance during ascending and descending blood alcohol concentrations. *Human Psychopharmacology* 29(4):370–383.

Stockwell, T., J. Zhao, M. Marzell, P. J. Gruenewald, S. Macdonald, W. R. Ponicki, and G. Martin. 2015. Relationships between minimum alcohol pricing and crime during the partial privatization of a Canadian government alcohol monopoly. *Journal of Studies on Alcohol and Drugs* 76(4):628–634.

Subramanian, R. 2002. *Transitioning to multiple imputation—A new method to estimate missing blood alcohol concentration (BAC) values in FARS*. Report no. DOT HS 809 403. Washington, DC: National Center for Statistics and Analysis.

Swedish Transport Administration. 2015. *Swedish Traffic Accident Data Acquisition (STRADA)*. https://www.trafikverket.se/en/startpage/operations/Operations-road/vision-zero-academy/Vision-Zero-and-ways-to-work/strada (accessed October 13, 2017).

Swedish Transport Administration. 2017. *The number of fatalities on Swedish roads is not decreasing*. http://www.trafikverket.se/en/visionzero/vision-zero-conference-2017/news/2017/2017-05/the-number-of-fatalities-on-swedish-roads-is-not-decreasing (accessed July 20, 2017).

Swedish Transport Administration. n.d. *Taking safety to new levels*. http://www.visionzeroinitiative.com/taking-safety-to-new-levels (accessed July 20, 2017).

Task Force on Community Preventive Services. 2000. Developing an evidence-based Guide to Community Preventive Services—Methods. *American Journal of Preventive Medicine* 18(1S):35–43.

Thorgeirsson, T., and I. Kawachi. 2013. Behavioral economics: Merging psychology and economics for lifestyle interventions. *American Journal of Preventive Medicine* 44(2):185–189.

Tingvall, C., and N. Haworth. 2000. Vision Zero: An ethical approach to safety and mobility. Paper read at 6th ITE International Conference Road Safety & Traffic Enforcement: Beyond 2000, Melbourne, Australia.

TZD (Toward Zero Deaths). 2015. *Background*. http://www.towardzerodeaths.org/strategy/background (accessed August 17, 2017).

Vision Zero Network. 2017. *Vision Zero cities map*. http://visionzeronetwork.org/resources/vision-zero-cities (accessed July 19, 2017).

Voas, R. B., and J. C. Lacey. 2011. *Alcohol and highway safety: A review of the state of knowledge*. Report no. DOT HS 811 374. Washington, DC: National Highway Traffic Safety Administration.

Wall, T. L., S. E. Luczak, and S. Hiller-Sturmhofel. 2016. Biology, genetics, and environment: Underlying factors influencing alcohol metabolism. *Alcohol Research* 38(1):59–68.

Weathermon, R., and D. W. Crabb. 1999. Alcohol and medication interactions. *Alcohol Research and Health* 23(1):40–54.

WHO (World Health Organization). n.d. *About social determinants of health*. http://www.who.int/social_determinants/sdh_definition/en (accessed October 6, 2017).

Williams, A. F. 2006. Alcohol-impaired driving and its consequences in the United States: The past 25 years. *Journal of Safety Research* 37(2):123–138.

Zaloshnja, E., T. R. Miller, and L. J. Blincoe. 2013. Costs of alcohol-involved crashes, United States, 2010. Paper read at 57th Annual Meeting of the Association for the Advancement of Automotive Medicine Conference, Quebec City, Canada.

Zimmerman, F. J. 2009. Using behavioral economics to promote physical activity. *Preventive Medicine* 49(4):289–291.

2

Current Environment: Alcohol, Driving, and Drinking and Driving

INTRODUCTION

To accelerate progress to reduce alcohol-impaired driving fatalities, it is important to understand the context in which these fatalities occur, as noted in the committee's conceptual framework (see Figure 1-5). This includes the trends and patterns of alcohol-impaired driving and the impacts and costs borne by society. For alcohol-impaired driving, there are two contexts that are especially salient and worth examining: the alcohol environment (e.g., social and cultural drinking norms, availability, pricing, and regulation) and the driving environment (e.g., road safety infrastructure, public transportation, and driving patterns). In this chapter, data on alcohol-impaired driving are discussed in depth, as well as the impacts and costs of crashes, injuries, and fatalities. The current alcohol and driving landscapes are discussed as the backdrop for alcohol-impaired driving. The chapter concludes with a high-level overview of the existing drinking- and driving-specific interventions in place for addressing alcohol-impaired driving.[1]

[1] The 2016 fatal traffic crash data became available late in the study process (October 2017); however, in-depth analyses had not yet been completed during the writing of this report. When 2016 analyses were not available, 2015 (or most recent) data were used.

THE ALCOHOL ENVIRONMENT

The alcohol environment today can be understood by examining drinking trends, social and cultural drinking norms, alcohol availability, promotion, pricing, regulation, and the policies and laws that shape these factors. The nature of this environment has important implications for drinking and driving behaviors (Bond et al., 2008; Huckle et al., 2006), as well as the relative success of interventions designed to reduce alcohol-impaired driving (Xuan et al., 2015a).

Drinking Behaviors and Trends

Alcohol consumption, while intertwined with many social and cultural norms in the United States, is not uniform across all populations (Babor, 2010a) and the overall prevalence of alcohol consumption varies. The 2015 National Survey on Drug Use and Health reported that of people 18 years or older, 86.4 percent have drunk alcohol at some time in their lives, 70.1 percent drank in the past year, and 56.0 percent drank in the past month (SAMHSA, 2016). These data run counter to the misperception that drinking is more widespread than it actually is, particularly among college-aged students, for whom drinking prevalence is commonly overestimated (Baer et al., 1991; Martens et al., 2006; Perkins et al., 2005). Research suggests that for those who do consume alcohol, drinking varies with respect to frequency, quantity, the rate at which people drink, and preferred alcoholic beverage and/or combination.

Despite standard drink sizes for beer, wine, and distilled spirits (see Chapter 1 for more information on standard drinks), it is often difficult for individuals to determine the amount of alcohol they have consumed because of variations in alcohol content per drink. While very little research has been done on the mean, distribution, and sources of variation in the alcohol content of drinks, some information is available. In regards to beer, draught beers tend to have higher alcohol by volume (ABV) than a standard drink (Kerr et al., 2008). Newer craft beers, typically with 7 to 9 percent ABV (compared to 5 percent ABV for a standard 12-ounce drink of beer), have also entered the market in recent years. Drinkers and bartenders may not be aware of these differences or pay much attention to them when serving and consuming alcohol, leading to greater levels of intoxication than intended. This is true for wine and distilled spirits as well. A Northern California focus group found that an average glass of wine and an average mixed drink served at a bar had 43 and 42 percent, respectively, more alcohol than a standard drink (Kerr et al., 2008). Not only is there wide variability in the alcohol content of drinks served in bars and restaurants, but there is also significant variability in the drinks served in people's homes (Kerr et al., 2005). A study conducted by Kerr and Stockwell (2012) found that drinkers have difficulty identifying and pouring standard drinks, with a propensity to overpour. As a result, it can be difficult to determine how much alcohol one has consumed based on the number of "drinks" they have had. Standard drink size also varies from country to country. The United Kingdom has a standard drink size of 8 grams of pure alcohol; in Australia a standard drink is 10 grams, in the United States it is 14 grams, and in Japan it is 19.75 grams (WHO, 2014).

Data from the 1975–2016 Monitoring the Future survey suggest that 32 percent of college students binge drink (Schulenberg et al., 2017).[2] Similarly, a review of studies on drinking among college students found a consistent national rate of binge drinking of about 40 percent (Wechsler and Nelson, 2008). In college settings, rates of drinking are highest among first-year students, athletes, and members of fraternities and sororities (Wechsler and Nelson, 2008). Additionally, almost one-quarter of college students who self-identify as current drinkers consume alcohol with energy drinks, putting themselves at a higher risk of serious consequences, as caffeine affects a drinker's ability to judge their level of impairment (O'Brien et al., 2008). Data from the 2005–2011 Monitoring the Future study also show that about one-fifth of high school seniors binge drink, and intensity of binge drinking is higher for students in rural areas (Patrick et al., 2013).

Recently published analyses from the National Epidemiologic Survey on Alcohol-Related Conditions (NESARC) found that alcohol consumption among U.S. adults rose substantially between 2001–2002 and 2012–2013, with annual use increasing by 11.2 percent (from 65.4 percent of the population 18 years or older in 2001–2002 to 72.7 percent in 2012–2013), and high-risk drinking increasing by 29.9 percent (from 9.7 in 2001–2002 to 12.6 percent in 2012–2013) (Grant et al., 2017).[3] The NESARC study also found the largest increases in alcohol consumption, alcohol-impaired driving, and alcohol use disorder in women, older adults, individuals of racial or ethnic minority, and individuals with lower income and educational attainment (Grant et al., 2017).[4]

Social and cultural norms of alcohol use vary by gender and among ethnic groups in the United States (Galvan and Caetano, 2003). For

---

[2] Binge drinking is defined in this study as consuming five or more drinks in a row on at least one occasion (i.e., typically over a period of 2 hours) in the past 2 weeks (Schulenberg et al., 2017).

[3] High-risk drinking is defined in this study as four or more drinks on any day among women and five or more drinks on any day among men (Grant et al., 2017).

[4] "Alcohol use disorder" as defined in the *Diagnostic and Statistical Manual of Mental Disorders* (DSM-IV).

example, men drink alcohol more often than women, including heavier drinking, and are more likely to experience drinking-related consequences (Rahav et al., 2006; Wilsnack et al., 2000, 2009). Furthermore, drinking alcohol has been linked with perceptions of masculinity (De Visser and Smith, 2007) and is strongly associated with the social aspect of sports and sporting events (Collins and Vamplew, 2011). In recent years, however, differences in patterns of drinking by gender have narrowed, particularly among adolescents and young adults (Jang et al., 2017). For example, research suggests an increase in binge drinking among younger and older women (Breslow et al., 2017; Dwyer-Lindgren et al., 2015). Drinking patterns across racial and ethnic groups are complex. In general, alcohol consumption is most common among non-Hispanic whites and people who report two or more races, and lowest among Asians (SAMHSA, 2014). Recent data from the National Longitudinal Survey of Youth reveal racial and ethnic differences in "aging out" of heavy drinking behaviors. African American and Hispanic men and women exhibited slower declines in heavy drinking frequency during their 20s than white men and women (Mulia et al., 2017). While life course trajectories of heavy drinking may show one pattern, age- and sex-adjusted estimates from the 2016 National Health Interview Survey demonstrate another. These findings showed that non-Hispanic white adults (31.2 percent) were more likely to have at least one heavy drinking day in the past year when compared to Hispanic and non-Hispanic Black adults (22.1 and 15.4 percent, respectively) (Clarke et al., 2017).

Beyond the physiological effects of alcohol, an individual's perceptions of his or her level of impairment can also affect his or her behavior. Alcohol metabolism facilitates the perception of impairment, and an individual is made aware of the effects of alcohol by biological cues or changes in his or her behavior (Laude and Fillmore, 2016). In studying the subjective view of impairment, researchers have found that the number of beverages a person thinks they can consume in 2 hours before their driving becomes impaired is 30 percent higher for African Americans and 26 percent higher for Hispanics compared to whites, indicating cultural disparities in drink preference (and therefore alcohol content) or subjective conception of impairment (Kerr and Greenfield, 2015; Kerr et al., 2006).

Generally, people are often not aware of how impaired they are because they misjudge the rates of alcohol absorption and elimination, or because they may not understand the relationship between the quantity of alcohol consumed and the resulting blood alcohol concentration (BAC) (Aston and Liguori, 2013).[5] This could lead drinkers to think they

---

[5] Some existing tools for understanding BAC include the National Highway Traffic Safety Administration's (NHTSA's) "ABCs of BAC."

are recovering from alcohol more quickly than they actually are. Drivers who underestimate their BAC are more willing to drive while above the limit set by state law compared to drivers who more correctly assess their BAC, and drivers who incorrectly estimate low BAC levels exhibit riskier driving (Laude and Fillmore, 2016). Furthermore, some impaired drivers exhibit riskier behaviors even while their psychomotor skills are not demonstrably compromised. Conversely, other drivers' risky behavior may not change but their psychomotor skills could be significantly impaired (Laude and Fillmore, 2016). A 2013 review noted nonalcoholic social drinkers were more capable than alcoholic drinkers at assessing changes in their BAC levels;[6] this population was also able to learn to estimate their BAC levels more accurately after training, while training was less effective in alcoholic drinkers (Aston and Liguori, 2013). Finally, stimulant drugs such as energy drinks and 3,4-Methylenedioxymethamphetamine (MDMA or Ecstasy) may reduce subjective views of intoxication and lead drinkers to think they are not impaired, but the effects of those drugs are not sufficient to overcome objectively measured alcohol impairment (Martin et al., 2013).

General Regulatory Framework for Alcohol

Historically, beer was the beverage of choice of the drinking driver (Berger and Snortum, 1985); more recent data are not available about which kinds of alcohol are most common among alcohol-impaired drivers today, but beer continues to claim the most consumer dollars of the three main types of alcohol beverages (beer, wine, and distilled spirits) (Impact Databank, 2017a,b). The Gallup poll also reports that beer is the most commonly consumed of the three beverage types (Beer Marketer's Insights, 2017). In the United States, 82 percent of the volume of beer sales are made for off-premise consumption (e.g., supermarkets, convenience stores, and stores selling distilled spirits),[7] while 53.7 percent of the dollar value of sales occur in on-premise establishments (e.g., bars and restaurants) (Beer Marketer's Insights, 2017). Prices of alcoholic beverages sold for off-premises consumption have become significantly more affordable

[6] Nonalcoholic social drinkers were defined in the study described by Aston and Liguori (2013) as moderate drinkers who (1) consumed 1 to 4 alcoholic beverages at least twice per week, with each drink containing the equivalent of 1 oz. of 80-proof (40 percent) alcohol; (2) consumed an average of 4 to 10 drinks at a party; (3) were able to consume at least 6 to 7 drinks on a single occasion (as required for the experimental procedure); and (4) had been intoxicated 2 to 12 times during the past year (Huber et al., 1976; Lansky et al., 1978).

[7] Off-premise outlets are establishments where alcohol can be sold, but not consumed (e.g., package stores and supermarkets), and on-premise outlets are establishments where alcohol can be sold and consumed (e.g., bars and restaurants).

from 1950 to 2011. One drink per day of the cheapest brand of spirits required 0.29 percent of U.S. mean per capita disposable income in 2011 versus 1.02 percent in 1980 and 4.46 percent in 1950 (Kerr et al., 2013a). This increase in affordability over this time period is reflected in beer and wine prices as well (Kerr et al., 2013a) (see Chapter 3 for more information on alcohol pricing and taxation).

Because of commercial speech protection afforded by judicial interpretations of the First Amendment, alcohol advertising is primarily self-regulated by the alcohol industry. One provision specifies that advertisements should not be directed at audiences in which 28.4 percent or more of the audience is under 21 years of age (FTC, 2013). Although the Federal Trade Commission has published occasional reports monitoring the effectiveness of the industry's self-regulatory codes and has generally been approving of them (FTC, 2013), independent researchers have found that violations of these codes in the media are frequent and that exposure of alcohol marketing to youth and other vulnerable populations is especially pervasive and often disproportionately large compared to adult populations (King et al., 2017).

Alcohol Industry

A crucial force in shaping the environments in which people make their decisions about drinking, which in turn affect their likelihood of drinking and driving, is the alcohol industry itself. By dint of its size and structure, it is a formidable political force. Its practices and innovations in product development, pricing, promotion, and making its products physically available essentially structure the context of drinking for Americans.

The U.S. alcohol industry is dominated by a small number of companies. Beer is the most concentrated segment in terms of ownership: As of 2016, two companies, Anheuser-Busch and MillerCoors, account for 67.3 percent of the market in terms of volume, while the top five companies sell 79.8 percent of beer (Advocates for Highway and Auto Safety, 2017). For both distilled spirits and wine, the top five producers account for more than half the volume of sales (Impact Databank, 2017a,b). While craft brewing and distilling have been increasingly visible, and the number of craft brewers and distillers has grown substantially in recent years, the largest "craft" segment, brewing, still only comprises a small percentage of the total beer market—less than 12 percent as of 2016. The craft brewing market itself is becoming more concentrated—the top ten craft brewers sold nearly 60 percent of craft beers in 2016, as opposed to 53 percent in 2011. Furthermore, craft beer brands that have been acquired by the largest beer companies are showing the strongest growth trends (Beer Marketer's Insights, 2017).

The oligopolistic structure of the alcohol industry creates the conditions for oligopolic profit-taking and the creation of high barriers to entry in the form of heavy spending on marketing. In 2016 alcohol producers spent approximately $2.2 billion on measured marketing (television, magazines, outdoor, radio, Internet, and newspapers). Unmeasured marketing activities include sports and other sponsorships, special events, discounting, and corporate "stakeholder" marketing. The latter category includes lobbying: in 2015 alcohol companies spent $13.2 million on lobbying in state legislatures (FollowTheMoney.org, n.d.); in 2016 they donated almost $27 million to members of Congress and reported 295 lobbyists working for them at the federal level (OpenSecrets.org, n.d.).

Stakeholder marketing also encompasses corporate social responsibility (CSR) activities such as efforts to prevent alcohol-impaired driving. However, global analyses of alcohol industry CSR activities have consistently found that the alcohol industry pursues and supports the least effective strategies and actively opposes the most effective (Babor et al., 2015, 2018; Esser et al., 2016; Pantani et al., 2017). Esser et al. (2016) performed a content analysis of 266 randomly sampled alcohol industry initiatives to decrease alcohol-impaired driving and found that insufficient evidence or no scientific evidence exists for 56.0 percent of these initiatives. Furthermore, two-thirds of the initiatives were rated as potentially harmful based on conflict with public health evidence (e.g., promoting the use of designated drivers, for which evidence of effectiveness is insufficient and suggests negative unintended consequences—see Chapter 4 and Finding 4-1 for more information), and 87.6 percent were found to be potential brand or company marketing activities (Esser et al., 2016). See Appendix C for more information on the alcohol industry's role in promoting alcohol-impaired driving interventions.

It is also important to recognize that there may be a basic conflict of interest for the alcohol industry between the need to maintain profitability and growth and efforts to reduce the prevalence of underage drinking and intoxication, both of which can lead to alcohol-impaired driving. Researchers estimated that in 2001 (the most recent year for which these estimates are available), underage and pathological drinking accounted for between 37.5 and 48.8 percent of consumer expenditures on alcohol (Foster et al., 2006). Thus, were the population to drink in a fully legal and nonpathological fashion, the industry could lose nearly half of its revenues, and the government would lose a large amount of its tax revenues as well.

Alcohol industry activities in product development, pricing, promotions and sponsorships, and physical availability of alcoholic beverages are briefly described below.

Product Development

Recent trends in alcoholic beverage development have presented particular risks for alcohol-impaired driving. Alcohol content in almost all types of alcoholic beverages has been steadily increasing, especially with the growing popularity of craft beverages (Kerr et al., 2013b; Mintel, 2015). In addition, the practice of mixing alcohol and caffeine, while effectively banned at the point of production at least for malt beverages (Babor et al., 2017), continues to be common, particularly among young binge drinkers (CDC, 2017a). Systematic reviews have found that young drinkers who consume mixtures of alcohol and energy drinks are at higher risk for binge drinking and driving, riding as a passenger in a vehicle with an intoxicated driver, and being arrested for driving while impaired (Babor et al., 2018; McKetin et al., 2015; Striley and Khan, 2014). Findings from a review of randomized controlled studies suggest that although energy drink consumption may deter small declines in cognitive function that result from alcohol consumption, such counteracting effects are not observed when driving (Babor et al., 2018; Lalanne et al., 2017). In addition, evidence suggests that consumption of drinks combining alcohol and energy drinks hinders a person's ability to estimate their level of impairment (Forward et al., 2017).

In 2015 Anheuser-Busch InBev (AB InBev) launched its Global Smart Drinking Goals, which include reducing harmful drinking by at least 10 percent in six pilot cities by 2020; implementing the best practices from pilot cities globally by 2025; influencing social norms and behaviors to reduce harmful drinking by investing in social marketing campaigns and programs by 2025; ensuring that no- or lower-alcohol beer products comprise at least 20 percent of all beer volume produced by the company; placing a guidance label on all beer products by 2020; and increasing alcohol health literacy by 2025 (AB InBev, n.d.). It is important to note that the AB InBev smart drinking goals have not yet been evaluated. Rehm et al. (2016) attempted to assess the potential effects of reducing alcoholic strength of available products on reducing harmful drinking. While the study authors cite one mechanism that may potentially reduce harmful drinking, they note there is not yet evidence to substantiate this. The smart drinking goals require rigorous evaluation and investigation into their potential for positive or negative impacts (Anderson and Rehm, 2016).

Pricing

Alcohol purchased at off-premises establishments is more affordable now than it has been in 60 years (Kerr et al., 2013a). Significant decreases in alcohol prices have resulted in large part from decreases in federal and state tax rates, particularly in the 1960s and 1970s (see Chapter 3 for more information on alcohol pricing and taxation) (Kerr et al., 2013a). More recently, product developments from the alcohol industry have led to lower priced options for consumers. Alcoholic energy drinks and premixed, ready-to-drink products, often with high alcohol and sugar contents, have been developed with younger and more cost-conscious populations (e.g., college students) in mind (Babor et al., 2018).

Promotions and Sponsorships

Alcohol industry marketing strategies have become increasingly more sophisticated and pervasive in media outlets, including television and print media. Exposure of youth to alcohol marketing is well documented in both traditional and digital media (Lobstein et al., 2017), and at least 25 longitudinal studies have found associations between youth exposure to alcohol marketing in various forms and subsequent youth drinking behavior (Jernigan et al., 2017). Evidence also suggests that alcohol marketing to youth is more likely to contain riskier content related to sexism and sexual activity; in one advertising study, advertisements with such content increased as the percentage of the advertisement audience that was under 21 increased (Rhoades and Jernigan, 2013).

The alcohol industry also promotes its products through sponsorships of sports events, music festivals, and other public events, many of which are likely to be more appealing to younger audiences (Babor et al., 2018). Alcohol industry promotion can be found in major U.S. professional sports leagues (all of which have at least one alcohol industry sponsor), particularly at professional motorsport racing events such as those held by NASCAR (Babor et al., 2018). In addition to encouraging greater alcohol consumption among younger audiences, the alcohol industry's marketing promotions and sponsorships may also target women and other high-risk and/or vulnerable populations (Babor et al., 2018).

Physical Availability

Alcohol as a retail product is widely available in the United States. There is strong evidence for the correlation between increased availability of alcohol and increased consumption and, as a result, increased alcohol-related problems (Ames and Grube, 1999; Babor, 2010b). Availability of alcohol to younger, often underage, populations is also widespread (Forster et al., 1995). The expansion of the alcohol beverage market by transnational producers is likely to result in increased and more widespread availability, sales, and consumption (Babor et al., 2018). Working alongside the aforementioned promotional and sponsorship activities, such market expansion has the potential to increase rates of alcohol-related problems including crashes and fatalities (Babor et al., 2018).

Conclusion 2-1: Alcoholic beverages as a commodity have changed significantly in the past 25 years. They are more affordable, of far greater variety, and more widely advertised and promoted than in earlier periods. In addition, inconsistent serving sizes and the combination of alcohol with caffeine and energy drinks undermine individuals' ability to estimate their level of impairment.

Shifts in Resources Allocated to Reducing Alcohol-Related Harm

Funding for federal programs aimed at reducing alcohol-related harm, particularly to minors, has significantly dwindled in recent years. The U.S. Department of Justice's Enforcing Underage Drinking Laws program is the sole federal initiative that exclusively addresses underage drinking and availability of alcohol to minors (DOJ, 2009). The program has provided funding in the form of block grants and discretionary awards as well as training and technical assistance to states to support local law enforcement agencies and community organizations in their efforts to decrease availability of alcohol to minors (DOJ, 2009). From its initiation in fiscal year (FY) 1998 through FY 2008, the program received $25 million in annual appropriations from Congress (NASADAD, 2016). Appropriation amounts decreased each year thereafter, with $2.5 million appropriated in FY 2014; in FYs 2015 and 2016 the program was not funded at all (NASADAD, 2016). Similarly, funding for the U.S. Department of Education's Safe and Drug-Free Families and Communities program was substantially decreased in FY 2011 and has remained completely unfunded since FY 2012 (HHS and SAMHSA, 2016). See Table 7-1 for funding of federal substance abuse prevention programs from 2009 to 2014.

ALCOHOL-IMPAIRED DRIVING TRENDS

In the United States an adult driver is considered to be alcohol impaired by state law when his or her BAC is 0.08 grams per deciliter (g/dL) or higher.[8] The term *driver* can refer to the operator of any motor vehicle, including motorcycles, passenger cars, light trucks, and large trucks. As discussed in Chapter 1, over the past four decades there have been significant reductions in alcohol-impaired driving, particularly from

[8] On March 23, 2017, Utah became the first state in the United States to pass a BAC law of 0.05% in the state (Utah State Legislature, 2017); however, the 0.05% limit set by state law will not take effect until December 30, 2018.

the 1980s to the early 2000s (Voas and Lacey, 2011). From 1973 to 2014, there was an 80 percent reduction in the proportion of drivers who were alcohol impaired during weekend nights (7.5 to 1.5 percent), a high-risk period for driving while impaired (Berning et al., 2015). Fatalities attributable to alcohol-impaired driving crashes also saw dramatic decreases over this period of time. Alcohol-impaired driving crash fatalities decreased by almost 40 percent from 1982 to 2015 (NCSA, 2016a; Voas and Lacey, 2011). As a function of vehicle miles traveled, the alcohol-related driving fatality rate per 100 million vehicle miles traveled declined by 63 percent compared to a 25 percent decline in non-alcohol-related fatalities from 1982 to 2003 (Voas and Lacey, 2011).[9] This reduction is noteworthy because during this time period, vehicle miles traveled increased substantially, indicating significant progress in past efforts to reduce alcohol-impaired driving fatalities.

Despite this progress, alcohol-impaired driving persists today, and alcohol-impaired driving fatalities have constituted almost 31 percent of overall motor vehicle crash fatalities in the last 10 years from 2006 to 2016 (Michael, 2017; NCSA, 2016a, 2017a). This fatality rate has held steady, with very little change, for more than 7 years (NCSA, 2016a, 2017a). Moreover, recent data reveal an increase in overall traffic fatalities from 2014 to 2016, including a rise in fatalities caused by alcohol-impaired driving crashes. NHTSA's National Center for Statistics and Analysis reported a 5.6 percent increase in motor vehicle crash fatalities in 2016 (37,461 deaths over the period of 1 year) and a 7.2 percent increase in 2015 (35,092 deaths in 2015 compared to 32,744 deaths in 2014), the largest percentage increase in nearly 50 years (NCSA, 2016b, 2017a). Among these fatalities in 2016, 10,497 were caused by alcohol-impaired driving crashes, a 1.7 percent increase from 2015 (NCSA, 2017a). The rate of alcohol-impaired driving fatalities in motor vehicle crashes per 100 million vehicle miles traveled, however, remained the same from 2014 to 2016 at a rate of 0.33 percent (NCSA, 2016a, 2017b). While alcohol-impaired driving fatalities decreased the most for crashes involving pickup truck drivers from 2007 to 2016 (5 percent decrease), the percentage increased by 1 percent for large trucks (NCSA, 2017b). Alcohol-related motorcyclist fatalities have also increased significantly, particularly for those ages 55 to 64 years old (DiMaggio et al., 2018).

Relative to other developed, high-income countries, the United States lags behind in terms of preventing alcohol-impaired driving fatalities (Sauber-Schatz et al., 2016). In an analysis of data from 2000 to 2013 collected by the World Health Organization and the Organisation for

[9] This rate includes alcohol-related crashes involving a driver with a BAC of 0.01% or greater.

Economic Co-operation and Development (OECD), the Centers for Disease Control and Prevention (CDC) found that the percentage of motor vehicle crash deaths involving alcohol-impaired driving in the United States, 31 percent, was the second highest among 19 OECD countries (Sauber-Schatz et al., 2016). Redelmeier and Detsky analyzed data from the OECD Road Safety 2015 Annual Report and found that alcohol-related traffic deaths per million population annually in the United States exceed those in Australia, Austria, Canada, France, Germany, Italy, the Netherlands, Spain, and the United Kingdom (Redelmeier and Detsky, 2017). CDC found that the United States consistently ranks poorly in rates of total crash fatalities compared to other high-income countries, even when taking into account population size (CDC, 2016). In a 2013 comparison of 10 high-income countries,[10] the United States had the most motor vehicle crash deaths per 100,000 people at 10.6 percent, while New Zealand and Canada[11] in second and third place trailed far behind at 6 percent (WHO, 2015a). This equaled about 90 people dying every day on U.S. roads (CDC, 2016). In the same report the United States came in second in percentage of crash deaths involving alcohol at 31 percent (WHO, 2015a). Canada ranked number one with 34 percent and New Zealand ranked third (WHO, 2015a). In 2016, 29 people died on U.S. roads every day from crashes involving alcohol-impaired drivers (NCSA, 2017b). While international comparisons may help to draw attention to progress made in reducing alcohol-impaired driving in similarly developed and motorized countries, there are many limitations for such comparisons (O'Neill and Kyrychenko, 2006).

While nationwide the number of alcohol-impaired driving fatalities increased from 2015 to 2016, a closer examination at the state level paints a more complex picture. Seventeen states and Puerto Rico saw reductions in alcohol-impaired driving fatalities, with Wyoming experiencing the largest decrease (40.7 percent). However, 29 states and the District of Columbia observed increases in fatalities, with the largest increase being in Vermont (80.0 percent) (NCSA, 2017a). In absolute terms, Mississippi saw the largest decrease in the number of alcohol-impaired driving fatalities (49 fewer deaths) and California experienced the largest increase (148 more deaths).

In 2016, among all alcohol-impaired driving crash fatalities,[12] 6,479 deaths (62 percent) were drivers who had BAC levels of 0.08% or higher,

---

[10] The 10 countries compared were Canada, France, Germany, Japan, New Zealand, Spain, Sweden, Switzerland, the United Kingdom, and the United States.

[11] Based on 2012 motor vehicle crash death data.

[12] The Fatal Analysis Reporting System (FARS) defines an alcohol-impaired driving crash to be one that involves a driver with a BAC of 0.08 g/dL or higher. Estimates of alcohol-

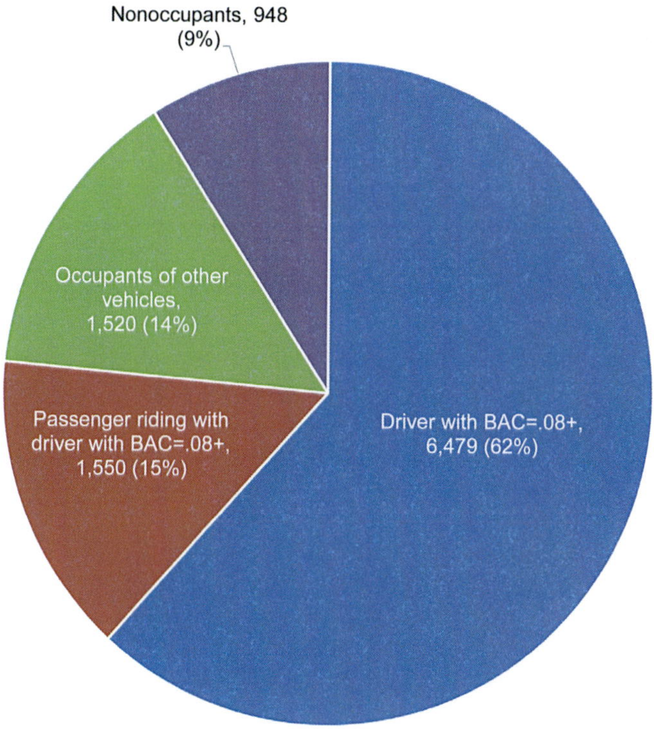

FIGURE 2-1 Fatalities, by role, in crashes involving at least one driver with a BAC ≥0.08%, 2016.
SOURCE: Data from NCSA, 2017b.

3,070 (29 percent) were motor vehicle occupants, and 948 (9 percent) were nonoccupants (NCSA, 2017b). See Figure 2-1 for more details on fatalities by role in alcohol-impaired driving crashes. Children are particularly vulnerable to alcohol-impaired driving crash fatalities. Among children ages 14 and younger who were killed in motor vehicle crashes in 2016, 17 percent died in alcohol-impaired driving crashes, 54 percent of whom were occupants of vehicles with drivers who had BAC levels of 0.08% or higher, 29 percent of whom were occupants in other vehicles, and 17 percent of whom were nonoccupants (pedestrians, cyclists, or others) (NCSA, 2017b). Most child passengers (61 percent) who were involved in

impaired driving are generated using BAC values reported to the FARS, and BAC values are estimated when not available.

an alcohol-impaired driving crash from 2001 to 2010 were unrestrained at the time of the collision (Quinlan et al., 2014). Data on pedestrian traffic fatalities in 2016 indicate that these are on the rise, and 15 percent of drivers involved in these crashes had a BAC of 0.08% or greater (Retting, 2017). In summary, alcohol-impaired driving fatalities are not limited to the drivers themselves; other vehicle occupants including children and nonoccupants such as cyclists and pedestrians are also victims of crashes caused by alcohol-impaired driving.

Alcohol-impaired drivers are more likely to drive at higher speeds and to be involved in motor vehicle crashes at excessive speeds, as impairment diminishes sensory motor function and increases (i.e., delays) reaction time. Evidence suggests that driving while impaired (DWI) enforcement, such as sobriety checkpoints and saturation patrols, in combination with enforcement of speeding laws is effective at decreasing alcohol-related driving crashes and resulting injuries and fatalities (Sanem et al., 2015). See Chapters 4 and 5 for information on these and other DWI enforcement efforts.

First-time DWI offenders comprise the majority of DWI convictions, and only a small number of fatally injured drivers have prior convictions on their driving records (Williams et al., 2007). Nonetheless, efforts to draw attention to "hardcore DWI offenders" (i.e. repeat offenders or those with excessively high BAC levels), as well as stricter sanctions for such persons, are common, particularly from the alcohol industry (Williams et al., 2007). Evidence suggests that interventions aimed at repeat offenders, such as ignition interlocks, may also be beneficial to first-time offenders by decreasing their likelihood of recidivism (Williams et al., 2007) (see Chapter 5 for information on ignition interlocks). Interventions to decrease alcohol-impaired driving are likely to be most effective when aimed at all groups of drivers (Williams et al., 2007).

Luoma and Sivak (2014) examined the differences in road safety among the Netherlands, Sweden, the United Kingdom, and the United States. The authors found that while the United States had the lowest average alcohol consumption per capita, it also reported the highest number of alcohol-related driving fatalities. These findings do not account for the differences in limits set by laws between countries and the underreporting of alcohol-related crashes, yet they highlight an important disparity in alcohol-related crash fatalities. Lower fatality rates in other high-income countries suggest that the United States needs to make significantly more progress in reducing motor vehicle crash deaths to catch up to its peer nations. Between 2000 and 2013 the United States reduced overall crash deaths by 31 percent, while the average reduction among comparable high-income countries was 56 percent (CDC, 2016).

Other Adverse Driving Behaviors

Alcohol-impaired driving exists among other forms of dangerous driving behaviors such as distracted driving, drowsy driving, and driving under the influence of other drugs (e.g., cannabis or prescription drugs). The increasing prevalence of these forms of risky driving and their associated consequences has drawn a considerable amount of attention in the news and public agenda (Fisher, 2018). These are dangerous driving behaviors that pose health and safety risks to the public, and they warrant systematic investigation and the implementation of tailored, evidence-based solutions. This is particularly relevant for states that are navigating the recent legalization of cannabis and how that change may affect their current systems to address problems related to driving while impaired (NHTSA et al., 2017), as the scope of the problems of drug-impaired driving as well as concurrent drug- and alcohol-impaired driving are not well understood. Increases in the use of cannabis and prescription drugs are necessitating current research efforts to examine crash risk associated with drug use (Gjerde et al., 2015; Strand et al., 2016), methods for identification of drug-impaired drivers, and countermeasures to reduce crashes and fatalities from drug-impaired driving. However, it is important to note that while these types of driving have garnered much of the public's attention, alcohol-impaired driving remains the most dangerous form of risky driving and constitutes the highest proportion of motor vehicle crash fatalities owing to human choices among distracted driving, restraint use, speeding, and drowsy driving (Compton and Berning, 2015; NCSA, 2016b). In addition, emerging evidence indicates that crash risk is highest for drivers impaired by both alcohol and drugs (AAA Foundation for Traffic Safety, 2016; WHO, 2015b, 2016). However, available data on driving fatalities due to impairment from drug use and impairment from co-use of drugs and alcohol is limited (see Chapter 6 for information on limitations in drug data collected by the FARS). Additional research will be needed to more fully understand the scope and extent of these problems.

Distracted driving occurs when drivers divert their attention from the driving task to another activity (e.g., texting, eating, talking to other passengers, or adjusting radio or climate controls). Talking and texting on cell phones are not only a distraction as manual tasks but also a cognitive distraction, and the combination of cognitive distraction with alcohol impairment increases the already heightened crash risk of either impairment alone. Distracted driving has increased over time and contributes to an increasing amount of motor vehicle crash fatalities per year (Wilson and Stimpson, 2010). In 2016, crash fatalities that involved distracted driving made up 9 percent of total crash fatalities (NCSA, 2017a). This is equivalent to almost one-third of the number of alcohol-impaired driving crash fatalities during that year. Furthermore, research suggests that alcohol is an increasingly significant factor to account for in the growing number of fatalities involving distracted driving. From 1999 to 2008 the proportion of distracted drivers involved in a fatal crash who were also drinking alcohol while driving increased from 26 to 30.8 percent (Wilson et al., 2013). The FARS collection of data on distracted driving has several gaps and weaknesses; see Chapter 6 for a detailed discussion of these limitations.

A similar pattern emerges when comparing alcohol- and drug-impaired driving. Data from the National Survey on Drug Use and Health show that in 2014 the prevalence of driving under the influence of alcohol was higher than the prevalence of driving under the influence of illicit drugs by twofold, and a high proportion of those driving under the influence of drugs were concurrently under the influence of alcohol (Lipari et al., 2016; SAMHSA, 2015) (see Figure 2-2). Drivers who test positive for drugs and have a BAC at or above 0.05% have 5.34 times the adjusted odds of crashing when compared to someone without any drugs or alcohol in their system (Compton and Berning, 2015). In addition, crash risk for drivers with a BAC at or above 0.05% without a drug presence was higher than for drivers with a BAC at or above 0.05% with a drug presence, although the difference was not significant. After controlling for demographic variables and alcohol presence, no significant risk associated with the presence of cannabis or other specific drugs was found, although sample sizes were small. A 2011 case-control study that assessed the risk

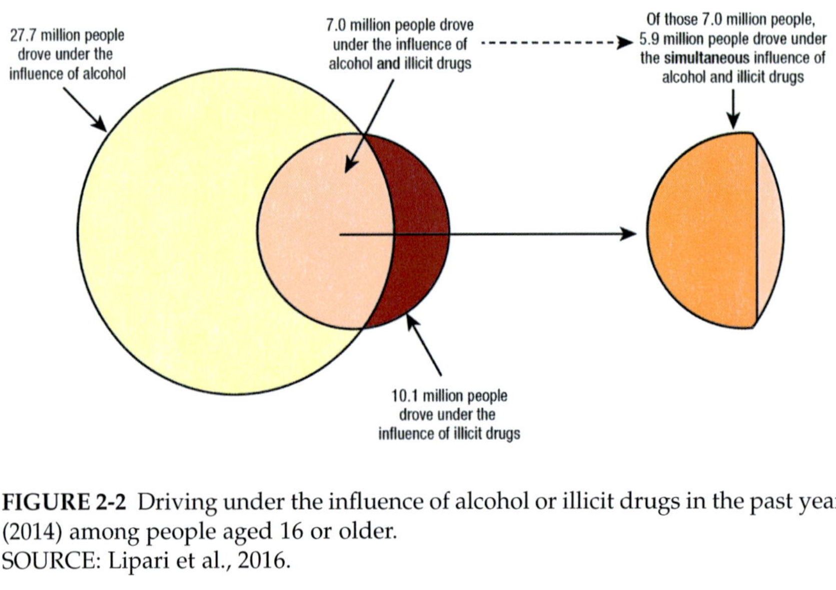

FIGURE 2-2 Driving under the influence of alcohol or illicit drugs in the past year (2014) among people aged 16 or older.
SOURCE: Lipari et al., 2016.

of driving under the influence of alcohol, illicit drugs, and medicines in European countries reported that the highest risk of serious injury or fatality was associated with driving with high BAC levels (above 0.12%) and driving with alcohol combined with other psychoactive substances (Hels et al., 2011). While the focus of this report is alcohol-impaired driving, targeting of both alcohol- and drug-related driving is needed.

PATTERNS OF ALCOHOL USE AND DEMOGRAPHICS

This section provides an overview of important demographics that need to be considered when approaching the problem of alcohol-impaired driving. First, based on the public health perspective outlined in Chapter 1, the importance of considering health equity and the social determinants of health is discussed. Relevant alcohol-related demographics are then provided.

The Importance of Applying a Health Equity Lens to the Issue

Because alcohol use and associated harms are unevenly distributed across populations, it is important to consider alcohol-related policies and interventions from an equity perspective (Roche et al., 2015a). While benefit to less advantaged populations is not a negative outcome, at times interventions may not benefit the population to which the intervention was intended to help or may disproportionately affect populations that were not the focus of the intervention. Researchers looking at public health strategies in general have found that some interventions may increase inequalities by disproportionately benefiting more advantaged groups (intervention-generated inequalities). Their findings are consistent with the idea that "downstream" preventive interventions are more likely to increase health inequities than "upstream" interventions (Lorenc et al., 2013). Unless consciously designed to avoid disparities, policies and actions that work for populations as a whole can inadvertently exacerbate inequalities (Smith and Foster, 2014).

The relationship between alcohol-related harm and social determinants may be bidirectional. For example, alcohol-related harms can contribute to loss of earnings, family disruption, interpersonal violence, mental health issues, and stigmatization, thus shaping social determinants (such as socioeconomic status) and exacerbating inequities. The resultant disadvantage may in turn compromise access to treatment (e.g., owing to cost or availability), heighten risk of co-occurring health problems, and perpetuate cycles of disadvantage (Schmidt et al., 2010). All alcohol-attributable mortality is in principle avoidable, and future alcohol policies are likely to be most effective if they take into consideration any differential effect on socioeconomic groups (Probst et al., 2014).

It is important to consider multiple levels of the social and physical environment in order to design multicomponent strategies that can be successful and change behavior. An important initial consideration is to understand the complexity of many interrelated influences on behavior to create policies and practices that are effective, while not increasing disparities among different populations. Important factors may include social norms and attitudes, social marginalization, education levels, socioeconomic status, geographic location, availability and cost of alcohol, and access to treatment resources.

Policy makers developing intervention strategies need to consider the local context in terms of knowledge, beliefs, and resources available to residents. For example, calls for enhanced enforcement, such as additional sobriety checkpoints, are unlikely to be effective without added financial resources or personnel and, more importantly, compassion for and cultural sensitivity toward populations of racial or ethnic minorities. Furthermore, a media campaign that urges impaired drivers to take a taxi or another form of public transportation home would be ineffective in rural areas where these resources are not available. Messaging composed in English in communities where a large number of residents do not speak English would be equally ineffective for that population. Public health campaigns that leverage local cultural beliefs and values to develop meaningful and relevant motivators to engage in certain behaviors may also be more effective. See Chapters 3 and 7 for more information on communication and messaging.

Social Determinants and Alcohol Use

Increasingly, health care policy makers and the public are understanding the link between social factors and health. There are many social factors that influence alcohol use patterns, including religious and cultural practices, peer groups, community and family relationships, social capital, poverty, education, advertising, economic conditions, the availability of alcohol, and the enforcement of alcohol laws (Dixon and Chartier, 2016; Roche et al., 2015b; Schor, 1996; Sudhinaraset et al., 2016). These factors are dynamic and intersect in myriad ways that are important to understand in a local context. They can contribute to differences in the burden of crashes, fatalities, injuries, and chronic health conditions that result from alcohol abuse and impaired driving among populations based on education, race and ethnicity, socioeconomic status, geography, and so on. In an effort to address alcohol use/abuse and impaired driving, it is important to move beyond the individual level and consider the social determinants of these behaviors to develop effective population-level strategies to mitigate the negative health consequences of these issues and to provide insight into interventions that are most likely to be effective and have the greatest reach.

Alcohol-Impaired Driver Demographics

Age

CDC reports that at all levels of BAC, the risk of being involved in a crash is greater for younger than for older people (CDC, 2017b). The prevalence of driving under the influence of alcohol increases with age through the young adult years and then generally declines thereafter. In 2014 self-reported driving under the influence of alcohol was highest among drivers ages 21 to 29 (Lipari et al., 2016). FARS estimates show that drivers ages 21 to 34 made up 55 percent of drivers with BAC levels of 0.08% or higher who were involved in fatal crashes in 2015 (NCSA, 2016a).

Sex

Among those aged 16 or older in 2014, with the exception of drivers ages 16–20,[13] men were more likely than women to have driven under the influence of alcohol in the past year; in addition, men aged 16 or older were more likely to drive under the influence of both alcohol and illicit drugs (Lipari et al., 2016). Of all drivers involved in fatal crashes in 2015, 21 percent of men and 14 percent of women had a BAC of 0.08% or higher (NCSA, 2016a). While this disparity has held constant for decades, there is limited research suggesting that female drivers are becoming increasingly involved in alcohol-impaired driving crashes (Vaca et al., 2014).

Race and Ethnicity

With respect to race and ethnicity, the groups that are consistently reported as having the highest risk of alcohol-impaired driving are American Indian or Alaska Native (AI/AN) and white drivers (Romano et al., 2010). For fatal crashes among AI/AN persons in 2012, 42 percent were alcohol related, while only 31 percent were alcohol related for other races overall (Letourneau and Crump, 2016). AI/AN persons had a substantially higher rate of alcohol-attributable deaths than whites from 2005

[13] The difference in percentages of men and women ages 16–20 who drove impaired was not found to be statistically significant (Lipari et al., 2016).

to 2009. In 2005 the age-adjusted motor vehicle-related death rate among AI/AN persons was twice as high as among all other races (Piontkowski et al., 2015). Cultural, socioeconomic, and alcohol availability differences between AI/AN groups have contributed to disparities in overall alcohol-related mortality (Landen et al., 2014).

Findings from the 2007 National Roadside Survey show that Asian and Hispanic or Latino drivers are less likely than white drivers to be drinking (Kelley-Baker et al., 2013). According to FARS data from 2000 to 2013, the majority of people (51.2 percent) who died in alcohol-impaired driving crashes were non-Hispanic whites (Hadland et al., 2017). However, there are inconsistencies across studies with respect to the disparities in alcohol-attributable injury mortality among black or African American and Hispanic or Latino groups that might be partially explained by methodological issues of the studies and/or other social determinants that affect the relationship between race and ethnicity and injury outcomes (Keyes et al., 2012).

Socioeconomic Status (SES)

Unlike many other behaviors that pose serious risks to health and safety (e.g., smoking and violence), alcohol consumption has a more complex relationship with SES (Jones et al., 2015). People with higher incomes and levels of education are more likely to drink alcohol and to drive while impaired when compared to lower income and less educated populations. However, alcohol consumption has a disproportionate effect on people with lower SES in terms of alcohol-attributable harm such as morbidity (e.g., cancer, stroke, hypertension, and liver disease) (Jones et al., 2015; Katikireddi et al., 2017; Scaglione et al., 2015) and mortality (Probst et al., 2014). Thus, a paradox exists between patterns of behavior and attributable harm when examining these through the lens of SES. Further research is needed to more critically assess the relationship among SES, alcohol consumption, and alcohol-attributable harms (Jones et al., 2015).

Patterns of drinking behavior are a significant factor with respect to alcohol-impaired driving. Esser et al. (2016) analyzed data from the National Survey on Drug Use and Health (2009–2011) and found that binge drinking was most common among those with household incomes of $75,000 or more, whereas alcohol dependence (DSM-IV) was more common among those with annual household incomes of less than $25,000. Findings from the 2006 Behavioral Risk Factor Surveillance System (BRFSS) showed that the prevalence of alcohol-impaired driving was high for binge drinkers across educational and income categories,[14] including those who had attended college and had high annual incomes (Flowers et al., 2008). More recent data from the 2012 BRFSS suggest that the likelihood of driving while alcohol impaired increases with income (Jewett et al., 2015). This is consistent with findings from the 2001–2002 National Epidemiologic Survey on Alcohol and Related Conditions, which indicated that hazardous use of alcohol (i.e., driving *after* drinking, drinking *while* driving, and other non-driving-related behaviors) was the only alcohol abuse criterion to have a significant positive relationship with income. More specifically, adjusted odds ratios showed that those in the highest income category ($70,000 or more past-year personal income) were about two times as likely to drive *after* drinking compared to those in the lowest income category (less than $20,000) and 2.46 times as likely to drink *while* driving compared to those in the lowest income group (Keyes and Hasin, 2008).

Urban and Rural Populations

Rural populations also suffer a much higher fatality rate from motor vehicle crashes (alcohol related and non-alcohol related) than urban residents. While 19 percent of the U.S. population lives in rural areas and rural areas account for 30 percent of total vehicle miles traveled, more than half of crash deaths occur there (FHWA, 2015; IIHS, 2016; U.S. Census Bureau, 2010). Crashes in rural areas tend to occur at higher speeds, head-on collisions are more common owing to the prevalence of two-lane roads with no median, and guardrails are less common. There are often fewer witnesses to call for help in rural locations, and help is often farther away. Rural hospitals often have less capacity to handle severe trauma. Fewer police officers covering larger areas are less likely to arrest alcohol-impaired drivers (Vock, 2013). Additionally, alternative and public transportation options are far fewer in rural areas (Mattson, 2016; TRB, 2016) (see Chapter 4 for information on alternative and public transportation). Safety and upkeep of rural transportation infrastructure is similarly lacking (TRIP, 2017).

Per Capita Alcohol Consumption

At the population level, alcohol consumption has historically been associated with the incidence of alcohol-related traffic fatalities (Voas and

---

[14] Binge drinking was defined in this study as five or more drinks for men and four or more drinks for women during one or more occasions (i.e., typically over a period of 2 hours) in the previous month (Flowers et al., 2008).

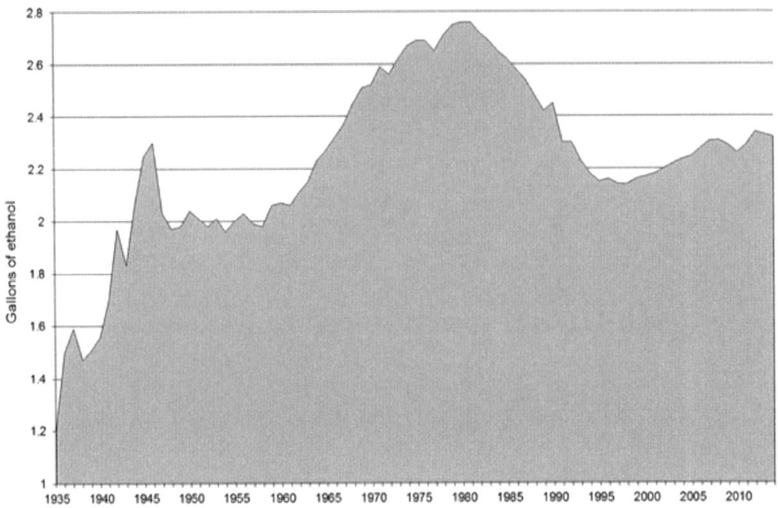

FIGURE 2-3 Total per capita ethanol consumption, United States, 1935–2014.
SOURCE: Haughwout et al., 2016.

Lacey, 2011). From 2011 to 2015, per capita alcohol consumption in the United States increased from 2.28 to 2.33 gallons (LaVallee et al., 2014). See Figure 2-3 for per capita alcohol consumption from 1935 to 2014. To meet the national goal set by Healthy People 2020 for per capita alcohol consumption to be no more than 2.1 gallons, a per capita decrease of 2.0 percent each year would need to take place for the next 5 years (Haughwout and Slater, 2017).

Patterns of Drinking

How people consume alcohol matters when it comes to consequences of alcohol-impaired driving. A substantial body of evidence indicates that binge drinking is strongly associated with alcohol-impaired driving (Flowers et al., 2008; Hingson et al., 2017; Naimi et al., 2009; Quinlan et al., 2005).[15] The 2012 BRFSS findings revealed that respondents who reported binge drinking accounted for 85 percent of alcohol-impaired

[15] The BRFSS definition for binge drinking was changed in 2006 from five or more drinks on one or more occasions (i.e., typically over a period of 2 hours) in the past month to sex-specific definitions of five or more drinks on one or more occasions in the past month for men and four or more drinks on one or more occasions in the past month for women (Chavez et al., 2011). Analysis by Naimi et al. (2009) and Quinlan et al. (2005) was based on

driving episodes, and the 4 percent who reported binge drinking at least four times per month accounted for 61 percent of all alcohol-impaired driving episodes (Jewett et al., 2015). In addition, early onset of drinking has been shown to be correlated with early onset of alcohol-impaired driving among young men (Zhang et al., 2014). Data on the prevalence of alcohol use disorders (AUDs) among DWI offenders are not consistently collected or reported (see Chapter 5 for information on screening for AUD among DWI offenders) (Lapham et al., 2004). From the data that are available, estimates suggest that alcohol use disorders are associated with having multiple DWI offenses (Lapham et al., 2011).

However, it is important to note that there is a large discrepancy between the amount of people who drink excessively but do not meet the diagnostic criteria for alcohol dependence and those who do. For example, national estimates of self-reported drinking behaviors from 138,100 adults who completed the National Survey on Drug Use and Health in 2009 to 2011 show that most people who drink excessively (90 percent) do not meet the criteria for alcohol dependence (Esser et al., 2014).[16] Flowers et al. (2008) analyzed data from the 2006 BRFSS and reported that binge drinking (i.e., high per occasion consumption) was more strongly associated with alcohol-impaired driving than heavy drinking (i.e., high average consumption).[17] Specifically, binge drinkers accounted for 84 percent of impaired drivers and 89 percent of impaired driving episodes, while heavy drinkers only accounted for 35 percent of impaired drivers and 52 percent of impaired driving episodes.

Furthermore, more than half of alcohol-impaired drivers who reported binge drinking were not classified as heavy drinkers based on their average daily consumption, yet they had more than twice the odds of driving impaired than those who were not binge drinkers or heavy drinkers, when adjusting for age, sex, marital status, education, and income (Flowers et al., 2008). In another study that examined BRFSS data from 2003 and 2004, drinking drivers who drank most of their alcohol in licensed establishments consumed an average of 8.1 alcoholic beverages

---

the non-sex-specific definition for binge drinking; analysis by Flowers et al. (2008) was based on the sex-specific definition for binge drinking.

[16] The study authors used the diagnostic criteria for alcohol dependence based on the DSM-IV, which has since changed in the DSM-5 to reflect varying degrees of severity of alcohol use disorder (e.g., mild, moderate, severe).

[17] At the time of the study, the BRFSS defined binge drinking as consumption of five or more drinks for men and four or more drinks for women on one or more occasions (i.e., typically over a period of two hours) in the past 30 days; the BRFSS defined heavy drinking as consumption in the past 30 days of an average of more than two drinks per day for men (i.e., greater than 60 drinks per month) and more than one drink per day for women (i.e., greater than 30 drinks per month) (Flowers et al., 2008).

on one occasion, and about one-fourth of this group consumed 10 or more drinks (Naimi et al., 2009). Cumulatively, these findings suggest that the risk of driving subsequent to binge drinking is substantial on a per-binge-drinking episode basis across the population.

The problem of alcohol-impaired driving fatalities is related to both excessive drinking and to driving after one is impaired. Given the hand-in-glove relationship between binge drinking and alcohol-impaired driving, it is easy to overlook the importance of interventions to reduce alcohol consumption, and binge drinking in particular, among the general population. Previous studies demonstrate that policies to reduce binge drinking are independently protective against alcohol-impaired driving and the odds of alcohol involvement in crash fatalities, even after accounting for policies designed to prevent driving after one is impaired (Naimi et al., 2009, 2017; Wagenaar et al., 2010). During the past 15 years, however, while states have adopted strategies to reduce alcohol-impaired driving, the adoption and implementation of population-based strategies to reduce binge drinking and related harms has not changed (Nelson et al., 2013). This may partly explain why the proportion of crash fatalities that are alcohol related has not declined during that period. Given the finding that alcohol-impaired driving is a binge drinking problem as well as a driving problem, the committee concludes:

> *Conclusion 2-2: Policies to reduce binge drinking are also protective against alcohol-impaired driving, and the adoption of a comprehensive set of effective interventions and population-based strategies that take advantage of synergies across interventions would further help to reduce binge drinking and related harms.*

Interventions and population-based strategies to reduce binge drinking and alcohol-impaired driving could include raising alcohol taxes, implementing policies to limit the physical availability of alcohol, and implementing policies to reduce the harmful effects of alcohol marketing (see Chapter 3 for more in-depth discussion of these policies).

SITUATIONAL FACTORS FOR ALCOHOL-IMPAIRED DRIVING

Day, Time, Distance, and Place of Last Drink

The findings of the 2013–2014 National Roadside Survey revealed substantial differences by day of the week and time of the day in the likelihood of drivers being alcohol impaired or having a BAC above the limit set by state law (Berning et al., 2015). Table 2-1 shows these differences. NHTSA's National Center for Statistics and Analysis reported that

TABLE 2-1 Alcohol Prevalence by Data Collection Period and BAC in the 2013 to 2014 National Roadside Survey

Time Period	% BAC >0.005%	% BAC >0.08%
Weekday daytime	1.1%	0.4%
Weekend nighttime	8.3%	1.5%

SOURCE: Berning et al., 2015.

in 2014 the rate of alcohol impairment among drivers involved in fatal crashes was almost four times higher at night than during the day (34 versus 9 percent).

The 2007 National Roadside Survey results revealed that drivers with positive BAC levels were most likely to be driving short distances (5 miles or less) and coming from a restaurant, club, tavern, or bar (Kelley-Baker et al., 2013). This is consistent with other research findings, which suggest that almost half of people arrested for alcohol-impaired driving are coming from a licensed establishment (Fell et al., 2010; Gallup, 2000; O'Donnell, 1985). See Chapter 6 for information on the importance of data on place of last drink.

Geographic Location

In 2012 the BRFSS results showed that the Midwest U.S. Census region had the highest annual alcohol-impaired driving rate at 573 per 1,000 people (Jewett et al., 2015). A recent analysis of FARS data showed that the majority of deaths from alcohol-impaired driving crashes from 2000 to 2013 occurred in the South (45.6 percent), followed by the West (21.9 percent) and the Midwest (21.0 percent) (Hadland et al., 2017). In 2014 the proportion of alcohol-impaired driving fatalities (caused by drivers with a BAC ≥0.08%) among total traffic fatalities in states ranged from a high of 41 percent (Massachusetts, North Dakota, and Texas) to a low of 20 percent (Vermont), compared to a national average of 31 percent (NCSA, 2015).

Rural and Urban Regions[18]

NHTSA reported that from 2005 to 2014, rural alcohol-impaired driving fatalities decreased by 34 percent (7,721 to 5,134) and urban

[18] Unless otherwise noted, the committee defines urban and rural areas using the 2010 Census Urban and Rural Classification: an urban area comprises a densely settled core of census tracts and/or census blocks that meet minimum population density requirements.

alcohol-impaired driving fatalities decreased by 19 percent (5,791 to 4,701) (NCSA, 2016c). In 2014, the relative proportions of alcohol-impaired driving fatalities were similar between rural and urban areas at 31 and 30 percent, respectively. However, among all alcohol-impaired driving fatalities in 2014, 52 percent occurred in rural areas and 47 percent occurred in urban areas. Vehicle miles traveled (VMT) per capita differ greatly in rural versus urban areas, with rural areas having far greater VMT per capita (Mattson, 2016). The most frequently recorded BAC among alcohol-impaired drivers in fatal crashes in rural areas was 0.19% and 0.14% for urban areas (NCSA, 2016c). DWI arrest rates also vary according to rural and urban composition, with arrests in nonmetropolitan areas outnumbering metropolitan arrests since the early 2000s (Huseth, 2012).

There are a number of important behavioral and environmental factors that contribute to higher fatality rates in rural areas. Some of these include differences in travel speed and speed limits; long distances between point of origin and destination, resulting in greater vehicle miles traveled (per capita); use of seatbelts; road conditions and aspects of road design; vehicle types; distance between point of sale or service of alcohol and place of residence; and delayed medical response and proximity of emergency care (Huseth, 2012; TRB, 2013). Decreasing use of seat belts, for example, has been found in rural areas (Beck et al., 2017). The unique challenges and characteristics of the rural environment will be discussed as important considerations in the design and implementation of interventions throughout the report.

Beverage of Choice of Alcohol-Impaired Drivers

The association of beer with alcohol-impaired driving is expected to be greater than for wine and distilled spirits, as there is greater general consumption of beer in the United States (WHO, 2011). However, research suggests that drinking beer also has a greater correlation than drinking wine or distilled spirits to alcohol-impaired driving because drivers underestimate intoxication from beer and perceive less risk from beer consumption (Greenfield and Rogers, 1999; Gruenewald and Ponicki, 1995; Walker et al., 2016). Beer consumption has also been shown to be correlated with higher rates of traffic fatalities (Rickard et al., 2013). Additional analyses would be needed to more critically analyze the higher

---

To qualify as an urban area, the territory identified must encompass at least 2,500 people, at least 1,500 of which reside outside institutional group quarters. The U.S. Census Bureau identifies two types of urban areas: (1) urbanized areas of 50,000 or more people and (2) urban clusters of at least 2,500 and less than 50,000 people. Rural areas are defined as all population, housing, and territory not included within an urban area (U.S. Census Bureau, 2010).

BOX 2-1
Key Findings

- Drivers ages 21–25 are disproportionately involved in fatal alcohol-impaired driving crashes when compared to other age groups. In 2015 this age group accounted for 28 percent of motor vehicle crashes where the driver had a BAC equal to or higher than 0.08%.
- Rural areas are disproportionally affected by alcohol-impaired driving crashes and fatalities.
- Per capita alcohol consumption and hazardous drinking are increasing.
- Binge drinking is strongly associated with alcohol-impaired driving.

association of beer with alcohol-impaired driving, such as analysis evaluating whether persons who exclusively drink beer (compared to those who exclusively drink wine and those who exclusively drink distilled spirits) are more likely drive impaired. Other variables to examine regarding the association with alcohol-impaired driving of beer versus wine versus distilled spirits include age, place of consumption, and quantity of alcohol consumed per drinking occasion. Additionally, differential beverage availability at drinking establishments has been shown to affect alcohol-impaired driving likelihood. A study in Western Australia[19] found that more alcohol-impaired drivers originated from drinking establishments selling more beer, including high alcohol content beer, and distilled spirits (Gruenewald et al., 1999). Beverage availability in on- and off-premises drinking establishments is an important consideration for alcohol pricing and taxation, which is discussed in Chapter 3. Box 2-1 summarizes some key findings presented in this chapter thus far.

THE DRIVING ENVIRONMENT

In addition to the alcohol environment, the driving environment includes equally important considerations for changing drinking and driving behaviors and for increasing the effectiveness of policies and interventions to reduce alcohol-impaired driving.

[19] A standard drink in Australia is 10 grams of pure alcohol, while in the United States it is 14 grams.

Driving Trends

As the size of the U.S. population increases, the number of drivers has also increased. With the exception of a brief leveling off beginning in 2009, the number of drivers and number of vehicles has generally followed the same trend as population growth (FHWA, 2017) (see Figure 2-4). In 2015 the total number of drivers was 218 million, an increase from 191 million in 2000; 49.4 percent of drivers were men and 50.6 percent of drivers were women (FHWA, 2017). Table 2-2 provides a distribution of drivers by age in 2015.

Vehicle miles traveled experienced a downturn in 2009—most likely from the financial crisis; it has since increased and is now at the highest level in U.S. history (FHWA, 2017). A recent study by the University of Michigan Transportation Research Institute found that from 2000 to 2016,

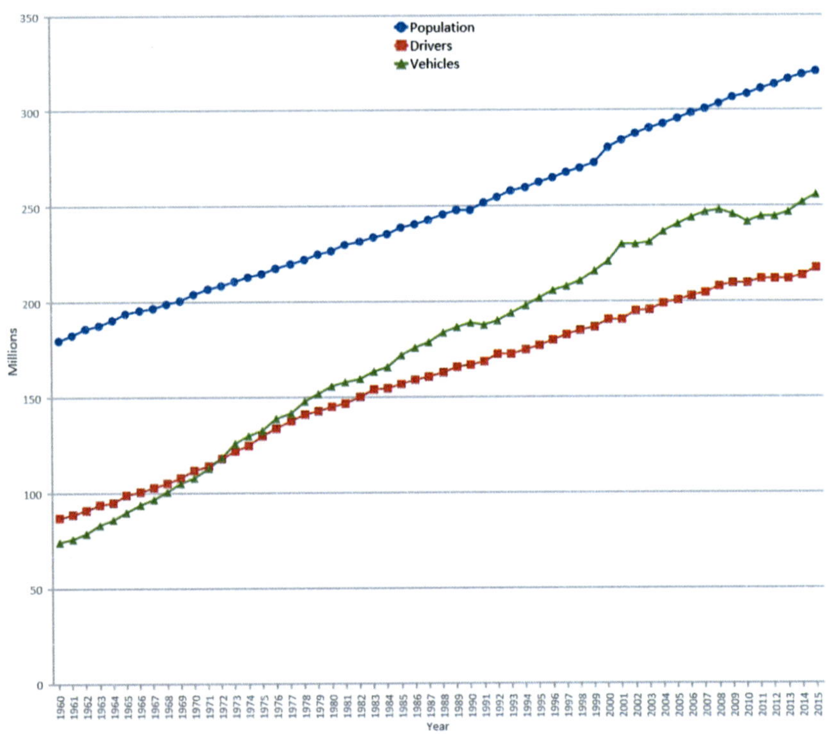

FIGURE 2-4 Licensed drivers, vehicle registrations, and resident population.
SOURCE: FHWA, 2017.

TABLE 2-2 Distribution of Licensed Drivers in 2015

Age	Percent
19 and under	3.9
20–24	8.1
25–34	17.6
35–44	16.6
45–54	18.1
55–64	17.3
65+	18.4

SOURCE: FHWA, 2016.

total vehicle miles traveled increased by 15 percent, an increase accounted for by the increase in the U.S. population in the same time period (Sivak and Schoettle, 2017). However, the same study found that while urban vehicle miles traveled increased by 33 percent, rural vehicle miles traveled decreased by 12 percent; changes in urban and rural populations did not account for changes in urban and rural vehicle miles traveled (Sivak and Schoettle, 2017).

Changes to the Physical Driving Environment

As urban and rural areas differ significantly by roadway environment, implementation of road safety countermeasures varies accordingly. Vehicle usage also varies; 4 percent of rural households do not have access to a vehicle compared to 10 percent of urban households (Mattson, 2016). Distinction between urban and rural areas can be problematic, however, as classification definitions often vary and roadway classifications may not reflect important differences. Traditionally, urban and rural roadways have been classified by roadway speeds and conditions.

Additionally, significant growth of suburban areas in recent years has contributed to several changes in the physical driving environment. Findings from a U.S. Department of Transportation study showed that 73 percent of overall motor vehicle crash fatalities took place in urban fringe areas—about 5 miles out from an urban boundary—suggesting that such "urban edge" transition zones are an important consideration for effective points for intervention (Subramanian, 2009). A possible explanation is that as residents of suburban areas are more dependent on automobiles to travel, more driving is necessary for suburban residents. As such, alternative modes of transportation, including taxis, public transportation, and smartphone-enabled transportation network ridesharing (see Chapter 4 for information), may be an important consideration to reduce crash fatalities in suburban and rural areas where greater distances of travel are necessary.

However, public transportation services in rural areas are particularly difficult to describe and catalogue, as availability changes significantly over time and can be difficult to track. Additionally, the existence of a transportation provider does not necessarily reflect access and ability to use it. Varying arrangements of public and private subsidies introduce additional complications.

Trends in traffic fatalities suggest that maintenance of transportation infrastructure is crucially important for safety. A general downward trend in traffic fatalities has taken place over the past decade; however, a slight increase occurred in 2012, and in 2016 there were 37,461 fatalities, the highest since 2008 (NCSA, 2017a), as well as an estimated 2.44 million injuries in 2015 (NCSA, 2016b).

Car Safety Features

Innovation in vehicle safety technology is rapidly expanding, with a range of technologies recently emerging that provide lane departure warnings, forward collision warnings, side view assists, adaptive cruise control, and many other features. Many hold promise to improve vehicle and road safety, although most are currently marketed not as safety features but as driver-assistance systems. Advanced vehicle technology in the form of the Driver Alcohol Detection System for Safety and autonomous vehicles are also in development (see Chapter 4 for more information). In addition to technological developments, recent efforts have focused on informing consumers about car safety features that are available and their capabilities.[20] Research will be needed to determine how drivers will interact with these technological systems and the effectiveness of these systems in reducing crash and fatality rates in real-world settings (effectiveness to date has mostly been defined as a function of crash types the systems are designed to avoid).

[20] For example, https://mycardoeswhat.org (accessed October 12, 2017).

IMPACTS OF ALCOHOL-IMPAIRED DRIVING

Impact on Health

As discussed in previous sections, alcohol-impaired driving crashes claim more than 10,000 lives per year. Driver and nondriver victims are among these deaths. Victims, including occupants of the same vehicle as the impaired driver, occupants of other vehicles, pedestrians, cyclists, and others on the road, make up 38 percent of alcohol-impaired driving crash fatalities (NCSA, 2017b). In addition to the loss of life as a result of alcohol-related crashes, victims often suffer from other consequences including pain, injury, and disability. Victims of alcohol-related crashes can also be subjected to emotional, psychological, and financial consequences that have the potential to greatly reduce their quality of life (Blincoe et al., 2015). The toll associated with injury, disability, and death that can affect victims of alcohol-related driving crashes can extend to their friends and family as well. These in part make up the secondhand effects of alcohol-impaired driving that are highlighted in Chapter 1.

Financial and Societal Costs

Driving under the influence of alcohol costs the nation significantly in financial and societal terms. Blincoe et al. (2015) estimate that the economic costs of alcohol-related crashes amounted to $52 billion in 2010. This estimate includes medical costs; emergency services, market productivity, household productivity, insurance administration, workplace costs, legal costs, congestion costs, and property damage (Blincoe et al., 2015). Their findings also indicated that in 2010 alcohol-related crashes accounted for 22 percent of all motor vehicle crash costs and that crashes involving drivers with a BAC of 0.08% or higher accounted for more than 90 percent of the economic costs and societal harm associated with alcohol-related crashes (Blincoe et al., 2015).

Taking overall societal costs into account, the effect of alcohol-related crashes is even greater. Zaloshnja et al. (2013) estimated that the total societal costs of alcohol-related crashes (where the driver's BAC was >0.05%) in 2010 amounted to $121.5 billion, including $113 billion for crashes where the driver had a BAC of 0.08% or higher (Zaloshnja et al., 2013). This estimate includes societal costs due to medical costs; earnings losses; household productivity losses; insurance administration costs; legal costs; traffic congestion; vehicle damage; roadside equipment costs; incident management; vocational rehabilitation; workplace costs; fire department services; police services; monetized quality-adjusted life years lost; victim mental health treatment; adjudication, sanctioning, and legal defense fees; and perpetrator productivity loss (Zaloshnja et al., 2013).

The costs of alcohol-impaired driving listed above affect many individuals beyond the victims. Productivity loss can be associated with lost work time or DWI conviction costs (e.g., fines, loss of driving privileges, difficulty securing or maintaining employment, and increased insurance costs) (Bouchery et al., 2011). The burden of alcohol-impaired driving crashes can affect employers as well. Zaloshnja et al. (2007) estimated employer costs attributable to all alcohol-involved injuries, including health fringe benefit costs, nonfringe costs (e.g., disruption costs preventing employees from working at full capacity), and wage premiums using data from FARS, the Crashworthiness Data System, and the General Estimate System (Zaloshnja et al., 2007). Annual employer costs of alcohol-impaired driving crashes from 1998 to 2000 were estimated to be $9.2 billion (Zaloshnja et al., 2007). Finally, the substantial time, personnel, and resources expended on the arrest and adjudication process for DWI offenders can be costly for local law enforcement and the court system (Goodwin et al., 2015). This can be especially problematic for law enforcement agencies that have many other competing priorities in the interest of public safety and health. The consequences of alcohol-impaired driving can be far reaching and have implications for costs across various actors and sectors.

Conclusion 2-3: The costs and consequences of alcohol-impaired driving extend beyond the driver to include health, economic, social, and emotional costs borne by other road users, their families and friends, social and medical institutions, and society at large.

ALCOHOL-IMPAIRED DRIVING INTERVENTIONS

Policies and interventions to reduce alcohol-impaired driving, crashes, and fatalities are discussed in detail in Chapters 3, 4, and 5. In examining different interventions and their effectiveness in different environments, an important consideration in reducing alcohol-impaired driving fatalities nationwide is the substantial variation in the types of policies and laws that exist in each state.[21] Below is a high-level overview.

---

[21] A table by the Governors Highway Safety Administration (last updated June 2017) with state laws on high BAC, administrative license suspension, limited driving privileges, ignition interlocks, vehicle and license plate sanctions, open container laws, repeat offender laws, and alcohol exclusion laws limiting treatment is available at http://www.ghsa.org/sites/default/files/2017-06/DrunkDrivingLaws_062617.pdf (accessed October 12, 2017).

State Variation in Laws and Policies

With the exceptions of 0.08% per se laws, zero tolerance laws for underage persons, and a minimum drinking age set by state law of 21, there is little uniformity in the policies that address alcohol-impaired driving across state lines; considerable intrastate variation in policies and regulations exists as well. Furthermore, how these policies are implemented (e.g., target population, penalties, and mandatory versus discretionary) and enforced are critical factors in determining their effectiveness for specific areas and at the national level. Such policies can be alcohol specific, driving specific, or alcohol-impaired driving specific, and they can affect any point of intervention illustrated in the committee's conceptual framework (see Figure 1-5) (e.g., alcohol consumption, drinking to impairment, and driving while impaired).

With respect to drinking-related policies, the variation in state regulation is a direct outcome of the Twenty-First Amendment. After the repeal of Prohibition, it was concluded that a uniform, nationwide alcohol control policy would not suit the heterogeneous makeup of the country (Fosdick and Scott, 1933). Moving forward, each state adopted the alcohol control policies and regulations most suitable for its respective local population. This is the underpinning of the patchwork of policies and regulation that is visible across the nation today (Schmidt, 2017). For example, after the repeal of Prohibition, the Illinois Control Act of 1934 gave voters in Chicago the right to vote specific precincts as "dry" (i.e., prohibiting liquor licenses within the precinct) through a local option referendum (Chicago Board of Election Commissioners, 2009). Other states, however, may completely preempt local control over alcohol availability.[22] Another alcohol-specific policy that varies from state to state is responsible beverage service and server training. As of 2016, 12 states plus the District of Columbia had mandatory service training laws, 20 had voluntary laws, 6 had a combination of mandatory and voluntary policies, and 12 had neither (APIS, 2016).

Other policies and laws related to alcohol-impaired driving also vary from state to state. Sobriety checkpoints, an effective countermeasure when conducted properly (Bergen et al., 2014), are not implemented uniformly from state to state. While some states authorize the use of sobriety checkpoints, others prohibit them or do not have any explicit statutory authority on checkpoints. For example, Texas bans checkpoints based on its interpretation of the Constitution, and Missouri state law authorizes checkpoints but prohibits funds from being spent on checkpoint programs

[22] See levels of preemption classified by state at http://www.camy.org/research-to-practice/place/alcohol-outlet-density/preemption-data-tool.html (accessed October 12, 2017).

(GHSA, 2016). Provisions of minimum drinking age laws also vary by state. One such provision concerns dram shop liability, which permits legal action against commercial establishments serving alcohol when illegal beverage service (i.e., to already-intoxicated adults or underage patrons) results in injury, death, or damages from alcohol-related vehicle crashes. Dram shop liability is enacted through statute in most states and through case law in others (Rammohan et al., 2011). The seven states that have neither dram shop liability laws nor statutes are Delaware, Kansas, Louisiana, Maryland, Nevada, South Dakota, and Virginia (Rammohan et al., 2011). In states in which dram shop liability is established through statute, additional legal hurdles, including limits to damages sought and strict requirements for evidence, may exist and create additional barriers that do not exist in states where liability is established through law (Rammohan et al., 2011).

There are inherent differences in how specific jurisdictions govern that shape the alcohol and driving policy environment. AI/AN territories, for example, have unique complexities of tribal sovereignty that have implications for how crimes such as alcohol-impaired driving are handled. Jurisdiction is complicated by "competing claims of federal, tribal, and state sovereignty manifested in a complex array of laws that create a system of jurisdiction based on location, type of crime, race of the perpetrator, and race of the victim" (*Harvard Law Review*, 2016, p. 1687).

In fact, in many states with AI/AN reservations, tribal law enforcement officers do not have the authority to stop a driver suspected of being impaired once the suspect crosses the border, leaving their jurisdiction. Such limitations are especially problematic for this population, since AI/ANs are at high risk for driving while impaired and sustaining injuries or fatalities from an alcohol-related crash (Letourneau and Crump, 2016). Additional differences in policies and laws will be discussed throughout the report as they apply to various interventions for alcohol-impaired driving.

Advocates for Highway and Auto Safety rates each state according to the implementation of what they deem as three optimal impaired driving laws: ignition interlock laws for all offenders, child endangerment laws, and open container laws (Advocates for Highway and Auto Safety, 2017) (see Figure 2-5). As of August 2017, 20 states and the District of Columbia have all three optimal laws enacted (good rating), 10 states have ignition interlocks for all offenders and one other optimal law enacted (caution rating), and 20 states had zero or one optimal impaired driving law (danger rating).

In addition to state-by-state variation in individual alcohol, driving, and alcohol-impaired driving policies, states' overall policy environments are also an important consideration for reducing alcohol-impaired driving

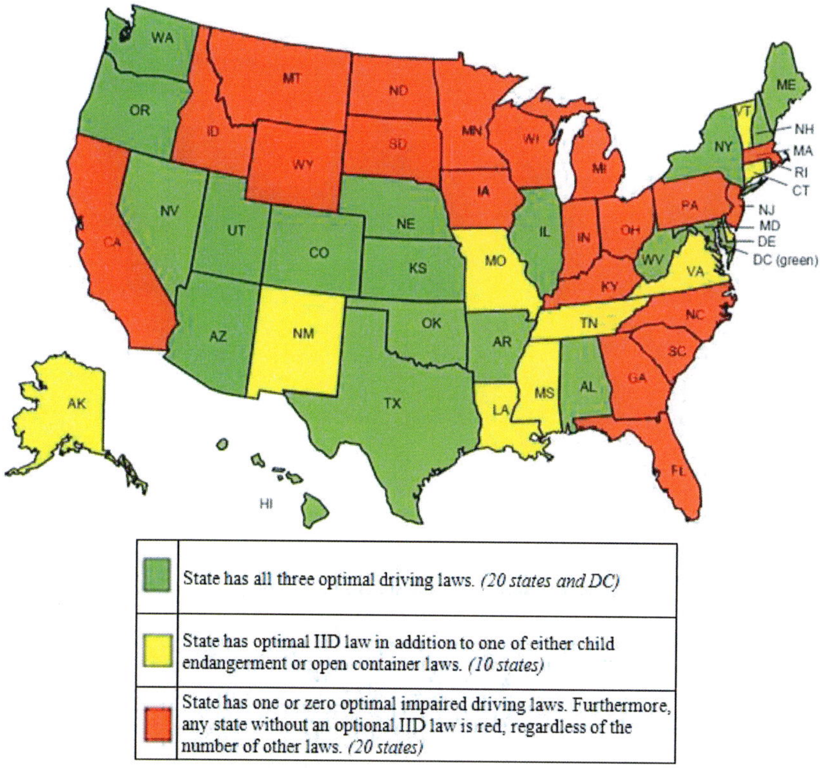

FIGURE 2-5 Rating of states based on implementation of optimal impaired driving laws by the Advocates for Highway and Auto Safety: (1) ignition interlock laws for all offenders, (2) child endangerment laws, (3) and open container laws.
NOTES: No credit is given for laws that are subject to secondary enforcement. This map reflects state impaired driving laws as of August 2017. IID = ignition interlock device.
SOURCES: Advocates for Highway and Auto Safety, 2017; Kennedy, 2017. Personal communication with Allison Kennedy, Advocates for Highway and Auto Safety on August 31, 2017. Available by request from the National Academies of Sciences, Engineering, and Medicine's Public Access Records Office (PARO@nas.edu).

fatalities. Studies have found that rates of binge drinking and self-reported alcohol-impaired driving are lower in states with more restrictive alcohol policy environments (Naimi et al., 2014; Xuan et al., 2015a,b). Furthermore, for those under 21 years of age, a 10 percent increase in the strength of a state's alcohol policy environment was found to be correlated with a 9 percent decrease in the risk of alcohol-impaired motor vehicle crash fatalities across age and sex for both drivers and passengers (Hadland et al., 2017). Although evidence on the effectiveness of states' overall policy environments to reduce alcohol-impaired driving fatalities among the general population is limited, implementation and enforcement of "a strong collection of alcohol control policies acting in concert in a state" is a promising strategy to accelerate progress (Hadland et al., 2017, p. 2). The lack of a comprehensive population-based strategy may partly explain why the proportion of crash fatalities that are alcohol impaired has not declined in the last decade and has plateaued and has begun to increase.

REFERENCES

AAA (American Automobile Association) Foundation for Traffic Safety. 2016. *Prevalence of marijuana involvement in fatal crashes: Washington, 2010–2014*. Washington, DC: AAA Foundation for Traffic Safety.

AB InBev (Anheuser-Busch InBev). n.d. *Global smart drinking goals*. http://www.ab-inbev.com/better-world/a-healthier-world/global-smart-drinking-goals.html (accessed December 6, 2017).

Advocates for Highway and Auto Safety. 2017. *Have we forgotten what saves lives?: 2017 roadmap of state highway safety laws*. Washington, DC: Advocates for Highway and Auto Safety.

Ames, G. M., and J. W. Grube. 1999. Alcohol availability and workplace drinking: Mixed method analyses. *Journal of Studies on Alcohol and Drugs* 60(3):383–393.

Anderson, P., and J. Rehm. 2016. Evaluating alcohol industry action to reduce the harmful use of alcohol. *Alcohol and Alcoholism* 51(4):383–387.

APIS (Alcohol Policy Information System). 2016. *Retail sales: Beverage service training and related practices*. https://alcoholpolicy.niaaa.nih.gov/Beverage_Service_Training_and_Related_Practices.html (accessed March 31, 2017).

Aston, E. R., and A. Liguori. 2013. Self-estimation of blood alcohol concentration: A review. *Addictive Behaviors* 38(4):1944–1951.

Babor, T. 2010a. *Alcohol: No ordinary commodity: Research and public policy*. New York: Oxford University Press.

Babor, T. 2010b. Alcohol: No ordinary commodity—A summary of the second edition. *Addiction* 105(5):769–779.

Babor, T. F., K. Robaina, and D. Jernigan. 2015. The influence of industry actions on the availability of alcoholic beverages in the African region. *Addiction* 110(4):561–571.

Babor, T. F., K. Robaina, and J. Noel. 2018. *The role of the alcohol industry in policy interventions for alcohol-impaired driving*. Paper commissioned by the Committee on Accelerating Progress to Reduce Alcohol-Impaired Driving Fatalities (see Appendix C).

Baer, J. S., A. Stacy, and M. Larimer. 1991. Biases in perception of drinking norms among college students. *Journal of Studies on Alcohol* 52(6):580–586.

Beck, L. F., J. Downs, M. R. Stevens, and E. K. Sauber-Schatz. 2017. Rural and urban differences in passenger-vehicle-occupant deaths and seat belt use among adults—United States, 2014. *Morbidity and Mortality Weekly Report Surveillance Summaries* 66(17):1–13.

Beer Marketer's Insights. 2017. *2017 beer industry update*. Suffern, NY: Beer Marketer's Insights.

Bergen, G., A. Pitan, S. Qu, R. A. Shults, S. K. Chattopadhyay, R. W. Elder, D. A. Sleet, H. L. Coleman, R. P. Compton, J. L. Nichols, J. M. Clymer, and W. B. Calvert. 2014. Publicized sobriety checkpoint programs: A community guide systematic review. *American Journal of Preventive Medicine* 46(5):529–539.

Berger, D. E., and J. R. Snortum. 1985. Alcoholic beverage preferences of drinking-driving violators. *Journal of Studies on Alcohol* 46(3):232–239.

Berning, A., R. Compton, and K. Wochinger. 2015. *Results of the 2013–2014 National Roadside Survey of Alcohol and Drug Use by Drivers.* DOT HS 812 118. Washington, DC: National Highway Traffic Safety Administration.

Blincoe, L., T. R. Miller, E. Zaloshnja, and B. A. Lawrence. 2015. *The economic and societal impact of motor vehicle crashes, 2010 (revised).* DOT HS 812 013. Washington, DC: National Highway Traffic Safety Administration.

Bond, J., T. K. Greenfield, and W. Kerr. 2008 (unpublished). *Variation in the relationship between alcohol beverage choice, risk perception, and self-reported drunk driving across the US states.* Emeryville, CA: Alcohol Research Group.

Bouchery, E. E., H. J. Harwood, J. J. Sacks, C. J. Simon, and R. D. Brewer. 2011. Economic costs of excessive alcohol consumption in the U.S., 2006. *American Journal of Preventive Medicine* 41(5):516–524.

Breslow, R. A., I. P. Castle, C. M. Chen, and B. I. Graubard. 2017. Trends in alcohol consumption among older Americans: National Health Interview Surveys, 1997 to 2014. *Alcoholism: Clinical and Experimental Research* 41(5):976–986.

CDC (Centers for Disease Control and Prevention). 2016. *Motor vehicle crash deaths: How is the US doing? CDC Vital Signs.* https://www.cdc.gov/vitalsigns/pdf/2016-07-vitalsigns.pdf (accessed August 7, 2017).

CDC. 2017a. *Fact sheets—Alcohol and caffeine.* https://www.cdc.gov/alcohol/fact-sheets/caffeine-and-alcohol.htm (accessed October 2, 2017).

CDC. 2017b. *Impaired driving: Get the facts.* https://www.cdc.gov/motorvehiclesafety/impaired_driving/impaired-drv_factsheet.html (accessed January 30, 2017).

Chavez, P. R., D. E. Nelson, T. S. Naimi, and R. D. Brewer. 2011. Impact of a new gender-specific definition for binge drinking on prevalence estimates for women. *American Journal of Preventive Medicine* 40(4):468–471.

Chicago Board of Election Commissioners. 2009. *Guideline for local option referenda.* https://chicagoelections.com/dm/general/document_51.PDF (accessed August 10, 2017).

Clarke, T. C., T. Norris, and J. S. Schiller. 2017. *Early release of selected estimates based on data from the 2016 National Health Interview Survey.* Hyattsville, MD: National Center for Health Statistics.

Collins, T., and W. Vamplew. 2011. *Mud, sweat and beers: A cultural history of sport and alcohol, Global sport cultures.* London, UK: Bloomsbury Academic.

Compton, R. P., and A. Berning. 2015. *Drug and alcohol crash risk.* Washington, DC: National Highway Traffic Safety Administration.

De Visser, R. O., and J. A. Smith. 2007. Alcohol consumption and masculine identity among young men. *Psychology and Health* 22(5):595–614.

DiMaggio, C., K. Wheeler-Martin, and J. Oliver. 2018. *Alcohol-impaired driving in the United States: Overview, review of data sources, and analyses.* Paper commissioned by the Committee on Accelerating Progress to Reduce Alcohol-Impaired Driving Fatalities (see Appendix A).

Dixon, M. A., and K. G. Chartier. 2016. Alcohol use patterns among urban and rural residents: Demographic and social influences. *Alcohol Research* 38(1):69–77.

DOJ (U.S. Department of Justice). 2009. *Enforcing underage drinking laws program.* https://www.ncjrs.gov/pdffiles1/ojjdp/227469.pdf (accessed August 23, 2017).

Dwyer-Lindgren, L., A. D. Flaxman, M. Ng, G. M. Hansen, C. J. Murray, and A. H. Mokdad. 2015. Drinking patterns in US counties from 2002 to 2012. *American Journal of Public Health* 105(6):1120–1127.

Esser, M. B., S. L. Hedden, D. Kanny, R. D. Brewer, J. C. Gfroerer, and T. S. Naimi. 2014. Prevalence of alcohol dependence among US adult drinkers, 2009–2011. *Preventing Chronic Disease* 11:E206.

Esser, M. B., J. Bao, D. H. Jernigan, and A. A. Hyder. 2016. Evaluation of the evidence base for the alcohol industry's actions to reduce drink driving globally. *American Journal of Public Health* 106(4):707–713.

Fell, J. C., S. Tippetts, and R. Voas. 2010. Drinking characteristics of drivers arrested for driving while intoxicated in two police jurisdictions. *Traffic Injury and Prevention* 11(5): 443–452.

FHWA (Federal Highway Administration). 2015. *Annual vehicle distance traveled in miles and related data-2014*. https://www.fhwa.dot.gov/policyinformation/statistics/2014/vm1.cfm (accessed October 31, 2017).

FHWA. 2016. *Highway statistics 2015. Distribution of licensed drivers—2015. By sex and percentage in each age group and relation to population*. https://www.fhwa.dot.gov/policyinformation/statistics/2015/dl20.cfm (accessed August 23, 2017).

FHWA. 2017. *Highway statistics series. Highway statistics 2015. Licensed drivers, vehicle registrations, and resident population (in millions)*. https://www.fhwa.dot.gov/policyinformation/statistics/2015/dv1c.cfm (accessed August 23, 2017).

Fisher, D. A. 2018. *Content analysis of alcohol-impaired driving stories in the news*. Paper commissioned by the Committee on Accelerating Progress to Reduce Alcohol-Impaired Driving Fatalities (see Appendix B).

Flowers, N. T., T. S. Naimi, R. D. Brewer, R. W. Elder, R. A. Shults, and R. Jiles. 2008. Patterns of alcohol consumption and alcohol-impaired driving in the United States. *Alcoholism, Clinical and Experimental Research* 32(4):639–644.

FollowTheMoney.org. n.d. *National Institute on Money in State Politics*. https://www.followthemoney.org (accessed October 2, 2017).

Forster, J. L., D. M. Murray, M. Wolfson, and A. C. Wagenaar. 1995. Commercial availability of alcohol to young people: Results of alcohol purchase attempts. *Preventive Medicine* 24(4):342–347.

Forward, J., J. Akhurst, R. Bruno, X. Leong, A. VanderNiet, H. Bromfield, J. Erny, T. Bellamy, and A. Peacock. 2017. Nature versus intensity of intoxication: Co-ingestion of alcohol and energy drinks and the effect on objective and subjective intoxication. *Drug and Alcohol Dependence* 180:292–303.

Fosdick, R. B., and A. L. Scott. 1933. *Toward liquor control*. New York: Harper and Brothers.

Foster, S. E., R. D. Vaughan, W. H. Foster, and J. A. Califano, Jr. 2006. Estimate of the commercial value of underage drinking and adult abusive and dependent drinking to the alcohol industry. *Archives of Pediatrics & Adolescent Medicine* 160(5):473–478.

FTC (Federal Trade Commission). 2013. *Alcohol advertising*. https://www.consumer.ftc.gov/articles/0391-alcohol-advertising (accessed September 20, 2017).

Gallup. 2000. *Volume I: Findings, racial and ethnic group comparisons, National Survey of Drinking and Driving, June 2000, attitudes and behaviors—1993, 1995, 1997*. DTNH22-96-c-05081. Washington, DC: National Highway Traffic Safety Administration.

Galvan, F. H., and R. Caetano. 2003. Alcohol use and related problems among ethnic minorities in the United States. *Alcohol Research & Health* 27(1):87–95.

GHSA (Governors Highway Safety Association). 2016. *Sobriety checkpoints*. http://www.ghsa.org/state-laws/issues/Sobriety-Checkpoints (accessed March 31, 2017).

Gjerde, H., M. C. Strand, and J. Morland. 2015. Driving under the influence of non-alcohol drugs—An update. Part I: Epidemiological studies. *Forensic Science Review* 27(2):89–113.

Goodwin, A., L. Thomas, B. Kirley, W. Hall, N. O'Brien, and K. Hill. 2015. *Countermeasures that work: A highway safety countermeasure guide for state highway safety offices*, 8th ed. DOT HS 812 202. Washington, DC: National Highway Traffic Safety Administration.

Grant, B. F., S. P. Chou, T. D. Saha, R. P. Pickering, B. T. Kerridge, W. J. Ruan, B. Huang, J. Jung, H. Zhang, A. Fan, and D. S. Hasin. 2017. Prevalence of 12-month alcohol use, high-risk drinking, and DSM-IV alcohol use disorder in the United States, 2001–2002 to 2012–2013: Results from the National Epidemiologic Survey on Alcohol and Related Conditions. *JAMA Psychiatry* 74(9):911–923.

Greenfield, T. K., and J. D. Rogers. 1999. Alcoholic beverage choice, risk perception and self-reported drunk driving: Effects of measurement on risk analysis. *Addiction* 94(11): 1735–1743.

Gruenewald, P. J., and W. R. Ponicki. 1995. The relationship of the retail availability of alcohol and alcohol sales to alcohol-related traffic crashes. *Accident Analysis & Prevention* 27(2):249–259.

Gruenewald, P. J., T. Stockwell, A. Beel, and E. V. Dyskin. 1999. Beverage sales and drinking and driving: The role of on-premise drinking places. *Journal of Studies on Alcohol* 60(1):47–53.

Hadland, S. E., Z. Xuan, V. Sarda, J. Blanchette, M. H. Swahn, T. C. Heeren, R. B. Voas, and T. S. Naimi. 2017. Alcohol policies and alcohol-related motor vehicle crash fatalities among young people in the US. *Pediatrics* 139(3):e20163037.

Harvard Law Review. 2016. Fresh pursuit from Indian country: Tribal authority to pursue suspects onto state land. *Harvard Law Review* 129(6):1685–1708.

Haughwout, S. P., and M. E. Slater. 2017. *Apparent per capita alcohol consumption: National, state, and regional trends, 1977–2015*. Surveillance report 108. Arlington, VA: CSR, Inc., National Institute on Alcohol Abuse and Alcoholism.

Haughwout, S. P., R. A. LaVallee, and I.-J. P. Castle. 2016. *Apparent per capita alcohol consumption: National, state, and regional trends, 1977–2014*. Surveillance report 104. Arlington, VA: CSR, Inc., National Institute on Alcohol Abuse and Alcoholism.

Hels, T., I. M. Bernhoft, A. Lyckegaard, S. Houwing, M. Hagenzieker, S.-A. Legrand, C. Isalberti, T. Van der Linden, and A. Verstraete. 2011. *Risk of injury by driving with alcohol and other drugs*. Driving under the Influence of Drugs, Alcohol and Medicines. Kongens Lyngby: Technical University of Denmark.

HHS and SAMHSA (U.S. Department of Health and Human Services and Substance Abuse and Mental Health Services Administration). 2016. Chapter 3: A coordinated federal approach to preventing and reducing underage drinking. In *September 2016 Report to Congress on the Prevention and Reduction of Underage Drinking*. Washington, DC: Interagency Coordinating Committee on the Prevention of Underage Drinking.

Hingson, R. W., W. Zha, and A. M. White. 2017. Drinking beyond the binge threshold: Predictors, consequences, and changes in the U.S. *American Journal of Preventive Medicine* 52(6):717–727.

Huber, H., R. Karlin, and P. E. Nathan. 1976. Blood alcohol level discrimination by nonalcoholics. The role of internal and external cues. *Journal of Studies on Alcohol* 37(1):27–39.

Huckle, T., M. Pledger, and S. Casswell. 2006. Trends in alcohol-related harms and offences in a liberalized alcohol environment. *Addiction* 101(2):232–240.

Huseth, A. 2012. *Alcohol-impaired driving: Common practices and performance*. Fargo: Rural Transportation Safety and Security Center, Upper Great Plains Transportation Institute, North Dakota State University.

IIHS (Insurance Institute for Highway Safety). 2016. *Urban/rural comparison*. http://www.iihs.org/iihs/topics/t/roadway-and-environment/fatalityfacts/roadway-and-environment (accessed October 31, 2017).

Impact Databank. 2017a. *The U.S. spirits market: Impact databank review and forecast*, 2017 ed. New York: Shanken Communications.

Impact Databank. 2017b. *The U.S. wine market: Impact databank review and forecast*, 2017 ed. New York: Shanken Communications.

Jang, J. B., M. E. Patrick, K. M. Keyes, A. D. Hamilton, and J. E. Schulenberg. 2017. Frequent binge drinking among US adolescents, 1991 to 2015. *Pediatrics* 139(6):e20164023.

Jernigan, D., J. Noel, J. Landon, N. Thornton, and T. Lobstein. 2017. Alcohol marketing and youth alcohol consumption: A systematic review of longitudinal studies published since 2008. *Addiction* 112(Suppl 1):7–20.

Jewett, A., R. A. Shults, T. Banerjee, and G. Bergen. 2015. Alcohol-impaired driving among adults—United States, 2012. *Morbidity and Mortality Weekly* 64(30):814–817.

Jones, L., G. Bates, E. McCoy, and M. A. Bellis. 2015. Relationship between alcohol-attributable disease and socioeconomic status, and the role of alcohol consumption in this relationship: A systematic review and meta-analysis. *BMC Public Health* 15:400.

Katikireddi, S. V., E. Whitley, J. Lewsey, L. Gray, and A. H. Leyland. 2017. Socioeconomic status as an effect modifier of alcohol consumption and harm: Analysis of linked cohort data. *Lancet Public Health* 2(6):e267–e276.

Kelley-Baker, T., J. H. Lacey, R. B. Voas, E. Romano, J. Yao, and A. Berning. 2013. Drinking and driving in the United States: Comparing results from the 2007 and 1996 national roadside surveys. *Traffic Injury and Prevention* 14(2):117–126.

Kerr, W. C., and T. K. Greenfield. 2015. Racial/ethnic disparities in the self-reported number of drinks in 2 hours before driving becomes impaired. *American Journal of Public Health* 105(7):1409–1414.

Kerr, W. C., and T. Stockwell. 2012. Understanding standard drinks and drinking guidelines. *Drug and Alcohol Review* 31(2):200–205.

Kerr, W. C., T. K. Greenfield, J. Tujague, and S. E. Brown. 2005. A drink is a drink? Variation in the amount of alcohol contained in beer, wine and spirits drinks in a US methodological sample. *Alcoholism: Clinical and Experimental Research* 29(11):2015–2021.

Kerr, W. C., T. K. Greenfield, and L. T. Midanik. 2006. How many drinks does it take you to feel drunk? Trends and predictors for subjective drunkenness. *Addiction* 101(10): 1428–1437.

Kerr, W. C., D. Patterson, M. A. Koenen, and T. K. Greenfield. 2008. Alcohol content variation of bar and restaurant drinks in northern California. *Alcoholism: Clinical and Experimental Research* 32(9):1623–1629.

Kerr, W. C., D. Patterson, T. K. Greenfield, A. S. Jones, K. A. McGeary, J. V. Terza, and C. J. Ruhm. 2013a. U.S. alcohol affordability and real tax rates, 1950–2011. *American Journal of Preventive Medicine* 44(5):459–464.

Kerr, W. C., D. Patterson, and T. K. Greenfield. 2013b. *The blurring of alcohol categories*. Alexandria, VA: National Alcohol Beverage Control Association.

Keyes, K. M., and D. S. Hasin. 2008. Socio-economic status and problem alcohol use: The positive relationship between income and the DSM-IV alcohol abuse diagnosis. *Addiction* 103(7):1120–1130.

Keyes, K. M., X. C. Liu, and M. Cerda. 2012. The role of race/ethnicity in alcohol-attributable injury in the United States. *Epidemiologic Reviews* 34:89–102.

King, C., 3rd, M. Siegel, C. S. Ross, and D. H. Jernigan. 2017. Alcohol advertising in magazines and underage readership: Are underage youth disproportionately exposed? *Alcoholism: Clinical and Experimental Research* 41(10):1775–1782.

Lalanne, L., P. E. Lutz, and F. Paille. 2017. Acute impact of caffeinated alcoholic beverages on cognition: A systematic review. *Progress in Neuro-Psychopharmacology & Biological Psychiatry* 76:188–194.

Landen, M., J. Roeber, T. Naimi, L. Nielsen, and M. Sewell. 2014. Alcohol-attributable mortality among American Indians and Alaska Natives in the United States, 1999–2009. *American Journal of Public Health* 104(Suppl 3):S343–S349.

Lansky, D., P. E. Nathan, S. M. Ersner-Hershfield, and T. R. Lipscomb. 1978. Blood alcohol level discrimination: Pre-training monitoring accuracy of alcoholics and nonalcoholics. *Addictive Behaviors* 3(3–4):209–214.

Lapham, S. C., J. C'de Baca, G. McMillan, and W. C. Hunt. 2004. Accuracy of alcohol diagnosis among DWI offenders referred for screening. *Drug and Alcohol Dependence* 76(2):135–141.

Lapham, S. C., R. Stout, G. Laxton, and B. J. Skipper. 2011. Persistence of addictive disorders in a first-offender driving while impaired population. *Archives of General Psychiatry* 68(11):1151–1157.

Laude, J. R., and M. T. Fillmore. 2016. Drivers who self-estimate lower blood alcohol concentrations are riskier drivers after drinking. *Psychopharmacology* 233(8):1387–1394.

LaVallee, R. A., T. Kim, and H.-Y. Yi. 2014. *Apparent per capita alcohol consumption: National, state, and regional trends, 1977–2012.* Surveillance report 98. Arlington, VA: CSR, Inc., National Institute on Alcohol Abuse and Alcoholism.

Letourneau, R. J., and C. E. Crump. 2016. *Tribal motor vehicle injury preventions (TMVIP) best practices guide 2016.* Atlanta, GA: Centers for Disease Control and Prevention.

Lipari, R. N., A. Hughes, and J. Bose. 2016. *Driving under the influence of alcohol and illicit drugs. The CBHSQ report: December 27, 2016.* Rockville, MD: Center for Behavioral Health Statistics and Quality, Substance Abuse and Mental Health Services Administration.

Lobstein, T., J. Landon, N. Thornton, and D. Jernigan. 2017. The commercial use of digital media to market alcohol products: A narrative review. *Addiction* 112(Suppl 1):21–27.

Lorenc, T., M. Petticrew, V. Welch, and P. Tugwell. 2013. What types of interventions generate inequalities? Evidence from systematic reviews. *Journal of Epidemiology and Community Health* 67(2):190–193.

Luoma, J., and M. Sivak. 2014. Why is road safety in the U.S. not on par with Sweden, the U.K., and the Netherlands? Lessons to be learned. *European Transport Research Review* 6(3):295–302.

Martens, M. P., J. C. Page, E. S. Mowry, K. M. Damann, K. K. Taylor, and M. D. Cimini. 2006. Differences between actual and perceived student norms: An examination of alcohol use, drug use, and sexual behavior. *Journal of American College Health* 54(5):295–300.

Martin, T. L., P. A. Solbeck, D. J. Mayers, R. M. Langille, Y. Buczek, and M. R. Pelletier. 2013. A review of alcohol-impaired driving: The role of blood alcohol concentration and complexity of the driving task. *Journal of Forensic Sciences* 58(5):1238–1250.

Mattson, J. 2016. *Rural transit fact book 2016.* Fargo: North Dakota State University. Upper Great Plains Transportation Institute. Small Urban and Rural Transit Center.

McKetin, R., A. Coen, and S. Kaye. 2015. A comprehensive review of the effects of mixing caffeinated energy drinks with alcohol. *Drug and Alcohol Dependence* 151:15–30.

Michael, J. 2017. Powerpoint presentation to the Committee on Accelerating Progress to Reduce Alcohol-Impaired Driving Fatalities in Washington, DC, February 16, 2017. http://www.nationalacademies.org/hmd/~/media/Files/Activity%20Files/AcceleratingProgresstoReduceAlcoholImpairedDrivingFatalities/16%20FEB%202017/1%20Michael.pdf (accessed September 26, 2017).

Mintel. 2015. *The craft effect: One in four beers launched globally in 2014 was high strength.* http://www.mintel.com/press-centre/food-and-drink/the-craft-effect-one-in-four-beers-launched-globally-in-2014-was-high-strength (accessed December 6, 2017).

Mulia, N., K. J. Karriker-Jaffe, J. Witbrodt, J. Bond, E. Williams, and S. E. Zemore. 2017. Racial/ethnic differences in 30-year trajectories of heavy drinking in a nationally representative US sample. *Drug and Alcohol Dependence* 170:133–141.

Naimi, T. S., D. E. Nelson, and R. D. Brewer. 2009. Driving after binge drinking. *American Journal of Preventive Medicine* 37(4):314–320.

Naimi, T. S., J. Blanchette, T. F. Nelson, T. Nguyen, N. Oussayef, T. C. Heeren, P. Gruenewald, J. Mosher, and Z. Xuan. 2014. A new scale of the U.S. alcohol policy environment and its relationship to binge drinking. *American Journal of Preventive Medicine* 46(1):10–16.

Naimi, T. S., Z. Xuan, V. Sarda, S. Hadland, M. Lira, T. Heeren, R. Voas, and M. H. Swahn. 2017. *Alcohol policies and alcohol-related motor vehicle crash fatalities among U.S. adults.* Paper presented at 43rd Annual Alcohol Epidemiology Symposium of the Kettil Bruun Society, Sheffield, England.

NASADAD (National Association of State Alcohol and Drug Abuse Directors). 2016. NASADAD *priority programs within the Department of Justice (DOJ).* http://nasadad.org/wp-content/uploads/2016/02/DOJ-Programs-Fact-Sheet-DRAFT-2016.pdf (accessed August 23, 2017).

NCSA (National Center for Statistics and Analysis). 2015. *Alcohol-impaired driving: 2014 data.* Traffic Safety Facts. DOT HS 812 231. Washington, DC: National Highway Traffic Safety Administration.

NCSA. 2016a. *Alcohol-impaired driving: 2015 data.* Traffic Safety Facts. Report No. DOT HS 812 350. Washington, DC: National Highway Traffic Safety Administration.

NCSA. 2016b. *2015 motor vehicle crashes: Overview.* Traffic Safety Facts. Report No. DOH HS 812 318. Washington, DC: National Highway Traffic Safety Administration.

NCSA. 2016c. *Rural/urban comparison: 2014 data.* Traffic Safety Facts. Report No. DOT HS 812 301. Washington, DC: National Highway Traffic Safety Administration.

NCSA. 2017a. *2016 fatal motor vehicle crashes: Overview.* Traffic Safety Facts Research Note. Report No. DOT HS 812 456. Washington, DC: National Highway Traffic Safety Administration.

NCSA. 2017b. *Alcohol-impaired driving: 2016 data.* Traffic Safety Facts. Report No. DOT HS 812 450. Washington, DC: National Highway Traffic Safety Administration.

Nelson, T. F., Z. Xuan, T. F. Babor, R. D. Brewer, F. J. Chaloupka, P. J. Gruenewald, H. Holder, M. Klitzner, J. F. Mosher, R. L. Ramirez, R. Reynolds, T. L. Toomey, V. Churchill, and T. S. Naimi. 2013. Efficacy and the strength of evidence of U.S. alcohol control policies. *American Journal of Preventive Medicine* 45(1):19–28.

NHTSA (National Highway Traffic Safety Administration), GHSA, and Volpe National Transportation Systems Center. 2017. *Impact of the legalization and decriminalization of marijuana on the DWI system: Highlights from the expert panel meeting.* Washington, DC: National Highway Traffic Safety Administration.

O'Brien, M. C., T. P. McCoy, S. D. Rhodes, A. Wagoner, and M. Wolfson. 2008. Caffeinated cocktails: Energy drink consumption, high-risk drinking, and alcohol-related consequences among college students. *Academic Emergency Medicine* 15(5):453–460.

O'Donnell, M. A. 1985. Research on drinking locations of alcohol-impaired drivers: Implications for prevention policies. *Journal of Public Health Policy* 6(4):510–525.

O'Neill, B., and S. Y. Kyrychenko. 2006. Use and misuse of motor-vehicle crash death rates in assessing highway-safety performance. *Traffic Injury Prevention* 7(4):307–318.

OpenSecrets.org. n.d. *Beer, wine, and liquor: Industry profile: Summary, 2016.* http://www.opensecrets.org/lobby/indusclient.php?id=N02&year=2016 (accessed October 2, 2017).

Pantani, D., R. Peltzer, M. Cremonte, K. Robaina, T. Babor, and I. Pinsky. 2017. The marketing potential of corporate social responsibility activities: The case of the alcohol industry in Latin America and the Caribbean. *Addiction* 112(Suppl 1):74–80.

Patrick, M. E., J. E. Schulenberg, M. E. Martz, J. L. Maggs, P. M. O'Malley, and L. D. Johnston. 2013. Extreme binge drinking among 12th-grade students in the United States: Prevalence and predictors. *JAMA Pediatrics* 167(11):1019–1025.

Perkins, H. W., M. P. Haines, and R. Rice. 2005. Misperceiving the college drinking norm and related problems: A nationwide study of exposure to prevention information, perceived norms and student alcohol misuse. *Journal of Studies on Alcohol* 66(4):470–478.

Piontkowski, S. R., J. S. Peabody, C. Reede, J. Velascosoltero, G. Tsatoke, T. Shelhamer, and K. R. Hicks. 2015. Reducing motor vehicle-related injuries at an Arizona Indian reservation: Ten years of application of evidence-based strategies. *Global Health: Science and Practice* 3(4):619–629.

Probst, C., M. Roerecke, S. Behrendt, and J. Rehm. 2014. Socioeconomic differences in alcohol-attributable mortality compared with all-cause mortality: A systematic review and meta-analysis. *International Journal of Epidemiology* 43(4):1314–1327.

Quinlan, K. P., R. D. Brewer, P. Siegel, D. A. Sleet, A. H. Mokdad, R. A. Shults, and N. Flowers. 2005. Alcohol-impaired driving among U.S. adults, 1993–2002. *American Journal of Preventive Medicine* 28(4):346–350.

Quinlan, K., R. A. Shults, and R. A. Rudd. 2014. Child passenger deaths involving alcohol-impaired drivers. *Pediatrics* 133(6):966–972.

Rahav, G., R. Wilsnack, K. Bloomfield, G. Gmel, and S. Kuntsche. 2006. The influence of societal level factors on men's and women's alcohol consumption and alcohol problems. *Alcohol and Alcoholism* 41(Suppl 1):i47–i55.

Rammohan, V., R. A. Hahn, R. Elder, R. Brewer, J. Fielding, T. S. Naimi, T. L. Toomey, S. K. Chattopadhyay, and C. Zometa. 2011. Effects of dram shop liability and enhanced overservice law enforcement initiatives on excessive alcohol consumption and related harms: Two community guide systematic reviews. *American Journal of Preventive Medicine* 41(3):334–343.

Redelmeier, D. A., and A. S. Detsky. 2017. Clinical action against drunk driving. *PLoS Medicine* 14(2):e1002231.

Rehm, J., D. W. Lachenmeier, E. J. Llopis, S. Imtiaz, and P. Anderson. 2016. Evidence of reducing ethanol content in beverages to reduce harmful use of alcohol. *The Lancet Gastroenterology & Hepatology* 1(1):78–83.

Retting, R. 2017. *Pedestrian traffic fatalities by state: 2016 preliminary data.* Washington, DC: Governors Highway Safety Association.

Rhoades, E., and D. H. Jernigan. 2013. Risky messages in alcohol advertising, 2003–2007: Results from content analysis. *Journal of Adolescent Health* 52(1):116–121.

Rickard, B. J., T. Garg, and M. Costanigro. 2013. Economic and social implications of regulating alcohol availability in grocery stores. *Applied Economic Perspectives and Policy* 35(4):613–633.

Roche, A., V. Kostadinov, J. Fischer, R. Nicholas, K. O'Rourke, K. Pidd, and A. Trifonoff. 2015a. Addressing inequities in alcohol consumption and related harms. *Health Promotion International* 30(Suppl 2):ii20–ii35.

Roche, A., V. Kostadinov, J. Fischer, and R. Nicholas. 2015b. *Evidence review: The social determinants of inequities in alcohol consumption and alcohol-related health outcomes.* Australian's National Research Centre on AOD Workforce Development and Flinders University.

Romano, E., R. B. Voas, and J. C. Lacey. 2010. *Alcohol and highway safety: Special report on race/ethnicity and impaired driving.* Washington, DC: National Highway Traffic Safety Administration.

SAMHSA (Substance Abuse and Mental Health Services Administration). 2014. *Results from the 2013 National Survey on Drug Use and Health: Summary of national findings.* NSDUH series H-48, HHS publication 14-4863. Rockville, MD: Substance Abuse and Mental Health Services Administration.

SAMHSA. 2015. *Behavioral health trends in the United States: Results from the 2014 National Survey on Drug Use and Health.* HHS publication 15-4927, NSDUH series H-50. https://www.samhsa.gov/data/population-data-nsduh (accessed April 27, 2017).

SAMHSA. 2016. *Results from the 2015 National Survey on Drug Use and Health: Detailed tables.* https://www.samhsa.gov/data/sites/default/files/NSDUH-DetTabs-2015/NSDUH-DetTabs-2015/NSDUH-DetTabs-2015.htm#tab2-41b (accessed March 31, 2017).

Sanem, J. R., D. J. Erickson, P. C. Rutledge, K. M. Lenk, T. F. Nelson, R. Jones-Webb, and T. L. Toomey. 2015. Association between alcohol-impaired driving enforcement-related strategies and alcohol-impaired driving. *Accident Analysis and Prevention* 78:104–109.

Sauber-Schatz, E. K., D. J. Ederer, A. M. Dellinger, and G. T. Baldwin. 2016. Vital signs: Motor vehicle injury prevention—United States and 19 comparison countries. *Morbidity and Mortality Weekly Report* 65(26):672–677.

Scaglione, S., S. Kliethermes, G. Cao, D. Shoham, R. Durazo, A. Luke, and M. L. Volk. 2015. The epidemiology of cirrhosis in the United States: A population-based study. *Journal of Clinical Gastroenterology* 49(8):690–696.

Schmidt, L. A., P. Mäkelä, J. Rehm, and R. Room. 2010. Alcohol: Equity and social determinants. In *Equity, social determinants and public health programs*, edited by E. Blas and A. S. Kurup. Geneva, Switzerland: World Health Organization.

Schmidt, S. 2017. PowerPoint presentation to the Committee on Accelerating Progress to Reduce Alcohol-Impaired Driving Fatalities. Washington, DC, March 22, 2017. http://nationalacademies.org/hmd/~/media/Files/Activity%20Files/AcceleratingProgresstoReduceAlcoholImpairedDrivingFatalities/22%20March%202017/1%20Steve%20Schmidt.pdf (accessed August 9, 2017).

Schor, E. L. 1996. Adolescent alcohol use: social determinants and the case for early family-centered prevention. Family-focused prevention of adolescent drinking. *Bulletin of the New York Academy of Medicine* 73(2):335–356.

Schulenberg, J. E., L. D. Johnston, P. M. O'Malley, J. G. Bachman, R. A. Miech, and M. E. Patrick. 2017. *Monitoring the future. National survey results on drug use, 1975–2016: Volume II, college students and adults ages 19–55.* Ann Arbor, MI: Institute for Social Research, University of Michigan.

Sivak, M., and B. Schoettle. 2017. *Recent diverging trends in the amount of urban and rural driving in the United States.* Ann Arbor: University of Michigan, Sustainable Worldwide Transportation.

Smith, K., and J. Foster. 2014. *Alcohol, health inequalities and the harm paradox: Why some groups face greater problems despite consuming less alcohol.* London, UK: Institute of Alcohol Studies.

Strand, M. C., H. Gjerde, and J. Morland. 2016. Driving under the influence of non-alcohol drugs—An update. Part II: Experimental studies. *Forensic Science Review* 28(2):79–101.

Striley, C. W., and S. R. Khan. 2014. Review of the energy drink literature from 2013: Findings continue to support most risk from mixing with alcohol. *Current Opinion in Psychiatry* 27(4):263–268.

Subramanian, R. 2009. *Geospatial analysis of rural motor vehicle traffic fatalities.* Report No. DOT HS 811 196. Washington, DC: National Highway Traffic Safety Administration.

Sudhinaraset, M., C. Wigglesworth, and D. T. Takeuchi. 2016. Social and cultural contexts of alcohol use: Influences in a socio-ecological framework. *Alcohol Research: Current Reviews* 38(1):35–45.

TRB (Transportation Research Board). 2013. *Emergency medical services response to motor vehicle crashes in rural areas.* Washington, DC: The National Academies Press.

TRB. 2016. *Between public and private mobility: Examining the rise of technology-enabled transportation services.* Washington, DC: The National Academies Press.

TRIP (The Road Improvement Program). 2017. *Rural connections: Challenges and opportunities in America's heartland.* Washington, DC: TRIP.

U.S. Census Bureau. 2010. *2010 census urban and rural classification and urban area criteria.* https://www.census.gov/geo/reference/ua/urban-rural-2010.html (accessed August 11, 2017).

Utah State Legislature. 2017. *H.B. 155 driving under the influence and public safety revisions.* http://le.utah.gov/~2017/bills/static/HB0155.html (accessed March 30, 2017).

Vaca, F. E., E. Romano, J. C. Fell, and E. Choo. 2014. Female drivers increasingly involved in impaired driving crashes: Actions to ameliorate the risk. *Academic Emergency Medicine* 21(12):1485–1492.

Voas, R. B., and J. C. Lacey. 2011. *Alcohol and highway safety: A review of the state of knowledge.* Washington, DC: National Highway Traffic Safety Administration.

Vock, D. C. 2013. *Rural states struggle to reduce road deaths.* http://www.pewtrusts.org/en/research-and-analysis/blogs/stateline/2013/03/12/rural-states-struggle-to-reduce-road-deaths (accessed October 2, 2017).

Wagenaar, A. C., A. L. Tobler, and K. A. Komro. 2010. Effects of alcohol tax and price policies on morbidity and mortality: A systematic review. *American Journal of Public Health* 100(11):2270–2278.

Walker, S., S. Higgs, and P. Terry. 2016. Estimates of the absolute and relative strengths of diverse alcoholic drinks by young people. *Substance Use & Misuse* 51(13):1781–1789.

Wechsler, H., and T. F. Nelson. 2008. What we have learned from the Harvard School of Public Health College Alcohol Study: Focusing attention on college student alcohol consumption and the environmental conditions that promote it. *Journal of Studies on Alcohol and Drugs* 69(4):481–490.

WHO (World Health Organization). 2011. *Global status report on alcohol and health.* Geneva, Switzerland: World Health Organization.

WHO. 2014. *Standard drink measures, in grams per unit. Data by country.* http://apps.who.int/gho/data/view.main.54180 (accessed March 30, 2017).

WHO. 2015a. *Global status report on road safety 2015.* Geneva, Switzerland: World Health Organization.

WHO. 2015b. *Report of the Second Technical Consultation on drug use and road safety. 16–17 December 2015.* Mallorca, Spain: World Health Organization.

WHO. 2016. *Drug use and road safety.* Geneva, Switzerland: World Health Organization.

Williams, A. F., A. T. McCartt, and S. A. Ferguson. 2007. Hardcore drinking drivers and other contributors to the alcohol-impaired driving problem: Need for a comprehensive approach. *Traffic Injury Prevention* 8(1):1–10.

Wilsnack, R. W., N. D. Vogeltanz, S. C. Wilsnack, and T. R. Harris. 2000. Gender differences in alcohol consumption and adverse drinking consequences: Cross-cultural patterns. *Addiction* 95(2):251–265.

Wilsnack, R. W., S. C. Wilsnack, A. F. Kristjanson, N. D. Vogeltanz-Holm, and G. Gmel. 2009. Gender and alcohol consumption: Patterns from the multinational GENACIS project. *Addiction* 104(9):1487–1500.

Wilson, F. A., and J. P. Stimpson. 2010. Trends in fatalities from distracted driving in the United States, 1999–2008. *American Journal of Public Health* 100(11):2213–2219.

Wilson, F. A., J. P. Stimpson, and M. K. Tibbits. 2013. The role of alcohol use on recent trends in distracted driving. *Accident Analysis & Prevention* 60(November):189–192.

Xuan, Z., J. G. Blanchette, T. F. Nelson, T. C. Heeren, T. H. Nguyen, and T. S. Naimi. 2015a. Alcohol policies and impaired driving in the United States: Effects of driving- vs. drinking-oriented policies. *International Journal of Alcohol and Drug Use* 4(2):119–130.

Xuan, Z., T. H. Nguyen, N. L. Oussayef, T. S. Naimi, J. G. Blanchette, T. S. Naimi, T. F. Nelson, S. E. Hadland, and T. C. Heeren. 2015b. Youth drinking in the United States: Relationships with alcohol policies and adult drinking. *Pediatrics* 136(1):18–27.

Zaloshnja, E., T. R. Miller, D. Hendrie, and D. Galvin. 2007. Employer costs of alcohol-involved injuries. *American Journal of Industrial Medicine* 50(2):136–142.

Zaloshnja, E., T. R. Miller, and L. J. Blincoe. 2013. Costs of alcohol-involved crashes, United States, 2010. Paper read at 57th Annual Meeting of the Association for the Advancement of Automotive Medicine Conference, Quebec City, Canada.

Zhang, L., W. F. Wieczorek, and J. W. Welte. 2014. The link between early onset drinking and early onset alcohol-impaired driving in young males. *American Journal of Drug and Alcohol Abuse* 40(3):251–257.

3

Interventions to Reduce Drinking to Impairment

INTRODUCTION

Most interventions to reduce alcohol-impaired driving have focused on decreasing the likelihood that someone will drive after already being impaired by alcohol. Conversely, less attention has been focused on reducing drinking to impairment before driving. This has been demonstrated in policy activity; during the past two decades the implementation of driving-oriented policies has increased among states, while the implementation of effective drinking-oriented policies has remained virtually unchanged (Nelson et al., 2015). However, there are a number of effective interventions to reduce drinking to the point of impairment (i.e., binge drinking[1]), and some of these interventions have an independent effect on reducing impaired driving and alcohol-impaired driving crashes (Elder et al., 2010; Fell et al., 2009; Hingson et al., 2008; McCartt et al., 2010; Rammohan et al., 2011; Xuan et al., 2015a). Therefore, increasing adoption of interventions that have been proven to reduce excessive drinking is an important and underused strategy to reduce morbidity and mortality from alcohol-impaired driving.

[1] Binge drinking is defined as drinking at or above levels during a drinking occasion/episode that typically results in impairment-level BACs (i.e., ≥0.08%) for most men and women drinking at typical drinking rates. This corresponds to drinking five or more drinks for men and four or more drinks for women in about 2 hours. Most public health and epidemiologic studies use five/four thresholds, and members of the general public interpret the *binge drinking* term to mean drinking to the point of impairment or intoxication.

As illustrated in the committee's conceptual framework (see Figure 1-5), the first two behaviors that the committee identified as points of intervention for reducing alcohol-impaired driving fatalities are alcohol consumption and drinking to impairment. Chapter 2 underscores the proximal relationship between binge drinking and alcohol-impaired driving. This chapter will highlight the drinking-oriented interventions (i.e., policies, programs, systems, and strategies) that have a strong evidence base supporting their population-level effectiveness, while other interventions discussed may be promising but underevaluated, or relatively ineffective but commonly used or familiar. These interventions will be examined within the context of the concepts and considerations for comparing interventions that were discussed in Chapter 1, as well as barriers to implementation and strategies to overcome them, lessons learned from other countries, and key research needs. This chapter is organized by the most salient intervention opportunities identified in the conceptual framework that target alcohol consumption (particularly consumption stemming from illegal sales to underaged or intoxicated persons) and interventions designed to reduce binge drinking, including policies and laws, enforcement, educational interventions, and technological interventions.

The chapter presents discussions of policies and laws that target the alcohol environment (e.g., policies to maintain or increase price of alcohol, limit physical availability, reduce illegal alcohol sales, and restrict alcohol marketing) and shape drinking behaviors that reduce alcohol-related harms (e.g., alcohol-impaired driving crashes). The committee applied an upstream, preventive approach to reducing alcohol-impaired driving fatalities and used the best available evidence to inform the selection of these specific policies and laws from an array of options for states and localities. However, it is important to recognize that some upstream interventions and policies have a broader reach than others. Some (e.g., social host liability) are targeted directly at preventing impaired driving, while others (e.g., enforcing underage drinking laws) target unlawful consumption. However, some of these polices (e.g., raising the price and reducing the number of alcohol outlets) operate further upstream and affect all consumers. The policy-relevant effect is that these actions reduce choice overall while aiming to reduce excessive or harmful alcohol consumption. The committee acknowledges that population-level policies may be more controversial than polices that are more precisely targeted at high-risk consumers, excessive consumption, or risky behavior. While these interventions have been shown to reduce most types of alcohol-related harm at the population level and achieve the desired public health benefits, they also have the potential to reduce liberties of responsible adult consumers. However, there are health benefits to these population-level policies beyond only reducing alcohol-impaired driving, for example, reducing violence and child abuse and neglect (Foran and O'Leary, 2008; Kuhns et al., 2014; Widom and Hiller-Sturmhofel, 2001). Ultimately, these considerations have to be balanced by policy makers in light of the values of their particular community. For purposes of this report, however, the committee believes the evidence shows that the trade-offs outweigh the potential reduction in individual choice.

Historically, the support for and enactment of effective policies and laws have been the impetus for reducing alcohol-impaired driving fatalities (Fell and Voas, 2006). Furthermore, these policies do not operate in siloes. As discussed in Chapter 1, progress in this area requires a comprehensive approach, which includes a set of complementary policies to reduce hazardous drinking, enhanced with enforcement. Throughout this chapter, the committee offers recommendations to all levels of government on which sets of policies and laws to adopt or improve to reduce alcohol-impaired driving. These are the policies and laws that the committee has determined will have the greatest effect on population health by reducing excessive drinking and ultimately, alcohol-impaired driving.

POLICIES TO MAINTAIN OR INCREASE PRICE

Raising Alcohol Taxes to Reduce Impaired Driving and Related Consequences

Overview

Alcohol taxes have perhaps the strongest and most consistent evidence base of any U.S. policy for reducing excessive drinking and related harms, and there is also strong evidence that higher alcohol taxes reduce alcohol-impaired driving and motor vehicle crash fatalities (Elder et al., 2010; Wagenaar et al., 2009, 2010). The 2016 *Surgeon General's Report on Alcohol, Drugs, and Health* identifies price and tax policies as an evidence-based policy to reduce alcohol misuse and related problems (HHS, 2016). Despite this, alcohol taxes do not cover alcohol-related costs and have declined in inflation-adjusted terms at both federal and state levels (Naimi et al., 2017; Sacks et al., 2015).

In the United States, alcohol taxes may be applied as *specific excise taxes*, which are based on a fixed dollar amount per volume and are sometimes referred to as *volume-based taxes*. This is the most common type of tax, and it is the only form of federal taxation on alcohol. Some states also have *ad valorem excise taxes*, which are based on a percentage of price. Most but not all states apply the general sales tax to alcohol (APIS, 2016c).

Higher alcohol taxes, which are imposed on the producers of alcohol, are typically passed through to consumers as higher prices. While the

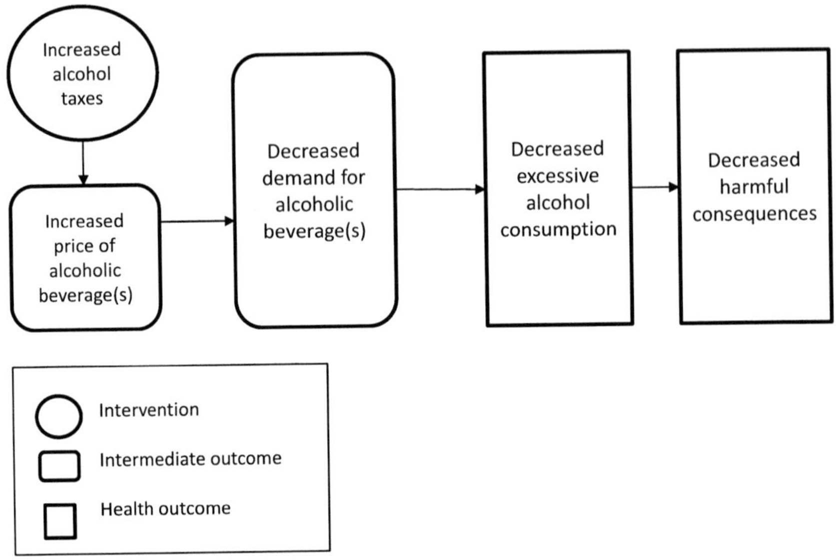

FIGURE 3-1 A conceptual model for the causal relationship between increased alcohol taxes and decreased excessive alcohol consumption and related harms.
SOURCE: Adapted from Elder et al., 2010.

industry could soften the effect of taxes by reducing their prices, alcohol taxes are typically passed on to consumers at an equal or even higher rate (Ally et al., 2014; Kenkel, 2005; Young and Bielinska-Kwapisz, 2002). Consequently, consumers face higher alcohol prices. The bulk of the evidence suggests that higher prices reduce both overall consumption and high-risk alcohol-related activities and adverse outcomes. The evidence base is strong, with consistent findings across a variety of study designs including quasi-experimental time series analyses and panel studies (see, for example, Elder et al., 2010; Wagenaar et al., 2009, 2010; Xuan et al., 2013). In addition, higher taxes are protective for a range of outcomes that are related to binge drinking, including interpersonal violence, sexually transmitted infections, and unintentional injuries including motor vehicle crashes (Wagenaar et al., 2010). See Figure 3-1 for a conceptual model that delineates the causal pathway by which an increase in alcohol taxes could reduce excessive alcohol consumption and harmful consequences.

Drinking, Binge Drinking, and Impaired Driving

Efforts to reduce the health, social, and economic costs of alcohol-impaired driving and alcohol-related crashes and crash fatalities depend on reducing the frequency and intensity of alcohol impairment in the population and on reducing the likelihood that those who are impaired will drive a motor vehicle. Overall, approximately 5 percent of drinkers report having driven after "having had perhaps too much to drink" during the past 30 days (Flowers et al., 2008). Binge drinking, which typically results in a level of blood alcohol concentration (BAC) that produces impairment, is therefore a precursor to alcohol-impaired driving among those who subsequently drive a motor vehicle. In addition, 12 percent of binge drinkers report having driven a motor vehicle during or within 2 hours of their most recent binge drinking episode. Those who reported binge drinking and subsequent driving consumed an average of 8 drinks, and 26 percent of them consumed 10 or more drinks (Naimi et al., 2009). In cross-sectional surveys, 84 percent of those who report having driven "after having perhaps too much to drink" also report binge drinking; self-reported binge drinkers account for 88 percent all of impaired driving episodes (Flowers et al., 2008). Because survey respondents may drink and binge drink less than the population as a whole, and because survey respondents may underreport their own consumption or related activities such as driving after binge drinking, it is likely these estimates are conservative.

Higher Taxes Reduce Alcohol Consumption and Binge Drinking

Higher prices for alcohol are related to lower consumption and reduced binge drinking among adults and youths (Elder et al., 2010; Wagenaar et al., 2009; Xuan et al., 2013). One summary measure of the effect of taxes on consumption is the price elasticity of demand; this is a proxy for the tax elasticity of demand. Across multiple studies, the average price elasticity of demand for alcohol is –0.65, which means that every 10 percent increase in price is associated with a 6.5 percent reduction in consumption (Wagenaar et al., 2009). Even among heavy drinkers the price elasticity for alcohol is –0.28 (Wagenaar et al., 2009). Furthermore, there is a strong inverse relationship between taxes and binge drinking (Xuan et al., 2015b) and taxes and outcomes related to binge drinking, which demonstrates that taxes still have a strong effect on those who drink excessively (Elder et al., 2010; Wagenaar et al., 2010).

Higher Taxes Reduce Impaired Driving and Motor Vehicle Crash Fatalities

There is also strong and direct evidence that higher taxes reduce impaired driving and fatal motor vehicle crashes. A meta-analysis by Wagenaar et al. (2010) examined effect sizes in studies that assessed a diverse set of alcohol-related outcome measures, including traffic crashes and alcohol-related driving measures. The study combined independent estimates in random-effects models to calculate aggregate effect estimates across 50 studies. Among the 21 studies that specifically examined effects of alcohol prices or taxes on traffic safety outcomes, all 34 independent estimates showed an inverse association, with 68 percent of those estimates reaching statistical significance. The average effect size for the 34 independent estimates was –0.112 ($p<0.001$). The authors concluded that doubling the alcohol tax would lead to an 11 percent reduction in traffic crash deaths (Wagenaar et al., 2010).

A systematic review by the Guide to Community Preventive Services convened by the Centers for Disease Control and Prevention (CDC) also found that alcohol-impaired driving was inversely related to the price of alcoholic beverages (Elder et al., 2010). The review included 11 studies that evaluated the effects of alcohol prices or taxes on motor vehicle crashes. Across the studies, the association between alcohol prices or taxes and motor vehicle injuries and fatalities was generally significant. Furthermore, the authors report that the magnitude was comparable to the relationship between alcohol prices or taxes and alcohol consumption. The elasticities reported in these studies were generally higher in the studies that examined outcomes more proximally related to alcohol consumption (e.g., alcohol-related crashes) when compared to those that are less directly related (e.g., overall crash fatalities). The authors also reviewed three studies that assessed the relationship between alcohol prices or taxes and price elasticities for self-reported alcohol-impaired driving. Price elasticities in samples from the United States and Canada (range of –0.50 to –0.81; all $p<0.05$) showed that there was consistent evidence of an inverse relationship between price and impaired driving.

A recent (2017) interrupted time series study investigated the effect of an increase in alcohol sales tax in Maryland on the rate of drivers involved in an injury crash who were "alcohol-positive" (i.e., drivers for which the investigating officer perceived any alcohol involvement or their BAC was above 0.00%). The authors found that the 2011 tax increase (from 6 percent to 9 percent) lead to a significant 12 percent reduction in alcohol-positive drivers aged 15–20 years ($p<0.007$) and 21–34 years ($p<0.001$). For drivers ages 55 and above, the rate of alcohol-positive drivers increased during the post-intervention period, which the authors posit could be related to this age group's average socioeconomic status in the state of Maryland and thus, decreased price sensitivity. Overall, the study also showed a 6 percent reduction ($p<0.03$) in the population-based rate of alcohol-positive drivers after the increase was enacted. The effect was modeled using three denominators—per population of Maryland, licensed drivers in Maryland, and vehicle miles traveled in Maryland—which all found similar results. The authors controlled for a number of factors (e.g., monthly unemployment prevalence in Maryland and annual state per-capita personal income) and included a proxy, alcohol-negative crashes, to control for external factors such as the economy, advancements in car safety, and highway design (Lavoie et al., 2017).

Cost-Effectiveness of Raising Alcohol Taxes

Raising taxes has been shown to reduce impaired driving and related consequences; these are important and valued benefits. Moreover, the additional, direct program costs of collecting the taxes are relatively small as the tax collecting infrastructure is already in place. Furthermore, the higher tax revenue raised by the government (i.e., federal or state) can more than offset these relatively small costs, depending on the size of the tax increase. Thus raising taxes is likely to generate government revenue. However, there may be a level of taxes beyond which taxes would no longer increase revenue; that is, if individuals reduced their consumption or price of alcohol consumed, or turned to untaxed black markets. Another potential cost would be the lost enjoyment (utility) to those drinkers who reduced their drinking levels. The committee considers that loss of utility to be small. Conversely, on a population level, this cost would be more than offset by reduced societal costs such as lost productivity and diminished utility (e.g., physical or emotional pain for victims or their friends and family) that result from excessive alcohol consumption and alcohol-impaired driving injuries and fatalities. In sum, considering all these costs leads the committee to the conclusion that raising taxes would be cost-beneficial.

Other Considerations in Raising Taxes, in Addition to Their Effectiveness

Despite evidence of effectiveness for reducing alcohol-impaired driving and alcohol-related crash fatalities, taxes are low and therefore represent an important "old" but neglected strategy that could be much more aggressively implemented. Thus, raising taxes represents an important public health opportunity. Currently, alcohol-specific excise taxes in states and at the federal level are low in absolute terms. Specifically, the federal tax on a standard drink (0.6 oz., or 14 grams of ethanol) of beer is $0.05, a standard drink of wine is $0.04, and a standard drink of distilled spirits is almost $0.13 (TTB, 2016). In 2015, the average state alcohol-specific excise tax per standard drink was $0.03 for beer, $0.03 for wine, and $0.05 for spirits. These taxes therefore account for a small percentage of the price of alcohol. Furthermore, federal and state taxes have eroded in inflation-adjusted terms relative to historical levels. Federal alcohol taxes have not been changed or adjusted for inflation since 1991. While alcohol taxes historically (late 1800s through early 1900s) accounted for more than one-third of federal government revenue, they now account for less than half of 1 percent of federal government revenue (Cook, 2007). Among states from 1991 to 2015, the average inflation-adjusted (in 2015 dollars) specific excise tax rate declined 30 percent for beer, 27 percent for wine, and 32 percent for spirits (see Figure 3-2). Alcohol tax erosion is not a new phenomenon. Average declines in specific excise taxes since their inception (which varied by state following the repeal of Prohibition) are more than twice as large as those from 1991 to 2015 (Naimi et al., 2018).

Taxes can be levied to reduce alcohol consumption, and/or to cover costs related to the use of alcohol, particularly those costs that are borne by those other than the drinker or alcohol-related businesses. These costs are sometimes referred to as *external* (or *secondhand* or *spillover* costs). Currently, alcohol taxes are considerably lower than the external costs or harms related to a standard drink of alcohol. For example, the external cost per one standard drink of alcohol is approximately $2.00, of which approximately 40 percent is paid by federal and state government (Sacks et al., 2015). This cost estimate includes health care costs (e.g., hospitalization, ambulatory care, specialty care for alcohol use disorder), lost productivity (e.g., impaired productivity at work, absenteeism), and other costs such as criminal justice corrections and alcohol-related crimes. By comparison, after factoring in federal and state alcohol taxes, the average tax per standard drink is less than $0.20 (Naimi, 2011, 2018).

Preventing medical and social harms to others is generally an important justification for public health interventions, and taxation in particular. Many of the adverse health effects and social harms from alcohol also include secondhand effects. In the case of alcohol-impaired driving, this would include all the effects on those other than the drinking driver, as evidenced by fatality data from comprehensive national and state level data sources (e.g., data from the Fatality Analysis Reporting System [FARS] and state highway safety offices) (NCSA, 2016; Quinlan et al., 2014; Retting, 2017). Other types of alcohol-related secondhand health effects include alcohol-related violence victimization, as demonstrated by high-quality meta-analytic reviews (Foran and O'Leary, 2008; Kuhns et al., 2014), and child abuse and neglect, for which the evidence is not yet conclusive (Widom and Hiller-Sturmhofel, 2001). In the case of tobacco policy, for example, adverse health outcomes from secondhand (e.g., external) smoke harms were an important consideration for adopting indoor smoking bans and other tobacco control policies (WHO and Task Force Initiative, 2007). Because of the effect of higher taxes on a number of other alcohol-related health outcomes, social problems, and economic costs, spillover effects from raising alcohol taxes would result in additional benefits beyond their impact on alcohol-related motor vehicle crash fatalities (e.g., reduced underage drinking, reduced alcohol-related violence).

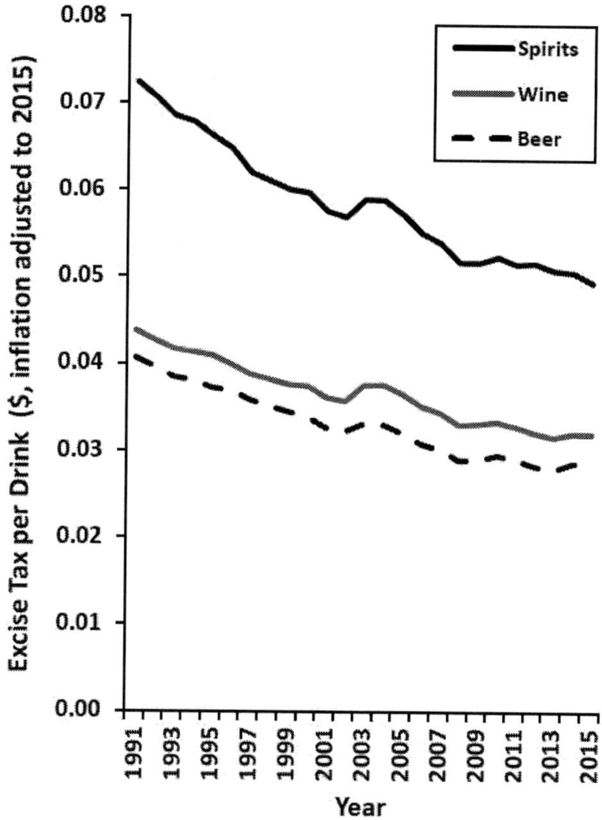

FIGURE 3-2 Average inflation-adjusted specific alcohol excise taxes among U.S. states from 1991 to 2015.
NOTE: The figure includes all 50 U.S. states for beer, and 32 states for distilled spirits and wine (those 32 states without any state monopoly on wholesale distribution or retail sales of either distilled spirits or wine).
SOURCE: Naimi et al., 2018. Reprinted with permission from Alcohol Research Documentation, Inc., publisher of the *Journal of Studies on Alcohol and Drugs*.

There are some concerns, however, about how increasing alcohol taxes will affect some drinkers and some special populations. The same tax per drink is paid by all drinkers, and thus drinkers who impose no harm on others will pay taxes. Yet, this is an inevitable side effect, and those who drink the most will pay the majority of increased alcohol-related costs. Specifically, those drinking in excess of recommended federal drinking guidelines would pay approximately five times as much in additional costs from tax increases compared to nonexcessive drinkers, and as a group heavy drinkers would pay at least 72 percent of aggregate additional costs. Furthermore, the total increase in alcohol-related costs (i.e., product plus tax) for most nonexcessive drinkers would be modest in absolute terms (Naimi et al., 2016).

There may be concern that increasing alcohol taxes could disproportionately burden disadvantaged or vulnerable populations. However, as a group, low-income persons tend to consume less alcohol than those with higher incomes—in part because low-income and minority groups are more likely to abstain from consuming alcohol (Esser et al., 2014). Therefore, additional costs from tax increases are actually higher for whites, for those with higher incomes, and for those who are employed (Naimi et al., 2016). A review that included nine studies assessing the relationship between price or taxes and drinking among young people found that alcohol taxes are also protective for underage drinking (Elder et al., 2010); this is important as underage drinkers constitute another important vulnerable population who are disproportionately likely to cause and incur harms from alcohol consumption.

Alcohol-related trade groups contend that alcohol taxes could adversely affect businesses that produce or sell alcohol (DISCUS, n.d.). However, research suggests that money diverted from alcohol production and consumption to other sectors of the economy could produce gains for those sectors. Additionally, the resulting reduction in excessive drinking could increase productivity. Economic modeling studies of the employment effects of alcohol taxes found that alcohol tax increases would actually lead to net increases in jobs at the state level, because of the transfer of jobs and spending from alcohol-related sectors to other, more labor-intensive sectors of the economy, such as government services or health care (Wada et al., 2017).

Increasing alcohol taxes raises revenue for whichever level of government imposes the taxes, such as state and federal governments. Raising alcohol taxes is thus a highly cost-effective policy intervention. Despite this, and the clear interest by government in additional revenue sources, taxes have been allowed to decline in inflation-adjusted terms over time. Increasing alcohol taxes is generally met with stiff opposition from alcohol-related trade groups and industries (Babor et al., 2018).

Public opinion polling has been used as a tool to measure support for alcohol taxes (Global Strategy Group, 2005; Gonzales Research & Marketing Strategies, 2009; Raabe, 2006; Richter et al., 2004). Jernigan et al. (2009, p. 13) assert that such "polling has consistently found substantial levels of support for increasing alcohol taxes, particularly if the proceeds or some portion thereof are dedicated to preventing and treating alcohol problems [e.g., increasing access to treatment] or expanding access to health care." Prior evidence suggests that public awareness of the efficacy of tax increases to reduce alcohol-related problems is low. Findings from a 1996 national survey showed that almost 80 percent of respondents did not believe alcohol tax increases would decrease injuries. Despite this, the respondents accurately assessed the role of alcohol in fatal falls, drowning, and poisoning, and overestimated its role in motor vehicle fatalities (Girasek et al., 2002). Interviews with policy makers in three states—Illinois, Maryland, and Massachusetts—that recently increased state alcohol taxes confirmed this finding: policy makers were both unaware and skeptical of the ability of alcohol tax increases to influence alcohol consumption or problems (Ramirez and Jernigan, 2017).

Increasing alcohol taxes is a highly effective strategy for reducing binge drinking and alcohol-related motor vehicle crash fatalities. In this section, the committee reviews a body of evidence including high-quality systematic reviews (e.g., Community Preventive Services Task Force[2] review by Elder et al., 2010) and meta-analyses (e.g., Wagenaar et al., 2009, 2010) that shows a consistent inverse relationship between alcohol taxes and alcohol consumption and binge drinking (see Chapter 2 for a discussion of the proximal relationship between binge drinking and alcohol-impaired driving), as well as motor vehicle crash fatalities. In addition to the empirical evidence that indicates the efficacy of increased prices and taxes for reducing binge drinking and alcohol-related motor vehicle crash fatalities, there are practical considerations that support the need for increased taxes. As discussed in this chapter, the erosion of alcohol taxes over the years, the cost-effectiveness of taxes as a population-based intervention, and the potential for wide reach provide additional rationale for increasing alcohol taxes. In addition, current alcohol excise taxes are very low, represent a small fraction of the price of alcohol, and do not cover alcohol-related costs. Drawing from the empirical evidence and the aforementioned considerations, the committee recommends:

Recommendation 3-1: Federal and state governments should increase alcohol taxes significantly.

By *significantly*, the committee means that alcohol taxes should be increased enough so that they have a meaningful impact on price, thence reducing alcohol-related crash fatalities. Increases should comprise a meaningful percent of the net-of-tax price (e.g., 30 percent or more) of

[2] The Community Preventive Services Task Force was formerly known as the Task Force on Community Preventive Services. Task Force publications prior to 2012 are cited as the latter, and those published after 2012 are cited as the former.

alcohol products, and cover the marginal external (i.e., secondhand) costs incurred by the sale of alcohol.[3]

These taxes can be levied as specific excise taxes (which in the United States are based on a fixed amount per unit volume of alcohol) or as ad valorem excise taxes (based on a percentage of price). Specific excise taxes may be preferred because it is the volume of ethanol that is associated with impaired driving. As a percentage of sale price-based taxes, ad valorem taxes are lower for less expensive alcohol products, which tend to be consumed by target groups, such as heavy drinkers and those who are more price sensitive (e.g., underage persons and young adults). However, volume-based excise taxes erode with inflation and therefore need to be indexed to inflation. Ideally, taxes would be based on ethanol content rather than beverage type. Taxes can be earmarked to support alcohol-related activities (e.g., funding sobriety checkpoints), which may enhance public support.

The Three-Tier System of Alcohol Distribution and Wholesale Pricing Policies

Since the end of Prohibition in 1933 most states have used a three-tier system to regulate the distribution of alcohol (Durkin, 2006). The first tier consists of producers and alcohol importers (NABCA, 2015; South Carolina Legislature, 2007). They sell directly to licensed wholesalers (tier two) who then sell to retailers who are licensed to sell alcohol to the public (tier three) (Durkin, 2006; South Carolina Legislature, 2007). Table 3-1 shows the distribution of the three tiers. The system was set up primarily to prevent organized crime from controlling alcohol sales as they did during Prohibition (Martin, 2001). In addition, the system was established to prevent alcohol producers from dominating community life, as they did during the period when saloons were the primary community institution and producers controlled the saloons (Aaron and Musto, 1981). To that end, each tier is regulated individually by the state, and no individual or company can invest in more than one tier (Martin, 2001). The system also helps to ensure orderly markets, prohibit the sales of alcohol to minors, and facilitate the collection of taxes (Martin, 2001).

---

[3] At the time this report was being finalized in December 2017, Congress passed a tax bill (Tax Cuts and Jobs Act of 2017, H.R.1, 115th Cong., 1st sess.) that would decrease federal alcohol excise taxes by about 16 percent. A recent analysis by the Urban-Brookings Tax Policy Center estimated the number of motor vehicle fatalities attributable to the reduction in alcohol taxes proposed by this legislation based on four empirical studies (Looney, 2017). The author concluded that the legislation would cause between 280 to 660 additional motor vehicle deaths and 1,550 total alcohol-related deaths from all causes per year.

TABLE 3-1 The Three-Tier System of Alcohol Distribution

Tier	Actors	Role
1. Producers	Wineries, breweries, distillers, and importers	Produce and sell alcoholic products to wholesalers
2. Wholesalers	Wine, beer, and distilled spirits distributors	Distribute alcohol to retailers
3. Retailers	On-premise (e.g., bars) and off-premise (e.g., package stores) retailers	Sell alcohol to the public

SOURCE: Information from NABCA, 2015.

A report from the National Alcohol Beverage Control Association discusses the economic, regulatory, commercial, and public health benefits of the three-tier system and cautions against the deregulation of the system (NABCA, 2015). Of note, one benefit is that the three-tier system maintains higher prices of alcohol products. In addition, the report cites industry actors, from manufacturers to wholesalers and distributors, who have expressed support for the three-tier system. Findings from a 2015 survey conducted by the Center for Alcohol Policy show that the majority of the public (89 percent) agrees that it is very important to keep the alcohol industry regulated. The key findings from the survey also indicate that the public supports the current system of alcohol regulation at the state level (CAP, 2015). However, recent changes in the alcohol market, such as the rise of Web-based commerce and other outlets, pose challenges to maintaining the current three-tier system (Schmidt, 2017).

The wholesalers within tier two are subject to pricing restrictions that are intended to maintain higher prices, reduce competition, corruption, and crime (APIS, 2016b). These laws can regulate wholesalers' ability to provide discounts based on the quantity of alcohol purchased, require them to establish a minimum markup or maximum discount for all products, require them to post their prices publicly and hold these prices for a set amount of time (i.e., post-and-hold laws), or restrict their ability to extend credit to retailers in the form of loans or deferred invoices (APIS, 2016b). These restrictions are implemented differently by state and by type of alcoholic beverage; for example, in Michigan the sale of beer and wine is regulated by the three-tier system and the sale of spirits is regulated by the state, while in Missouri all three types of alcohol are regulated by the tier system but volume discounts and post-and-hold laws only apply to wine and spirits (APIS, 2016b). Those states that did not set up a three-tier system for alcohol distribution after Prohibition chose to operate as monopolies, regulating the distribution and sales of alcohol themselves (for more information see the section "Policies to Address Physical Availability") (Foust, 1999; McGowan, 1997).

Retail Price Restrictions

Happy hours, two-for-one specials, unlimited drinks, and free drinks are examples of alcoholic drink specials that are available over a specified period of time, during which alcohol is sold at a discounted price and/or higher volume at an on-premises location such as a bar or restaurant. The laws restricting these kinds of drink specials vary by state. For example, in Alaska happy hours are prohibited but free beverage specials and unlimited beverages for a fixed price or period are allowed, while in South Carolina happy hours are permitted between 4:00 pm and 8:00 pm and specials that provide multiple servings for a single serving price are allowed (APIS, 2016a). Currently there are 18 states that have no laws placing restrictions on drink specials (APIS, 2016a).

Studies have found that these kinds of drink specials are associated with increased excessive alcohol consumption (Babor et al., 1978, 1980; Thombs et al., 2008, 2009), especially among young drinkers (Baldwin et al., 2014; Kuo et al., 2003; Van Hoof et al., 2008). Research also shows that about half of drinkers who drive impaired are coming from a licensed establishment (e.g., bars, restaurants, or clubs) (Naimi et al., 2009). One study assessed the relationship between banning drink specials and alcohol consumption in Ontario, Canada, but owing to study design limitations the results were inconclusive (Babor, 2010; NHTSA, 2005a; Smart, 1996; Smart and Adlaf, 1986). More research is needed to determine the effects of introducing these policies on alcohol consumption and alcohol-impaired driving specifically. Enforcement and adjudication of these laws are time-consuming, as they require observation, surveillance, and undercover operations, and tend to be a low priority for enforcement officials (NHTSA, 2005a). Collecting place of last drink (POLD) data from alcohol-impaired driving offenders could help target enforcement at problematic establishments, thereby increasing the effectiveness of policies restricting drink specials (NHTSA, 2005a).

Minimum Alcohol Pricing

Minimum alcohol pricing typically sets a minimum price per standard drink based on ethanol. In the event of a price increase (e.g., alcohol tax increase), drinkers can consume less, purchase cheaper products, or a combination thereof. Substituting lower price for quality can mitigate the effects of policies that increase alcohol prices (Gruenewald et al., 2006). Thus, the premise of minimum pricing is to limit substituting lower priced alcohol for quality and excessive consumption by placing a limit on how low alcohol beverage prices can be. Minimum alcohol pricing has been shown to reduce hazardous alcohol consumption (Gruenewald et al., 2006; Holmes et al., 2014; Purshouse et al., 2010) and related harms (Stockwell et al., 2013; Zhao et al., 2013) in countries such as Canada and the United Kingdom. The available evidence indicates that less expensive products demonstrate higher price sensitivities than higher-priced products and that less expensive products are preferred by hazardous drinkers (Stockwell et al., 2015). Therefore, these policies have an effect on hazardous drinkers, including low-income drinkers (Holmes et al., 2014), and potentially underage persons, as they do not have a great deal of discretionary income and are relatively price sensitive.

POLICIES TO ADDRESS PHYSICAL AVAILABILITY

Regulating Outlet Density

Policies to address the physical availability of alcohol to reduce excessive alcohol consumption and related harms often target outlet density, the number of establishments within a given area where alcohol may be legally sold to be consumed on-premise (e.g., bars, clubs, restaurants) or off-premise (e.g., package stores) (Campbell et al., 2009). There is evidence that increased alcohol outlet density is associated with increased alcohol-related crashes (Scribner et al., 1994; Treno et al., 2007) and self-reported impaired driving (Gruenewald et al., 2002), including among underage persons (Reboussin et al., 2011; Treno et al., 2003). An ecological study conducted in New Mexico found that areas within the highest tertile of distilled spirits outlet density were associated with a 50 percent increase in alcohol-related crash rates and a two-fold increase in alcohol-related crash fatalities when compared with the lowest tertile of outlet density (Escobedo and Ortiz, 2002).[4] While there is a body of literature that documents the positive relationship between outlet density and subsequent drinking and alcohol-impaired driving, there is less research examining reductions in alcohol outlet density.

The Community Preventive Services Task Force found that there is sufficient evidence to recommend the regulation of alcohol outlet density based on the positive association between outlet density and excessive alcohol consumption, as well as related harms (Task Force on Community Preventive Services, 2009). However, it is important to note that the authors concluded that the available studies specifically evaluating the

[4] Distilled spirits outlet density rates were calculated for each county, and counties were divided into three groups: low, middle, and high.

relationship between alcohol outlet density and motor vehicle crashes have produced mixed results (Campbell et al., 2009).

More recently, Ponicki et al. (2013) conducted a spatial panel analysis of all California zip codes from 1999 to 2008, and the results showed that local bar density was positively associated with the likelihood that motor vehicle crashes were alcohol related. Other research points to traffic flow as a moderator of the relationship between outlet density and single-vehicle nighttime crashes; that is, crashes were more likely to occur in areas with higher on-premise outlet density and highway traffic flow (i.e., motor vehicles per day). These findings have implications for local transportation and planning decisions, and the authors suggest that the effects of alcohol outlets on crashes are context dependent (Gruenewald and Johnson, 2010).

There are a number of challenges to regulating alcohol outlet density. Similar to other alcohol policies, commercial and financial consequences can prompt the alcohol industry (manufacturers, distributers, and retailers) to actively oppose policies to limit or reduce outlet density (Campbell et al., 2009; Giesbrecht, 2000). In addition, state preemption laws can limit local governments' ability to regulate outlet density (Mosher, 2001). Despite these barriers, there is evidence that employing tools such as health impact assessments can help drive policy changes to reduce outlet density (Thornton et al., 2013). Another potential challenge with addressing outlet density is the measurement of outlet density in a given state or community. CDC provides guidance on how to measure alcohol outlet density and identifies three main approaches: container-based, distance-based, and spatial access-based (CDC, 2017). Such public health surveillance approaches can identify high-risk areas and provide data to make the case for regulating outlet density in a given area.

Regulating Hours and Days of Sale

Policies that regulate when alcohol can be sold vary by state and retail setting (i.e., on- or off-premise) and can also vary within states that allow local jurisdictions to set their own restrictions (Hahn et al., 2010). On-premise alcohol outlets are allowed to operate for a median of 19 hours per day on weekdays and Saturdays and 17 hours per day on Sundays; nine states have no restrictions on limits of hours of sale (Hahn et al., 2010). All U.S. policies that limit days of off-premise sales target Sundays,[5] but these policies vary from state to state. As of 2016, 12 states

[5] Sunday bans on alcohol sales originate from "blue" laws, some of which date back to pre-Revolution-era policies that prohibited working, shopping, or consuming alcohol on Sundays (APIS, 2016d).

had full bans or minor exceptions (e.g., selling at wineries or on special events); other states have reduced hours, bans on spirits, or no bans at all (APIS, 2016d).

In 2010 the Community Preventive Services Task Force (Task Force) reviewed the evidence on regulating hours and days of sale. Hahn et al. (2010) examined studies assessing the effects of increased hours of sale in on-premise settings on excessive alcohol consumption and related harms. The authors concluded that limiting hours of alcohol sales in on-premises settings was effective in reducing alcohol-related harms (no studies were found on the effects of sales in off-premises settings) (Hahn et al., 2010). The Task Force reviewed studies conducted in high-income countries, but no research was available on how limiting hours of sales would affect alcohol-impaired driving fatalities in the United States specifically. The Task Force also found that an increase in 2 or more hours of sale led to an increase in harm, while there was insufficient evidence to determine the effect of increasing hours of sale by less than 2 hours (Hahn et al., 2010).

The Task Force also synthesized the evidence on maintaining or reducing days of sale. The authors reported that maintaining existing limits on days of sale is effective at preventing alcohol-related harms, and increasing days of sale leads to increased alcohol-related harms and decreasing days of sale leads to decreased alcohol-related harms (Middleton et al., 2010). Another study on days of sale and alcohol-related crash fatalities used a quasi-experimental approach to assess the effect of repealing or scaling back bans on Sunday sales in 14 states (Stehr, 2010). The results demonstrated an effect in New Mexico only, where Sunday sales were associated with a 3.7 percent increase in alcohol-related traffic fatalities. Stehr (2010) posits that this finding is related to a corresponding increase in alcohol consumption in New Mexico (14.1 percent and 8 percent increases in the sale of beer and spirits, respectively—much higher than what was reported in the other states).

A 2017 systematic review of policies regulating hours and days of alcohol sales included studies that assessed the effect on motor vehicle crashes and fatalities from a number of countries including Australia, Canada, the United Kingdom, and the United States (Sanchez-Ramirez and Voaklander, 2017). The authors reported mixed results on the effect of extended hours of sale on motor vehicle crashes and fatalities. This included a study that found that the extension of bar hours in the United Kingdom was associated with a decrease in motor vehicle crashes (Green et al., 2014). The authors of the review conclude that the relationship between these policies and motor vehicle outcomes is complex, and more research is needed in this area.

There are a number of barriers to maintaining or imposing limits on hours and days of sale. This type of regulation could affect alcohol sales, which would beget opposition from the alcohol manufacturing, distribution, and retail industry (DISCUS, 2017; Hahn et al., 2010; Middleton et al., 2010). According to the Community Preventive Services Task Force, state preemption laws could also undermine local efforts to regulate the sale of alcohol (Hahn et al., 2010), which has been a common barrier for local public health prevention efforts (IOM, 2011).

State Monopolization of Alcohol Sales

There are currently 17 states[6] as well as several jurisdictions in Alaska, Maryland, Minnesota, and South Dakota in which government agencies control the sale of beer, wine, and/or spirits (NABCA, 2017). The government monopoly standardizes the price of alcohol throughout a state and the profits are kept by the state (Simon, 1966). Overall, privatization of alcohol sales is associated with an increase in the price of alcohol (Simon, 1966). However, Hahn et al. (2012) theorize that privatized systems may offer a wider array of low-priced products that could appeal to high-volume or high-risk drinkers. A study conducted in Iowa found that after privatization only 37.4 percent of those surveyed who purchased spirits in the past month noticed that sales prices had increased since privatization (Fitzgerald and Mulford, 1993). In its evidence review, the Community Preventive Services Task Force concluded that the privatization of alcohol sales increases per capita alcohol consumption, and by proxy, alcohol-related harm (Hahn et al., 2012). The review also found that remonopolization of alcohol sales is associated with decreased alcohol consumption (Hahn et al., 2012). The median increase in per capita sales of alcohol of the studies reviewed was 44.4 percent (Hahn et al., 2012). Trolldal (2005) evaluated the effects of the privatization of alcohol sales in Alberta, Canada, on fatal motor vehicle crashes and found a nonsignificant decrease. The author speculated that there may not have been a great effect because alcohol wholesales were still monopolized and that private alcohol sales were confined to distilled spirits stores. Another study conducted in Iowa after the privatization of wine and spirit sales also found no significant decrease in motor vehicle crashes (Fitzgerald and Mulford, 1992). The privatization of alcohol sales, however, does result in higher alcohol outlet density, which may account for some of the harmful effects (Hahn et al., 2012).

[6] These states are Alabama, Idaho, Iowa, Maine, Michigan, Mississippi, Montana, New Hampshire, North Carolina, Ohio, Oregon, Pennsylvania, Utah, Vermont, Virginia, West Virginia, and Wyoming.

Alcohol Sales Concurrent with Driving

One important yet understudied feature of the alcohol environment is the sale of alcohol that is concurrent with or very proximal to driving. This includes the concurrent sale of alcohol and gasoline, the sale of consumption-ready single-serving drinks, drive-through package stores, and the sale of alcohol in fast-food establishments. In many cases this also includes the marketing of alcohol, such as beer, with the sale of gasoline. While there is not a substantial evidence base to draw from in this area, it is important to address because the nature of these sales often involve driving shortly after purchase.

There is some limited evidence on the relationship between drive-through package stores and alcohol-related motor vehicle crashes. One study explored alcohol purchase locations among convicted impaired drivers in New Mexico. For offenders who bought the alcohol they drank prior to their arrest, drive-through stores were the preferred outlet of purchase. The authors found a statistically significant relationship between purchase at drive-through package stores and screening as high-risk problem drinkers ($p<0.01$) and drinking in the vehicle prior to arrest ($p<0.01$) (Lewis et al., 1998). Another study conducted in New Mexico examined the spatial relationship between drive-through package store locations and alcohol-related crashes before and after the state banned drive-through alcohol sales using cross-sectional and longitudinal regression analyses. The authors found an increasing trend of alcohol-related crashes relative to total crashes prior to the ban and a decreasing trend after the ban. However, there was no statistically significant relationship between the number of drive-through outlets and the rate of alcohol-related crashes (Lapham et al., 2004).

Some states have implemented restrictions on the sale of alcohol concurrent with or proximal to driving, such as bans on drive-through package stores. These are often presented as common sense measures to reduce alcohol-related harm. More research is needed to determine the effects of the sale of alcohol concurrent with driving on alcohol-impaired driving.

Open Container Laws

Related to alcohol sales concurrent with driving are open container laws, which were designed to reduce alcohol-impaired driving by prohibiting the possession or consumption of open alcoholic beverage containers in a motor vehicle.[7] As part of the 1998 Transportation Equity Act for the

[7] An open container is defined as "any bottle, can, or other receptacle that contains any amount of alcoholic beverage, and that is open or has a broken seal, or the contents of which are partially removed" (APIS, 2016e).

21st Century, Congress stipulated that states enact open container laws that meet six specific criteria or have a portion of their federal highway funds allocated to alcohol-impaired driving countermeasure programs, law enforcement, and/or hazard elimination (APIS, 2016f).[8] These criteria require that state law prohibit possession of alcoholic beverage containers and consumption of alcohol in motor vehicles; cover the entire passenger area; apply to all types of alcoholic beverages; apply to all vehicle occupants; apply to all vehicles on public highways; and provide for primary enforcement of the law. While the parameters of the law vary by state, 40 states and the District of Columbia are in compliance with federal requirements (Advocates for Highway and Auto Safety, 2017). As of 2016, six states had no form of open container law. In addition to the open container laws that have been passed by most states, as of 2013, 39 states currently have laws that allow on-premise establishments to re-seal an opened, but unfinished bottle of wine so that it can be transported in a vehicle without violating the open container law (NCSL, 2013).

There is a limited body of evidence that examines the relationship between open container laws and drinking while driving or alcohol-impaired driving (Goodwin et al., 2015). Stuster et al. (2002) conducted pre- and post-analyses of four states (Iowa, Maine, Rhode Island, and South Dakota) that passed open container laws in 1999. The authors found a decline in alcohol-related crashes among the states that passed the law over the 6-month period following enforcement when compared to the same 6-month period of the prior year. The decline was not statistically significant. However, the findings also showed that states with no open container laws had significantly greater proportions of alcohol-related fatal crashes than states with partially or fully compliant laws. Furthermore, the states that had enacted fully compliant laws had the lowest proportions of alcohol-related crashes among the four states examined. Two other studies have also found a relationship between open container laws and reduced alcohol-related fatalities (Benson et al., 2000; Eisenberg, 2003), while one multivariate regression analysis found no significant effect (Chang et al., 2012). More recent research suggests that while having an open container law is not related to alcohol-impaired driving, enforcement of open container prohibitions is associated with reduced self-reported alcohol-impaired driving (Lenk et al., 2016). Given the limited available evidence and the high number of states that have open container laws, there is an opportunity to further investigate the effects of these laws and their levels of enforcement.

This chapter discusses how the alcohol environment can shape alcohol-related outcomes such as excessive drinking (a precursor to impaired

[8] 23 U.S.C. § 154.

driving) and alcohol-impaired driving. One important feature of this environment is the physical availability of alcohol (e.g., outlet density and hours and days of sale), which can vary by community or state. In this section, the committee presents an overview of the recent literature on outlet density and hours and days of sale from high-quality systematic reviews by the Community Preventive Services Task Force (e.g., Campbell et al., 2009; Hahn et al., 2010; Middleton et al., 2010) and individual studies with a variety of methodologies and outcome data sources (e.g., telephone surveys, hospital discharge data, state forensic data, and state highway and transportation department data) (Escobedo and Ortiz, 2002; Gruenewald et al., 2002; Treno et al., 2003, 2007). Collectively, this body of evidence suggests a strong, positive association between physical availability of excessive alcohol consumption and alcohol-related harms. Although this relationship is more clearly demonstrated by the evidence for other alcohol-related harms, alcohol-impaired driving and crashes are also affected by physical availability and have a strong link to excessive consumption (Flowers et al., 2008). This evidence indicates a need to limit physical availability in areas that have not already done so. It is important to note that more research is needed to determine optimal physical availability policies to reduce alcohol-impaired driving specifically. Furthermore, each state and locality will have different concentrations of physical availability and existing policies, thus requiring a tailored approach based on that area's needs and available policy levers. Therefore, the committee recommends:

Recommendation 3-2: State and local governments should take appropriate steps to limit or reduce alcohol availability, including restrictions on the number of on- and off-premises alcohol outlets, and the days and hours of alcohol sales.

In addition, states should consider restricting or eliminating alcohol sales in locations in which the customer is driving or may drive shortly after purchasing alcohol (i.e., potentially high-risk outlets with respect to drinking and driving), such as at drive-through windows at package stores, gasoline stations, and fast-food restaurants.

POLICIES TO REDUCE ILLEGAL ALCOHOL SALES

Minimum Legal Drinking Age Laws and Enforcement

Federal legislation encouraging a minimum legal drinking age (MLDA) of 21 was passed in 1984, and by 1988 all states and the District of Columbia had enacted a minimum legal age of 21 for the purchase and possession of alcohol (Fell et al., 2008). Most states enforce laws against the sale of alcohol to minors through local law enforcement agencies and alcohol beverage control agencies (Elder et al., 2007). Both types of agencies often lack resources to effectively carry out their enforcement duties. The federal Enforcement of Underage Drinking Laws Program aimed to help alleviate such resource constraints, allocating $25 million in federal block grants to all states and the District of Columbia. Since 2010, funding for this program decreased and eventually dissipated (see Table 7-1 for funding of this and other federal substance abuse prevention programs).

MLDA Laws

There is a robust evidence base that supports the passage and maintenance of MLDA laws based on the effects they have had on decreasing alcohol-related harm in persons under age 21. Based on strong evidence for the effectiveness of MLDA laws of 21 in decreasing alcohol-related vehicle crashes and injuries among 18- to 20-year-olds, the Community Preventive Services Task Force recommended maintaining current MLDA laws (Shults et al., 2001). A systematic review of 49 studies examining the effects of raising and lowering the MLDA indicated 10 to 16 percent decreases in alcohol-related crashes when the MLDA was raised and increases of similar magnitude when it was lowered (Shults et al., 2001). Wagenaar and Toomey (2002) published a review of the effects of MLDA laws based on 79 studies published from 1960 to 2000. Among the studies, 58 percent found an inverse relationship between the age 21 MLDA and traffic crashes; none found an opposite association (Wagenaar and Toomey, 2002). DeJong and Blanchette (2014) conducted a review of the evidence on the age 21 MLDA from 2006 to 2013 and concluded that this research has reinforced the finding that the federal MLDA law has led to a reduction in alcohol-related crashes and consumption among youth, with other positive effects for this population in the long term.

Enforcement of MLDA Laws

While MLDA laws have been found to be effective (HHS, 2016), strict and consistent enforcement is needed to optimize the effect of these laws. Elder et al. (2007) reviewed eight studies analyzing the effects of programs implemented by local law enforcement or alcohol beverage control agencies that aimed to increase compliance checks in community retailers. When enhanced enforcement programs were in place, including high intensity and publicity, successful purchases of alcohol by decoys who lacked identification proving their age decreased by an average of 42 percent (range of 17 to 57 percent decrease). Results of two studies indicated that the effects of enhanced enforcement decreased when enforcement programs were discontinued (Scribner and Cohen, 2001; Wagenaar et al., 2005). One study indicated that enhanced enforcement was correlated with a 20 percent reduction in self-reported alcohol consumption and binge drinking among high school students (Barry, 2004). Publicized enforcement of MLDA and driving while impaired (DWI) laws has also been shown to reduce drinking and driving in a college community as measured by roadside surveys (McCartt et al., 2009).

Enforcement programs, which include age-related compliance checks, are underutilized and require improvements. The National Research Council (NRC) and the Institute of Medicine (IOM) report *Reducing Underage Drinking: A Collective Responsibility* (2004) discusses the need for enhanced enforcement against retailers who sell to minors. The report explores this issue in the context of the success of tobacco control and youth smoking, citing the Synar Amendment[9] as a model to inform underage alcohol sales enforcement. This amendment mandates tobacco sales compliance checks and ties the enactment and enforcement of laws prohibiting the sale of tobacco to minors to state block grant funding for substance abuse prevention. Ultimately, the committee recommended that states bolster compliance check programs using media campaigns and license revocation (NRC and IOM, 2004).

Enforcement programs may be ineffective if perception of a lack of support from the community is high, as law enforcement agencies may not have sufficient incentive to carry out enforcement efforts (Elder et al., 2007). A study of 17,830 students surveyed in the 2007 Oregon Health Teens Survey found that perceived community disapproval of adolescents' alcohol use and adolescents' personal beliefs were positively associated with perceived local law enforcement of MLDA laws (Lipperman-Kreda et al., 2010). Enforcement programs that solely target retailers for reducing sales to minors may result in minors substituting retailers with social providers such as friends, family, and strangers (Elder et al., 2007). Therefore, preventing alcohol sales to minors depends on a series of complementary policies and practices that target prevention of purchase, possession, consumption, and internal possession,[10] such as compliance checks, social host laws, dram shop liability laws, and others. These poli-

---

[9] The Synar Amendment was enacted with the Alcohol, Drug Abuse, and Mental Health Administration Reorganization Act (Public Law 102-321) in 1992 with the goal of reducing youth access to tobacco. The amendment mandates that all states enact and enforce laws that prohibit the sale and distribution of tobacco to individuals under the age of 18. In order for states to receive their Substance Abuse Prevention and Treatment Block Grant, they must comply with the Synar Amendment (SAMHSA, 2017).

[10] A minor-in-possession charge requires "evidence of alcohol in the minor's body, as determined by a blood, breath, or urine test, but does not otherwise require any specific

cies and practices will be discussed as strategies to reduce illegal sales to minors in the following sections.

Dram Shop Liability Laws

Dram shop liability laws permit legal action against commercial establishments serving alcohol to underage persons or already intoxicated persons regardless of age (Scherer et al., 2015). (For the history of dram shop liability and insurance, see Sloan et al.'s [2000] *Drinkers, Drivers, and Bartenders.*) Owners and servers may be held liable when illegal beverage service (i.e., to intoxicated or underage patrons) results in injury, death, or damages from alcohol-related vehicle crashes (Rammohan et al., 2011). Survey data of commercial servers suggest an association between a state's status of dram shop laws (i.e., strictness) and perceived risk of liability (Sloan et al., 2000). Dram shop liability laws, in combination with enhanced enforcement documenting alcohol service violation history, provide important data for connecting injury caused by intoxicated drivers and the drinking establishment at which they were served (Graham et al., 2014).

The Community Preventive Services Task Force recommends the use of dram shop liability laws to prevent and reduce alcohol-related harms (Rammohan et al., 2011; Task Force on Community Preventive Services, 2011). Using methodology from the *Guide to Community Preventive Services*, Rammohan et al. (2011) examined 11 studies and found that dram shop liability laws were correlated with a 6.4 percent average decrease in alcohol-related driving fatalities (values ranged from 3.7 to 11.3 percent). Reductions were also found across all studies for other measured outcomes, including all-cause motor vehicle fatalities, alcohol consumption, alcohol-related violence, and alcohol-related diseases.

Using FARS data, Scherer et al. (2015) found that dram shop liability laws were correlated with a 2.4 percent decrease in the ratio of drinking to nondrinking drivers under age 21 involved in fatal crashes (Scherer et al., 2015). The authors estimated that 64 lives had been saved in the jurisdictions that have the law and that 9 more lives could be saved each year if the six states without the law were to adopt it. The authors also found that strong dram shop liability laws were significantly correlated with lower per capita beer consumption.

In 1983 and 1984, two widely publicized server liability cases took place in Texas. Analysis of single-vehicle nighttime crashes in the state from 1978 through 1988 indicated significant decreases of 6.5 and 5.3

---

evidence of possession or consumption (e.g., through witness observation or an admission on the part of the minor)" (APIS, 2016g).

percent following the 1983 and 1984 case filings, respectively. As the decreases were found to have taken place at the time the lawsuits were filed and not when the courts issued their decisions 3 to 4 years later, increased awareness of server liability laws and concern from retail alcohol establishment owners generated through newspaper publicity are likely to have contributed to the reductions (Holder et al., 1990).

The Community Preventive Services Task Force did not find any studies examining the cost-benefit of dram shop liability laws. However, Rammohan et al. (2011) note that litigation may not be cost-effective or achievable in certain cases, as establishing proof that illegal beverage service took place (and resulted in injury) may be difficult (Martineau et al., 2013). Obtaining legal services may also be especially burdensome for those of low socioeconomic status. Most of the studies examined in the systematic review were conducted prior to widespread enactment of dram shop liability laws in the late 1990s (Rammohan et al., 2011; Task Force on Community Preventive Services, 2011). More research is needed to analyze the effectiveness of these laws, especially as states have enacted shorter statutes of limitation and more stringent requirements for legal evidence.

Social Host Liability

Another complementary policy that is designed to reduce underage and hazardous drinking is social host liability. Social host laws assign criminal or civil liability for providing alcohol to someone under the legal drinking age and/or to an obviously intoxicated adult if damages or injury are caused by that individual (e.g., in a motor vehicle crash) (NHTSA, 2016; Voas and Lacey, 2011). The primary purpose is to hold individuals or noncommercial providers of alcohol liable, whereas dram shop liability applies to licensed establishments. As of 2016, 21 states had general hosting laws, 10 states had social host laws specific to underage parties, and 19 states and the District of Columbia had no social host laws (APIS, 2016h). The purpose of such laws is to deter adults from hosting parties where underage drinking occurs, purchasing alcohol for underage drinkers, providing alcohol for underage persons, and overserving alcohol (Voas and Lacey, 2011). The majority of adolescents obtain alcohol from social sources (Pemberton et al., 2008); thus, they are an important point of intervention to reduce underage drinking and subsequent impaired driving. Additionally, there has been public support for assigning liability to social hosts for alcohol-related injuries (Wagenaar et al., 2001).

Social host liability laws differ from state to state, and implementation is an important factor that requires investigation. Findings from California suggest that social host laws with strict liability and swift, administrative civil penalties could reduce underage drinking in private settings, especially among youth who have already initiated alcohol use (Paschall et al., 2014). While social host laws may send a powerful message, effective dissemination of that message is required for effectiveness (Grube and Stewart, 2004; Holder and Treno, 1997; Voas and Lacey, 2011). In the 2004 NRC and IOM report on underage drinking, the authors posit that the mixed findings on social host laws could be attributable to the lack of a comprehensive program that ensures that the public is aware of potential liability exposure. To that end, the report discusses media campaigns as an integral component of implementing social host liability laws.

Over the past few decades, there has not been a substantial amount of evidence on social host laws and alcohol-impaired driving, and the existing evidence is conflicting (Goodwin et al., 2015; NRC and IOM, 2004; Voas and Lacey, 2011). Early study findings using data from the Behavioral Risk Factor Surveillance System showed that social host laws had a deterrent effect with respect to binge drinking and drinking and driving (Sloan et al., 2000; Stout et al., 2000). More recently, Fell et al. (2014) examined the effects of social host laws on the ratio of drinking drivers under age 21 to nondrinking drivers under age 21 involved in fatal crashes from 1982 to 2010. Social host civil liability laws (allow suing social hosts for injuries caused by underage drinking guests) had a negative but nonsignificant ($p = 0.054$) effect, and social host prohibitions (prohibit hosting underage drinking parties) had no effect on the ratio of drinking to nondrinking drivers under age 21 in a fatal crash. Dills (2010) investigated the effect of the presence of a social host liability law on self-reported driving after drinking and alcohol-impaired driving fatalities at the state level from 1975 to 2005 among 18- to 20-year-olds. The author found significant reductions of 5 to 9 percent and 3 percent in alcohol-related traffic fatalities and driving after drinking, respectively (Dills, 2010). Given the insufficient body of research around social host laws and alcohol-impaired driving, more research is needed in this area (Hingson and White, 2014; Wagoner et al., 2013).

Responsible Beverage Service and Server Training

Responsible beverage service (RBS) has been studied as a potential point of intervention to reduce excessive drinking and subsequent alcohol-impaired driving (Fell et al., 2017; Graham, 2000; Linde et al., 2016; Rammohan et al., 2011; Saltz, 1987; Scherer et al., 2015; Shults et al., 2001). Research indicates that approximately half of drivers arrested for alcohol-impaired driving had their last drink at a licensed establishment (Fell et al., 2010; Gallup, 2000; O'Donnell, 1985), and this is consistent with self-reported data on driving after binge drinking (Naimi et al., 2009).

The training for servers typically focuses on serving procedures, signs of intoxication, methods for verifying age, and intervention strategies. There are also aspects of manager training that incorporate the abovementioned, in addition to policy and procedure development and staff supervision (APIS, 2016e). Public acceptance has been relatively high for RBS policies, with a national survey indicating that 89 percent of the population was in favor of policies mandating server training (Wagenaar et al., 2000).

Programs for server training can be mandatory, voluntary, or a combination of both. States with voluntary beverage service training programs typically provide incentives for retailers (e.g., defense in dram shop liability lawsuits, discounts for dram shop liability insurance, or mitigation of fines or other penalties for service violations). It is important to note that incentives such as protection from dram shop liability can have unintended consequences. These protections can hinder the effectiveness of dram shop laws, which have been shown to be effective in reducing alcohol-related harm (Rammohan et al., 2011), as discussed previously. As of 2016, 12 states and the District of Columbia had mandatory service training laws, 20 had voluntary laws, 6 had a combination of mandatory and voluntary policies, and 12 had neither (APIS, 2016e). In the past, there have been federal incentive grants for states that engage in specific server training activities,[11] such as training point-of-sale personnel to recognize signs of intoxication, but those have since been rescinded.

In *Countermeasures That Work*, Goodwin et al. (2015) review the evidence on RBS and conclude that the findings on the effectiveness of server training have been mixed. They note that few studies have examined the effect of RBS on alcohol-impaired driving crashes specifically. The Community Preventive Services Task Force conducted a review of interventions to reduce alcohol-impaired driving, including training programs for servers of alcoholic beverages. Shults et al. (2001) concluded that, based on the rules of evidence presented in *The Community Guide*, there was sufficient evidence that intensive, high-quality, face-to-face server training (when supplemented with active management support) is effective in reducing the level of intoxication among patrons (and is therefore likely to have an effect on impaired driving if the affected patrons cease drinking or continue elsewhere in a safe environment after leaving). Shults et al. (2001) also noted that optimally, server training would be established in all licensed establishments in a community to have a community-wide effect. However, research on such community-wide alcohol server interventions is limited (Shults et al., 2001). A recent study of demonstration projects that incorporated RBS and enhanced alcohol enforcement for

[11] 23 U.S.C. § 410, https://www.gpo.gov/fdsys/pkg/USCODE-2006-title23/pdf/USCODE-2006-title23-chap4-sec410.pdf (accessed October 2, 2017).

problem bars in two communities also produced mixed findings (Fell et al., 2017). Jones et al. (2011) completed a systematic review of multiple countries (including the United States) and found that server intervention programs designed to reduce alcohol use in drinking environments had mixed effects on patrons' alcohol consumption. The observed effects on patron drinking were minimal, except where training was mandated (Jones et al., 2011). In summary, more research is needed to determine the critical elements that contribute to the effectiveness of RBS policies and training.

Sales to Intoxicated Persons

Sales to intoxicated persons (SIP) laws make it illegal to sell alcohol to an obviously intoxicated person. These laws, which can be criminal or administrative, exist in every state except Florida and Nevada. In Wyoming, it is only illegal to sell alcohol to an intoxicated person at a drive-through window at a package store. There is substantial variation in state SIP laws with respect to the state's definition of intoxication, who is held liable (e.g., licensees, servers, or social hosts), the evidence required to establish a SIP violation, and subsequent penalties (Mosher et al., 2009). SIP laws are an example of another alcohol-related policy for which the overall effectiveness likely depends on the quality and consistency of enforcement practices.

Alcohol Law Enforcement

As discussed previously, enforcement is a crucial determinant of adherence to the policies to reduce illegal alcohol sales. Alcohol law enforcement aims to increase compliance with laws by increasing perceived likelihood of arrest among those who are subject to legal restrictions (NHTSA, 2005b). Enforcement approaches can include compliance checks for underage sales, bar inspections, undercover operations, and educational programs (Ramirez, 2017). There is research that suggests the enforcement of policies to limit alcohol service to underage persons and intoxicated patrons reduces alcohol-related harm and improves public safety (McKnight and Streff, 1994; Ramirez, 2017; Ramirez et al., 2008).

Lenk et al. (2014) conducted a survey of randomly selected local and state alcohol enforcement agencies to gather information on enforcement of sales to obviously intoxicated patrons. The findings, which reflected responses from 1,082 local and 49 state agencies, showed that only about 20 percent of local and 60 percent of state agencies conducted enforcement activities to reduce SIP in their jurisdictions. Furthermore, less than half of the agencies employed specific enforcement strategies at least monthly, and for local agencies, enforcement activities were more common when there was a full-time officer who was specifically assigned to such activities.

For alcohol law enforcement agencies, the number of licensed establishments that require monitoring and enforcement varies from state to state. In most states (e.g., Alabama, Utah, Virginia), there are 250 licensees or less per one alcohol law enforcement agent, but in some states (e.g., Missouri, Wisconsin) there are more than 1,000 premises per agent (Ramirez, 2017). Levy and Miller (1995) conducted a cost-benefit analysis of increased enforcement of laws forbidding service to intoxicated patrons, based on a case study in Michigan, and found that the benefits greatly outweighed the costs. Their study findings also demonstrated a 22 percent increase in the number of intoxicated patrons who were refused service after implementing a program that used undercover police officers to monitor service in licensed establishments.

The 2017 County Health Rankings included a review of the evidence on SIP law enforcement. The key finding was that the available evidence indicates that efforts to enforce SIP laws can reduce overservice and alcohol-impaired driving, especially when implemented in areas at risk for excessive alcohol consumption (County Health Rankings, 2017). Another key element of enforcement is the administration of sanctions or legal charges for evidenced violations. States have a number of penalties for violations including fines, license suspensions, and revocations (Mosher et al., 2009), yet these penalties are often reduced or appealed.

Challenges for Enforcement

While promising, enforcement of policies to reduce illegal alcohol sales is largely lacking (Goodwin et al., 2015; Mosher et al., 2009) because of a number of the following factors: cultural norms, lack of political will, lack of a systematic approach to enforcement (Graham et al., 2014; Mosher et al., 2009; NHTSA, 2005a,b; Ramirez, 2017), and lack of resources to detect and track violations (Mosher et al., 2002, 2009; NHTSA, 2005b). For example, in some states, the number of licensed establishments outnumbers the amount of available law enforcement personnel (Ramirez, 2017). Alcohol law enforcement agents have many responsibilities in addition to enforcing alcohol laws (e.g., gaming, tobacco, drugs, and human trafficking) (Ramirez, 2017).

Promising Strategies

Despite the barriers that exist for effective enforcement of alcohol policies, there are promising strategies that have emerged from common practices and the literature that can be applied to enhance enforcement efforts. For example, some states collect data on POLD when an individual is arrested for DWI and then target those establishments (NHTSA, 2005a). In 2012 the National Transportation Safety Board made a safety recommendation to the 50 states, the District of Columbia, and Puerto Rico to require law enforcement agencies to collect POLD data as part of any arrest or crash investigation involving an alcohol-impaired driver (NTSB, 2012) (see Chapter 6 for more discussion of POLD data). In addition to data collection, it is important to publicize enforcement efforts to ensure that there is a high perceived risk of being apprehended and receiving a sanction. Furthermore, developing political will to support ongoing enforcement through research and media fosters sustainability of efforts. Mosher et al. (2009) emphasize the importance of interagency collaboration and adopting a structure of enforceable consequences for violations and adequate penalties that cannot be negotiated or made eligible for exemption for specific licensees (e.g., licensees who have completed RBS training).

As discussed in this chapter, the illegal sale of alcohol subsumes sales to already-intoxicated adults and to underage persons. The available research indicates that both types of illegal sales are related to binge drinking and to increased risk of alcohol-impaired driving. The committee discusses a number of interventions that can reduce illegal sales, binge drinking, and alcohol-impaired driving with varying degrees of evidence. Among some of these policies, the evidence of effectiveness is strong (i.e., informed by high-quality systematic reviews and studies across multiple contexts). This includes MLDA laws (see, for example, DeJong and Blanchette, 2014; Shults et al., 2001; Wagenaar and Toomey, 2002), enforcement of MLDA laws (see, for example, Barry, 2004; Elder et al., 2007; Scribner and Cohen, 2001; Wagenaar et al., 2005), and dram shop liability laws (see, for example, Holder et al., 1990; Rammohan et al., 2011; Scherer et al., 2015). For other illegal sales-related policies, there is a good theoretical justification but mixed evidence of effectiveness depending on the type of policy and degree of enforcement. These include social host liability laws (see, for example, Fell et al., 2014; Paschall et al., 2014; Wagoner et al., 2013) and responsible beverage service practices and policies (see, for example, Fell et al., 2017; Jones et al., 2011; Shults et al., 2001). For laws preventing SIP, there is a strong theoretical basis for their implementation, yet a relative lack of empirical evidence on these policies, in part because most states have them, which limits opportunities for well-designed evaluations.

Research also indicates that enforcement programs are underutilized and require more resources to be effective. To reach the below conclusion the committee relied on evidence ranging from empirical studies evaluating enforcement programs and systematic reviews of studies to legal, administrative, and qualitative data. These include, but are not limited to, the NRC and IOM (2004) report *Reducing Underage Drinking: A Collective Responsibility*, a Community Preventive Services Task Force review of enhanced enforcement laws prohibiting sales to minors (Elder et al., 2007), a NHTSA (2005b) research report that uses legal and interview data to inform its findings on the role of alcohol beverage control agencies in enforcing alcohol laws, and data from the National Liquor Law Enforcement Association (Ramirez, 2017; Ramirez et al., 2008). The decline in federal funding for the enforcement of underage drinking programs further demonstrates the diminishing resources allocated to such programs (see Table 7-1). It is also noteworthy that the evidence from empirical studies and qualitative data show that quality of implementation and complementary activities (e.g., media publicity and collection of POLD data) to enhance enforcement are important (Elder et al., 2007; McCartt et al., 2009; NRC and IOM, 2004; NTSB, 2012). Furthermore, to reduce excessive alcohol consumption prior to driving at the population level, there is a need for a comprehensive set of policies that minimize the illegal sale of alcohol to underage persons and already-intoxicated persons. Given the evidence presented in this chapter on the effectiveness of policies to reduce illegal alcohol sales and the need for enhanced enforcement of these policies, the committee offers the following recommendation and conclusion:

> **Recommendation 3-3: Federal, state, and local governments should adopt and/or strengthen laws and dedicate enforcement resources to stop illegal alcohol sales (i.e., sales to already-intoxicated adults and sales to underage persons).**
>
> *Conclusion 3-1: Some policies to reduce illegal alcohol sales are not effective due to a lack of enforcement activities. In addition, a systematic approach to enforcement (i.e., increased resources, data collection and sharing, multisector collaboration, and publicity) is needed to optimize the effects of such alcohol policies.*
>
> Recommendation 3-3 includes the following laws and actions:
>
> - Strong penalties for licensees who engage in illegal alcohol sales to already-intoxicated adults;
> - Dram shop liability laws without caps;
> - High-quality mandatory responsible beverage service training for managers and sellers;

- Strong social host laws and other laws to limit adults from providing alcohol to underage persons;
- Improvement of enforcement of MLDA laws, including passing laws to permit compliance checks using underage decoys and conducting such compliance checks;
- Collection of POLD data; and
- Adequate enforcement personnel to enforce existing laws in this area.

POLICIES TO REDUCE THE HARMFUL EFFECTS OF ALCOHOL MARKETING

At least 25 longitudinal studies have found associations between young people's exposure to alcohol marketing in a variety of forms—from traditional marketing to online marketing to sponsorships and alcohol-branded merchandise—and their subsequent drinking behavior (Anderson et al., 2009b; Jernigan et al., 2016; Smith and Foxcroft, 2009). Another study, completed before the dramatic increase in alcohol advertising on cable television, looked at the effect of alcohol advertising on motor vehicle traffic fatalities and concluded that a complete ban on broadcast alcohol advertising could save between 2,000 and 3,000 lives per year, and ending the tax deductibility of alcohol advertising could prevent approximately 1,300 deaths per year (Saffer, 1997).

One of the distinguishing features of alcohol advertising since 2000 has been the dramatic expansion of advertising, especially for distilled spirits, on cable television. Distillers maintained a voluntary ban on television advertising in general until 1996, and in 2001 struck an agreement with NBC to begin advertising on that broadcast network (Elliott, 2001). However, outcry from Congress and from public health advocates led NBC to back away from the agreement, and distillers in response moved rapidly onto cable networks (Jernigan and O'Hara, 2004). In 2000, distillers spent $4.3 million, or 1.2 percent of their measured advertising budgets, on television; by 2016, this amount had grown to $227.6 million, or 56.8 percent of their budgets (Impact Databank, 2017).

Marketing does not only consist of advertising, but rather rests on the "four Ps" of product, place, price, and promotion (Hastings et al., 2005). (See Chapter 2 for discussions of industry activities within the four Ps.) Other sections of this report have discussed policy options to address the first three Ps. Since commercial speech enjoys strong protection from the First Amendment in the United Sates, alcohol marketing has been primarily governed by industry self-regulation. Findings from a systematic review show that numerous peer-reviewed studies have found this self-regulation to be ineffective (Noel et al., 2016), and there have been significant debates in the United States about how it could be improved. In 2004, the NRC and IOM recommended that the industry move from its then-current voluntary standard of only advertising where at least 70 percent of the viewing, reading, or listening audience was of legal purchase age (that is, over age 21) to a 25 percent maximum for underage audiences immediately, and eventually to a 15 percent maximum for underage audiences. This was based roughly on the proportion of the underage population at greatest risk of initiating drinking—the 12- to 20-year-old group (NRC and IOM, 2004). In 2011, 24 state and territorial attorneys general added their endorsements to the 15 percent standard (Shurtleff et al., 2011). In that same year, alcohol industry trade associations announced a lowering of their standard to 28.4 percent, based on the 2010 census numbers. In 2007, one company—Beam Global Spirits—adopted the 25 percent maximum; an independent evaluation of that standard concluded that, even with imperfect implementation, it led to a reduction in youth exposure to alcohol advertising for that company's brands compared to its competitors, and at the same time it did not result in an increase in the company's advertising costs for reaching adult audiences (Ross et al., 2016). The authors concluded that other alcohol companies should consider adopting a similar standard to the 25 percent maximum.

However, the lack of voluntary movement toward a stricter standard by most alcohol companies has resulted in continued disproportionate youth exposure to alcohol advertising. One study examined magazine advertising of alcohol brands most likely to be consumed by young people (determined through a national survey of youth alcohol consumption by brand [Siegel et al., 2013]), and found that such brands were more likely than other brands to advertise in magazines with higher youth readerships, demonstrating the inadequacy of the industry's voluntary guidelines in protecting youth from disproportionate exposure compared to adults (King et al., 2017).

The industry's voluntary guidelines also include numerous provisions regarding the content of alcohol advertising. However, independent evaluation of the implementation of these guidelines has found them to be ineffective (Babor et al., 2013). Enforcement of content regulations is also more likely to raise First Amendment issues, which helps to explain why much of the policy debate regarding alcohol industry self-regulation has focused on placement guidelines.

While much of the regulatory authority over alcohol advertising lies at the federal level, and specifically in the U.S. Department of the Treasury, an agency without an explicit public health or safety mission, state and local governments have also demonstrated that they can play a role in reducing both youth and population-level exposure to alcohol advertising. The Center on Alcohol Marketing and Youth's (2012) report *State*

Laws to Reduce the Impact of Alcohol Marketing on Youth: Current Status and Model Policies identifies the following specific actions that states can take:

- Prohibit false and misleading alcohol advertising;
- Prohibit advertising that targets minors;
- Claim state jurisdiction over electronic media, at least theoretically permitting them to require, for instance, higher audience standards for advertising placed in media such as radio that originate locally;
- Restrict outdoor alcohol advertising in locations where children are likely to be present;
- Prohibit outdoor alcohol advertising near schools, public playgrounds, and churches;
- Restrict alcohol advertising on alcohol retail outlet windows and outside areas;
- Prohibit alcohol advertising on college campuses; and
- Restrict alcohol industry sponsorship of civic events (e.g., fairs, music concerts, and sporting events).

While no state has employed all of these powers, the fact that they all exist in state law in at least one and often numerous states suggests that there is more potential at the state and local levels for reducing exposure to alcohol advertising than has yet been used.

Another promising strategy regarding alcohol marketing is the use of countermarketing. Countermarketing campaigns are a form of media campaigns that seek to offset pro-alcohol influences and promote health promotion messages (CDC, 2003). They often emphasize the harmful and/or deceptive strategies companies use to market a product that can be harmful for particular audiences (e.g., youth) in an effort to neutralize these influences and promote healthier behavior. While there is very little experience and no studies of effectiveness regarding this for alcohol use, it has been an effective strategy for reducing tobacco use (Apollonio and Malone, 2009). Several well-funded, high-profile tobacco countermarketing media campaigns in California, Florida, and nationally (e.g., the truth campaign) have contributed to reduced rates of youth smoking and adult cigarette consumption in these areas (Farrelly et al., 2002; Hu et al., 1995; Sly et al., 2002). (For more on media campaigns, see the following section, "Education and Awareness.")

One important consideration in assessing the impact of alcohol marketing and developing interventions to reduce the harmful effects of such marketing is the changing media landscape, particularly for youth. Traditional means of watching television (e.g., cable or satellite television) are being replaced with online streaming services. Of note, Pew Research

Center's survey data from 2017 show that 61 percent of adults ages 18–29 use streaming services as their primary means of watching television (Raine, 2017). Such changes in television consumption could potentially have implications for the frequency, duration, and intensity for which youth are exposed to alcohol marketing. Therefore, updated research is needed on the effects of such changes in media consumption on exposure to alcohol marketing among youth.

In this section, the committee has presented an overview of the empirical and historical evidence around alcohol marketing exposure and regulation. To examine the link between alcohol marketing and consumption among underage persons, the committee drew from peer-reviewed systematic reviews of longitudinal studies on youth exposure to alcohol marketing and drinking outcomes (Anderson et al., 2009b; Jernigan et al., 2016; Smith and Foxcroft, 2009). While there is only one study cited that examines and demonstrates a positive relationship between alcohol advertising and motor vehicle crash fatalities (Saffer, 1997), there is a strong theoretical basis for this association, particularly for youth. Given that young people (ages 21–24) are at high risk of alcohol-impaired driving (Lipari et al., 2016; NCSA, 2016) and the available research strongly indicates that they are influenced by alcohol marketing, as evidenced by the systematic reviews cited above, the committee has identified alcohol marketing as an important point of intervention to reduce alcohol consumption, and by extension, alcohol-impaired driving among underage persons. Furthermore, numerous studies have found the alcohol industry's self-regulation of its marketing to be ineffective and insufficient because the voluntary standards are permissive and vague, not consistently followed, and without penalties for violations (Babor et al., 2013; King et al., 2017; Noel and Babor, 2016; Noel et al., 2016; Siegel et al., 2013). Therefore, the committee recommends:

Recommendation 3-4: Federal, state, and local governments should use their existing regulatory powers to strengthen and implement standards for permissible alcohol marketing content and placement across all media, establish consequences for violations, and promote and fund countermarketing campaigns.

EDUCATION AND AWARENESS

School-Based Education Programs

School-based alcohol education programs aim to prevent or delay youth drinking as well as prevent related risky activities such as drinking and driving and/or riding with drinking drivers. Although educational programs are popular with policy makers, the public, and alcohol-related economic operators, in general school-based educational programs have limited evidence of producing change, particularly at the population level. The available evidence is inconsistent or shows no effect on behavior change related to alcohol alone or in combination with driving (Elder et al., 2005; Foxcroft and Tsertsvadze, 2012; NRC and IOM, 2004; Mann et al., 1986; Shope et al., 2001). However, more research is needed as many education programs have not been evaluated (Anderson et al., 2009a; Goodwin et al., 2015; Lee et al., 2016; Mann et al., 1986; NRC and IOM, 2004; Stigler et al., 2011; Washington Traffic Safety Commission, 2014). In addition, education programs can be costly since they are delivered to relatively small groups of individuals, and their effects degrade quickly unless actively maintained. Anderson et al. (2009a) concluded in *The Lancet* that while school-based programs are not effective in modifying behavior, they can play an important role in increasing visibility of alcohol on public agendas. Other intermediate outcomes of programs include the promotion of social and emotional competencies and resilience among youth participants (Stigler et al., 2011).

There are a number of limitations with school-based programs and the current literature that examines them. Programs have been criticized for having weak evaluation designs and short follow-up times while only measuring intermediate outcomes such as alcohol knowledge, attitudes, and intent (Mann et al., 1986; Washington Traffic Safety Commission, 2014). There is a documented need for additional robust studies with alcohol-impaired driving outcome measures such as DWIs and alcohol-related crashes; for example, examining driving behaviors of students after an education program and measuring more specific traffic safety outcomes (Elder et al., 2005; Mann et al., 1986; Shope et al., 2001; Washington Traffic Safety Commission, 2014). Some of the alcohol education programs studied have been successful in increasing youth knowledge about alcohol and alcohol misuse, as well as influencing attitudes and intent toward alcohol, but these positive effects usually dissipate after 6 months to 1 year. Therefore, intensity, duration, and quality of the program are key elements that require further investigation.

Despite the limitations and inconsistent evidence on school-based programs, there are some positive spillover effects. For example, school-based programs can engage groups such as Students Against Destructive Decisions (SADD) and parent–teacher associations to raise awareness about alcohol-impaired driving. Elder et al. (2005) cite a number of positive effects of participation in peer organizations such as SADD, including personal growth, social support, and a sense of citizenship in the school community. At the school level, such effects include stronger attitudes against alcohol-impaired driving and riding with an impaired driver, increased knowledge of alternatives, and increased access to alcohol-free events (Elder et al., 2005).

Alcohol Warning Labels

Legislation requiring alcohol warning labels was enacted in 1989, which stated that all alcoholic beverage containers sold in the United States must display the following warning label.

> GOVERNMENT WARNING: (1) According to the Surgeon General, women should not drink alcoholic beverages during pregnancy because of the risk of birth defects. (2) Consumption of alcohol impairs your ability to drive a car or operate machinery, and may cause health problems.[12]

As of 2012, the United States is 1 of 31 countries that require warning labels on alcoholic beverages (WHO, 2014). The scientific evidence on whether warning labels are effective in decreasing excessive drinking is inconclusive. A cross-sectional survey occurring 6 months after implementation of the alcohol warning labels in the United States found that 16 percent of respondents remembered the message about the risks of driving impaired, and about 25 percent of the respondents who reported being heavy drinkers and who had driven under the influence of alcohol in the past had seen the label (Greenfield and Kaskutas, 1993). However, it is important to note that such cross-sectional data do not lend themselves to causal inferences. Another study also found that those who reported driving under the influence of alcohol in the past were more likely to remember the warning label than those who had not (Parker et al., 1994). Other studies found alcohol warning labels to be ineffective in changing behavior and encouraged different approaches (Creyer et al., 2002; Stockley, 2001). For example, the use of color, icons, increasing clarity, contrast, shape and/or size of the message, simplicity, and specificity of the message are all factors that can contribute to consumer awareness.

Research also suggests that providing standard drink labels on alcoholic beverage containers increases the drinker's accuracy in assessing alcohol content (Stockwell, 1993; Stockwell et al., 1991). Some argue that this would help responsible drinkers moderate their consumption (Kerr and Stockwell, 2012). Others argue against standard drink labels, citing an Australian study that found that young drinkers use standard drink labels in order to select stronger drinks (Jones and Gregory, 2009). Other cues beyond labels, however, can be used to assess alcohol content such as IPA, imperial, or double. Standard drink labels therefore might not provide new information to consumers.

---

[12] 27 CFR § 16.21 subpart C sec 16.21(1).

In the United States, beer and distilled spirits advertisements are self-regulated by the alcohol industries and do not require that a warning be included in ads (Beer Institute, 2015; DISCUS, 2011). Often, however, consumers are told to "drink responsibly" or "drink in moderation" in these ads. An analysis of advertisements appearing in magazines found that 87 percent of them included a responsibility message but that these messages did not define *responsibility* and were often used to promote the product rather than convey information (Smith et al., 2014). Not only is the information provided in the responsibility messages vague, but an eye-tracking study found that the responsibility messages in print advertising did not capture the attention of teenage viewers (Thomsen and Fulton, 2007). These findings suggest that ambiguous responsibility messages are ineffective in capturing the attention of consumers, providing helpful public health information, or encouraging drinkers to be responsible and/or moderate in their alcohol consumption. Guidelines for the size, content, and placement of alcohol warning labels are needed in order to increase effectiveness.

Media Campaigns

There is strong evidence, based on findings from a variety of high-quality systematic reviews across numerous health behavior domains, that mass media campaigns can promote meaningful changes in health behavior at the population level when implemented alongside broader, community-level interventions (Hornik, 2002; Wakefield et al., 2010). This work further identifies a variety of factors that increase or decrease the likelihood of success in changing behavior at the population level. Effective campaigns are typically characterized by the following:

- High levels of exposure among the target audience over an extended period of time;
- Implementation alongside other complementary interventions (e.g., tax increases or enforcement of legal sanctions against an unhealthy and illegal behavior);
- Widespread availability and access to relevant products and services (e.g., smoking cessation aids, condoms for safer sex); and
- Use of formative research and behavior change theory to guide their design (Hornik, 2002; Noar, 2006; Randolph and Viswanath, 2004; Snyder et al., 2004; Wakefield et al., 2010).

The strongest evidence in support of mass media campaign effectiveness in changing behavior stems from evaluations of well-funded mass media campaigns to reduce tobacco use (Wakefield et al., 2010). Work in this area further suggests that behavior change campaigns can have complementary effects on creating a public opinion and a policy climate that supports the passage of stronger tobacco control policies (Niederdeppe et al., 2007, 2017b).

Evidence of Media Campaign Effectiveness in Reducing Alcohol-Related Fatal Crashes

Several systematic and meta-analytic reviews have attempted to assess the causal effect of media campaigns to reduce alcohol-impaired driving and its consequences, both with and without accompanying interventions. Efforts to reduce alcohol-related traffic fatalities in the United States face a variety of challenges to campaign effectiveness (Wakefield et al., 2010). Social norms around alcohol use in general are much more permissive than social norms around drinking and driving (Greenfield and Room, 1997). The alcohol industry spends an enormous amount of resources to promote the sale and use of alcohol. Alcohol use disorder is a widespread problem, as alcohol is an addictive substance. In light of this context, it is perhaps no surprise that several systematic reviews find only limited evidence that alcohol control campaigns are associated with reduced alcohol-related harm (Anderson et al., 2009a; Chisholm et al., 2004; Doran et al., 2008; Spoth et al., 2008), often noting limitations in the breadth and quality of the studies assessing their effects. Several of these reviews, however, note that media campaigns are likely an integral component of multipolicy interventions to reduce alcohol-related harm in general because they support awareness and compliance with policies and may enhance public and policy maker commitment to laws and regulations (e.g., Anderson et al., 2009a; Doran et al., 2008).

Campaigns specific to preventing traffic crashes and fatalities paint a more optimistic picture. Elder et al.'s (2004) systematic review concluded that carefully planned and well-funded media campaigns, when implemented alongside other prevention activities (including increased legal enforcement of drunk driving laws), are associated with a 13 percent decline in alcohol-related traffic crashes. Another study found that strategic efforts to increase news media coverage of efforts to reduce alcohol-impaired driving, combined with other community mobilization and enforcement activities, reduced alcohol-related injury crashes relative to a control community (Holder et al., 2000). Furthermore, Bergen et al. (2014) concluded that sobriety checkpoint programs are effective when well publicized with mass media campaigns to promote awareness of these enforcement initiatives. While Yadav and Kobayashi (2015) did not find sufficient evidence that media campaigns alone or concurrent with increased enforcement reduced alcohol-related fatal crashes, these authors featured different inclusion criteria than several previous reviews, were unable to account for the volume of media campaign exposure achieved by the interventions, and concluded that the heterogeneity of study design and quality precluded definitive conclusions about media campaign effect. Finally, while there is a lack of rigorous evaluation data on the campaign, the Ad Council and the U.S. Department of Transportation's "Friends don't let friends drive drunk" campaign that aired in the 1980s is often credited with contributing to a cultural shift that countered the norm of drinking and driving (Ad Council, 2016; Glascoff et al., 2013).

Systematic reviews of the evidence supporting (non-alcohol-related) traffic safety campaigns further underscore the value of media campaigns in conjunction with increased enforcement or other policy interventions. Two reviews found strong evidence that public education campaigns, when combined with enhanced legal enforcement, increase use of child safety seats and reduce related fatal injuries (Zaza et al., 2001) and increase use of safety belts and reduce traffic-related fatalities (Dinh-Zarr et al., 2001; Williams et al., 1996). The public's perception of the risk of legal consequences is important in determining the effectiveness of media campaigns. This is reflected in the likelihood that a person will drive while impaired (WHO, 2016) and intervene as a bystander (Guerette et al., 2013).

These studies make a strong case that campaigns against alcohol-impaired driving, combined with increased enforcement, have strong potential as a strategy to reduce alcohol-related fatal crashes. Some important caveats are in order, however. The only available study included in a systematic review of designated driver interventions (Ditter et al., 2005) failed to find evidence of behavioral changes in response to a modestly funded designated driver campaign in Australia (Boots and Midford, 1999). This suggests that the content and target of mass media campaigns is likely an important consideration, a conclusion that echoes findings from other behavioral contexts highlighting the importance of using formative research and behavior change theory to guide campaign design (e.g., Noar, 2006; Randolph and Viswanath, 2004). Recent evidence also underscores the need for significant funding to generate widespread levels of campaign exposure in this context (Niederdeppe et al., 2017a).

These findings emphasize the need for well-funded media campaigns that are able to achieve widespread exposure among target audiences (see Hornik, 2002; Wakefield et al., 2010). The definition of a "well-funded" campaign has not been standardized for alcohol-impaired driving, but has been operationalized for anti-tobacco campaigns. For example, CDC cites gross ratings points (GRPs) as an indicator for the recommended budget level and makes the case that between 1,600 and 2,800 GRPs, which equates to about five to seven exposures per month, are sufficient (CDC, 2014). More importantly, this is a rate of exposure that donated time is not likely to achieve. Unfortunately, most recent campaigns against alcohol-impaired driving appear to have relied on donated airtime from broadcasters (Ad Council, 2013, 2016). Sustained, well-funded media campaigns in other behavioral contexts have been funded from one of three sources: tax revenue (e.g., NCI, 2008), industry litigation (e.g., Farrelly et al., 2009), or acts of Congress (Hornik et al., 2008). It therefore seems unlikely that the typical model of relying on donated air time to generate exposure to alcohol-impaired driving related media campaigns is likely to achieve levels of exposure needed to have a large-scale effect on alcohol-related fatal crashes.

Furthermore, the changing nature of the media landscape warrants consideration in the development of media campaigns to reduce alcohol-impaired driving. As highlighted in the section "Policies to Reduce the Harmful Effects of Alcohol Marketing," traditional means of watching television are changing to online streaming services (Raine, 2017). Given the shifting landscape of media consumption, research into the most effective media by which to disseminate campaigns could optimize efforts to increase exposure to messages that run counter to alcohol-impaired driving.

Cost-Effectiveness Estimates

There are some cost-effectiveness studies on the effect of mass media campaigns on alcohol-related crash fatalities, although these assessments have the same causal evaluation challenges as noted above. Several cost-effectiveness reports that assess mass media campaigns conclude that media campaigns do not affect health outcomes and thus are not considered to be cost-effective (Anderson et al., 2009a; Chisholm et al., 2004; Cobiac et al., 2009). This may be attributable to the variability of mass media campaign studies, as heterogeneity among studies makes it difficult to make any conclusions on the effectiveness of these campaigns and, therefore, the cost-effectiveness of them (Yadav and Kobayashi, 2015).

Some studies demonstrate that these campaigns may be cost-effective under some circumstances, although these conclusions are based on a small subset of the population. Elder et al. (2004) evaluated several alcohol-impaired driving media campaigns in the United States and Australia for cost savings and found three of them to be cost-effective. Effectiveness was measured in terms of the following outcomes: drinking and driving behavior, alcohol-related crashes, and crash-related injuries or fatalities.

Several studies (see Bergen et al., 2014, for a review) also examined mass media campaigns to make drivers aware of upcoming sobriety checkpoints. These studies found that a combination of sobriety checkpoints and mass media campaigns have the potential to reduce the burden of alcohol-related traffic injuries, and that high coverage of mass media campaigns and a very low frequency of sobriety checkpoints is cost-effective and more efficient than sobriety checkpoints alone.

In summary, there appears to be little research and few clear findings on the cost-effectiveness of media campaigns with respect to alcohol-related fatalities. In many of the studies mentioned above, media campaigns (largely considered in isolation) have not been found to be effective overall, and as a result are not found to be cost-effective. Nevertheless, systematic reviews by both Elder et al. (2004) and Bergen et al. (2014) conclude that media campaigns plus increased enforcement (for Bergen et al. in the context of increased sobriety checkpoints) are both effective and can serve as cost-effective interventions to reduce alcohol-impaired driving and related crash fatalities. Wakefield et al.'s (2010) comprehensive review of systematic reviews makes clear that well-designed and well-funded media campaigns can influence behavior when combined with broader community-level interventions.

In this section, the committee reviews a body of evidence including systematic reviews specific to alcohol-impaired driving (e.g., Community Preventive Services Task Force review by Elder et al., 2004; more recent reviews by Bergen et al., 2014, and Yadav and Kobayashi, 2015), systematic reviews on media effects on other driving-related interventions (e.g., Zaza et al., 2011, on child safety seat use; Dinh-Zarr et al., 2001, on more general use of safety belts), and a comprehensive synthesis of systematic review evidence across a wide variety of behavioral domains (Wakefield et al., 2010). The committee assesses this evidence, along with other recent and relevant studies that were not included in these reviews, with the recognition that media campaigns are rarely conducted in isolation, vary considerably in size and quality, and typically lack randomized designs that permit unambiguous causal inference. Nevertheless, the committee argues that the accumulated body of evidence permits the following conclusion:

Conclusion 3-2: There is sufficient evidence to conclude that well-funded media campaigns are an important component of alcohol-impaired driving enforcement policy interventions to ensure their successful adoption and impact. Campaigns are more likely to be effective when rigorous formative research and behavioral change theories inform their design and dissemination.

TECHNOLOGICAL INTERVENTIONS

Personal Devices and Technology for Estimating BAC

Interventions that allow drinkers to estimate their BAC levels accurately, and thus better assess their risk, have the potential to reduce alcohol-impaired driving fatalities. There is good evidence that drinkers, and specifically those with high BAC levels, are poor at estimating their BAC (Beirness, 1987; Beirness et al., 1993; Martin et al., 2016; Thombs et al., 2003). Individuals who underestimate their BAC are more likely to judge they are fit to drive when they are over the BAC limit set by state law (Beirness, 1987; Beirness et al., 1993)[13] and they are more likely to take more risks while driving (Laude and Fillmore, 2016). Recent work has shown that one's perception of intoxication has a bigger effect on risk taking than actual physiological levels of intoxication (Corazzini et al., 2015; Proestakis et al., 2013). Making individuals aware of their level of intoxication might reduce risk taking.

There has been research and policy interest since the 1970s in determining whether BAC feedback through breath-testing devices could be used as an intervention to prevent alcohol-impaired driving (Oates, 1978; Russ et al., 1988). Breath-testing devices have been validated against blood alcohol levels (Kriikku et al., 2014; Schechtman and Shinar, 2011; Van Tassel et al., 2004). Theorized positive benefits of BAC feedback include decreasing alcohol consumption to not exceed the BAC limit set by state law and increasing the likelihood of opting not to drive (Russ et al., 1988).

Despite the theoretical benefits, providing BAC feedback through breath-testing devices was not shown to reduce alcohol-impaired driving in a review of studies conducted in the 1970s and 1980s (Russ et al., 1988). The majority of these studies were conducted on the premises of drinking establishments in Canada, New Zealand, and the United States. A more recent study from 2008 found that self-administered BAC feedback enabled individuals leaving drinking establishments to more accurately determine whether they could legally drive, but it did not change individuals' perceived fitness to drive (Johnson et al., 2008). The lack of behavioral change when presented with information on risk (communicated as BAC) underscores the predictable irrationality of those who repeatedly drive after drinking to above the limit set by state law (Ariely, 2008). For example, individuals who drive after drinking, compared to those who do not, understand DWI laws better but are poorer planners, more

[13] In these two studies, estimation of BAC was measured during a simulated naturalistic social drinking situation (Beirness, 1987) and a voluntary roadside survey of nighttime drivers (Beirness et al., 1993).

impulsive, and myopic decision makers (Sloan et al., 2014). Some studies have even suggested that BAC feedback has the potential to *increase* driving after drinking among those with BAC levels less than 0.05% (Bullers and Ennis, 2006; Johnson and Voas, 2004; Johnson et al., 2008). At or below this level, drinkers tend to overestimate their BAC in this range. Therefore, there is concern that BAC feedback in this range could lead to these individuals to decide it is safe to drive since they are under the limit set by state law, despite feeling some effects of impairment. More research is greatly needed to determine the net benefit and unintended consequences of BAC feedback on decisions to drive after moderate drinking.

Although personal breath-testing devices have existed since the 1980s, data are very sparse on who uses them, their accuracy, and their effect on public health.[14] Despite variability in accuracy of personal breath-testing devices (Ashdown et al., 2014), these devices do not currently require FDA approval to be marketed to consumers.

Personal breath-testing devices appear to be more common in European countries. One survey estimated 11 percent of Finnish households with licensed drivers owned a personal breath-testing device in 2007 (Radun et al., 2009). In this survey, more men than women reported owning a breath-testing device; 24 percent of those who owned one did not use it. The respondents reported 77 percent used it the day/morning following drinking, rather than while drinking (18 percent) or just before driving home after drinking (6 percent). In 2012, France passed a law requiring a breath-testing device to be carried in every vehicle (BBC, 2012). The law was suspended a year later because of shortages and reported test inaccuracy of the device. The effort was later criticized because of commercial financial conflicts of interest with the breath-testing kit manufacturer. Independent analyses of outcomes are not currently available (Radun et al., 2014).

In the last 5 years, there have been two major innovations that have led to a new generation of personal breath-testing devices marketed to consumers. The first is new fuel cell sensors that can maintain consistent measurements for up to 1 year of use without needing to be professionally calibrated. The second innovation is smartphone connectivity via Bluetooth or a headphone jack connection (Andrews, 2013). Smartphone applications associated with personal breath-testing devices can now provide an automated interpretation of BAC levels and cautionary messages, as well as the estimated time to return to BAC levels less than 0.02%. These apps track levels over time, and can be used to prompt safety measures such as hailing a rideshare or sending alerts to social contacts. For those

[14] For a list of approved evidential breath-testing devices, see https://www.transportation.gov/odapc/approved-evidential-breath-testing-devices (accessed October 13, 2017).

with alcohol use disorders, these smartphone-connected breath-testing devices can be used for remote alcohol monitoring via notifications to submit breath samples within a certain time frame. The smartphone camera can be used to verify the identity of the individual submitting the sample, and the submitted samples can be time-stamped and geocoded. A recent, small randomized controlled trial demonstrated that contingency management with financial incentives using this smartphone-enabled remote monitoring approach reduces alcohol consumption among those with alcohol use disorders (Alessi and Petry, 2013). Furthermore, aggregated data collected from smartphone-paired breath-testing devices are able to provide a novel source of data on alcohol consumption, as well as BAC levels among the population who uses them.[15] The costs of smartphone-paired breath-testing devices range from $30 to $100 and they are now available in major household, electronic, and online retail outlets.

There is very little scientific literature on the use of newer generation personal and smartphone-paired breath-testing devices for purposes of moderating drinking and reducing alcohol-impaired driving. Industry data indicate there are two main factors cited by users for using smartphone-paired breath-testing devices: (1) making sure their BAC is under the limit set by state law before they drive, and (2) avoiding a DWI. A 2016 survey study by the Colorado Department of Transportation in which 225 bar patrons were given a smartphone-paired breath-testing device reported that using a breath-testing device lowered their risk of a DWI and that the patrons were much less likely to drive impaired compared to prior to using a breath-testing device (Colorado DOT, 2016).[16]

A major limitation of breath-testing devices is that they require active use and engagement and only provide point-in-time estimates of BAC levels. This could potentially be dangerous if an individual's BAC is ascending, and they receive a reading that is below the limit set by state law, indicating that it would be safe to drive. Therefore, there is great potential and interest in having passively collected, continuous estimates of BAC as could be collected through transdermal alcohol sensors that measure alcohol content in skin sweat. Starting in the early 2000s, transdermal alcohol sensors have been used for remote monitoring in the criminal justice system (see Chapter 5 for a discussion of monitoring alcohol use among DWI offenders). These devices have included a tamper-resistant ankle bracelet and a wrist-wearable device (Swift et al., 1992).

---

[15] See, for example, the BACtrack consumption report, https://www.bactrack.com/pages/bactrack-consumption-report (accessed October 13, 2017).

[16] The Colorado DOT has since partnered with BACtrack, a personal breath-testing device company, to offer their products to Colorado residents for a discounted price (Colorado DOT, 2017). This partnership and its outcomes have not yet been evaluated.

These devices capture the presence of alcohol consumption in a continuous, passive fashion (Marques and McKnight, 2007; Sakai et al., 2006) and have been used for contingency management in treatment of those with alcohol use disorder (Dougherty et al., 2014).

However, compared with breath-testing devices, there are more challenges to providing real-time BAC estimates owing to lag time in skin accumulation of alcohol. The mathematical translation of transdermal alcohol content to estimated BAC in real time is an area of active research (Leffingwell et al., 2013). In addition, smartphone-paired transdermal alcohol sensors that could be integrated with smart watches are in development (Gutierrez et al., 2015). Finally, there is emerging research on passively monitoring alcohol intoxication based on how individuals use their smartphone with the ability to accurately detect light drinking and heavy drinking episodes with 96 percent accuracy (Bae et al., 2017).

Like other smartphone-enabled personal monitoring applications and devices, breath and alcohol sensors have the potential to facilitate changes in health behavior, but they are not likely to change behavior in isolation (Patel et al., 2015). These devices will need to be coupled with theoretically guided and evidence-based behavioral engagement strategies to reduce alcohol-impaired driving. These engagement strategies can be made more effective by incorporating feedback loops and concepts from behavioral economics that shape decision making, such as lottery-based designs that offer rewards combined with anticipated regret associated with not securing the reward (Patel et al., 2015). Future research and development is needed to determine whether coupling alcohol monitoring with behavioral strategies that take advantage of smartphone connectivity can lead to reductions in alcohol-impaired driving (Sahabiswas et al., 2016). Promising strategies include ongoing feedback support, real-time notifications of peers and loved ones, leveraging social norms, contingency management, prompting the use of ridesharing services, and pairing with in-vehicle devices and smartphone applications that monitor driving.

In this section, the committee reviews the literature on drinkers' self-estimates of BAC and whether BAC feedback from personal breath testing reduces decisions to drive at levels consistent with impairment. There is good evidence from multiple studies that drinkers with high BAC levels underestimate their BAC and that those who underestimate their BAC perceive they are fit to drive when their BAC is over the limit set by state law (e.g., Beirness, 1987; Beirness et al., 1993; Martin et al., 2016; Thombs et al., 2003). However, there is a lack of evidence from studies conducted in the 1970s to early 2000s to support that personal BAC feedback reduces alcohol-impaired driving. Starting in 2013, a new generation of consumer-marketed smartphone-paired breath-testing devices has emerged, presenting several opportunities to facilitate novel interventions based on the interpretation and sharing of the data generated by these devices. From a policy perspective, given that breath and transdermal alcohol sensors are increasingly being marketed to consumers and are being used to make decisions about driving after drinking, there is a need for peer-reviewed, objective evidence to verify their accuracy, including research into unintended consequences related to binge drinking and alcohol-impaired driving, before recommending widespread adoption. If it is found that some consistently underestimate BAC, there is a need for more regulatory oversight of this market such as by requiring FDA 510(k) premarket clearance before marketing to consumers.[17]

Conclusion 3-3: Consumer marketed personal breath-testing devices are an emerging technology with the potential to reduce alcohol-impaired driving by promoting more accurate BAC self-estimation. However, these technologies require further investigation of their accuracy and effects on behavior before promoting widespread use.

Other BAC Estimation Tools

Traditionally, BAC estimation tools have existed in the form of wallet-size cards, often titled "know your limit" and distributed to patrons of a licensed establishment. While "know your limit" cards do not have sufficient evidence to determine their effectiveness, they have been widely used for decades (Johnson and Clapp, 2011). As discussed with the personal breath-testing devices, the limitations and potential pitfalls of estimation tools have been explored in the literature (Johnson and Voas, 2004; Johnson et al., 2008). Another related tool that has emerged with the advent of smartphones and other handheld devices is mobile applications that allow individuals to gauge their BAC levels. Similarly to the "know your limit" cards, these applications allow users to input information on their sex, weight, and the number of drinks consumed during a fixed period of time to calculate their BAC. Some of these applications include an estimated time frame for reaching a BAC of 0.00%. It is important to note that these mobile application estimation tools have not been well evaluated. Nonetheless, they have potential for widespread use given the common platform on which they are offered, which warrants systematic investigation of their effectiveness and potential negative consequences.

[17] A 510(k) is a premarket submission made to FDA to demonstrate that the device to be marketed is at least as safe and effective, that is, substantially equivalent, to a legally marketed device (21 CFR § 807.92(a)(3)) that is not subject to premarket approval (FDA, 2017).

CONCLUDING OBSERVATIONS

Throughout this chapter, the committee has identified a number of areas that require further investigation to inform the implementation and design of drinking-oriented interventions. Addressing these evidence gaps would allow for more targeted and evidence-based interventions to reduce alcohol-impaired driving fatalities. The following subjects indicate research areas for which investigation would benefit the field of alcohol-impaired driving:

- Effects of introducing retail price restrictions on excessive alcohol consumption and alcohol-impaired driving;
- Specific effects of social host laws on underage alcohol consumption and alcohol-impaired driving;
- Key elements of effectiveness for responsible beverage service training and policies;
- Effect of permitting alcohol sales concurrent with or proximal to driving (e.g., drive-through package stores, sale of alcohol at gasoline marts, sale of alcohol at fast-food restaurants) on alcohol-impaired driving and related crashes and fatalities, including spatial analyses;
- Effectiveness of various strategies to reduce the effect of alcohol advertising on underage drinking and alcohol-impaired driving;
- Design, messaging, and placement of effective alcohol warning labels; and
- Effectiveness of BAC estimation tools, such as personal breath-testing devices and mobile applications, in addition to potential consequences or misuse.

While the country has made great strides in adopting alcohol-related policies, programs, and strategies, a revised and comprehensive approach is needed to once again achieve progress in reducing alcohol-impaired driving. It is important to note that progress will require a multicomponent approach, encompassing multilevel interventions that work synergistically. This could include maintaining and enhancing the enforcement of alcohol policies to influence price, availability, illegal sales, and responsible marketing; increasing the use of underused strategies such as age-related compliance checks; and more. This chapter examines the evidence-based and promising interventions that shape the likelihood of drinking to impairment and makes recommendations for how to inform, implement, and optimize these interventions. This is a crucial phase in the sequence of behaviors that lead to alcohol-impaired driving. The next chapter will explore interventions that reduce the act of alcohol-impaired driving itself.

REFERENCES

Aaron, P., and D. Musto. 1981. Temperance and prohibition in America: An historical overview. In *Alcohol and public policy: Beyond the shadow of prohibition*, edited by M. Moore and D. Gerstein. Washington, DC: National Academy Press.

Ad Council. 2013. *Project roadblock: Local TV puts the brakes on drunk driving for ninth holiday season*. http://www.adcouncil.org/News-Events/Press-Releases/ProjectRoadblock-Local-TV-Puts-the-Brakes-on-Drunk-Driving-for-Ninth-Holiday-Season (accessed September 29, 2017).

Ad Council. 2016. *Drunk driving prevention*. http://www.adcouncil.org/Our-Campaigns/The-Classics/Drunk-Driving-Prevention (accessed June 7, 2017).

Advocates for Highway and Auto Safety. 2017. *Have we forgotten what saves lives?: 2017 Roadmap of state highway safety laws*. Washington, DC: Advocates for Highway and Auto Safety.

Alessi, S. M., and N. M. Petry. 2013. A randomized study of cellphone technology to reinforce alcohol abstinence in the natural environment. *Addiction* 108(5):900–909.

Ally, A. K., Y. Meng, R. Chakraborty, P. W. Dobson, J. S. Seaton, J. Holmes, C. Angus, Y. Guo, D. Hill-McManus, A. Brennan, and P. Meier. 2014. Alcohol tax pass-through across the product and price range: Do retailers treat cheap alcohol differently? *Addiction* 109(12):1994–2002.

Anderson, P., D. Chisholm, and D. C. Fuhr. 2009a. Effectiveness and cost-effectiveness of policies and programmes to reduce the harm caused by alcohol. *The Lancet* 373(9682): 2234–2246.

Anderson, P., A. De Bruijn, K. Angus, R. Gordon, and G. Hastings. 2009b. Impact of alcohol advertising and media exposure on adolescent alcohol use: A systematic review of longitudinal studies. *Alcohol and Alcoholism* 44(3):229–243.

Andrews, T. M. 2013. *Breathalyzers of the future today*. https://www.theatlantic.com/health/archive/2013/06/breathalyzers-of-the-future-today/277249 (accessed October 13, 2017).

APIS (Alcohol Policy Information System). 2016a. *Alcohol beverages pricing: Drink specials*. https://alcoholpolicy.niaaa.nih.gov/alcohol_beverages_pricing_drink_specials.html (accessed March 31, 2017).

APIS. 2016b. *Alcohol beverages pricing: Wholesale pricing practices and restrictions*. https://alcoholpolicy.niaaa.nih.gov/alcohol_beverages_pricing_wholesale_pricing_practices_and_restrictions.html (accessed March 31, 2017).

APIS. 2016c. *Alcohol beverages taxes: Beer*. https://alcoholpolicy.niaaa.nih.gov/Taxes_Beer.html (accessed October 11, 2017).

APIS. 2016d. *Retail sales: Bans on off-premises Sunday sales*. https://alcoholpolicy.niaaa.nih.gov/Bans_on_Off-Premises_Sunday_Sales.html (accessed March 31, 2017).

APIS. 2016e. *Retail sales: Beverage service training and related practices*. https://alcoholpolicy.niaaa.nih.gov/Beverage_Service_Training_and_Related_Practices.html (accessed March 31, 2017).

APIS. 2016f. *Transportation: Open containers of alcohol in motor vehicles*. https://alcoholpolicy.niaaa.nih.gov/Open_Containers_of_Alcohol_in_Motor_Vehicles.html (accessed March 31, 2017).

APIS. 2016g. *Underage drinking: Possession/consumption/internal possession of alcohol*. https://alcoholpolicy.niaaa.nih.gov/Underage_Possession_Consumption_Internal_Possession_of_Alcohol.html (accessed September 1, 2017).

APIS. 2016h. *Underage drinking: Prohibitions against hosting underage drinking parties*. https://alcoholpolicy.niaaa.nih.gov/Prohibitions_Against_Hosting_Underage_Drinking_Parties.html (accessed September 21, 2017).

Apollonio, D. E., and R. E. Malone. 2009. Turning negative into positive: Public health mass media campaigns and negative advertising. *Health Education Research* 24(3):483–495.

Ariely, D. 2008. *Predictably irrational: The hidden forces that shape our decisions.* New York: HarperCollins.

Ashdown, H. F., S. Fleming, E. A. Spencer, M. J. Thompson, and R. J. Stevens. 2014. Diagnostic accuracy study of three alcohol breathalysers marketed for sale to the public. *BMJ Open* 4(12):e005811.

Babor, T. 2010. *Alcohol: No ordinary commodity: Research and public policy.* New York: Oxford University Press.

Babor, T. F., J. H. Mendelson, I. Greenberg, and J. Kuehnle. 1978. Experimental analysis of the "happy hour": Effects of purchase price on alcohol consumption. *Psychopharmacology* 58(1):35–41.

Babor, T. F., J. H. Mendelson, B. Uhly, and E. Souza. 1980. Drinking patterns in experimental and barroom settings. *Journal of Studies on Alcohol* 41(7):635–651.

Babor, T. F., Z. Xuan, D. Damon, and J. Noel. 2013. An empirical evaluation of the US Beer Institute's self-regulation code governing the content of beer advertising. *American Journal of Public Health* 103(10):e45–e51.

Babor, T., K. Robaina, and J. Noel. 2018. *The role of the alcohol industry in policy interventions for alcohol-impaired driving.* Paper commissioned by the Committee on Accelerating Progress to Reduce Alcohol-Impaired Driving Fatalities (see Appendix C).

Bae, S., D. Ferreira, B. Suffoleto, J.-C. Puyana, R. Kurtz, T. Chung, and A. K. Dey. 2017. Detecting drinking episodes in young adults using smartphone-based sensors. *Proceedings of the ACM on Interactive, Mobile, Wearable and Ubiquitous Technologies* 1(2):Article 5.

Baldwin, J. M., J. M. Stogner, and B. L. Miller. 2014. It's five o'clock somewhere: An examination of the association between happy hour drinking and negative consequences. *Substance Abuse Treatment, Prevention, and Policy* 9(1):1.

Barry, R. 2004. Enhanced enforcement of laws to prevent alcohol sales to underage persons—New Hampshire, 1999–2004. *Morbidity and Mortality Weekly Report* 53(21):452–454.

BBC (British Broadcasting Corporation). 2012. *France orders breathalyser for motorists.* http://www.bbc.com/news/world-europe-18662555 (accessed October 13, 2017).

Beer Institute. 2015. *Advertising and marketing code.* Washington, DC: Beer Institute.

Beirness, D. J. 1987. Self-estimates of blood alcohol concentration in drinking-driving context. *Drug and Alcohol Dependence* 19(1):79–90.

Beirness, D. J., R. D. Foss, and R. B. Voas. 1993. Drinking drivers' estimates of their own blood alcohol concentration. *Journal of Traffic Medicine* 21(2):73–78.

Benson, B. L., B. D. Mast, and D. W. Rasmussen. 2000. Can police deter drunk driving? *Applied Economics* 32(3):357–366.

Bergen, G., A. Pitan, S. L. Qu, R. A. Shults, S. K. Chattopadhyay, R. W. Elder, D. A. Sleet, H. L. Coleman, R. P. Compton, J. L. Nichols, J. M. Clymer, W. B. Calvert, and Community Preventive Services Task Force. 2014. Publicized sobriety checkpoint programs: A community guide systematic review. *American Journal of Preventive Medicine* 46(5):529–539.

Boots, K., and R. Midford. 1999. "Pick-a-skipper": An evaluation of a designated driver program to prevent alcohol-related injury in a regional Australian city. *Health Promotion International* 14(4):337–345.

Bullers, S., and M. Ennis. 2006. Effects of blood-alcohol concentration (BAC) feedback on BAC estimates over time. *Journal of Alcohol and Drug Education* 50(2):66.

Campbell, C. A., R. A. Hahn, R. Elder, R. Brewer, S. Chattopadhyay, J. Fielding, T. S. Naimi, T. Toomey, B. Lawrence, and J. C. Middleton. 2009. The effectiveness of limiting alcohol outlet density as a means of reducing excessive alcohol consumption and alcohol-related harms. *American Journal of Preventive Medicine* 37(6):556–569.

CAMY (Center on Alcohol Marketing and Youth). 2012. *State laws to reduce the impact of alcohol marketing on youth: Current status and model policies.* http://www.camy.org/_docs/research-to-practice/promotion/legal-resources/state-ad-laws/CAMY_State_Alcohol_Ads_Report_2012.pdf (accessed September 28, 2017).

CAP (Center for Alcohol Policy). 2015. *2015 alcohol regulation policy national survey.* http://www.centerforalcoholpolicy.org/wp-content/uploads/2015/08/2015-CAP-National-Survey-Alcohol-Regulatory-Policy.pdf (accessed August 31, 2017).

CDC (Centers for Disease Control and Prevention). 2003. *Designing and implementing an effective tobacco counter-marketing campaign.* Atlanta, GA: National Center for Chronic Disease Prevention and Health Promotion.

CDC. 2014. *Best practices for comprehensive tobacco control programs—2014.* Atlanta, GA: National Center for Chronic Disease Prevention and Health Promotion, Office on Smoking and Health.

CDC. 2017. *Guide for measuring alcohol outlet density.* Atlanta, GA: Centers for Disease Control and Prevention, U.S. Department of Health and Human Services.

Chang, K., C.-C. Wu, and Y.-H. Ying. 2012. The effectiveness of alcohol control policies on alcohol-related traffic fatalities in the United States. *Accident Analysis & Prevention* 45(1):406–415.

Chisholm, D., J. Rehm, M. Van Ommeren, and M. Monteiro. 2004. Reducing the global burden of hazardous alcohol use: A comparative cost-effectiveness analysis. *Journal of Studies on Alcohol* 65(6):782–793.

Cobiac, L., T. Vos, C. Doran, and A. Wallace. 2009. Cost-effectiveness of interventions to prevent alcohol-related disease and injury in Australia. *Addiction* 104(10):1646–1655.

Colorado DOT (Department of Transportation). 2016. *Smartphone breathalyzers lower risk of DUI, say 84 percent of CDOT program participants.* https://www.codot.gov/news/2016-news-releases/10-2016/smartphone-breathalyzers-lower-risk-for-dui (accessed October 12, 2017).

Colorado DOT. 2017. *CDOT and BACtrack announce partnership to reduce impaired driving.* https://www.codot.gov/news/2017-news/august/cdot-and-bactrack-announce-partnership-to-reduce-impaired-driving (accessed October 12, 2017).

Cook, P. J. 2007. *Paying the tab: The costs and benefits of alcohol control.* Princeton, NJ: Princeton University Press.

Corazzini, L., A. Filippin, and P. Vanin. 2015. Economic behavior under the influence of alcohol: An experiment on time preferences, risk-taking, and altruism. *PLoS ONE* 10(4):e0121530.

County Health Rankings. 2017. *Sales to intoxicated persons (SIP) law enforcement.* http://www.countyhealthrankings.org/policies/sales-intoxicated-persons-sip-law-enforcement (accessed August 31, 2017).

Creyer, E. H., J. C. Kozup, and S. Burton. 2002. An experimental assessment of the effects of two alcoholic beverage health warnings across countries and binge-drinking status. *Journal of Consumer Affairs* 36(2):171–202.

Dejong, W., and J. Blanchette. 2014. Case closed: Research evidence on the positive public health impact of the age 21 minimum legal drinking age in the United States. *Journal of Studies on Alcohol and Drugs, Supplement* (S17):108–115.

Dills, A. K. 2010. Social host liability for minors and underage drunk-driving accidents. *Journal of Health Economics* 29(2):241–249.

Dinh-Zarr, T. B., D. A. Sleet, R. A. Shults, S. Zaza, R. W. Elder, J. L. Nichols, R. S. Thompson, D. M. Sosin, and Community Preventive Services Task Force. 2001. Reviews of evidence regarding interventions to increase the use of seatbelts. *American Journal of Preventive Medicine* 21(4):48–65.

DISCUS (Distilled Spirits Council of the United States). 2011. *Code of responsible practices for beverage alcohol advertising and marketing*. http://jamanetwork.com/journals/jamapediatrics/fullarticle/2089643 (accessed July 7, 2017).

DISCUS. 2017. *Sunday alcohol sales: Rolling back the blue laws*. http://www.discus.org/policy/sunday (accessed August 28, 2017).

DISCUS. n.d. *Increasing alcohol taxes punishes the entire hospitality industry*. http://www.discus.org/policy/taxes (accessed October 2, 2017).

Ditter, S. M., R. W. Elder, R. A. Shults, D. A. Sleet, R. Compton, J. L. Nichols, and Community Preventive Services Task Force. 2005. Effectiveness of designated driver programs for reducing alcohol-impaired driving: A systematic review. *American Journal of Preventive Medicine* 28(5):280–287.

Doran, C., T. Vos, L. Cobiac, W. Hall, I. Asamoah, A. Wallace, S. Naidoo, J. Byrnes, G. Fowler, and K. Arnett. 2008. *Identifying cost-effective interventions to reduce the burden of harm associated with alcohol misuse in Australia*. Brisbane, Old Australia: University of Queensland.

Dougherty, D. M., N. Hill-Kapturczak, Y. Liang, T. E. Karns, S. E. Cates, S. L. Lake, J. Mullen, and J. D. Roache. 2014. Use of continuous transdermal alcohol monitoring during a contingency management procedure to reduce excessive alcohol use. *Drug and Alcohol Dependence* 142:301–306.

Durkin, G. E. 2006. What does Granholm v. Heald mean for the future of the twenty-first amendment, the three-tier system, and efficient alcohol distribution? In *Washington and Lee Law Review* 63:1095–1130.

Eisenberg, D. 2003. Evaluating the effectiveness of policies related to drunk driving. *Journal of Policy Analysis and Management* 22(2):249–274.

Elder, R. W., R. A. Shults, D. A. Sleet, J. L. Nichols, R. S. Thompson, W. Rajab, and Community Preventive Services Task Force. 2004. Effectiveness of mass media campaigns for reducing drinking and driving and alcohol-involved crashes: A systematic review. *American Journal of Preventive Medicine* 27(1):57–65.

Elder, R. W., J. L. Nichols, R. A. Shults, D. A. Sleet, L. C. Barrios, and R. Compton. 2005. Effectiveness of school-based programs for reducing drinking and driving and riding with drinking drivers: A systematic review. *American Journal of Preventive Medicine* 28(5 Suppl):288–304.

Elder, R. W., B. A. Lawrence, G. Janes, R. D. Brewer, T. L. Toomey, R. W. Hingson, T. S. Naimi, S. Wing, and J. Fielding. 2007. Enhanced enforcement of laws prohibiting sale of alcohol to minors: Systematic review of effectiveness for reducing sales and underage drinking. *Transportation Research Circular* 2007(E-C123):181–188.

Elder, R. W., B. Lawrence, A. Ferguson, T. S. Naimi, R. D. Brewer, S. K. Chattopadhyay, T. L. Toomey, J. E. Fielding, and Community Preventive Services Task Force. 2010. The effectiveness of tax policy interventions for reducing excessive alcohol consumption and related harms. *American Journal of Preventive Medicine* 38(2):217–229.

Elliott, S. 2001. The media business: Advertising; NBC, with conditions, to accept ads for liquor. *New York Times*. http://www.nytimes.com/2001/12/14/business/the-media-business-advertising-nbc-with-conditions-to-accept-ads-for-liquor.html (accessed October 2, 2017).

Escobedo, L. G., and M. Ortiz. 2002. The relationship between liquor outlet density and injury and violence in New Mexico. *Accident Analysis & Prevention* 34(5):689–694.

Esser, M. B., S. L. Hedden, D. Kanny, R. D. Brewer, J. C. Gfroerer, and T. S. Naimi. 2014. Prevalence of alcohol dependence among U.S. adult drinkers, 2009–2011. *Preventing Chronic Disease* 11:E206.

Farrelly, M. C., C. G. Healton, K. C. Davis, P. Messeri, J. C. Hersey, and M. L. Haviland. 2002. Getting to the truth: Evaluating national tobacco countermarketing campaigns. *American Journal of Public Health* 92(6):901–907.

Farrelly, M. C., J. Nonnemaker, K. C. Davis, and A. Hussin. 2009. The influence of the national truth campaign on smoking initiation. *American Journal of Preventive Medicine* 36(5):379–384.

FDA (U.S. Food and Drug Administration). 2017. *510(k) Premarket notification*. https://www.accessdata.fda.gov/scripts/cdrh/cfdocs/cfPMN/pmn.cfm (accessed December 21, 2017).

Fell, J. C., and R. B. Voas. 2006. Mothers Against Drunk Driving (MADD): The first 25 years. *Traffic Injury Prevention* 7(3):195–212.

Fell, J. C., D. A. Fisher, R. B. Voas, K. Blackman, and A. S. Tippetts. 2008. The relationship of underage drinking laws to reductions in drinking drivers in fatal crashes in the United States. *Accident Analysis & Prevention* 40(4):1430–1440.

Fell, J. C., D. A. Fisher, R. B. Voas, K. Blackman, and A. S. Tippetts. 2009. The impact of underage drinking laws on alcohol-related fatal crashes of young drivers. *Alcoholism, Clinical and Experimental Research* 33(7):1208–1219.

Fell, J. C., S. Tippetts, and R. Voas. 2010. Drinking characteristics of drivers arrested for driving while intoxicated in two police jurisdictions. *Traffic Injury Prevention* 11(5):443–452.

Fell, J. C., M. Scherer, S. Thomas, and R. B. Voas. 2014. Effectiveness of social host and fake identification laws on reducing underage drinking driver fatal crashes. *Traffic Injury Prevention* 15(Suppl 1):S64–S73.

Fell, J. C., D. A. Fisher, J. Yao, and A. S. McKnight. 2017. Evaluation of a responsible beverage service and enforcement program: Effects on bar patron intoxication and potential impaired driving by young adults. *Traffic Injury Prevention* 18(6):557–565.

Fitzgerald, J., and H. Mulford. 1992. Consequences of increasing alcohol availability: The Iowa experience revisited. *Addiction* 87(2):267–274.

Fitzgerald, J., and H. Mulford. 1993. Privatization, price and cross-border liquor purchases. *Journal of Studies on Alcohol* 54(4):462–464.

Flowers, N. T., T. S. Naimi, R. D. Brewer, R. W. Elder, R. A. Shults, and R. Jiles. 2008. Patterns of alcohol consumption and alcohol-impaired driving in the United States. *Alcoholism: Clinical and Experimental Research* 32(4):639–644.

Foran, H. M., and D. O'Leary. 2008. Alcohol and intimate partner violence: A meta-analytic review. *Clinical Psychology Review* 28:1222–1234.

Foust, J. 1999. State power to regulate alcohol under the twenty-first amendment: The constitutional implications of the twenty-first amendment enforcement act. *Boston College Law Review* 41(3):659–697.

Foxcroft, D. R., and A. Tsertsvadze. 2012. Cochrane review: Universal school-based prevention programs for alcohol misuse in young people. *Evidence-Based Child Health: A Cochrane Review Journal* 7(2):450–575.

Gallup. 2000. *Volume I: Findings, racial and ethnic group comparisons, National Survey of Drinking and Driving, June 2000, attitudes and behaviors—1993, 1995, 1997*. DTNH22-96-c-05081. Washington, DC: National Highway Traffic Safety Administration.

Giesbrecht, N. 2000. Roles of commercial interests in alcohol policies: Recent developments in North America. *Addiction* 95(12):581–595.

Girasek, D. C., A. C. Gielen, and G. S. Smith. 2002. Alcohol's contribution to fatal injuries: A report on public perceptions. *Annals of Emergency Medicine* 39(6):622–630.

Glascoff, M. A., J. S. Shrader, and R. K. Haddock. 2013. Friends don't let friends drive drunk, but do they let friends drive high? *Journal of Alcohol and Drug Education* 57(1):66–84.

Global Strategy Group. 2005. *Summary of study findings: National alcohol tax*. http://www.cspinet.org/new/pdf/alcohol_poll.pdf (accessed June 21, 2009).

Gonzales Research & Marketing Strategies. 2009. *Conducted for National Council on Alcoholism and Drug Dependence-Maryland, Maryland Development Disabilities Coalition*. Annapolis, MD: Gonzales Research & Marketing Strategies.

Goodwin, A., L. Thomas, B. Kirley, W. Hall, N. O'Brien, and K. Hill. 2015. *Countermeasures that work: A highway safety countermeasure guide for state highway safety offices.* 8th ed. DOT HS 812 202. Washington, DC: National Highway Traffic Safety Administration.

Graham, K. 2000. Preventive interventions for on-premise drinking: A promising but under-researched area of prevention. *Contemporary Drug Problems* 27(3):593–668.

Graham, K., P. Miller, T. Chikritzhs, M. A. Bellis, J. D. Clapp, K. Hughes, T. L. Toomey, and S. Wells. 2014. Reducing intoxication among bar patrons: Some lessons from prevention of drinking and driving. *Addiction* 109(5):693–698.

Green, C. P., J. S. Heywood, and M. Navarro. 2014. Did liberalising bar hours decrease traffic accidents? *Journal of Health Economics* 35:189–198.

Greenfield, T. K., and L. A. Kaskutas. 1993. Early impacts of alcoholic beverage warning labels: National study findings relevant to drinking and driving behavior. *Safety Science* 16(5–6):689–707.

Greenfield, T. K., and R. Room. 1997. Situational norms for drinking and drunkeness: Trends in the U.S. adult population 1979-1990. *Addiction* 92(1):33–47.

Grube, J. W., and K. Stewart. 2004. Preventing impaired driving using alcohol policy. *Traffic Injury Prevention* 5(3):199–207.

Gruenewald, P. J., and F. W. Johnson. 2010. Drinking, driving, and crashing: A traffic-flow model of alcohol-related motor vehicle accidents. *Journal of Studies on Alcohol and Drugs* 71(2):237–248.

Gruenewald, P. J., F. W. Johnson, and A. J. Treno. 2002. Outlets, drinking and driving: A multilevel analysis of availability. *Journal of Studies on Alcohol* 63(4):460–468.

Gruenewald, P. J., W. R. Ponicki, H. D. Holder, and A. Romelsjo. 2006. Alcohol prices, beverage quality, and the demand for alcohol: Quality substitutions and price elasticities. *Alcoholism: Clinical and Experimental Research* 30(1):96–105.

Guerette, R. T., J. L. Flexon, and C. Marquez. 2013. Instigating bystander intervention in the prevention of alcohol-impaired driving: Analysis of data regarding mass media campaigns. *Journal of Studies on Alcohol and Drugs* 74(2):205–211.

Gutierrez, M. A., M. L. Fast, A. H. Ngu, and B. J. Gao. 2015. Real-time prediction of blood alcohol content using smartwatch sensor data. Paper read at International Conference on Smart Health, Phoenix, AZ.

Hahn, R. A., J. L. Kuzara, R. Elder, R. Brewer, S. Chattopadhyay, J. Fielding, T. S. Naimi, T. Toomey, J. C. Middleton, and B. Lawrence. 2010. Effectiveness of policies restricting hours of alcohol sales in preventing excessive alcohol consumption and related harms. *American Journal of Preventive Medicine* 39(6):590–604.

Hahn, R. A., J. C. Middleton, R. Elder, R. Brewer, J. Fielding, T. S. Naimi, T. L. Toomey, S. Chattopadhyay, B. Lawrence, and C. A. Campbell. 2012. Effects of alcohol retail privatization on excessive alcohol consumption and related harms: A community guide systematic review. *American Journal of Preventive Medicine* 42(4):418–427.

Hastings, G., S. Anderson, E. Cooke, and R. Gordon. 2005. Alcohol marketing and young people's drinking: A review of the research. *Journal of Public Health Policy* 26(3):296–311.

HHS (U.S. Department of Health and Human Services). 2016. *Facing addiction in America: The Surgeon General's report on alcohol, drugs, and health.* Washington, DC: Office of the Surgeon General.

Hingson, R., and A. White. 2014. New research findings since the 2007 Surgeon General's call to action to prevent and reduce underage drinking: A review. *Journal of Studies on Alcohol and Drugs* 75(1):158–169.

Hingson, R. W., M. H. Swahn, and D. A. Sleet. 2008. Interventions to prevent alcohol-related injuries. In *Handbook of injury and violence prevention.* New York: Springer. Pp. 295–310.

Holder, H., and A. J. Treno. 1997. Media advocacy in community prevention: News as a means to enhance policy change. *Addiction* 92(Suppl. 2):S189–S199.

Holder, H., A. Wagenaar, R. Saltz, J. Mosher, and K. Janes. 1990. *Alcoholic beverage server liability and the reduction of alcohol-related problems: Evaluation of dram shop laws.* DOT HS 807 628. Washington, DC: National Highway Traffic Safety Administration.

Holder, H. D., P. J. Gruenewald, W. R. Ponicki, A. J. Treno, J. W. Grube, R. F. Saltz, R. B. Voas, R. Reynolds, J. Davis, and L. Sanchez. 2000. Effect of community-based interventions on high-risk drinking and alcohol-related injuries. *JAMA* 284(18):2341–2347.

Holmes, J., Y. Meng, P. S. Meier, A. Brennan, C. Angus, A. Campbell-Burton, Y. Guo, D. Hill-McManus, and R. C. Purshouse. 2014. Effects of minimum unit pricing for alcohol on different income and socioeconomic groups: A modelling study. *The Lancet* 383(9929):1655–1664.

Hornik, R. 2002. Evaluation design for public health communication programs. In *Public health communication*, edited by R. Hornick. Mahwah, NJ: Lawrence Erlbaum Associates. Pp. 385–408.

Hornik, R., L. Jacobsohn, R. Orwin, A. Piesse, and G. Kalton. 2008. Effects of the national youth anti-drug media campaign on youths. *American Journal of Public Health* 98(12): 2229–2236.

Hu, T., H. Sung, and T. E. Keeler. 1995. Reducing cigarette consumption in California: Tobacco taxes vs an anti-smoking media campaign. *American Journal of Public Health* 85(9):1218–1222.

Impact Databank. 2017. *The U.S. spirits market: Impact databank review and forecast.* New York: Shanken Communications.

IOM (Institute of Medicine). 2011. *For the public's health: Revitalizing law and policy to meet new challenges.* Washington, DC: The National Academies Press.

Jernigan, D., and J. O'Hara. 2004. Alcohol advertising and promotion. In *Reducing underage drinking: A collective responsibility*, edited by R. J. Bonnie and M. E. O'Connell. Washington, DC: The National Academies Press.

Jernigan, D., and H. Waters. 2009. *The potential benefits of alcohol excise tax increases in Maryland.* Baltimore, MD: Johns Hopkins Bloomberg School of Public Health.

Jernigan, D., J. Noel, J. Landon, N. Thornton, and T. Lobstein. 2016. *Alcohol marketing and youth alcohol consumption: A systematic review of longitudinal studies published since 2008. Addiction* 112(Suppl 1):7–20.

Johnson, M. B., and J. D. Clapp. 2011. Impact of providing drinkers with "know your limit" information on drinking and driving: A field experiment. *Journal of Studies on Alcohol and Drugs* 72(1):79–85.

Johnson, M. B., and R. B. Voas. 2004. Potential risks of providing drinking drivers with BAC information. *Traffic Injury Prevention* 5(1):42–49.

Johnson, M. B., R. B. Voas, T. Kelley-Baker, and C. D. M. Furr-Holden. 2008. The consequences of providing drinkers with blood alcohol concentration information on assessments of alcohol impairment and drunk-driving risk. *Journal of Studies on Alcohol and Drugs* 69(4):539–549.

Jones, L., K. Hughes, A. M. Atkinson, and M. A. Bellis. 2011. Reducing harm in drinking environments: A systematic review of effective approaches. *Health and Place* 17(2):508–518.

Jones, S. C., and P. Gregory. 2009. The impact of more visible standard drink labelling on youth alcohol consumption: Helping young people drink (ir)responsibly? *Drug and Alcohol Review* 28(3):230–234.

Kenkel, D. S. 2005. Are alcohol tax hikes fully passed through to prices? Evidence from Alaska. *AEA Papers and Proceedings* 95(2):273–277.

Kerr, W. C., and T. Stockwell. 2012. Understanding standard drinks and drinking guidelines. *Drug and Alcohol Review* 31(2):200–205.

King, C., M. Siegel, C. Ross, and D. Jernigan. 2017. Alcohol advertising in magazines and underage readership: Are underage youth disproportionately exposed? *Alcoholism: Clinical and Experimental Research* 41(10):1775–1782.

Kriikku, P., L. Wilhelm, S. Jenckel, J. Rintatalo, J. Hurme, J. Kramer, A. W. Jones, and I. Ojanperä. 2014. Comparison of breath-alcohol screening test results with venous blood alcohol concentration in suspected drunken drivers. *Forensic Science International* 239:57–61.

Kuhns, J. B., M. L. Exum, T. A. Clodfelter, and M. C. Bottia. 2014. The prevalence of alcohol-involved homicide offending: A meta-analytic review. *Homicide Studies* 18(3):251–270.

Kuo, M., H. Wechsler, P. Greenberg, and H. Lee. 2003. The marketing of alcohol to college students: The role of low prices and special promotions. *American Journal of Preventive Medicine* 25(3):204–211.

Lapham, S. C., P. J. Gruenwald, L. Remer, and L. Layne. 2004. New Mexico's 1998 drive-up liquor window closure. Study I: Effect on alcohol-involved crashes. *Addiction* 99(5): 598–606.

Laude, J. R., and M. T. Fillmore. 2016. Drivers who self-estimate lower blood alcohol concentrations are riskier drivers after drinking. *Psychopharmacology* 233(8):1387–1394.

Lavoie, M.-C., P. Langenberg, A. Villaveces, P. C. Dischinger, L. Simoni-Wastila, K. Hoke, and G. S. Smith. 2017. Effect of Maryland's 2011 alcohol sales tax increase on alcohol-positive driving. *American Journal of Preventive Medicine* 53(1):17–24.

Lee, N. K., J. Cameron, S. Battams, and A. Roche. 2016. What works in school-based alcohol education: A systematic review. *Health Education Journal* 75(7):780–798.

Leffingwell, T. R., N. J. Cooney, J. G. Murphy, S. Luczak, G. Rosen, D. M. Dougherty, and N. P. Barnett. 2013. Continuous objective monitoring of alcohol use: Twenty-first century measurement using transdermal sensors. *Alcoholism: Clinical and Experimental Research* 37(1):16–22.

Lenk, K. M., T. L. Toomey, T. F. Nelson, R. Jones-Webb, and D. J. Erickson. 2014. State and local law enforcement agency efforts to prevent sales to obviously intoxicated patrons. *Journal of Community Health* 39(2):339–348.

Lenk, K. M., T. F. Nelson, T. L. Toomey, R. Jones-Webb, and D. J. Erickson. 2016. Sobriety checkpoint and open container laws in U.S.: Associations with reported drinking-driving. *Traffic Injury Prevention* 17(8):782–787.

Levy, D. T., and T. R. Miller. 1995. A cost-benefit analysis of enforcement efforts to reduce serving intoxicated patrons. *Journal of Studies on Alcohol* 56(2):240–247.

Lewis, N. O., S. C. Lapham, and B. J. Skipper. 1998. Drive-up liquor windows and convicted drunk drivers: A comparative analysis of place of purchase. *Accident Analysis & Prevention* 30(6):763–772.

Linde, A. C., T. L. Toomey, J. Wolfson, K. M. Lenk, R. Jones-Webb, and D. J. Erickson. 2016. Associations between responsible beverage service laws and binge drinking and alcohol-impaired driving. *Journal of Alcohol and Drug Education* 60(2):35.

Lipari, R. N., A. Hughes, and J. Bose. 2016. *Driving under the influence of alcohol and illicit drugs. The CBHSQ report: December 27, 2016.* Rockville, MD: Center for Behavioral Health Statistics and Quality, Substance Abuse and Mental Health Services Administration.

Lipperman-Kreda, S., J. W. Grube, and M. J. Paschall. 2010. Community norms, enforcement of minimum legal drinking age laws, personal beliefs and underage drinking: An explanatory model. *Journal of Community Health* 35(3):249–257.

Looney, A. 2017. *Measuring the loss of life from the Senate's tax cuts for alcohol producers.* https://www.brookings.edu/research/measuring-the-loss-of-life-from-the-senates-tax-cuts-for-alcohol-producers/?utm_campaign=Brookings%20Brief&utm_source=hs_email&utm_medium=email&utm_content=58721243#fn1 (accessed December 11, 2017).

Mann, R. E., E. R. Vingilis, G. Leigh, L. Anglin, and H. Blefgen. 1986. School-based programmes for the prevention of drinking and driving: Issues and results. *Accident Analysis and Prevention* 18(4):325–337.

Marques, P. R., and A. S. McKnight. 2007. *Evaluating transdermal alcohol measuring devices.* Washington, DC: National Highway Traffic Safety Administration.
Martin, R. J., B. H. Chaney, J. Cremeens-Matthews, and K. Vail-Smith. 2016. Perceptions of breath alcohol concentration (BrAC) levels among a sample of bar patrons with BrAC values of 0.08% or higher. *Psychology of Addictive Behaviors* 30(6):680.
Martin, S. L. 2001. Changing the law: Update from the wine war. *Journal of Law and Politics* 17(1):63–98.
Martineau, F., E. Tyner, T. Lorenc, M. Petticrew, and K. Lock. 2013. Population-level interventions to reduce alcohol-related harm: An overview of systematic reviews. *Preventive Medicine* 57(4):278–296.
McCartt, A. T., L. A. Hellinga, and J. K. Wells. 2009. Effects of a college community campaign on drinking and driving with a strong enforcement component. *Traffic Injury and Prevention* (2):141–147.
McCartt, A. T., L. A. Hellinga, and B. B. Kirley. 2010. The effects of minimum legal drinking age 21 laws on alcohol-related driving in the United States. *Journal of Safety Research* 41(2):173–181.
McGowan, R. 1997. *Government regulation of the alcohol industry: The search for revenue and the common good.* Westport, CT: Greenwood Publishing Group.
McKnight, A. J., and F. M. Streff. 1994. The effect of enforcement upon service of alcohol to intoxicated patrons of bars and restaurants. *Accident Analysis & Prevention* 26(1):79–88.
Middleton, J. C., R. A. Hahn, J. L. Kuzara, R. Elder, R. Brewer, S. Chattopadhyay, J. Fielding, T. S. Naimi, T. Toomey, and B. Lawrence. 2010. Effectiveness of policies maintaining or restricting days of alcohol sales on excessive alcohol consumption and related harms. *American Journal of Preventive Medicine* 39(6):575–589.
Mosher, J. F. 2001. *Alcohol issues: The perils of preemption.* Chicago, IL: American Medical Association.
Mosher, J. F., T. L. Toomey, C. Good, E. Harwood, and A. C. Wagenaar. 2002. State laws mandating or promoting training programs for alcohol servers and establishment managers: An assessment of statutory and administrative procedures. *Journal of Public Health Policy* 23(1):90–113.
Mosher, J., A. Hauck, M. Carmona, R. Treffers, D. Reitz, C. Curtis, R. Ramirez, A. Moore, and S. Saetta. 2009. *Legal research report: Laws prohibiting alcohol sales to intoxicated persons.* Washington, DC: National Highway Traffic Safety Administration.
NABCA (National Alcohol Beverage Control Association). 2015. *The 3 tier system: A modern view.* Alexandria, VA: National Alcohol Beverage Control Association.
NABCA. 2017. *Beverage alcohol control agency info sheet.* http://www.nabca.org/page/one_pagers (accessed August 28, 2017).
Naimi, T. S. 2011. The cost of alcohol and its corresponding taxes in the U.S.: A massive public subsidy of excessive drinking and alcohol industries. *American Journal of Preventive Medicine* 41(5):546–547.
Naimi, T. S. 2018. *State alcohol taxes in the U.S.: Types, amounts, and comparison to alcohol-related costs.* Paper presented at the Alcohol Policy Conference 18, Washington, DC.
Naimi, T. S., D. E. Nelson, and R. D. Brewer. 2009. Driving after binge drinking. *American Journal of Preventive Medicine* 37(4):314–320.
Naimi, T. S., J. I. Daley, Z. Xuan, J. G. Blanchette, F. J. Chaloupka, and D. H. Jernigan. 2016. Who would pay for state alcohol tax increases in the United States? *Preventing Chronic Disease* 13.
Naimi, T. S., J. G. Blanchette, Z. Xuan, and F. J. Chaloupka. 2018. Erosion of state alcohol excise taxes in the U.S. *Journal of Studies on Alcohol and Drugs* 79(1):43–48.
NCI (National Cancer Institute). 2008. *The role of the media in promoting and reducing tobacco use. Tobacco control monograph 19.* NIH publication 07-6242. Bethesda, MD: National Cancer Institute.

NCSA (National Center for Statistics and Analysis). 2016. *Alcohol-impaired driving: 2015 data.* Traffic Safety Facts. DOT HS 812 350. Washington, DC: National Highway Traffic Safety Administration.

NCSL (National Conference of State Legislatures). 2013. *Open container and open consumption of alcohol state statutes.* http://www.ncsl.org/research/financial-services-and-commerce/open-container-and-consumption-statutes.aspx (accessed December 5, 2017).

Nelson, T. F., Z. Xuan, J. G. Blanchette, T. C. Heeren, and T. S. Naimi. 2015. Patterns of change in implementation of state alcohol control policies in the United States, 1999–2011. *Addiction* 110(1):59–68.

NHTSA (National Highway Traffic Safety Administration). 2005a. *Preventing over-consumption of alcohol—sales to the intoxicated and "happy hour" (drink special) laws.* Washington, DC: U.S. Department of Transportation.

NHTSA. 2005b. *The role of alcohol beverage control agencies in the enforcement and adjudication of alcohol laws.* DOT HS 809 877. Washington, DC: U.S. Department of Transportation.

NHTSA. 2016. *Digest of impaired driving and selected beverage control laws.* 29th ed. DOT HS 812 267. Washington, DC: U.S. Department of Transportation.

Niederdeppe, J., M. C. Farrelly, and D. Wenter. 2007. Media advocacy, tobacco control policy change, and teen smoking in Florida. *Tobacco Control* 16(1):47–52.

Niederdeppe, J., R. Avery, and E. N. Miller. 2017a. Alcohol-control public service announcements (PSAs) and drunk-driving fatal accidents in the United States, 1996-2010. *Preventive Medicine* 99:320–325.

Niederdeppe, J., M. Kellogg, C. Skurka, and R. J. Avery. 2017b. Market-level exposure to state antismoking media campaigns and public support for tobacco control policy in the United States, 2001–2002. *Tobacco Control.* doi: 10.1136/tobaccocontrol-2016-053506.

Noar, S. M. 2006. A 10-year retrospective of research in health mass media campaigns: Where do we go from here? *Journal of Health Communication* 11(1):21–42.

Noel, J. K., and T. F. Babor. 2016. Does industry self-regulation protect young persons from exposure to alcohol marketing? A review of compliance and complaint studies. *Addiction* 112(Suppl 1):51–56.

Noel, J. K., T. F. Babor, and K. Robaina. 2016. Industry self-regulation of alcohol marketing: A systematic review of content and exposure research. *Addiction* 112(Suppl 1):28–50.

NRC (National Research Council) and IOM. 2004. *Reducing underage drinking: A collective responsibility.* Washington, DC: The National Academies Press.

NTSB (National Transportation Safety Board). 2012. *Safety recommendation H-12-032.* https://www.ntsb.gov/about/employment/_layouts/ntsb.recsearch/Recommendation.aspx?Rec=H-12-032 (accessed June 26, 2017).

Oates, J. F. 1978. *Study of self test devices.* Washington, DC: National Highway Traffic Safety Administration.

O'Donnell, M. A. 1985. Research on drinking locations of alcohol-impaired drivers: Implications for prevention policies. *Journal of Public Health Policy* 6(4):510–525.

Parker, R. N., R. F. Saltz, and M. Hennessy. 1994. The impact of alcohol beverage container warning labels on alcohol-impaired drivers, drinking drivers and the general population in northern California. *Addiction* 89(12):1639–1651.

Paschall, M. J., S. Lipperman-Kreda, J. W. Grube, and S. Thomas. 2014. Relationships between social host laws and underage drinking: Findings from a study of 50 California cities. *Journal of Studies on Alcohol and Drugs* 75(6):901–907.

Patel, M. S., D. A. Asch, and K. G. Volpp. 2015. Wearable devices as facilitators, not drivers, of health behavior change. *JAMA* 313(5):459–460.

Pemberton, M. R., J. D. Colliver, T. M. Robbins, and J. C. Gfroerer. 2008. *Underage alcohol use: Findings from the 2002–2006 National Surveys on Drug Use and Health.* SMA 08-4333, Analytic Series A-30. Rockville, MD: Substance Abuse and Mental Health Services Administration, Office of Applied Studies.

Ponicki, W. R., P. J. Gruenewald, and L. G. Remer. 2013. Spatial panel analyses of alcohol outlets and motor vehicle crashes in California: 1999–2008. *Accident Analysis and Prevention* 55:135–143.

Proestakis, A., A. M. Espín, F. Exadaktylos, A. Cortés Aguilar, O. A. Oyediran, and L. A. Palacio. 2013. The separate effects of self-estimated and actual alcohol intoxication on risk taking: A field experiment. *Journal of Neuroscience, Psychology, and Economics* 6(2):115.

Purshouse, R. C., P. S. Meier, A. Brennan, K. B. Taylor, and R. Rafia. 2010. Estimated effect of alcohol pricing policies on health and health economic outcomes in England: An epidemiological model. *The Lancet* 375(9723):1355–1364.

Quinlan, K., R. A. Shults, and R. A. Rudd. 2014. Child passenger deaths involving alcohol-impaired drivers. *Pediatrics* 133(6):966–972.

Raabe, S. 2006 (unpublished). *Memorandum to Diana Morris, Director, Open Society Institute-Baltimore*. OpinionWorks.

Radun, I., H. Summala, and J. E. Radun. 2009. Drinking and driving "safely": Who uses a breathalyzer and when? *Transportation Research Part F: Traffic Psychology and Behaviour* 12(2):155–158.

Radun, I., J. Kaistinen, and T. Lajunen. 2014. Public-private partnership in traffic safety research and injury prevention. *International Journal of Epidemiology* 44(1):364–365.

Raine, L. 2017. *About 6 in 10 young adults in the U.S. primarily use online streaming to watch TV.* http://www.pewresearch.org/fact-tank/2017/09/13/about-6-in-10-young-adults-in-u-s-primarily-use-online-streaming-to-watch-tv (accessed November 30, 2017).

Ramirez, R. 2017. PowerPoint presentation to the Committee on Accelerating Progress to Reduce Alcohol-Impaired Driving Fatalities. Washington, DC, February 16, 2017. http://nationalacademies.org/hmd/~/media/Files/Activity%20Files/AcceleratingProgress-toReduceAlcoholImpairedDrivingFatalities/16%20FEB%202017/5%20Ramirez.pdf (accessed April 24, 2017).

Ramirez, R. L., and D. H. Jernigan. 2017. Increasing alcohol taxes: Analysis of case studies from Illinois, Maryland, and Massachusetts. *Journal of Studies on Alcohol and Drugs* 78(5):763–770.

Ramirez, R., D. Nguyen, C. Cannon, M. Carmona, and B. Freisthler. 2008. *A campaign to reduce impaired driving through retail-oriented enforcement in Washington state.* Washington, DC: National Highway Traffic Safety Administration.

Rammohan, V., R. A. Hahn, R. Elder, R. Brewer, J. Fielding, T. S. Naimi, T. L. Toomey, S. K. Chattopadhyay, C. Zometa, and Community Preventive Services Task Force. 2011. Effects of dram shop liability and enhanced overservice law enforcement initiatives on excessive alcohol consumption and related harms: Two community guide systematic reviews. *American Journal of Preventive Medicine* 41(3):334–343.

Randolph, W., and K. Viswanath. 2004. Lessons learned from public health mass media campaigns: Marketing health in a crowded media world. *Annual Review of Public Health* 25:419–437.

Reboussin, B. A., E. Y. Song, and M. Wolfson. 2011. The impact of alcohol outlet density on the geographic clustering of underage drinking behaviors within census tracts. *Alcoholism: Clinical and Experimental Research* 35(8):1541–1549.

Retting, R. 2017. *Pedestrian traffic fatalities by state: 2016 preliminary data.* Washington, DC: Governors Highway Safety Association.

Richter, L., R. D. Vaughan, and S. E. Foster. 2004. Public attitudes about underage drinking policies: Results from a national survey. *Journal of Public Health Policy* 25(1):58–77.

Ross, C. S., A. Sparks, and D. H. Jernigan. 2016. Assessing the impact of stricter U.S. advertising standards: The case of Beam Global Spirits. *Journal of Public Affairs* 16(3):245–254.

Russ, N. W., E. S. Geller, and L. S. Leland. 1988. Blood-alcohol level feedback: A failure to deter impaired driving. *Psychology of Addictive Behaviors* 2(3):124.

Sacks, J. J., K. R. Gonzales, E. E. Boucher, L. E. Tomedi, and R. D. Brewer. 2015. 2010 national and state costs of excessive alcohol consumption. *American Journal of Preventive Medicine* 49(5):e73–e79.

Saffer, H. 1997. Alcohol advertising and motor vehicle fatalities. *Review of Economics and Statistics* 79(3):431–442.

Sahabiswas, S., S. Saha, P. Mitra, R. Chatterjee, R. Ray, P. Saha, R. Basu, S. Patra, P. Paul, and B. A. Biswas. 2016. Drunken driving detection and prevention models using internet of things. Paper read at Information Technology, Electronics and Mobile Communication Conference (IEMCON), 2016 IEEE 7th Annual, Vancouver, BC.

Sakai, J. T., S. K. Mikulich-Gilbertson, R. J. Long, and T. J. Crowley. 2006. Validity of transdermal alcohol monitoring: Fixed and self regulated dosing. *Alcoholism: Clinical and Experimental Research* 30(1):26–33.

Saltz, R. F. 1987. The roles of bars and restaurants in preventing alcohol-impaired driving: An evaluation of server intervention. *Evaluation and Health Professions* 10(1):5–27.

SAMHSA (Substance Abuse and Mental Health Services Administration). 2017. *About the Synar Amendment and program.* https://www.samhsa.gov/synar/about (accessed November 14, 2017).

Sanchez-Ramirez, D. C., and D. Voaklander. 2017. The impact of policies regulating alcohol trading hours and days on specific alcohol-related harms: A systematic review. *Injury Prevention* 24:94–100. doi: 10.1136/injuryprev-2016-042285.

Schechtman, E., and D. Shinar. 2011. An analysis of alcohol breath tests results with portable and desktop breath testers as surrogates of blood alcohol levels. *Accident Analysis & Prevention* 43(6):2188–2194.

Scherer, M., J. C. Fell, S. Thomas, and R. B. Voas. 2015. Effects of dram shop, responsible beverage service training, and state alcohol control laws on underage drinking driver fatal crash ratios. *Traffic Injury Prevention* 16(Suppl 2):S59–S65.

Schmidt, S. 2017. PowerPoint presentation to the Committee on Accelerating Progress to Reduce Alcohol-Impaired Driving Fatalities in Washington, DC, March 22, 2017. http://nationalacademies.org/hmd/~/media/Files/Activity%20Files/AcceleratingProgresstoReduceAlcoholImpairedDrivingFatalities/22%20March%202017/1%20Steve%20Schmidt.pdf (accessed November 14, 2017).

Scribner, R., and D. Cohen. 2001. The effect of enforcement on merchant compliance with the minimum legal drinking age law. *Journal of Drug Issues* 31(4):857–866.

Scribner, R. A., D. P. MacKinnon, and J. H. Dwyer. 1994. Alcohol outlet density and motor vehicle crashes in Los Angeles County cities. *Journal of Studies on Alcohol and Drugs* 55(447–453).

Shope, J. T., M. R. Elliott, T. E. Raghunathan, and P. F. Waller. 2001. Long-term follow-up of a high school alcohol misuse prevention program's effect on students' subsequent driving. *Alcoholism: Clinical and Experimental Research* 25(3):403–410.

Shults, R. A., R. W. Elder, D. A. Sleet, J. L. Nichols, M. O. Alao, V. G. Carande-Kulis, S. Zaza, D. M. Sosin, R. S. Thompson, and Community Preventive Services Task Force. 2001. Reviews of evidence regarding interventions to reduce alcohol-impaired driving. *American Journal of Preventive Medicine* 21(4):66–88.

Shurtleff, M., D. Gansler, T. Horne, G. Jepsen, J. R. I. Biden, L. Rapadas, D. Louie, L. Wasden, L. Madigan, T. Miller, M. Coakley, J. Hood, C. Cortez Masto, M. Delaney, G. King, E. Schneiderman, S. Pruitt, J. Kroger, P. Kilmartin, A. Wilson, R. E. Cooper, W. H. Sorrell, R. McKenna, and G. Phillips. 2011. *Re: Alcohol reports, paperwork comment; Project P114503. A communication from the chief legal officers of the following states: Arizona, Connecticut, Delaware, Guam, Hawaii, Idaho, Illinois, Iowa, Maryland, Massachusetts, Mississippi, Nevada, New Hampshire, New Mexico, New York, Oklahoma, Oregon, Rhode Island, South Carolina, Tennessee, Utah, Vermont, Washington, Wyoming.* https://www.ftc.gov/sites/default/files/documents/public_comments/alcohol-reports-project-no.p114503-00071%C2%A0/00071-58515.pdf (accessed September 29, 2017).

Siegel, M., W. DeJong, T. S. Naimi, E. K. Fortunato, A. B. Albers, T. Heeren, D. L. Rosenbloom, C. Ross, J. Ostroff, S. Rodkin, C. King, D. L. Borzekowski, R. N. Rimal, A. A. Padon, R. H. Eck, and D. H. Jernigan. 2013. Brand-specific consumption of alcohol among underage youth in the United States. *Alcoholism: Clinical and Experimental Research* 37(7):1195–1203.

Simon, J. L. 1966. The economic effects of state monopoly of packaged-liquor retailing. *Journal of Political Economy* 74(2):188–194.

Sloan, F. A., E. M. Stout, K. Whetten-Goldstein, and L. Liang. 2000. *Drinkers, drivers, and bartenders: Balancing private choices and public accountability.* Chicago and London: The University of Chicago Press.

Sloan, F. A., L. M. Eldred, and Y. Xu. 2014. The behavioral economics of drunk driving. *Journal of Health Economics* 35:64–81.

Sly, D. F., E. Trapido, and S. Ray. 2002. Evidence of the dose effects of an antitobacco counteradvertising campaign. *Preventive Medicine* 35(5):511–518.

Smart, R. G. 1996. The happy hour experiment in North America. *Contemporary Drug Problems* 23(2):291–300.

Smart, R. G., and E. M. Adlaf. 1986. Banning happy hours: The impact on drinking and impaired-driving charges in Ontario, Canada. *Journal of Studies on Alcohol* 47(3):256–258.

Smith, K. C., S. Cukier, and D. H. Jernigan. 2014. Defining strategies for promoting product through "drink responsibly" messages in magazine ads for beer, spirits and alcopops. *Drug and Alcohol Dependence* 142:168–173.

Smith, L. A., and D. R. Foxcroft. 2009. The effect of alcohol advertising, marketing and portrayal on drinking behaviour in young people: Systematic review of prospective cohort studies. *BMC Public Health* 9:51.

Snyder, L., M. Hamilton, E. Mitchell, J. Kiwanuka-Tondo, F. Fleming-Milici, and D. Proctor. 2004. A meta-analysis of the effect of mediated health communication campaigns on behavior change in the United States. *Journal of Health Communication* 9(Suppl 1):71–96.

South Carolina Legislature. 2007. *Alcohol and alcoholic beverages.* Chapter 4: Beer, ale, porter, and wine: Article 1 general provisions. In *61.* Columbia, SC.

Spoth, R., M. Greenberg, and R. Turrisi. 2008. Preventive interventions addressing underage drinking: State of the evidence and steps toward public health impact. *Pediatrics* 121(Suppl 4):S311–S336.

Stehr, M. F. 2010. The effect of Sunday sales of alcohol on highway crash fatalities. *The BE Journal of Economic Analysis & Policy* 10(1).

Stigler, M. H., E. Neusel, and C. L. Perry. 2011. School-based programs to prevent and reduce alcohol use among youth. *Alcohol Research and Health* 34(2):157–162.

Stockley, C. S. 2001. The effectiveness of strategies such as health warning labels to reduce alcohol-related harms—an Australian perspective. *International Journal of Drug Policy* 12(2):153–166.

Stockwell, T. 1993. Influencing the labelling of alcoholic beverage containers: Informing the public. *Addiction* 88(S1):53S–60S.

Stockwell, T., D. Blaze-Temple, and C. Walker. 1991. The effect of "standard drink" labelling on the ability of drinkers to pour a "standard drink." *Australian Journal of Public Health* 15(1):56–63.

Stockwell, T., J. Zhao, G. Martin, S. Macdonald, K. Vallance, A. J. Treno, W. R. Ponicki, A. Tu, and J. Buxton. 2013. Minimum alcohol prices and outlet densities in British Columbia, Canada: Estimated impacts on alcohol-attributable hospital admissions. *American Journal of Public Health* 103(11):2014–2020.

Stockwell, T., J. Zhao, M. Marzell, P. J. Gruenewald, S. Macdonald, W. R. Ponicki, and G. Martin. 2015. Relationships between minimum alcohol pricing and crime during the partial privatization of a Canadian government alcohol monopoly. *Journal of Studies on Alcohol and Drugs* 76(4):628–634.

Stout, E. M., F. A. Sloan, L. Liang, and H. H. Davies. 2000. Reducing harmful alcohol-related behaviors: Effective regulatory methods. *Journal of Studies on Alcohol* 61(3):402–412.

Stuster, J., M. Burns, and D. Fiorentino. 2002. *Open container laws and alcohol involved crashes: Some preliminary data.* Washington, DC: National Highway Traffic Safety Administration.

Swift, R. M., C. S. Martin, L. Swette, A. Laconti, and N. Kackley. 1992. Studies on a wearable, electronic, transdermal alcohol sensor. *Alcoholism: Clinical and Experimental Research* 16(4):721–725.

Task Force on Community Preventive Services. 2009. Recommendations for reducing excessive alcohol consumption and alcohol-related harms by limiting alcohol outlet density. *American Journal of Preventive Medicine* 37(6):570–571.

Task Force on Community Preventive Services. 2011. Recommendations on dram shop liability and overservice law enforcement initiatives to prevent excessive alcohol consumption and related harms. *American Journal of Preventive Medicine* 41(3):344–346.

Thombs, D. L., R. S. Olds, and B. M. Snyder. 2003. Field assessment of BAC data to study late-night college drinking. *Journal of Studies on Alcohol* 64(3):322–330.

Thombs, D. L., V. Dodd, S. B. Pokorny, M. R. Omli, R. O'Mara, M. C. Webb, D. M. Lacaci, and C. Werch. 2008. Drink specials and the intoxication levels of patrons exiting college bars. *American Journal of Health Behavior* 32(4):411–419.

Thombs, D. L., R. O'Mara, V. J. Dodd, W. Hou, M. L. Merves, R. M. Weiler, S. B. Pokorny, B. A. Goldberger, J. Reingle, and C. E. Werch. 2009. A field study of bar-sponsored drink specials and their associations with patron intoxication. *Journal of Studies on Alcohol and Drugs* 70(2):206–214.

Thomsen, S. R., and K. Fulton. 2007. Adolescents' attention to responsibility messages in magazine alcohol advertisements: An eye-tracking approach. *Journal of Adolescent Health* 41(1):27–34.

Thornton, R. L. J., A. Greiner, C. M. Fichtenberg, B. J. Feingold, J. M. Ellen, and J. M. Jennings. 2013. Achieving a healthy zoning policy in Baltimore: Results of a health impact assessment of the Transform Baltimore zoning code rewrite. *Public Health Reports* 128(6 Suppl 3):87–103.

Treno, A. J., J. W. Grube, and S. E. Martin. 2003. Alcohol availability as a predictor of youth drinking and driving: A hierarchical analysis of survey and archival data. *Alcoholism: Clinical and Experimental Research* 27(5):835–840.

Treno, A. J., F. W. Johnson, L. G. Remer, and P. J. Gruenewald. 2007. The impact of outlet densities on alcohol-related crashes: A spatial panel approach. *Accident Analysis & Prevention* 39(5):894–901.

Trolldal, B. 2005. An investigation of the effect of privatization of retail sales of alcohol on consumption and traffic accidents in Alberta, Canada. *Addiction* 100(5):662–671.

TTB (Alcohol and Tobacco Trade and Tax Bureau). 2016. *Tax and fee rates.* https://www.ttb.gov/tax_audit/atftaxes.shtml (accessed October 2, 2017).

Van Hoof, J., M. Van Noordenburg, and M. De Jong. 2008. Happy hours and other alcohol discounts in cafés: Prevalence and effects on underage adolescents. *Journal of Public Health Policy* 29(3):340–352.

Van Tassel, W., M. Dennis, and M. Parker. 2004. Pocket model, numerical readout breath alcohol measurement devices: A laboratory- and in-vivo based evaluation. Paper read at Proceedings of the 17th International Conference on Alcohol, Drugs and Traffic Safety. Glasgow, Scotland.

Voas, R. B., and J. C. Lacey. 2011. *Alcohol and highway safety: A review of the state of knowledge.* Washington, DC: National Highway Traffic Safety Administration.

Wada, R., F. J. Chaloupka, L. M. Powell, and D. Jernigan. 2017. Employment impacts of alcohol taxes. *Preventive Medicine.* doi: 10.1016/j.ypmed.2017.08.013. [Epub ahead of print.]

Wagenaar, A. C., and T. L. Toomey. 2002. Effects of minimum drinking age laws: Review and analyses of the literature from 1960 to 2000. *Journal of Studies on Alcohol* (Suppl 14):206–225.

Wagenaar, A. C., E. H. Harwood, T. L. Toomey, C. E. Denk, and K. M. Zander. 2000. Public opinion on alcohol policies in the United States: Results from a national survey. *Journal of Public Health Policy* 21(3):303–327.

Wagenaar, A. C., C. E. Denk, P. J. Hannan, H. Chen, and E. M. Harwood. 2001. Liability of commercial and social hosts for alcohol-related inujuries: A national survey of accountability norms and judgments. *Public Opinion Quarterly* 65(3):344–368.

Wagenaar, A. C., T. L. Toomey, and D. J. Erickson. 2005. Preventing youth access to alcohol: Outcomes from a multi-community time-series trial. *Addiction* 100(3):335–345.

Wagenaar, A. C., M. J. Salois, and K. A. Komro. 2009. Effects of beverage alcohol price and tax levels on drinking: A meta-analysis of 1003 estimates from 112 studies. *Addiction* 104(2):179–190.

Wagenaar, A. C., A. L. Tobler, and K. A. Komro. 2010. Effects of alcohol tax and price policies on morbidity and mortality: A systematic review. *American Journal of Public Health* 100(11):2270–2278.

Wagoner, K. G., M. Sparks, V. T. Francisco, D. Wyrick, T. Nichols, and M. Wolfson. 2013. Social host policies and underage drinking parties. *Substance Use and Misuse* 48(1-2):41–53.

Wakefield, M. A., B. Loken, and R. C. Hornik. 2010. Use of mass media campaigns to change health behaviour. *The Lancet* 376(9748):1261–1271.

Washington Traffic Safety Commission. 2014. *Effectiveness of school-based alcohol misuse and drinking/driving programs.* http://wtsc.wa.gov/wp-content/uploads/2016/05/School-Based-Prevention-Programs_May2014.pdf (accessed June 20, 2017).

WHO (World Health Organization). 2014. *Global status report on alcohol and health - 2014.* http://www.who.int/substance_abuse/publications/global_alcohol_report/msb_gsr_2014_1.pdf?ua=1 (accessed October 9, 2017).

WHO. 2016. *Road safety mass media campaigns: A toolkit.* Geneva, Switzerland: World Health Organization.

WHO and Task Force Initiative. 2007. *Protection from exposure to second-hand tobacco smoke: Policy recommendations.* Geneva, Switzerland: World Health Organization.

Widom, C. S., and S. Hiller-Sturmhofel. 2001. Alcohol abuse as a risk factor for and consequence of child abuse. *Alcohol Research & Health* 25(1):52–57.

Williams, A., D. Reinfurt, and J. Wells. 1996. Increasing seat belt use in North Carolina. *Journal of Safety Research* 27(1):33–41.

Xuan, Z., T. F. Nelson, T. Heeren, J. Blanchette, D. E. Nelson, P. Gruenewald, and T. S. Naimi. 2013. Tax policy, adult binge drinking, and youth alcohol consumption in the United States. *Alcoholism: Clinical and Experimental Research* 37(10):1713–1719.

Xuan, Z., J. G. Blanchette, T. F. Nelson, T. C. Heeren, T. H. Nguyen, and T. S. Naimi. 2015a. Alcohol policies and impaired driving in the United Sstates: Effects of driving- vs. drinking-oriented policies. *International Journal of Alcohol and Drug Research* 4(2):119–130.

Xuan, Z., F. J. Chaloupka, J. G. Blanchette, T. H. Nguyen, T. C. Heeren, T. F. Nelson, and T. S. Naimi. 2015b. The relationship between alcohol taxes and binge drinking: Evaluating new tax measures incorporating multiple tax and beverage types. *Addiction* 110(3):441–450.

Yadav, R.-P., and M. Kobayashi. 2015. A systematic review: Effectiveness of mass media campaigns for reducing alcohol-impaired driving and alcohol-related crashes. *BMC Public Health* 15(1):1.

Young, D. J., and A. Bielinska-Kwapisz. 2002. Alcohol taxes and beverage prices. *National Tax Journal* 55(1):57–73.

Zaza, S., D. Sleet, R. Thompson, D. Sosin, J. Bolen, and Community Preventive Services Task Force. 2001. Reviews of evidence regarding interventions to increase use of child safety seats. *American Journal of Preventive Medicine* 21(4 Suppl):31–47.

Zhao, J., T. Stockwell, G. Martin, S. Macdonald, K. Vallance, A. Treno, W. R. Ponicki, A. Tu, and J. Buxton. 2013. The relationship between minimum alcohol prices, outlet densities and alcohol-attributable deaths in British Columbia, 2002–09. *Addiction* 108(6): 1059–1069.

4

Alcohol-Impaired Driving Interventions

INTRODUCTION

The committee's conceptual framework for preventing alcohol-impaired driving crash fatalities was presented in Chapter 1 (see Figure 1-5). This framework illustrates the pathway from initially consuming alcohol to drinking to impairment and to driving while impaired, and shows how these actions can lead to motor vehicle crashes and the risk of serious injuries or death. Along the continuum between initial alcohol consumption and the occurrence of a fatal or serious motor vehicle crash, there are numerous opportunities for interventions that could reduce or eliminate alcohol-impaired driving incidents. This chapter examines several intervention opportunities for reducing alcohol-impaired driving, including changes in policies, laws, and enforcement; technological advances and vehicle features that could offer protections to drivers, occupants, and others; and programs or policies that could affect the sociocultural environment. These interventions offer promising approaches for improving the safety of drivers, passengers, and the public at large. A research needs section outlining gaps in the knowledge base for alcohol-impaired driving interventions is included at the end of the chapter.

POLICIES AND LAWS

A reexamination of, or modification to, existing policies and laws could provide opportunities for reducing the incidence of alcohol-impaired driving crashes. Interventions discussed in this section include changes to blood alcohol concentration (BAC) laws, zero tolerance laws, graduated licensing laws, and child endangerment laws.

Blood Alcohol Concentration (BAC) Laws

Overview

Laws limiting permissible BAC among operators of motor vehicles are important interventions for reducing alcohol-impaired driving and related injuries and fatalities. Currently, in each state in the United States, drivers 21 years of age and older are prohibited from driving with a BAC that exceeds 0.08%, which is the limit proscribed in state per se laws for alcohol-impaired drivers (APIS, 2016).[1] In December 2018, however, Utah will be the first state to lower its BAC per se law to 0.05%. Commercial drivers cannot exceed a BAC of 0.04%,[2] and drivers under the age of 21 are restricted to a BAC varying from 0.00% to 0.02% (Fell et al., 2016; so-called zero tolerance laws, discussed later in this chapter), depending on the state where they are licensed to drive. Any individual, regardless of age or type of license, who drives with a BAC in excess of that proscribed by state law can be subject to punishments, including fines, license revocation, vehicle impoundment or restrictions, mandatory treatment, or arrest.

The following section provides information about how BAC affects the human body and an overview of the history and context of BAC laws in the United States and internationally. The section also reviews relevant scientific evidence, including laboratory and epidemiological studies of crash risk at measured BAC levels of less than 0.08%, to determine the point at which alcohol impairment occurs. Potential barriers to adopting laws lowering BAC limits and information on overcoming those barriers are also discussed. Based on its review of the evidence on the effectiveness of 0.05% BAC laws, the committee ends the section with a recommendation to state governments to lower the BAC limit set by state laws from 0.08% to 0.05%. Based on recent literature reviews and estimates by the committee and others, adoption of 0.05% per se laws nationally could save more than 1,500 lives annually (Fell and Scherer, 2017).

---

[1] A per se law means that the act in question is illegal and a crime.

[2] For more information, see Federal Motor Carrier Safety Administration: BAC Standards. https://www.fmcsa.dot.gov/registration/commercial-drivers-license/states (accessed December 6, 2017).

Background

Blood alcohol (i.e., ethanol) concentration is based on the number of grams of alcohol per every 100 milliliters (1 deciliter) of blood, and it is commonly used to quantify an individual's level of alcohol impairment or intoxication for medical or legal purposes. When an individual consumes alcohol, up to 20 percent of the alcohol is absorbed into the bloodstream from the stomach, while 80 percent or more is absorbed from the small intestine (Levine, 2006). Once alcohol is absorbed, an individual's BAC can be measured in blood, urine, saliva, breath, perspiration, and vitreous humor, or tissues of the liver and spleen. BAC testing usually takes place at a hospital or, if a driver has been fatally injured, during an autopsy. In some cases, such as during a crash investigation or after a driver fatality, an individual's BAC will be estimated using back (or retrograde) extrapolation, which uses a driver's physical characteristics (sex, weight, height); absorption rate, amount, and location of alcohol in bodily tissues; and the rate of elimination to help determine an individual's BAC when he or she was driving. Back extrapolation provides an estimate of BAC, but it is not as accurate as direct measurement from biological samples since the actual conditions under which alcohol was consumed, such as the number of drinks and time span, cannot be accounted for (Kelly and Mozayani, 2012).

After consuming alcohol, the human body undergoes multiple changes that can affect an individual's perception and performance. Such changes include a loss of inhibition or judgment and a decrease in self-awareness, emotional stability, and coordination (Kelly and Mozayani, 2012). These deficits become more evident as the amount of alcohol ingested increases and, as a result, an individual's ability to operate a motor vehicle safely can be negatively affected (see Chapter 1 for more details on alcohol impairment). As shown in Table 4-1, each increase in BAC is accompanied by physiological effects and inherent predictable effects on an individual's driving capability.

Alcohol tolerance decreases the sedative effects of alcohol, making the drinker feel more alert and less intoxicated (Roehrs and Roth, n.d.; Williams and Salamy, 1972); however, tolerance has been shown to have no effect on cognitive accuracy (Schweizer and Vogel-Sprott, 2008), inhibition (Fillmore et al., 2005), executive functions (Cromer et al., 2010), short-term memory (Cromer et al., 2010), or motor impairment (García Moreno et al., 2004). In addition, the effects of alcohol tolerance can cause drinkers to underestimate the dangers of driving with a high BAC, making them think that they are not as impaired as they actually are (Amlung et al., 2014; Lapham, 2010). Similarly, mixing caffeine with alcohol has been shown to decrease awareness of impairment without decreasing the actual level of impairment (Lalanne et al., 2017; Weldy, 2010), potentially keeping a person awake longer and giving them the opportunity to drink

TABLE 4-1 Blood Alcohol Concentration (BAC) Levels and Physiological Effects, Effects on Driving

Blood Alcohol Concentration	Typical Physiological Effects	Typical Effects on Driving
0.02%	• Some loss of judgment • Relaxation • Slight body warmth • Altered mood	• Decline in visual functions (rapid tracking of a moving target) • Decline in ability to perform two tasks at the same time (divided attention)
0.05%	• Exaggerated behavior • May have loss of small-muscle control (e.g., focusing the eyes) • Impaired judgment • Usually good feeling • Lowered alertness • Release of inhibition	• Reduced coordination • Reduced ability to track moving objects • Difficulty steering • Reduced response to emergency driving situations
0.08%	• Muscle coordination becomes poor (e.g., balance, speech, vision, reaction time, and hearing) • Harder to detect danger • Judgment, self-control, reasoning, and memory are impaired	• Decline in ability to concentrate • Short-term memory loss • Decline in control of speed • Reduced information processing capability (e.g., signal detection, visual search) • Impaired perception
0.10%	• Clear deterioration of reaction time and control • Slurred speech, poor coordination, and slowed thinking	• Reduced ability to maintain lane position and brake appropriately
0.15%	• Far less muscle control than normal • Vomiting may occur (unless this level is reached slowly or a person has developed a tolerance for alcohol) • Major loss of balance	• Substantial impairment in vehicle control, attention to driving task, and in necessary visual and auditory information processing

SOURCE: Adapted from NHTSA, n.d.-a.

more alcohol and/or drive (De Sanctis et al., 2017). Typically, an *alcoholic drink* is defined on the basis of ethanol content in a beverage. In the United States, the standard serving size for an alcoholic drink is defined as 14 grams of ethanol or 0.6 ounces of ethanol, which is equivalent to

- 12 ounces of beer (5 percent alcohol by volume [ABV]),
- 8 ounces of malt liquor (7 percent ABV),
- 5 ounces of wine (12 percent ABV), or
- 1.5 ounces or a "shot" of 80-proof (40 percent ABV) distilled spirits, such as gin, rum, vodka, or whiskey (NIAAA, 2017).

Chapter 2 provides more information on the variety of alcoholic products available on the market.

After consuming an alcoholic beverage, the absorption and elimination rates of the ethanol will determine the peak BAC. Consuming alcohol while fasting will result in a more rapid absorption of alcohol from gastric elimination, while alcohol consumed with a liquid or solid meal or while the stomach is filled will be absorbed into the body more slowly. Time to peak BAC also varies according to how much alcohol is consumed. It takes vodka (a distilled spirit) and tonic 36 minutes (±10 minutes) to reach peak BAC, wine takes 54 minutes (±14 minutes), and beer takes 62 minutes (±10 minutes) (Mitchell et al., 2014). Time to peak BAC is especially important when considering factors affecting alcohol-impaired driving since peak BAC can be reached well after a person has consumed their last alcoholic beverage but within a period of time when they may be driving a vehicle.

After ingesting alcohol, the rate of elimination from the body varies depending on the amount of alcohol and the circumstances in which it was consumed, as well as factors such as sex and weight (Wall et al., 2016) (see Figure 4-1). Approximately 90 percent of alcohol in the body is metabolized by the liver. The remaining alcohol is excreted via urine, breath, and perspiration (NHTSA, 2013a). After consuming equivalent doses of alcohol, women reach higher peak BAC levels than men (Mumenthaler et al., 1999); however, alcohol elimination per hour tends to be slightly faster among women (0.018 g/dL) than men (0.015 g/dL) (Levine, 2006; Mishra et al., 1989; NIAAA, 1999; Thomasson, 2000). One possible explanation for this disparity is that women typically have higher liver volume per unit body mass (Kwo et al., 1998; Li et al., 1998), enabling women to metabolize alcohol faster than men (Levitt et al., 1997).

Because of the relationship between BAC and impairment, law enforcement officials have used BAC measurements to estimate whether a driver's alcohol consumption has impaired his or her capacity to drive. Of the many ways to determine an individual's BAC, the most convenient and noninvasive—and therefore the easiest for law enforcement officials—is with a breath-testing device. The amount of alcohol (ethanol) in an individual's breath is proportional to that in the blood; a blood alcohol reading of 0.100 g/100 mL in blood is roughly equivalent to 0.100 g/210 L in a deep-lung breath (Borkenstein et al., 1974). Police officers administer

A

Drinks	Body Weight (lbs)								
	100	120	140	160	180	200	220	240	
0	0	0	0	0	0	0	0	0	Only Safe Limit
1	.05	.04	.03	.03	.03	.02	.02	.02	.01–.03 Impairment begins
2	.09	.08	.06	.06	.05	.05	.04	.04	
3	.14	.11	.10	.09	.08	.07	.06	.06	.04–.07 Driving skills deteriorating; driver can be arrested for DWI
4	.18	.15	.13	.11	.10	.09	.08	.08	
5	.23	.19	.16	.14	.13	.11	.10	.09	
6	.27	.23	.19	.17	.15	.14	.12	.11	.08 Illegal to drive, immediately lose license; subject to criminal penalties, fines, and/or jail
7	.32	.27	.23	.20	.18	.16	.14	.13	
8	.36	.30	.26	.23	.20	.18	.17	.15	

B

Drinks	Body Weight (lbs)									
	100	120	140	160	180	200	220	240	260	
0	0	0	0	0	0	0	0	0	0	Only Safe Limit
1	.04	.03	.03	.02	.02	.02	.02	.02	.01	.01–.03 Impairment begins
2	.07	.06	.05	.05	.04	.04	.03	.03	.03	
3	.11	.09	.08	.07	.06	.06	.05	.05	.04	.04–.07 Driving skills deteriorating; driver can be arrested for DWI
4	.15	.12	.11	.09	.08	.07	.07	.06	.06	
5	.19	.16	.13	.12	.10	.09	.08	.08	.07	
6	.22	.19	.16	.14	.12	.11	.10	.09	.09	.08 Illegal to drive, immediately lose license; subject to criminal penalties, fines, and/or jail
7	.26	.22	.19	.16	.15	.13	.12	.11	.10	
8	.30	.25	.21	.19	.17	.15	.14	.12	.12	

FIGURE 4-1 Average relationship between alcohol consumption (based on number of standard drinks and body weight) and BAC: (A) for women and (B) for men.
SOURCE: Moore and Pierce, 2016.

standardized field sobriety tests or a preliminary breath test using a portable device to help determine if an individual has been driving under the influence of alcohol. If warranted, additional breath tests or testing of blood samples may be conducted at a police station or a hospital by a trained professional; the results of these tests could be admissible in a court of law (Moore and Pierce, 2016). Studies have shown that urinary ethyl glucuronide (EtG) and ethyl sulfate (EtS) biomarkers can detect recent consumption of alcohol in urine samples from 24 hours and up to 5 days after ingestion, depending on the amount of alcohol consumed (Høiseth et al., 2008, 2010; Schmitt et al., 1995; Wurst et al., 2006); however, measurements of EtG or EtS biomarkers would be unlikely to be admissible in court. Securing court-admissible test results that meet the legal requirements to be used as admissible evidence in a courtroom can sometimes be challenging (see Chapter 5).

U.S. Laws Regarding BAC

A per se law means that the act in question is illegal and a crime; with regard to impaired driving, if a driver's BAC exceeds the limit set by state law no further proof of impairment is required, regardless of other evidence of sobriety (APIS, 2016). These laws make it easier to prosecute offenders in court if these laws are violated (LII, n.d.). In the United States, the vast majority of BAC laws fall under the jurisdiction of state courts, although an existing federal BAC per se law prohibits driving at a BAC of ≥0.08% on federal land—including, for example, military bases, national parks or forests, and court houses—and some localities have enacted local traffic codes that regulate BAC limits. Administrative license suspension (ALS) and administrative license revocation (ALR) laws authorize law enforcement officials to confiscate or revoke a driver's license from any driver who refuses or is unable to pass a sobriety test. The suspensions or revocation occur at the time of the failed test or refusal; subsequent fines or sanctions, such as mandatory educational programs or assessment/treatment, may be levied against the offender (Chamberlain and Solomon, 2002). This is consistent with the behavioral psychology theory of deterrence, which states that laws are most effective when consequences to breaking them are delivered with certainty and celerity (Nagin, 2013). ALS/ALR laws have proven to be effective for both general and specific deterrence effects, and the laws reduce alcohol-impaired driving crashes and convictions. To date, 41 states and the District of Columbia have enacted ALS/ALR laws, which are discussed in greater detail in Chapter 5.

Rogers (1997) examined recidivism and alcohol-related crashes among driving-while-impaired (DWI) offenders in California between

1989 and 1991. This time period included two legal changes related to alcohol-impaired driving. The BAC per se law was reduced to 0.08% on January 1, 1990, and administrative per se (APS) pre-conviction license suspension on arrested DWI offenders was imposed on July 1, 1990. The probability of alcohol-related crash risk as well as the probability of DWI conviction 1 year subsequent to original arrest decreased among both first and repeat DWI offenders from 1989 (pre-law changes) to 1991 (post-law changes). While the contribution of lowered BAC versus the contribution of license suspension cannot be separated in the study design, in totality these results indicated that lowering BAC in conjunction with administrative and other sanctions is an effective deterrent among high-risk drivers.

The first state law penalizing drivers for driving while "under the influence of alcohol" was passed in New York State in 1920; however, prosecution of alcohol-impaired drivers was limited because law enforcement officers used behavioral observations alone to determine impairment, resulting in convictions that could be easily challenged in court (Voas and Lacey, 1990). This began to change in the 1930s with the development of breath-testing devices that could measure an individual's BAC and the advent of laws being passed that standardized what it meant to be "impaired" (Voas and Lacey, 1990). In 1941 New York State was the first to allow a BAC of ≥0.15% (tested by breath, blood, urine, or saliva) to stand as proof of intoxication in a court of law (King and Tipperman, 1975).

Despite these early developments, decades passed before alcohol-impaired driving began to be seen as an important public health issue (Fell and Voas, 2006). In the 1970s, the National Highway Traffic Safety Administration (NHTSA) was officially established and began advocating for stricter laws and penalties for alcohol-impaired driving; soon after, Mothers Against Drunk Driving (MADD) was founded in 1980 (Fell and Voas, 2006). The efforts of these two organizations influenced the passage of many laws, including zero tolerance laws, which prohibit underage drivers from operating a vehicle after consuming any alcohol (Fell and Voas, 2006). The minimum legal drinking age of 21, which prohibits those under 21 years of age from purchasing or publicly consuming alcohol, was adopted by all states by 1988 (APIS, n.d.). Despite these successes, enacting nationwide laws focused on lowering BAC levels has been challenging.

In 1992 NHTSA released a report recommending that Congress reduce the BAC limit to 0.08% for all drivers 21 years of age and older (Snyder, 1992). In response, Congress passed the Transportation Equity Act for the 21st Century, which included $500 million of incentive grants to states enacting and enforcing a 0.08% BAC per se law (DOT, 1998). The incentives were not effective. When the act was passed in 1998, 34 states and the District of Columbia had a BAC per se law of 0.10%, and 2 years later only two additional states had adopted the change (APIS, 2016). In 2000 the Community Preventive Services Task Force recommended lowering the BAC limit set by state law to 0.08%, making it clear that it was an effective public health countermeasure (Community Preventive Services Task Force, 2000). That same year the Department of Transportation Appropriations Act was passed; it specified that states that failed to pass a 0.08% per se law by 2004 would begin losing federal highway construction funds.[3] With the threat of losing funds looming, more states adopted lower BAC levels. By 2004, 45 states had passed BAC 0.08% per se laws, and only 5 states remained with a BAC per se law of 0.10% (APIS, 2016). Minnesota was the last state to lower its BAC per se law to 0.08% in August 2005 (APIS, 2016).

Should BAC Laws Be Lowered in the United States?

Today, although 0.08% BAC per se laws have become widely accepted in the United States, pressure is mounting in some states to further reduce the BAC allowed by law. In 1983 Utah became the first state in the nation to pass a criminal per se law lowering the BAC limit from 0.10% to 0.08% (Chamberlain and Solomon, 2002). Now Utah is set to lead the country again with new BAC legislation. On March 23, 2017, Utah became the first state to pass a BAC per se law of 0.05%, and the bill is set to take effect on December 30, 2018 (Utah State Legislature, 2017). Currently Washington State and Hawaii are also considering similar legislation (Hawaii State Legislature, 2017; Washington State Legislature, 2017).

Several prominent organizations, such as the U.S. National Transportation Safety Board and the World Health Organization (WHO), have recommended lowering the BAC limit to 0.05% (NTSB, 2013; Peden et al., 2004). Although current BAC limits allowed by different countries for drivers range from 0.0% (in Uruguay and in many Middle Eastern countries, including Afghanistan, Egypt, and Saudi Arabia) to 0.15% (in some West African countries, including Equatorial Guinea and Guinea-Bissau), most countries have a limit of 0.05% or 0.08% (WHO, 2014). As of 2015, 34 countries—representing 2.1 billion people—had laws limiting a driver's BAC to 0.05% or less and to 0.0% to 0.02% for young or novice drivers. These BAC limits, considered to be best practice by WHO, are imposed by many industrialized, high-income countries such as Australia, France, Germany, and Italy. Approximately 57.7 percent of countries have a national BAC limit lower than 0.08% (WHO, 2014, 2015).

---

[3] Department of Transportation and Related Agencies Appropriations Act of 2001, Public Law 106-346, 106th Cong. (October 23, 2000).

Laboratory Studies of Impairment

Researchers have used motor vehicle or motorcycle simulators in laboratory settings to measure alcohol's effects at various BAC levels on factors such as response or reaction time, standard deviation of speed, peripheral detection, divided-attention task performance, and the ability to maintain a consistent position in a driving lane or standard deviation of lane position. Standard deviation of lane position measurements are considered one of the best indicators of impaired driving (Irwin et al., 2017). Such tests allow researchers to examine impairment and its potential effect on motor vehicle or motorcycle crashes by recreating real-world scenarios in controlled environments. Although some laboratory studies examine differences between alcohol-consuming subjects and controls, most studies examine the magnitude of impairment by measuring differences in performance measures before and after alcohol consumption in test subjects acting as their own control.

The committee reviewed a number of individual laboratory studies published since 2000 that examined alcohol consumption and subsequent driving. All of the reviewed studies were relatively small (8–40 subjects). The majority of studies used automobile simulators (Breitmeier et al., 2007; Calhoun et al., 2004; Cheng et al., 2010; Freydier et al., 2014; Friedman et al., 2011; Liu and Ho, 2010; Meskali et al., 2011; Mets et al., 2011; Parks et al., 2002; Ronen et al., 2010; Rupp et al., 2007; Tremblay et al., 2015; Verster et al., 2009); three studies were restricted to relatively inexperienced drivers and/or young adults (Freydier et al., 2014; Rudin-Brown et al., 2013; Verster et al., 2009). Examples of automobile simulator outcomes that were related to BAC levels of 0.05% or less included delayed reaction time, increased driving speed, more lane deviation, and greater inattention (Cheng et al., 2010; Freydier et al., 2014; Moskowitz et al., 2000; Parks et al., 2002). Overall the committee found consistent evidence for impairment at BAC levels of 0.05% on the basis of experimental motor vehicle driving simulator studies. Three laboratory studies used motorcycle simulator measurements for their analysis (Creaser et al., 2009; Filtness et al., 2013; Rudin-Brown et al., 2013). Outcomes adversely affected in motorcycle simulator studies at BAC levels of 0.05% or less included impaired static balance, increased standard deviation of driver position, and reduced hazard avoidance. Reaction times to visual or auditory stimuli were adversely affected in a stimuli-related study (Cheng et al., 2010).

A recent review and meta-analysis by Irwin et al. (2017) analyzed alcohol-impaired driving studies that were conducted with the use of driving simulators. After excluding studies that lacked precise performance measures, 48 different acute alcohol consumption trials—37 placebo-controlled trials and 11 trials with no control—were included in the analysis. The studies estimated BAC levels measured at the start and finish of simulated driving tasks using breath-testing instruments. Meta-analysis results showed that acute alcohol consumption, as indicated by BAC levels ranging from 0.023% to 0.10%, significantly increased standard deviation of lane position and standard deviation of speed.

A report by NHTSA reviewed 112 studies published prior to 2000 that examined the effect of alcohol consumption on driving-related skills (Moskowitz and Fiorentino, 2000). The reviewed studies assessed the effect of alcohol consumption by measuring a range of BAC levels and performance on tasks in 13 categories of driving-related behaviors. Based on the studies reviewed, Moskowitz and Fiorentino (2000) concluded that, at a BAC of 0.05%, experimental studies reported significant impairment across a range of simulator outcomes related to vision, vigilance and drowsiness, psychomotor skills, attention, and information processing. Specifically, BAC levels in 27 percent of studies reported significant impairment by 0.039%, 47 percent of the studies by 0.049%, and 92 percent by 0.079%.

Laboratory studies allow for an assessment of the effects of various BAC levels on driving-related tasks in a controlled setting. To learn how these effects translate into real-world settings, however, reviewing the findings of epidemiological studies is imperative.

Epidemiological Studies of Crash Risk by BAC

Despite state laws mandating a limit of 0.08% BAC in the United States, evidence shows that a substantial proportion of alcohol-related crashes and fatalities occur when drivers have BAC levels below 0.08%. In 2015 there were 10,265 alcohol-impaired driving fatalities (BAC ≥0.08) in the United States and 1,808 fatalities involved a driver with a BAC between 0.01% and 0.07% (NHTSA, 2015). Because the presence of alcohol does not mean that crashes and related fatalities are necessarily attributable to alcohol consumption, in addition to reviewing the evidence from simulator studies (above), the committee also reviewed epidemiological studies that examined the risks of fatal crashes involving driver BACs below 0.08%. The best epidemiological evidence of the relationships between driver BAC levels and the risk of a crash are case-control studies in which BAC levels in drivers involved in crashes (cases) are compared with BAC levels in drivers not involved in crashes (controls). Case-control studies match controls with cases using drivers from the same geographic areas and ideally during the same day of the week and time of day. Some studies also obtain controls from cars traveling on the same roadways in the same direction in which case fatalities occurred. Studies conducted in the United States and abroad have consistently found an increased risk of fatal crashes among drivers with BAC levels from 0.05% to 0.079% compared to having a BAC of zero (no alcohol), both overall and across a range of gender and age groups. In fact, crash risk begins to increase below 0.05%, but this chapter focuses on this range because it is a prevalent policy-related threshold in other parts of the developed world. The analyses below present a range of expected reductions in lives saved or lost at differing BAC levels owing to variations in types of implementation (i.e., sanctions, enforcement, publicity) and research methodologies.

Borkenstein et al. (1974) conducted one of the earliest case-control studies of the relationship between alcohol use and alcohol-related crashes. Crash data collected between May 1, 1959, and April 30, 1962, by the Grand Rapids (Michigan) Police Department formed the basis for the identification of control subjects who were matched to drivers involved in crashes by their proximity to the same date, time, and location of the crash. Researchers conducted four interviews with non-crash drivers at 2,000 former crash sites between July 1962 and 1963. They found that drivers with BAC levels in excess of 0.04% had an increased rate of crashes while drivers with BAC levels over 0.08% were significantly more likely to have single-vehicle crashes and crashes that were more severe and costly than those involving sober drivers. Drivers with BAC levels between 0.04% and 0.08% had a positive, steadily increasing risk of being involved in a crash.

An update to the Borkenstein et al. (1974) study was conducted by Blomberg et al. (2005). Similar in design to the study by Borkenstein et al., researchers interviewed and collected breath tests from a sample of crash and non-crash drivers from crashes of all severities that occurred in Long Beach, California, and Fort Lauderdale, Florida, during a 12-month period between June 1997 and September 1999. The final analyses of interview data collected from 4,919 crash-involved drivers (2,422 from Long Beach, 2,497 from Fort Lauderdale) and 10,066 control non-crash drivers matched to crash cases by location, day of the week, and time of day 1 week after the initial crash, found relative risks (RRs) began to increase in drivers whose BAC levels were in the range 0.05–0.06% (RR = 1.38), and those risks continued to climb with increasing BAC. The adjusted RR for drivers with a BAC of 0.06% was 1.63, 0.07% was 2.09, and 0.08% was 2.69.

Data from Blomberg et al. (2005) were reanalyzed by Peck et al. (2008) to evaluate the relationship between BAC, a driver's age, and the risk of being in a crash. Data were evaluated according to specific age ranges—under 21, 21–24, 25–54, and 55 and older—to determine how age and a driver's BAC affect the risk of a crash. While BAC alone was highly correlated with crash risk, Peck at al. (2008) also found that drivers under the age of 21 years had an elevated risk of being involved in a crash at all BAC levels greater than 0.0%, and those risks continued to rise with each increase in BAC (e.g., a BAC of 0.05% yielded a RR of 2.75; 0.08% BAC, RR = 7.4; and 0.10% BAC, RR = 16.0). Drivers in this age group with BAC levels of 0.08% were 27.4 times more likely to be involved in a crash when compared to same-age drivers who had not been drinking (0.0% BAC). Elevated RRs were observed for drivers from all four age groups when BAC levels reached 0.05% or higher. Among drivers 21 and over the risk of being in a crash started increasing at a BAC of 0.05% (RR = 1.07), and those risks continued to increase at 0.08% (RR = 1.64) and 0.10% (RR = 2.43) but on a less steep curve than for drivers under 21.

A study of BAC and fatal crash risk was conducted by Zador (1991) and reanalyzed by Zador et al. (2000). In the original study, Zador (1991) used data from the Fatality Analysis Reporting System (FARS) collected in 1985 and 1986 and exposure data from the second National Roadside Breath-Testing Survey to analyze single-vehicle fatal crashes using drivers' age, sex, and BAC. Researchers found that fatal crash risk increased with increasing BAC for all drivers, regardless of sex and age group (16–20, 21–24, and 25 and older). Risk of crash doubled with each 0.02% increase in a driver's BAC above 0.0%. Drivers with BAC levels of 0.05–0.09%, regardless of age group, were nine times more likely to have a fatal crash than drivers who had a BAC of 0.0%. Male and female drivers with BAC levels between 0.05% and 0.09% had an increased risk of being killed in a single-car crash compared to comparable drivers with BAC levels ≤0.01% (RRs ranged from 9 to 54). When compared to drivers 25 years of age and older with similar BAC levels, female drivers between 16 and 21 years of age with BAC levels between 0.05% and 0.09% were at the greatest risk of dying in a single-vehicle crash (RR = 21.3); males in the same age range and with comparable BAC levels had a lower but still elevated risk (RR = 12.3).

Zador et al. (2000) updated the 1991 study using FARS data from 1996 and exposure data from the 1996 National Roadside Survey of Drivers to evaluate BAC levels in drivers of single-vehicle and two-vehicle fatal crashes. Age (16–20, 21–34, and 35 and older) and sex were evaluated in relation to BAC levels in drivers involved in crashes with fatalities. For both males and females, the fatal-crash risk was inversely proportional to the driver's age, and increasing BAC levels consistently elevated the fatal crash risk. Contrary to the findings reported in Zador (1991), young males between 16 and 20 years of age with BAC levels between 0.05% and 0.079% had a higher likelihood of being involved in a single-car or two-car fatal crash (RR = 17.32 versus 9.94, respectively) than comparable females (RR = 7.04 versus 6.53). Among drivers 16 to 20 years of age, males had a consistently higher fatal-crash rate than females, regardless of BAC; however, these differences were not evident for drivers 21 years of age or older. Drivers between 21 and 34 years of age with BAC levels between

0.05% and 0.079% had a higher risk of being involved in a fatal crash than drivers 35 years of age and older. This finding was consistent for all males and females with BAC levels over 0.02%.

In 2012, Voas et al. updated the Zador et al. (2000) analysis by comparing the 1996 data to 2006 and 2007 FARS crash data (cases; n = 6,863); control blood-alcohol data were obtained from 2007 U.S. National Roadside Survey results (n = 6,823). Crash data—age, gender, type of crash (single-vehicle fatal crash versus all fatal vehicle crashes in which the driver survived), and BAC—were used to compare changes in RR between 1996 and 2007. The percentage of alcohol-impaired drivers involved in fatal crashes remained largely unchanged between 1996 and 2007 (~22 percent); assessment of gender differences indicated that underage women were increasingly at risk of alcohol-impaired driving between the two study periods, yet underage men were increasingly likely to crash even at BAC of 0.0%. Nevertheless, overall, the relative risk for being involved in a fatal crash increased steadily with increasing BAC. Among drivers 16 to 20 years of age, compared to BAC of 0.0% the relative risk of fatalities in single-vehicle crashes was 1.47, 3.84, and 12.18 at BAC levels of 0.001–0.019%, 0.02–0.049%, and 0.05–0.079%, respectively. Among all drivers, compared to BAC of 0.0%, relative risks were 1.33, 2.68, and 6.24 at BAC levels of 0.001–0.019%, 0.02–0.049%, and 0.05–0.079%, respectively. Above age 21, all age groups with a BAC of ≥0.02 were at a significantly increased risk of single-vehicle and multiple-vehicle crash fatalities. Taken together, these data indicate that BAC above 0.02%, and for underage drivers BAC above 0.001% is associated with increased crash risk in a dose-response fashion.

Lacey et al. (2016) conducted a case-control study in Virginia Beach, Virginia, that estimated how a driver's use of alcohol, drugs, or a combination of the two contributed to crash risk. Biological samples were collected from more than 3,000 drivers from local crash scenes (cases) and 6,000 non-crash drivers (controls) matched 1 week later according to the time and location of the initial crash. Drivers were found to be 2.07 more likely to be involved in a crash if they had a BAC of 0.05% when compared to controls, and drivers who had a BAC of 0.08% were 3.93 times more likely to be involved in a crash.

More recently, Phillips and Brewer (2011) analyzed severity of crash risk by BAC among decedents in the FARS data from 1994 to 2008. The FARS codes injury severity from most to least severe as fatal injury, incapacitating injury, nonincapacitating injury, possible injury, and no injury. The ratio of serious versus nonserious driver injuries for each BAC was reported for all automobile crashes involving at least one fatality. There was a monotonic increase in the ratio of serious to nonserious injuries with increasing BAC in an involved driver. Even among those crashes with driver BAC of 0.01%, there were four times as many serious injuries as nonserious, compared with three times as many serious as nonserious injuries when vehicle drivers had a BAC level of 0.0%. Inference is limited, however, given that to be in the FARS data, there had to be at least one fatality. Nevertheless, findings held true for the 14-year time period analyzed, for both single- and multiple-vehicle crashes, and after excluding the potentially confounding variables of inattention and fatigue, suggesting that BAC, even at low levels, increases not only the risk of being in a crash, but also the risk of serious injury for each crash that occurs.

With respect to BAC levels below 0.08% and the increased risk of a fatal crash, findings from U.S. studies are generally consistent with those from other developed countries. A case-control study conducted by Connor et al. (2004) in Auckland, New Zealand, evaluated the effect of alcohol consumption on vehicle crashes in which at least one occupant was seriously injured or killed. Researchers interviewed and collected breath or blood tests from 571 drivers involved in serious crashes (cases) and 588 representative drivers (controls). If those involved in the crash were unable to partake in the interview, their next of kin or a proxy was interviewed instead. After controlling for confounders, drivers with a BAC level of 0.03–0.05% were 10 times more likely to be involved in a fatal crash than drivers who did not drink. Furthermore, the researchers estimated from their models that 34 to 35 percent of fatal crashes could be eliminated if drivers with BAC levels of at least 0.03% could be prevented from driving.

Another international study by Krüger and Vollrath (2004) used data from the German Roadside Survey conducted from 1992 to 1994 (Krüger et al., 1995) and weighted those data according to a study of representative drivers to calculate the risk of alcohol-related crashes in Germany. For drivers with BAC levels between 0.05% and 0.079%, there was an increased risk of being in a crash (odds ratio [OR] = 3.6, 95 percent confidence interval [CI] 2.3–5.7).

A recent empirical nonrandomized study by Byrne et al. (2016) evaluated the deterrent effectiveness of countermeasures put in place in Ontario in 2009 and 2010 that included implementation of administrative sanctions for drivers with BAC levels between 0.05% and 0.08%. With the new administrative sanctions in place, alcohol-impaired drivers with BAC levels in this range were subject to immediate license suspensions and administrative fines, and repeat offenders could be required to attend alcohol educational classes or install an ignition interlock on their vehicle. To evaluate the effectiveness of these new sanctions, researchers analyzed data from the Ontario Ministry of Transportation's Accident Data System and performed time series analyses. Between the time administrative sanctions were introduced and December 31, 2012, Byrne et al. estimated that the sanctions resulted in a 15 to 17 percent reduction in all alcohol-related driving crashes and a 12 percent reduction in major injuries and fatalities caused by alcohol-related driving crashes.

Effect of Lowering Blood Alcohol Limits for Driving

Lowering blood alcohol limits for driving to 0.05% Although there may be increased risk of a crash at BACs above 0.05%, that does not necessarily mean that lowering the legal limit to 0.05% would reduce crashes or crash fatalities. Therefore, the committee also evaluated international studies that assessed whether or the degree to which reducing the BAC limit to 0.05% is effective in decreasing alcohol-related crashes. Overall, the majority of international evidence suggests that lowering the BAC limit to 0.05% reduces alcohol-related crashes and driving fatalities, and those effects are greatest among those groups at highest risk. An international review by Mann et al. (2001) analyzed the effect of introducing or lowering the BAC limit on traffic safety measures. A total of 27 studies conducted between 1973 and 2000 were reviewed and, of those, 13 specifically looked at countries that had reduced or introduced a BAC limit of 0.05% (Bartl and Esberger, 2000; Bernhoft and Behrensdorff, 2003; Brooks and Zaal, 1992; Desapriya and Iwase, 1996; Henstridge et al., 1997; Kloeden and McLean, 1994; McLean et al., 1995; Mercier-Guyon, 1998; Noordzij, 1977, 1994; Smith, 1986; Van Ooijen, 1977; Vingilis et al., 1988). The remainder of the studies reviewed focused on the effects of BAC levels lowered to limits other than 0.05%.

The 13 studies on the effects of introducing or reducing the BAC limit to 0.05% were epidemiological time series analyses and pre-post comparisons that examined the changes in Australia, Austria, Canada, Denmark, France, Japan, and the Netherlands. Mann and colleagues found that the studies reviewed varied in rigor and results. The pre-post comparison studies were subject to the most confounding factors, but even complex time series analyses could sometimes be influenced by confounding variables. Nevertheless, all areas that lowered the BAC limit to 0.05% or that introduced a new BAC limit of 0.05% saw reductions in alcohol-related crashes, injuries, or fatalities, although some of these effects were temporary. In South Australia decreasing the BAC limit from 0.08% to 0.05% led to a 14.1 percent reduction in the proportion of drivers with a positive BAC compared to 2 years prior (Vingilis et al., 1988). In Austria, the same reduction in the BAC limit resulted in a 0.6 percent decline in the proportion of injuries caused by alcohol-impaired driving crashes nationwide (Bartl and Esberger, 2000). The review suggests that the overall significant decreases in alcohol-impaired driving are caused by a general deterrence effect as opposed to a targeted effect on drivers with a BAC of 0.05–0.079% because reductions in crash fatalities have been observed across a range of

BAC levels, not just those from 0.05% to 0.079%. The jurisdictions that had the most success in reducing traffic crashes by lowering the BAC broadly publicized the new law (e.g., publicity and education) and conducted highly visible sobriety checkpoints, thereby increasing the perceived risk of being caught. Some of the reviewed studies found that the beneficial effects of the new law declined over time, which the authors posited may have been attributable to the public's belief that, over time, the actual risk of apprehension was not as high as the perceived risk when the BAC limit was first lowered.

Albalate (2008) evaluated the effectiveness of lowering the BAC limit to 0.05% in eight European countries that changed their policies between 1991 and 2003 (Austria, Belgium, Denmark, France, Germany, Greece, Italy, and Spain), using a differences-in-differences estimation procedure in which the change in road traffic fatality rates in the country with the policy change was compared to the change in fatality rates of a control country that had not lowered its BAC. By using this approach the author was able to control for many possibly confounding variables, including socioeconomic factors such as unemployment and GDP growth rates, increasing use of motor vehicles in a country, the proportion of roads in the country that are highways and national roads, and the minimum legal drinking age. Albalate found that lowering the BAC limit to 0.05% was effective in reducing fatality rates by 4.3 percent and reducing fatality rates per kilometer driven by 6.1 percent. Among 20- to 40-year-olds, the BAC policy change reduced fatality rates by 10.5 percent, and among 40- to 50-year-olds, the BAC policy change led to an 8 percent reduction in fatality rates. No significant effect was found in females or in nonurban areas, although the authors suggested that this may be because the fatality rate among females was already low and other factors or road conditions may play a larger role in fatalities in rural areas. Among males the policy led to a 5.7 percent decrease in fatality rates and among urban males a 9.5 to 10.9 percent decrease. Lowering the BAC limit was only effective if paired with increased enforcement measures such as sobriety checkpoints. Positive effects of lowering the BAC limit were usually seen more than 2 years after the new policy went into effect.

Two recent studies evaluating the effect of lowering the BAC limit in Canada showed similar reductions in alcohol-related crashes and fatalities. Blais et al. (2015) studied the effectiveness of Canadian 0.05% administrative BAC laws by using data from the Traffic Injury Research Foundation and Statistics Canada to determine how newly instituted alcohol and driving measures may have affected alcohol-related crashes over a 24-year period. Blais and colleagues found that between 1987 and 2010, 0.05% administrative BAC laws were responsible for reducing the number of fatally injured drivers with BAC levels of 0.05% or higher by

4.1 percent (95 percent CI 0.8–7.5). A 3.5 percent reduction (95 percent CI 0.10–6.9) was also estimated in the number of fatally injured drivers with BAC levels exceeding 0.08%, and a 4.9 percent reduction (95 percent CI 1.35–8.51) was estimated in the number of fatally injured drivers with BAC levels exceeding 0.15%. Byrne et al. (2016) conducted a study in the province of Ontario to evaluate the deterrent effectiveness of new countermeasures, including lowering the BAC limit from 0.08% to 0.05%. The researchers found that the implementation of roadside suspensions for drivers with BAC levels between 0.05% and 0.08% resulted in a 17 percent decrease in injuries and fatalities related to alcohol-related crashes.

Recently, Fell and Scherer (2017) conducted a review and meta-analysis that included 36 empirical journal articles on international studies that analyzed the effects of lowering the BAC limit to 0.08% or lower. The authors calculated a pooled variance to standardize the changes observed in the different studies and determined an estimated effect size based on their results. They estimated that lowering the BAC limit from 0.08% to 0.05% in the United States would result in a decline in fatal alcohol-related crashes of 11.1 percent and save approximately 1,800 lives annually.

Lowering blood alcohol limits for driving to levels other than 0.05% (both lower and higher) The committee also reviewed evidence of the effect of laws lowering permissible BAC limits for driving to levels other than 0.05%. These studies find evidence of protective effects of lowering BAC limits to values higher and lower than 0.05%, which is important corroborating evidence that demonstrates consistency with studies where BAC limits are lowered to 0.05% specifically. Several studies provide a global perspective on the different levels of restriction that have been adopted throughout the past few decades—such as the 1990 BAC limit decrease in Sweden from 0.05% to 0.02% (Norstrom, 1997) and the 2002 BAC limit decrease in Japan from 0.05% to 0.03% (Desapriya et al., 2007; Nagata et al., 2006), both of which were effective in reducing alcohol-related driving fatalities. The evidence also finds that lowering the BAC limit from 0.10% to 0.08% for drivers in the United States was an effective policy for reducing alcohol-impaired traffic fatalities—particularly among young drivers, the age group at the highest risk for alcohol-related driving fatalities (Dee, 2001; Wagenaar et al., 2007). The majority of evidence on the effectiveness of lowering the BAC limit to levels other than 0.05% is based on time series studies and other pre-post designs that do not have a control population or quasi-experimental estimator. Of those that do, a meta-analysis shows a reduction in traffic fatalities (Wagenaar et al., 2007), but two other studies show limited effects (Freeman, 2007; Tippetts et al., 2005). Almost all available time series studies are suggestive of benefits to lowering the BAC limit (Andreuccetti et al., 2011; Apsler et al., 1999; Bernat et al., 2004; Blomberg, 1992; Dee, 2001; Foss et al., 2001; Freeman, 2007; Gorman et al., 2006; Nagata et al., 2008; Norstrom, 1997; Otero and Rau, 2017; Rogers, 1995; Tippetts et al., 2005; Voas et al., 2000, 2002; Wagenaar et al., 2007). There is also variation in the size and consistency of the effect, and these variations may be related to public knowledge of the laws and enforcement (Andreuccetti et al., 2011; Bernat et al., 2004; Nakahara et al., 2013; Schwartz and Davaran, 2013; Tippetts et al., 2005).

Summary of Evidence

The available evidence can be summarized as follows. In the United States, all states currently have per se regulations that it is criminal for adults to drive with a BAC over 0.08%; lower BAC cut-points are criminal for commercial drivers and underage drivers. Yet, alcohol impairs motor vehicle operation at BACs below 0.08%, with the preponderance of experimental driving simulator evidence suggesting that BAC levels above 0.02–0.03% are associated with impairment for most people (Irwin et al., 2017; Moskowitz and Fiorentino, 2000). With regard to crash risk, the preponderance of evidence indicates that risk of crash increases monotonically with alcohol consumption, especially for underage drivers, and for all drivers at BACs beginning around 0.03% (Blomberg et al., 2005; Peck et al., 2008; Voas et al., 2012; Zador, 1991; Zador et al., 2000). Thus, the committee concludes that alcohol consumption impairs motor vehicle safety at BACs above 0.03%, and increases crash risk monotonically at this level as well.

Due to this evidence, many countries around the world have decreased the BAC limit to drive to 0.05%. This allows for an assessment of the efficacy of lowering BAC to 0.05% on driving outcomes, acknowledging that generalization from other countries to the potential experience in the United States should be done with caution. Nevertheless, the preponderance of evidence indicates that lowering the BAC limit to 0.05% significantly and substantially reduces crash and fatality risk (Albalate, 2008; Blais et al., 2015; Byrne et al., 2016; Mann et al., 2001). Importantly, crash and fatality risks are reduced not only among those drivers at or around a BAC of 0.05% or in the range 0.05–0.079%, but also at *all BAC levels*. This is indicative of the general *deterrent* effect of lowering allowable BAC to drive, or of increased awareness of impaired driving across consumption levels. The impact of lower BAC laws is observable whether enforced through administrative or criminal sanctions, and seems enhanced when introduced alongside high-visibility enforcement, sobriety checkpoints, and publicity activities (Mann et al., 2001). For the United States, Fell and Scherer (2017) estimated an 11 percent decrease in fatal alcohol-related crashes, or approximately 1,800 fewer fatalities, if the BAC limit was lowered to 0.05%.

Based on the magnitude of effect and consistency of the evidence, the committee concludes that reducing the BAC limit to 0.05% is an effective strategy for reducing alcohol-impaired driving fatalities. The committee recommends BAC per se laws at 0.05% rather than another cutoff as it is the standard in many countries throughout the world, including most western countries, and thus has a solid evidence base for effective reductions in impaired driving.

Recommendation 4-1: State governments should enact per se laws for alcohol-impaired driving at 0.05% blood alcohol concentration (BAC). The federal government should incentivize this change, and other stakeholders should assist in this process. The enactment of 0.05% per se laws should be accompanied by media campaigns and robust and visible enforcement efforts.

The effectiveness of lowering the per se laws from 0.08% to 0.05% will be supported by legislation that currently applies to 0.08% per se laws, including, but not limited to, use of sobriety checkpoints, administrative license revocation, and penalties for refusing preliminary breath tests or blood tests that are equal to or greater than penalties for alcohol-impaired driving offenses. This means that the same laws and sanctions that currently apply to 0.08% per se laws could remain in place but would be enforceable at the 0.05% BAC limit. Effectiveness will also be enhanced by efforts to publicize 0.05% per se laws through mass media campaigns, by strong and sustained enforcement efforts, and through the implementation and enforcement of laws and policies to prevent illegal alcohol sales to underage or intoxicated persons (e.g., underage compliance checks with alcohol licensees, dram shop liability laws). Incentives from the federal government could include incentive grants to states or, if necessary, the threat of losing highway funding, as was done with the passage of the 0.08% per se laws. Countries with a 0.05% BAC limit implement the law through either administrative sanctions (a traffic citation with sanctions that may include insurance company notification, license suspension, and/or fines) or criminal offenses with various sanctions for drivers with a BAC between 0.05% and 0.079%. The committee offers this recommendation with the understanding that alcohol impairment and increased crash risk begin at BAC levels well below 0.08%. The primary intent of this recommendation is to reduce serious injuries and fatalities caused by alcohol-related crashes, as well as to align with other developed nations and their impaired-driver laws.

Potential Barriers to Adoption and Opportunities

Lowering the BAC limit in the United States from 0.08% to 0.05% will present several challenges. While many other countries have demonstrated reductions in injuries and fatalities after lowering driving BAC limits to 0.05%, variations in population characteristics, the constitutional rights of citizens, and law enforcement strategies make it difficult to draw direct correlations between experiences in those countries and potential effectiveness in the United States. There is an opportunity, however, to learn from the experiences of other countries that lowered the BAC limit and prepare for any challenges they faced. Moreover, implementation on a state-by-state basis would likely occur over time and assessments of the impacts could be conducted to inform decisions in other states.

Critics of lowering the BAC limit from 0.08% to 0.05% have argued that adoption of lower BAC limits may be onerous for police officers to enforce and could place an undue burden on the court system; however, this has not been demonstrated in studies conducted in other countries where the BAC limit has been lowered. While it is true that lowering the BAC limit to 0.05% would increase the number of drivers who fit the legal definition of being alcohol impaired, studies in other countries have shown that when the BAC limit was lowered—especially when accompanied by a well-publicized marketing campaign—there was a greater perceived risk of sanctions for drivers, which resulted in fewer alcohol-impaired drivers on the roads and a reduction in alcohol-related crashes (Albalate, 2008; Blais et al., 2015; Kloeden and McLean, 1994; Mann et al., 2001; Otero and Rau, 2017). Lowering the BAC limit also had a deterrent effect for young and new drivers, as well as drivers with no prior alcohol-related violations (Byrne et al., 2016).

Although lowering the BAC limit may result in fewer alcohol-impaired drivers on the roads, law enforcement officials would still require special training and equipment to allow them to detect impaired drivers, as is currently the case for 0.08% laws. Enforcement of a 0.05% per se law will depend on the amount of available resources for, among other things, conducting trainings, increasing police presence, and accurately conducting frequent sobriety checkpoints. It should be noted, however, that these concerns currently exist for enforcement of 0.08% laws.

Advocacy and special interest groups can have a significant effect on the public's perception or acceptance of new public policies (Molnar et al., 2017). An example of this was seen in Utah with the passage of the first U.S. law lowering the BAC limit from 0.08% to 0.05%, which is scheduled to go into effect on December 30, 2018 (Utah State Legislature, 2017). Although a recent poll found that 51 percent of Utah residents opposed the bill, support by members of the Church of Jesus Christ of Latter-Day Saints, a group that prohibits the use of alcohol as part of their church doctrine, has been credited with being instrumental for passage of the new state law (UtahPolicy.com, 2017). Despite the support that the new law received in Utah, other advocacy groups have been largely silent on the issue or have opposed it outright. MADD, arguably the most vocal proponent of reducing alcohol-impaired driving and a leading advocate in the fight to lower the BAC limit from 0.10% to 0.08%, has chosen to maintain their support of a BAC limit of 0.08% and did not support the new Utah legislation (MADD, 2017). The American Automobile Association (AAA) also has focused on other issues such as distracted, drowsy, aggressive, and impaired (defined broadly) driving (AAA, 2017). Garnering the support of MADD, AAA, and other safe driving advocacy groups would help to increase support for decreasing the BAC limit to 0.05%. Opposition to decreasing the BAC limit to 0.05% has come from distilled spirits lobbying groups, such as the American Beverage Institute (ABI). When the new BAC legislation was pending in Utah, ABI used aggressive marketing campaigns in Utah and neighboring states, and online petitions, to try to defeat the legislation (ABI, 2017a,b,c,d).

Collecting and marketing accurate information to the public is an important component of any plan to increase support for new laws lowering the BAC limit to 0.05%. As with any successful campaign, it is important for advocacy and research groups to work in concert to present a unified message and clearly counter any misleading or inaccurate information. Research into the best practices for launching, focusing, and running a successful campaign to increase support of new laws lowering BAC limits would advance the likelihood of passing new legislation and decreasing the number of alcohol-related crashes, injuries, and fatalities.

Despite the success in Utah of passing the first BAC 0.05% law and the submission of similar bills in Washington State (Washington State House of Representatives, 2017) and Hawaii (Hawaii State Legislature, 2017), support for changing U.S. laws more broadly has been lacking. Political leaders will typically act on behalf of constituents who cast their votes, and constituents have been largely silent on this issue. Alternatively, some individuals may oppose the legislation because of erroneous information such as that the law will unfairly target social drinkers or that having one drink will result in a BAC that exceeds the limit set by state law, neither of which are true (see Figure 4-1 for BAC calculation). To overcome misunderstandings among politicians and the general public, advocates for change will have to be clear and consistent with their message regarding exactly what the laws mean for drivers and the potential lives that could be saved by lowering the BAC limit across the country (Eby et al., 2017). To succeed with lowering the BAC would require a groundswell of support from grassroots organizations and voters to research and understand the issues, have access to the most credible data available from which to make policy decisions, and be motivated to work on behalf of adopting strategies and legislation that can potentially save lives (see Chapter 7 on generating action for more information and a recommendation on model legislation to improve uniformity and the adoption of effective policies nationwide).

What Would It Take to Pass a 0.05% BAC Law?

The evidence reviewed by the committee suggests that lowering BAC per se laws is an effective policy in reducing alcohol-impaired driving fatalities, nonfatal injuries, and crashes. By studying the process of lowering the BAC limit from 0.10% to 0.08% in the United States, there are insights to be learned regarding what it might take to lower it further to 0.05%. Opposition against lowering the BAC per se law from 0.10% to 0.08% was strongest among the alcohol and hospitality industries and opposing legislators (Rodriguez-Iglesias et al., 2001). At that time, the main arguments in opposition to the bill were that it was unnecessary because the states already had administrative sanctions at 0.08% or that other interventions, such as increased penalties for repeat offenders, would have a greater effect on reducing alcohol-impaired driving and would not target "social" drinkers (i.e., those with BAC levels between 0.08% and 0.099%) (Rodriguez-Iglesias et al., 2001).

A study funded by NHTSA in 2001 analyzed the process of lowering the BAC per se law to 0.08% in six states, four of which had passed the law at the time of the study (Illinois, Texas, Virginia, and Washington) and two of which had not (Maryland and Minnesota) (Rodriguez-Iglesias et al., 2001). Through in-depth interviews with those involved in the process, the authors identified the following five components that were essential for getting the law passed: strong influential leadership from a key individual who is committed to the issue; the formation of strong advocacy coalitions with public and private support; bipartisan support for the bill; an effective mass media campaign; and a strong working relationship between advocates and opponents. As noted earlier, the effectiveness of lowering the per se laws to 0.05% will be supported by legislation that currently applies to 0.08% per se laws.

Laws Pertaining to Young and Inexperienced Drivers

Although motor vehicle crashes remain at the top of the list of leading causes of death for U.S. teens, the number of fatalities from crashes involving teen drivers, persons 15–20 years of age, has steadily declined from 3,490 fatalities in 2006 to 1,886 in 2015 (NHTSA, 2017a). Two laws that have been proven to be effective interventions for reducing crashes and fatalities in drivers under the age of 21 are zero tolerance laws and graduated driver licensing (GDL) laws.

Zero Tolerance Laws

Zero tolerance laws, enacted in all 50 states and the District of Columbia, make it illegal for drivers under the age of 21 to drive with alcohol in their system (BAC levels in excess of 0.0–0.02%, to allow for variance in testing results). Studies of these laws have found them to be highly effective for reducing the number of young drivers who get behind the wheel after consuming alcohol (CDC, 2012; Fell et al., 2009, 2016; Haegerich et al., 2016; Liang and Huang, 2008; Shults et al., 2001).

Graduated Driver Licensing Laws

All 50 states and the District of Columbia have some form of GDL systems in place for teen drivers (CDC, 2016). These systems restrict driving privileges for teens depending on their age, the length of time they have been driving, or the time of day when they are allowed to drive a vehicle. Although specific regulations vary by state, different stages of licensure include:

- Teens with a *learners permit* can only drive with a licensed, adult driver in the vehicle, and the teens may have to meet a minimum age requirement for eligibility (McCartt et al., 2010);
- A *provisional license* allows a teen to drive without an adult in the vehicle, but the teen's driving may be restricted to certain hours of the day or night or the teen may be prohibited from driving with teenage passengers in their vehicle; and
- An *unrestricted license* allows a driver to drive a vehicle without time or passenger restrictions (CDC, 2016).

GDL systems have been found to be effective for reducing the number of crashes involving young, inexperienced drivers (Curry et al., 2017; Fell et al., 2011, 2016; Masten et al., 2011; McCartt et al., 2010; Salam et al., 2016; Williams et al., 2016). States with GDL systems rated as "good"—based on unsupervised driving restrictions, minimum age requirements for obtaining learners permits, and driving restrictions after licensing for a period of time or until a certain age—were associated with a 30 percent reduction in fatal crashes involving 15- to 17-year-old drivers (McCartt et al., 2010), and, although findings were not uniform for all teens, stronger GDL programs were significantly associated with a decrease in fatal crash risk for 16-year-old drivers (rate ratio = 0.74; 95 percent CI 0.65–0.84)

(Masten et al., 2011). In a study looking at long-term effects of the North Carolina GDL program, 16-year-old drivers who received their license under the GDL system had a lower incidence of first crashes than pre-GDL system drivers, and 16- to 17-year-old drivers' crash incidence was 10 percent lower than comparable drivers who received their driver's license prior to the adoption of the GDL system (Masten and Foss, 2010). The largest reductions in fatal crashes among teen drivers were seen in states with stricter nighttime driving restrictions and states that restricted new drivers to zero or one passenger for a designated period of time after receiving their driver's license (McCartt et al., 2010).

It should be noted that many teens opt to delay obtaining a driver's license until the age of 18, thereby exempting themselves from GDL restrictions. Some of the primary reasons cited for delaying licensure include a lack of time, money, or interest; limited or no access to a vehicle; or choosing alternate transportation options that do not require a driver's license such as riding with friends, biking, walking, or ride-sharing options; however, gender, race, and socioeconomic status have also been shown to impact the likelihood of obtaining a driver's license (Romano et al., 2011; Schoettle and Sivak, 2013; Tefft et al., 2013, 2014). It is possible that some teens may opt to delay obtaining a driver's license until they are beyond the age when they would be subject to GDL restrictions, but, although this could happen, studies have not identified this as a significant concern (Shoettle and Sivak, 2013; Tefft et al., 2013).

Any alcohol use by a teen driver is a serious and dangerous offense. Of the teen drivers killed in 2015, 26 percent had BAC levels of 0.01% or higher and 80 percent of those killed had BAC levels that equaled or exceeded 0.08%, the limit set by state law for drivers over the age of 21 (NHTSA, 2017a). Drinking by novice drivers over the legal drinking age is a further concern, especially since drivers over the age of 18 are not subject to the GDL restrictions and therefore can drive at any hour, without passenger restrictions. More research is needed to investigate how to restrict teen and novice drivers from getting behind the wheel after consuming alcohol. Efforts should also be made to develop strategies for restricting passengers from riding in a vehicle driven by an impaired driver, including vehicles driven by teen or novice drivers (Li et al., 2013; Walker et al., 2003).

Summary of Zero Tolerance Laws and Graduated Licensing Laws

Studies of zero tolerance and graduated licensure laws have found that the creation of high-visibility enforcement programs targeting young drivers (Johnson, 2016), increasing or strengthening existing state licensing restrictions (Williams et al., 2016), further restricting the hours when young drivers can operate a motor vehicle (Curry et al., 2017; Shults and Williams, 2016), or promoting awareness of license restrictions to parents of teens (Naz and Scott-Parker, 2017) could increase the effectiveness of existing laws. More research is needed to identify how new drivers over the age of 18 fare without GDL restrictions and whether driving restrictions should be compulsory for all novice drivers. Research is also needed into further limiting alcohol-impaired driving among teens and new drivers, and strategies for preventing passengers from riding with those drivers.

DWI Child Endangerment Laws

DWI child endangerment laws target alcohol-impaired drivers who are found driving with children in their vehicles. Currently in the United States, all but three states—New Mexico, South Dakota, and Vermont—have some form of DWI child endangerment law and 42 states subject alcohol-impaired drivers to additional penalties if they are caught driving with children in their vehicle at the time of their arrest (NDAA, 2015). There is a great deal of variation between states regarding the ages of drivers and/or children who are covered by these laws, and punishments can vary from fines to community service, installation of an ignition interlock device, or imprisonment depending on details of the arrest and the state where the offense took place. Despite existing DWI child endangerment laws, children continue to be killed in crashes involving alcohol-impaired drivers. Of the 1,132 children ages 14 and younger who were killed in motor vehicle traffic crashes in 2015, 16 percent, or 181 children, were killed in alcohol-impaired driving crashes. Just over half of those children killed—92 out of 181—were passengers in vehicles driven by individuals with BAC levels that met or exceeded the limit set by state law for DWI (NHTSA, 2016a).

There is limited research regarding the efficacy of child endangerment laws as they pertain to alcohol-impaired driving, and what data exist suggest that these laws have not been effective in reducing child fatalities (Kelley-Baker and Romano, 2014, 2016; Quinlan et al., 2000; Thomas et al., 2014). Researchers have suggested that examining the effectiveness and impact of current laws, collecting and studying more granular data regarding detailed crash information and the age and gender of drivers and victims, or increasing public awareness of existing DWI child endangerment laws may lead to a greater understanding of how to increase the effectiveness of DWI child endangerment laws and eventually help to reduce the likelihood of future child fatalities in alcohol-related crashes (Kelley-Baker and Romano, 2014, 2016; Thomas et al., 2014).

ENFORCEMENT AND ARREST

Interventions for reducing alcohol-impaired driving fatalities can take many forms. One intervention in the area of enforcement and arrest that shows promise is the use of sobriety checkpoints.

Sobriety Checkpoints

Background

Sobriety checkpoints are a high-visibility prevention and enforcement strategy that aims to prevent alcohol-impaired driving. Law enforcement officers can conduct breath testing at sobriety checkpoints selectively or randomly. For selective breath testing, which is used in the United States, law enforcement officers stop vehicles and conduct a breath test on the driver only when they observe and suspect impairment (Bergen et al., 2014a). For random breath testing, which is used in many European countries and Australia but illegal in the United States, officers breath test all stopped drivers (Bergen et al., 2014a). Among states in which conducting sobriety checkpoints is legal, 58 to 72 percent of law enforcement and state patrol agencies conduct sobriety checkpoints (Eichelberger and McCartt, 2016; Erickson et al., 2015).

Although the legality of sobriety checkpoints was challenged when law enforcement agencies in the United States began using them in the early 1980s, the Supreme Court ruled that they present "a minimal and acceptable intrusion given the benefit of preventing impaired driving and the small amount of time required of nonimpaired drivers" (Bergen et al., 2014a). Currently 37 states, the District of Columbia, and 2 U.S. territories (the Northern Mariana Islands and the Virgin Islands) conduct sobriety checkpoints; states that do not allow sobriety checkpoints include Idaho, Iowa, Michigan, Minnesota, Oregon, Rhode Island, Texas, Washington, Wisconsin, and Wyoming (GHSA, n.d.; IIHS and HLDI, 2017).

Evidence

The Community Preventive Services Task Force found strong evidence for the effectiveness of publicized sobriety checkpoint programs based on the results of a systematic review of studies published between 2000 and 2012 (Bergen et al., 2014a). Based on 10 studies that reported the number of alcohol-related crash fatalities, the median relative decrease in alcohol-related crash fatalities was 8.9 percent (interquartile interval: –16.5, –3.4). Fatality decreases were attributed to publicized sobriety checkpoint programs implemented at city, county, state, and national levels as well as in rural, urban, and both rural and urban areas, indicating their effectiveness across a wide range of settings. Two considerations described by the authors are the importance of including media campaigns in sobriety checkpoint programs and of implementing multiple checkpoints over a relatively long period of time (e.g., 1 to 3 years). The findings of the review are consistent with a previous review conducted by the Task Force, which found that sobriety checkpoints decreased alcohol-related crashes by 20 percent with selective breath testing and by 18 percent with random breath testing (Shults, 2001). A meta-analysis found that sobriety checkpoints decreased alcohol-related crashes by 17 percent (14 percent when controlling for publication bias) and all-cause crashes by 10 to 15 percent (Erke et al., 2009). The effectiveness of sobriety checkpoints was also found to increase when breath testing was performed on all stopped drivers, as is standard practice in several countries, including Australia and New Zealand. More recently, Lenk et al. (2016) found that states in which conducting sobriety checkpoints is legal had an 18.2 percent lower rate of alcohol-impaired driving; of these, the states that conduct sobriety checkpoints at least monthly had a 40.6 percent lower rate of alcohol-impaired driving. Additionally, Hingson et al. (1996) found that combining the use of sobriety checkpoints with enforcement of speeding laws can be an effective strategy for enforcing DWI laws since alcohol-impaired drivers are more likely to drive at excessive speeds.

Some state and local jurisdictions employ saturation patrols either in conjunction with sobriety checkpoints or on their own. When conducting saturation patrols, law enforcement officials carry out alcohol-impaired driving enforcement efforts within specific geographic areas rather than at one specific location. In some cases these patrols may be used when state or local laws restrict the use of sobriety checkpoints. A recent study by Erickson et al. (2015) found that 95.8 percent of state patrol agencies and 62.7 percent of local law enforcement agencies used saturation patrols. Saturation patrols have been shown to be inversely associated with self-reported alcohol-impaired driving; however, they are more effective when combined with other enforcement strategies (such as sobriety checkpoints or seatbelt enforcement) and when advertised through a media campaign (Sanem et al., 2015).

NHTSA's *Countermeasures That Work* rates the effectiveness of sobriety checkpoints as high and notes that implementation time can be short when law enforcement officers are appropriately trained (Goodwin et al., 2015). Costs are rated as medium,[4] as checkpoints with at least 15 officers typically cost between \$5,000 and \$7,000 and publicity through paid media exposure can significantly increase costs (e.g., budgets for

[4] Costs in the medium category (designated as \$\$ in the study) are defined as requiring some additional staff time, equipment, facilities, and/or publicity (Goodwin et al., 2015).

a specific sobriety checkpoint program's media exposure ranged from $25,000 to $433,000 depending on the state). However, costs can be realistically managed with smaller numbers of staff, which can cost as little as $500 to $1,500 (Goodwin et al., 2015) (and for which NHTSA offers a planning, operation, and evaluation guidance) (NHTSA, 2006), and with earned media exposure.

State-level publicized enforcement demonstration programs in seven states realized an 11 to 20 percent decrease in alcohol-related fatalities in states where checkpoints or other highly visible impaired driving enforcement operations were carried out and where enforcement activities were covered by intensive publicity, including paid advertising (Fell et al., 2008). Evaluations of statewide campaigns in Connecticut (Zwicker et al., 2007a) and West Virginia (Zwicker et al., 2007b), which included sobriety checkpoints along with extensive paid media, realized declines in alcohol-related fatalities following the campaigns and fewer drivers who had positive BAC levels at roadside surveys. Researchers have also examined effective sobriety checkpoint programs in Georgia, Louisiana, Pennsylvania, Tennessee (Fell et al., 2005), and Maryland (Beck and Moser, 2004).

Barriers

One of the primary barriers to a more widespread use of sobriety checkpoints is a shortage of law enforcement staff and financial resources available to devote to these efforts (Bergen et al., 2014a; Fell et al., 2003; Goodwin et al., 2015). The greatest costs for sobriety checkpoint implementation are officer time and publicity (Goodwin et al., 2015). In some states law enforcement agencies also face legal obstacles that prevent sobriety checkpoints and breath testing (Voas and Fell, 2013). While some states have authorized sobriety checkpoint use through state law, state law or interpretations of federal law prohibit use of and/or funding for sobriety checkpoints in other states (GHSA, n.d.). Driver privacy is also a concern, as drivers stopped at sobriety checkpoints may find the breath-testing process to be intrusive (Bergen et al., 2014a). However, as previously mentioned, such concerns were addressed by the U.S. Supreme Court, which deemed sobriety checkpoints a minimally intrusive inconvenience to non-alcohol-impaired drivers and acceptable given their potential to detect alcohol-impaired drivers (Bergen et al., 2014a).

A strategy that may increase the effectiveness and visibility of sobriety checkpoint programs is to implement and advertise "No Refusal" nights and/or weekends, during which law enforcement officials may quickly obtain a search warrant for a blood sample from a driver suspected of alcohol-impaired driving who refuses a breath test. "No Refusal" nights and weekends are typically implemented during national holidays (such as Fourth of July and New Year's Eve) and on days of large events (such as St. Patrick's Day and Super Bowl Sunday). In jurisdictions that have implemented "No Refusal" initiatives, officers may request search warrants from on-call judges by phone to obtain blood test results legally and more swiftly for conviction (NHTSA, n.d.-b). These search warrants, usually issued as electronic warrants, are discussed in more detail in Chapter 5.

The first "No Refusal" effort to be implemented was the "No Refusal Weekends" initiative that has existed in certain jurisdictions in Texas since 2005. In one county the program led to a decrease in breath test refusal rates at sobriety checkpoints from 50 percent in 2005 to 10 percent in 2010; in addition, DWI conviction rates have significantly increased and case dismissal rates have decreased (NHTSA, n.d.-b). Funding from the Texas Department of Transportation pays for additional time required of prosecutors and for nurses to obtain blood for BAC testing and has enabled an increase in the number of "No Refusal" nights each year from 16 to 56 (GHSA, 2011).

A limitation of "No Refusal" initiatives is that the additional resources and personnel needed to obtain search warrants may be burdensome for jurisdictions already working with limited resources (Winkler, 2012). In addition, the legality of "No Refusal" programs has been challenged in several states as a violation to the Fourth Amendment; however, courts have maintained that it is only unconstitutional to obtain a blood test when done so without a warrant (Solomon, 2014). Other criticisms include that "No Refusal" laws do not specify how long prosecutors may keep blood samples in their possession and that judges are quick to sign search warrants and rarely, if ever, turn them down (Winkler, 2012). Nonetheless, "No Refusal" laws in some states have successfully increased both the proportion of drivers who agree to a breath test and rates of DWI convictions (Sommer, 2016). However, stronger evidence will be needed to more accurately ascertain their effect.

A toolkit of informational and promotional materials for implementing and advertising "No Refusal" programs is available online from NHTSA (2017b). Information from the toolkit's website states that nine states (Arizona, Florida, Idaho, Illinois, Kansas, Louisiana, Missouri, Texas, and Utah) have implemented "No Refusal" programs; of those that have not, 21 states have the "necessary legal authority" in place to do so (NHTSA, n.d.-b).

Unintended Consequences

Evidence suggests that racial profiling and targeting of undocumented immigrants are two potential unintended consequences of sobriety checkpoint programs in the United States. In 2010 law enforcement officers in Escondido, California, enlisted the help of U.S. Immigration and Customs Enforcement to screen for immigration status at sobriety checkpoints; 10 unlicensed drivers (a majority of unlicensed drivers are undocumented immigrants) were discovered for every alcohol-impaired driver (Cavanaugh et al., 2012). The potential for law enforcement agencies and towing companies to profit financially from sobriety checkpoint programs has also contributed to racial profiling and targeting of undocumented immigrants. In 2009 sobriety checkpoints in the California cities of Oakland, San Jose, San Rafael, Hayward, and Redwood City generated about $40 million from towing and law enforcement fines; the majority of impounded motor vehicles were taken from persons of racial or ethnic minority, many of whom were undocumented immigrants (Gabrielson, 2010). In stark comparison, the California Highway Patrol does not collect revenue from motor vehicle seizures and in 2008 arrested four alcohol-impaired drivers for every vehicle seized (Gabrielson, 2010).

Racial profiling and financial profitability could undermine the success of sobriety checkpoint programs in detecting alcohol-impaired drivers and reducing resulting crashes and fatalities. To minimize the risk of racial profiling, Bergen et al. (2014a) encourage systematic selection and standardized methodology to select vehicles and drivers for breath testing so driver selection is not left to the discretion of individual law enforcement officers. See Chapter 2 for a discussion on the importance of health equity considerations specific to the implementation of interventions to reduce alcohol-impaired driving.

Cost-Effectiveness

A number of studies were identified that explicitly examined the cost-effectiveness or cost-benefit of sobriety checkpoints. Among these, results varied somewhat owing to differences between countries and/or states analyzed, measurements of costs, time periods covered and duration of follow-up periods, variation in study populations, and outcomes analyzed (fatalities only and injuries). An analysis of various studies by the Community Preventive Services Task Force found that the benefits of sobriety checkpoints outweighed the costs (Ditter et al., 2005); however, because of gaps in the literature, competing policies and perspectives, cost differences, and differences in outcome measurements, accurately measuring and comparing the cost-effectiveness of these interventions can be difficult. The same studies are also reviewed and summarized by Bergen et al. (2014a) and this review again concluded that publicized sobriety checkpoints are cost-effective and suggest that the cost-effectiveness may increase when operated at a higher scale. Of the five studies reviewed by the Community Preventive Services Task Force (Ditter et al., 2005) and Bergen et al. (2014a), a study by Stuster and Blowers (1995) conducted in California would be most applicable to U.S. policy making. The other cost-benefit studies included in the reviews were conducted in the Netherlands (Wesemann, 1989), New Zealand (Miller et al., 2004), and South Wales (Arthurson, 1985), which makes them less instructive for the United States since the impact and cost-effectiveness is based on driving patterns, road structure, and other interventions and policies that are time and place specific. Since some of these dimensions also vary between states, the findings from the California study may not be applicable across all U.S. states. Overall, although the conclusions reached by the Community Preventive Services Task Force (Ditter et al., 2005) and Bergen et al. (2014a) suggest that sobriety checkpoints would likely be cost-effective, the reviewed studies may be outdated, and most occur in countries other than the United States and have somewhat weak methods and measures. For these reasons, confidence in these findings is not high.

Taking a different approach, Miller et al. (1998) modeled potential monetary benefits of a sobriety checkpoint in a hypothetical community. Using information from a sobriety checkpoint program in Tennessee to model outcomes, the study authors predicted that the program saved the community $6 for every $1 spent. Costs and estimated monetary benefits in the study were defined in terms of potential cost reductions or savings—measured in the categories of medical care, public programs, property damage, future earnings, and quality of life—resulting from a sobriety checkpoint program. However, the calculations may not be generalizable because of the study's focus on one specific program, the use of a hypothetical community, and the length of time that has passed since the study was conducted.

In summary, the evidence across multiple studies weakly suggests that sobriety checkpoints could be cost-effective depending on how they are conducted (randomized or selective), how often they occur, the scale or intensity (high or low level) with which they are carried out, and whether they are accompanied by media campaigns. In order to be confident of the cost-effectiveness of sobriety checkpoints, new and more rigorous studies are needed.

International Perspective

There is strong evidence for the effectiveness of publicized sobriety checkpoint programs in other countries, including Australia, Canada, New Zealand, Spain, Taiwan, and Thailand (Alcañiz et al., 2014; Chang and Shih, 2012; Chuliá et al., 2016; Ditsuwan et al., 2015; Erke et al., 2009; Miller et al., 2004; Solomon et al., 2011).

In addition to the selective and random breath-testing methods used in these countries, Sweden has recently piloted a sobriety checkpoint program with automated breath testing. A Swedish traffic safety non-profit, MHF, has developed and implemented an automated sobriety checkpoint that is currently in use in Stockholm. Known as Alco Gates, the checkpoint is located in Frihamnen, a harbor where large cruise ships dock to enter Stockholm. Passengers traveling with vehicles disembark by driving to the checkpoint and blowing into a noncontact breath testing device, after which a boom gate lifts if the driver is found to be sober (Ascarelli, 2014). The checkpoint is operated by a control station and traffic management center that monitors the system with 16 cameras and 30 sensors and is capable of communicating with drivers in 12 different languages. The checkpoint is compliant with Swedish law and reported 244 alcohol-impaired drivers out of 46,553 passengers over a trial interval of 12 months (Sjöström and Jonsson, n.d.). Following evaluation and reporting of results from the trial in 2015, the Swedish government implemented Alco Gates at several additional ports. Implementation of Alco Gates has been a collaborative effort between MHF and the Swedish Transport Administration, the Swedish Police Authority, the Swedish Customs Service, the Swedish Coast Guard, Ports of Stockholm, and shipping companies whose cruise services access the port (Sjöström and Jonsson, n.d.).

Special Populations

Low-staff, weekly sobriety checkpoint programs can be effective at reducing alcohol-impaired driving in small rural communities (Lacey et al., 2006) and well-publicized, highly visible sobriety checkpoints have been credited with reducing injuries from alcohol-impaired driving in American Indian/Alaska Native reservations (Piontkowski et al., 2015). Box 4-1 describes a successful motor vehicle injury prevention program implemented in a tribal community in Arizona that combined sobriety checkpoints with culturally appropriate social marketing methods, emphasizing the importance of publicity and high visibility for sobriety checkpoints to be effective. In addition to benefiting rural populations, sobriety checkpoints have also been effective at reducing alcohol-related crashes in high-risk populations including men and young people 21 to 34 years (Bergen et al., 2014a).

The University of Wisconsin Population Health Institute's *What Works for Health* evidence review on strategies to improve rural health identifies sobriety checkpoints as a scientifically supported strategy (defined as having been tested in multiple robust studies with consistently positive results) (Bergum et al., 2016). Rural law enforcement agencies may be particularly lacking in personnel to staff sobriety checkpoints. However,

BOX 4-1
San Carlos Apache Motor Vehicle Injury Prevention Program

Setting: The San Carlos Apache Indian Reservation in central Arizona is home to roughly 11,000 tribal members. The tribe's unemployment rate in 2010 was 64 percent, and nearly 42 percent of the population lives below the federal poverty line. The Motor-Vehicle Injury Prevention Program was funded through the Tribal Injury Prevention Cooperative Agreement Program (TIPCAP) and the Indian Health Service from 2004 to 2009. Because of its success, it was again funded in 2010 to 2015 by another TIPCAP award. The goal of the project was to reduce alcohol-impaired driving and increase occupant protection by expanding seat belt usage.

Strategies: The project coordinators used a social marketing approach to get the word out about the program and its activities, and to disseminate messages about the problem of alcohol-impaired driving. Focus groups with tribal members were conducted to tailor culturally appropriate messaging about the program and the problem of alcohol-impaired driving. The marketing logos incorporated local, culturally significant designs. Messaging was also increased on tribal holidays and used evidence-based slogans to ensure that the most appropriate messages were reaching the target audience.

The program used numerous high-visibility DWI checkpoints across the reservation on strategically planned days and times based on anecdotal evidence and crash report data. The program coordinators used creative and meaningful incentives for police officers to encourage participation in the program. The police department increased patrols at high-risk times in high-risk areas. The tribe passed laws that lowered the blood alcohol concentration limit from 0.10% to 0.08% and made seat belt violations a stoppable offense.

Outcomes: Seat belt use increased from 19 percent in 2011 to 47 percent in 2013. Motor vehicle crashes decreased significantly by about 5 to 7 percent per year over the 10 years the program was funded. Community attitudes about DWI prevention and seat belt use also changed over the course of the program, as did their knowledge about appropriate designated driver usage.

SOURCE: Piontkowski et al., 2015.

low-staff sobriety checkpoints do not require the amount of personnel and resources that are commonly deployed (i.e., 12 to 15 police officers on site) (IIHS, 2005; Stuster and Blowers, 1995). Lacey et al. (2006) examined the effectiveness of weekly, low-staffed sobriety checkpoints (three to five police officers) in two rural counties in West Virginia over a 1-year period and estimated a 70 percent reduction in drivers with BAC levels ≥0.05% in the experimental counties relative to the control counties. Interestingly, the proportion of drivers who had been drinking at all (BAC ≥0.01%) only declined by 5 percent. Residents were surveyed at baseline and postintervention on whether they had seen or heard about a police checkpoint in the past 30 days and the proportion that responded yes increased significantly between baseline and postintervention periods (41 versus 62 percent).

When low-staff checkpoints were integrated into West Virginia's statewide comprehensive program to reduce traffic crashes, the state saw a 17.3 percent reduction in alcohol-related driving fatalities the following year and an 8.1 percent decrease the year after that (Neil, 2006). West Virginia continues to conduct low-staff checkpoints as indicated by its 2017 Highway Safety Plan (Tomblin et al., 2016).

Passive alcohol sensors can be used during checkpoints to assist officers in detecting drinking drivers. The passive alcohol sensor is a device, usually integrated into an officer's flashlight or clipboard, that measures whether alcohol is detected in the air where the driver is breathing. They can be used without notifying the driver and without probable cause because they are considered "an extension of the officer's nose" and are nonintrusive. Detection of alcohol using a passive alcohol sensor can give the officer probable cause to request standard field sobriety tests. Passive alcohol sensors are generally reliable and effective at detecting alcohol in ambient air, especially during checkpoints, where officers have very little time to screen drivers (they can increase detection of drivers with BAC levels ≥0.10% by up to 50 percent) (Fell and Compton, 2007). A major barrier to the common use of passive alcohol sensors is the lack of acceptance among law enforcement. Some reasons include requiring the officer to be closer than they would like to the drivers; requiring a portion of the officer's attention, which may need to be focused on more pertinent things like their personal safety; keeping them from having one of their hands free; and some officers believe they do not need the device to detect alcohol (Goodwin et al., 2005; Preusser, 2000).

Conclusion

Evidence indicates that publicized sobriety checkpoints are effective at decreasing alcohol-impaired driving and resulting crashes and fatalities. As described in this section, two systematic reviews conducted by the Community Preventive Services Task Force (Bergen et al., 2014a; Shults, 2001) and a meta-analysis conducted by Erke et al. (2009) found that publicized sobriety checkpoint programs with selective or random breath testing were effective at decreasing alcohol-impaired driving and resulting crashes and fatalities in rural and urban areas as well as at city, county, state, and national levels. More recently, Lenk et al. (2016) found that states that conduct sobriety checkpoints at least monthly had a 40.6 percent lower rate of alcohol-impaired driving. In addition, NHTSA has supported the effectiveness of sobriety checkpoints in its *Countermeasures That Work*. Results from studies of sobriety checkpoint programs in several states also indicate that they are effective when paired with publicity and advertising efforts (Beck and Moser, 2004; Fell et al., 2005, 2008; Zwicker et al., 2007a,b) or enforcement of speeding laws (Hingson et al., 1996). Evidence also suggests that sobriety checkpoints are effective among specific, often high-risk, populations including small rural communities (Lacey et al., 2006), American Indian/Alaska Native reservations (Piontkowski et al., 2015), and for men and young people 21 to 34 years of age (Bergen et al., 2014a). In addition, there is some evidence to suggest that sobriety checkpoints are cost-effective; however, results from these studies indicate that the cost-effectiveness of sobriety checkpoints depends on several factors related to their implementation. Updated studies with more rigorous methods are needed to more accurately and confidently assess the cost-effectiveness of sobriety checkpoints. Based on its review of a strong body of evidence supporting the effectiveness of sobriety checkpoints at decreasing alcohol-impaired driving in a variety of geographical environments and for a range of specific populations, the committee recommends:

> **Recommendation 4-2: States and localities should conduct frequent sobriety checkpoints in conjunction with widespread publicity to promote awareness of these enforcement initiatives.**

The ideal frequency of sobriety checkpoints requires additional research. When full-scale sobriety checkpoints are not feasible (due to staffing, cost, or other limitations), low-staff checkpoints have been shown to be an effective alternative. The committee makes this recommendation despite the fact that sobriety checkpoints are currently illegal in several states. To maximize the potential benefits of publicized sobriety checkpoints, these restrictive laws would need to be changed. Data on where and when fatal and serious physical injury crashes occur should be leveraged to ensure strategic placement of the checkpoints. (See Chapter 6 for information on using big data and predictive analytics to help determine effective interventions, including their geographic placement, to reduce alcohol-impaired driving.)

TECHNOLOGY AND VEHICLE FACTORS

In the areas of technology and vehicle factors, the committee focused on existing and emerging interventions that have reduced—or shown promise of reducing—alcohol-impaired driving and alcohol-related crashes. Passenger restraints and existing vehicle safety technology are discussed, as well as emerging and promising interventions such as the Driver Alcohol Detection System for Safety (DADSS) program and other developing technologies, such as autonomous vehicles. Alternative transportation and ridesharing opportunities using smartphone technology have also shown promise for providing alcohol-impaired drivers with a safe transportation option. Smartphone technologies are discussed in the Alternative Transportation section located at the end of this chapter.

Passenger Restraints

Primary Seat Belt Laws

Seat belt use and infant and child restraints provide a means for drivers and passengers in cars or trucks to reduce their risk of injury or death during a crash. According to NHTSA data, drivers and front seat passengers who use seat belts (lap/shoulder) reduce their risk of fatal injury by 45 percent and are 50 percent more likely to avoid moderate to critical injury (Kahane, 2015; NCSA, 2017). In 2015 alone, seat belts were credited with saving nearly 14,000 individuals 5 years of age and older, and 266 infants and children (up to 4 years of age) were saved by child restraints (including all types of car seats). NHTSA estimates that since 1975, approximately 345,000 lives have been saved because of the use of seat belts (NCSA, 2017).

Alcohol-impaired drivers are less likely to use seat belts relative to nonimpaired drivers. A study of nighttime Minnesota drivers found that drivers with a BAC of 0.10% or higher were significantly less likely (OR = 2.17) to be using seat belts (Foss et al., 1994). Another study examining seat belt use found that relative to fatally injured teenage drivers with low or zero probability of a BAC at or greater than 0.10%, those with a high probability of a BAC at or above 0.10% were 60 percent less likely to use seat belts (McCartt and Northrup, 2004). More recently, analysis of data from the 2012 Behavioral Risk Factor Surveillance System survey found that the rate of alcohol-impaired driving among persons who reported not always wearing a seat belt (1,321) was three times higher than for those who reported always wearing a seat belt (398) (Jewett et al., 2015). Evidence also indicates that persons who consume alcohol more frequently are less likely to use seat belts (Kweon and Kockelman, 2006).

Although some form of seat belts were installed in all vehicles as early as 1964 (lap belts, shoulder belts, or a combination of the two), two decades passed before the nation's first seat belt law was passed in New York State in 1984 (Goodwin et al., 2015). Currently 34 states and the District of Columbia have *primary* seat belt laws in effect, meaning that law enforcement officials are permitted to stop vehicles if drivers or passengers are not wearing seat belts. Fifteen states have *secondary* laws, which prohibit law enforcement officials from stopping vehicles for seat belt violations, but allow officials to ticket drivers for noncompliance if the vehicles are first pulled over for another offense (NCSA, 2017). Occupant restraint laws, including those for infant and child restraints, vary from state to state. Some states have primary or secondary laws requiring certain vehicle occupants to wear seat belts according to their location in the vehicle (driver, or front seat or backseat passengers), while other states regulate seat belt use according to the ages of the occupants (e.g., children 18 years of age and younger).

Several different factors—primary versus secondary seat belt law, time of day, urban versus rural driving, and strength of seat belt reminder system—can affect seat belt use. In 2016, seat belt use in states with primary seat belt laws reached a compliance rate of 92.1 percent while seat belt use in states without primary laws reached 83 percent (Pickrell and Li, 2016). States that moved from secondary seat belt laws to primary laws saw an increase in seat belt use during both daytime and nighttime hours, and motorist fatality rates decreased by an estimated 7 percent (Farmer and Williams, 2005; Tison et al., 2010). A 4-year study conducted by Lange and Voas (1998) found that after California changed the state seat belt laws from secondary to primary, the rate of compliance with seat-belt laws increased from 73 to 95.6 percent. During this same period, the authors found that seat belt use increased from 53.4 to 92.1 percent among drivers with BAC levels ≥0.10%. In 2010, Tison et al. (2010) analyzed FARS data on motor vehicle fatalities (1998–2007) and found that nighttime seat belt use (between the hours of 9 p.m. and 3:59 a.m.) is approximately 18 percent lower than during daytime hours (from 4 a.m. to 8:59 p.m.). Furthermore, only 26 percent of alcohol-impaired drivers—versus 52 percent of nighttime drivers in the zero BAC group—were wearing seat belts at the time of their fatal crash. Seat belt use is lowest in the Midwest (85.5 percent) and highest in the West, and seat belt use in rural areas is slightly lower than in urban areas (89.5 versus 90.5 percent, respectively) (Pickrell and Li, 2016). As required by federal safety standards, seat belt reminder systems provide a warning light and sound lasting 4 to 8 seconds (IIHS, 2017). Enhanced belt reminder systems have been found to increase the rate of seat belt use by about 3 percent (Farmer and Wells, 2010; Freedman et al., 2007).

Seat belt laws are not without controversy. Some opponents to seat belt laws believe that they infringe upon personal choice and individual rights (Advocates for Highway and Auto Safety, 2017), while others are concerned that these laws provide a mechanism by which members of minority populations can be unfairly targeted and subjected to harassment by law enforcement officials (ACLU, 2016; Factor et al., 2013). While the committee is cognizant that these concerns have been raised, the benefits afforded by seat belt use have been well documented. Seat belt use has been shown to be an effective intervention for saving lives and protecting individuals from harm and although the equitable implementation of seat belt laws has been a concern, the committee does not believe the controversy negates the need for, or enforcement of, these laws. Based on the evidence described in this section, the committee concludes:

> *Conclusion 4-1: Seat belts are highly effective in reducing serious injuries and fatalities caused by motor vehicle crashes. Given the low rates of seat belt use and high rates of crashes in rural areas, universal adoption of primary seat belt laws for all occupants and child restraints, combined with enhanced enforcement, could reduce alcohol-related crash injuries and fatalities, particularly in these high-risk areas.*

Vehicle Safety Technology

Contemporary cars offer several vehicle safety features; however, the extent to which these features may prove to be especially helpful for individuals who drive under the influence of alcohol is largely unknown. Of the new technology available in vehicles—traction control, backup cameras, pedestrian detection, parking assist, and vehicle speed limiters, to name a few—the advances that may show the most promise for aiding alcohol-impaired drivers are lane departure warnings (sometimes referred to as *lane keeping assist systems*) and the forward collision warning. Studies have shown that an alcohol-impaired driver's ability to maintain lane position and vehicle control is compromised, thus making these drivers a hazard to themselves and others (Irwin et al., 2017; Rakauskas et al., 2008). Although functionality of motor vehicle warning systems may vary from vehicle to vehicle, most systems use auditory alerts, vibrations of the steering wheel or driver's seat, or visual cues on the dashboard to alert a driver to unintentional lane drift or risk of collision. Some systems also provide autonomous braking and steering to help drivers regain control of their vehicle.

To test whether these warning systems could have prevented or mitigated vehicle crashes and reduced injuries, Kusano and Gabler (2015) ran computational models using nationally representative crash data from 1,042 rear-end collisions from 1997 to 2013 to simulate crashes with and without forward collision and lane departure warning systems. Their analysis found that up to 67 percent of all crashes and between 2 and 69 percent of injuries (moderate to fatal) could have been prevented if these warning systems had been in use at the time of the initial crashes. A study in Sweden by Sternlund (2017) had similar findings after an analysis of 104 fatal car crashes from 2010 that potentially involved lane departures (52 head-on crashes, 48 single-car crashes, and 4 crashes while passing other cars). Lane departure-related crashes were determined to be responsible for half of all head-on and single-vehicle crashes, of which 33 to 38 percent could potentially have been prevented if lane departure warning systems were used at the time of the initial crash.

The benefits that these systems may have for alcohol-impaired drivers, however, are unknown. A recent study by Cicchino and Zuby (2017) accessed data from NHTSA's 2005–2007 National Motor Vehicle Crash Causation Survey to analyze 631 lane-drift crashes that occurred between 6 a.m. and midnight to determine the proportion of drivers who might have been able to regain control of their vehicle if a lane departure warning system had been used at the time of the crash. The study found that the full potential of lane departure warning systems may not be realized because even if the warning system had been used in the lane-drift crashes analyzed by the researchers, 34 percent of all drivers and 42 percent of drivers involved in serious or fatal injuries would have been unable to fully regain control of their vehicles because they were asleep at the wheel or otherwise incapacitated at the time of the crash. An additional 13 to 14 percent of crashes were affected by the driver experiencing a nonincapacitating medical condition, a BAC ≥0.08%, or another physical factor.

Although lane departure and forward collision warning systems seem to show promise for all drivers, research is lacking regarding how beneficial and effective these systems may prove to be for alcohol-impaired drivers. As more cars are manufactured that contain these new technology features, it would be informative to study how effective they can be for reducing the incidence of alcohol-related crashes or mitigating crash severity. If these or other new and innovative advances (such as automated braking) are shown to be effective, they may provide additional opportunities to help reduce the occurrence of alcohol-related crashes and related injuries or fatalities.

Driver Alcohol Detection System for Safety (DADSS)

The DADSS program is a public–private partnership between NHTSA and the Automotive Coalition for Traffic Safety (ACTS)[5] to develop noninvasive, vehicle-integrated technology that prevents a vehicle from moving

[5] ACTS represents motor vehicle manufacturers responsible for about 99 percent of light vehicle sales in the United States (Zaouk et al., 2015).

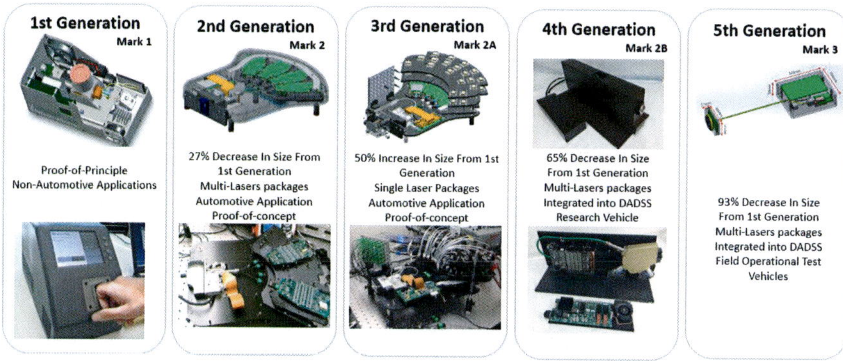

FIGURE 4-2 Evolution of touch-based DADSS device.
SOURCE: Zaouk et al., 2015.

when the driver's BAC exceeds the limit of 0.08% set by state law. The program also focuses on understanding public policy challenges associated with the implementation of such technology and developing strategies to overcome these challenges. The two technologies currently in development are the TruTouch touch-based device and the SenseAir breath-based device. DADSS technologies were introduced to the general public in 2011 at a press conference held by the U.S. Secretary of Transportation and then NHTSA Administrator.[6] The first two research test vehicles were created in 2013 and 2015, respectively, and the third test vehicle, which is being used for pilot field testing, was created in 2017.[7] To further its mission, ACTS will license DADSS technology to any entity with the capability of manufacturing, deploying, and supporting DADSS technologies.[8]

Touch-Based Technology

The touch-based DADSS device uses spectrometry to measure alcohol concentration in the driver's skin tissue (DADSS, 2016a; Zaouk et al., 2015) (see Figure 4-2). Once the driver's finger is in contact with the device's optical touch pad, near-infrared light propagates into the skin tissue and the touch pad collects a sample of the light reflected back to the tissue surface, from which the unique chemical and tissue structure

---

[6] Personal communication with Robert Strassburger, Automotive Coalition for Traffic Safety. Available by request from the National Academies of Sciences, Engineering, and Medicine's Public Access Records Office (PARO@nas.edu).

[7] Ibid.

[8] Ibid.

information contained in the light can be read and alcohol concentration determined (DADSS, 2016a; Zaouk et al., 2015). The device focuses on analyzing 40 discrete wavelengths that indicate alcohol presence and is expected to be capable of performing multiple BAC readings in less than 1 second (DADSS, 2016a). The technology is envisioned to be integrated into the push button of new vehicles so that a driver's BAC will be measured when they use their fingertip to start their vehicle (DADSS, 2016a); if the driver's BAC is at or above 0.08%, DADSS will prevent the car from moving.

Breath-Based Technology

The breath-based DADSS device uses spectrometry to measure alcohol concentration in the driver's exhaled breath (DADSS, 2016b; Zaouk et al., 2015) (see Figure 4-3). The device transmits midinfrared light toward the driver and assesses the alcohol concentration of the driver's exhaled breath by analyzing the reflected and absorbed spectrum (DADSS, 2016b; Zaouk et al., 2015). Blood and breath alcohol concentrations are closely correlated, but breath from around the driver's face or within the vehicle cabin is diluted with cabin air; the degree of dilution can be calculated from measuring carbon dioxide and alcohol at the same point (the concentration of carbon dioxide in ambient air and the concentration of carbon

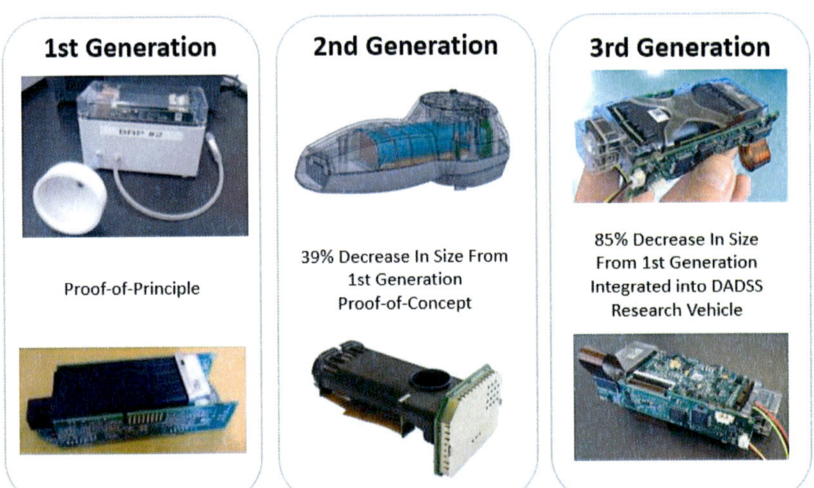

FIGURE 4-3 Evolution of breath-based DADSS device.
SOURCE: Zaouk et al., 2015.

dioxide in alveolar air are known and predictable), and using the ratio of measured carbon dioxide and alcohol concentrations and the known concentration of carbon dioxide in alveolar air, the alveolar air alcohol concentration can be determined (Zaouk et al., 2015). The breath-based device does not require skin contact to assess the driver's BAC, and the vehicle will not move if the driver's BAC is higher than the limit set by state law. Possible locations for the device that are being researched include the driver's side door and the steering column as well as multiple other locations within the vehicle cabin (DADSS, 2016b).

Background

Funding for the DADSS program is made via annual appropriations by NHTSA and ACTS. Funding for the now-concluded cooperative agreement begun in 2008 totaled $12.3 million.[9] Federal funding for the cooperative agreement begun in 2013 was authorized by the Moving Ahead for Progress in the 21st Century Act (MAP-21)[10] and covered fiscal years 2013 through 2016 (NHTSA, 2013b).[11] Total funding provided by NHTSA and ACTS for these fiscal years totaled $26.8 million.[12] Authorization for the DADSS program was extended by the Fixing America's Surface Transportation (FAST) Act[13] to include fiscal years 2017 through 2020.[14] The total amount of funding authorized is $21.2 million.[15] In addition to the funding provided by NHTSA and ACTS, General Motors provided funds to be used in the Pilot Field Operational Trial of DADSS technologies that will begin in fiscal year 2018.[16]

Recently, NHTSA began to allow states to use certain grant funds to support some DADSS-related projects, particularly the trial deployment of DADSS technologies. Beginning in fiscal year 2017, the Commonwealth of Virginia was the first state to dedicate a portion of its federal grant

---

[9] Ibid.

[10] MAP-21 is the 2-year transportation reauthorization bill signed into law by President Obama in July 2012 (FMCSA, n.d.).

[11] Personal communication with Robert Strassburger, Automotive Coalition for Traffic Safety. Available by request from the National Academies of Sciences, Engineering, and Medicine's Public Access Records Office (PARO@nas.edu).

[12] Ibid.

[13] The FAST Act is the 5-year highway reauthorization bill signed into law by President Obama in December 2015 (FHWA, n.d.).

[14] Personal communication with Robert Strassburger, Automotive Coalition for Traffic Safety. Available by request from the National Academies of Sciences, Engineering, and Medicine's Public Access Records Office (PARO@nas.edu).

[15] Ibid.

[16] Ibid.

funds received from NHTSA to DADSS projects; such funding determinations are made annually (DADSS, 2016c; NHTSA, 2016b).

The 5-year cooperative agreement begun in 2008 consisted of two phases (Zaouk et al., 2015). During phase 1, which was completed in early 2011, two breath-based and one touch-based prototype were tested; one of the breath-based prototypes and the touch-based prototype yielded promising results and were chosen for further research and development, which began in late 2011 and finished in late 2013 (phase 2). With the cooperative agreement's extension in 2013, phase 3 (currently ongoing) has involved further technological refinement and research to understand how the technologies might interact with humans and be integrated into and operate in vehicles. If the technologies are determined to have commercial potential, the private sector is expected to continue product development and vehicle integration efforts (Zaouk et al., 2015).

To assess reliability, accuracy, and precision, as well as speed of measurement, ACTS developed performance specifications and standard calibration devices to measure accuracy and precision of both systems and to ensure that the devices meet specified performance requirements (Zaouk et al., 2015). The accuracy and speed requirements adopted by the DADSS program are far more rigorous than current alcohol measurement devices are capable of achieving. For example, the amount of time for a DADSS device to provide a BAC reading is expected to be no longer than the current industry standard to activate a vehicle's motive power, 325 milliseconds, while current breath-based alcohol measurement devices can take at least 30 seconds to provide a BAC estimate (Zaouk et al., 2015). Papers detailing validation studies have been presented at Enhanced Safety of Vehicles conferences. Additionally, the program has partnered with the Commonwealth of Virginia to test the technology in controlled settings, such as limited fleet testing, and refine performance specifications. The DADSS program also aims to increase awareness of the technology by having a presence at university sporting events, a NASCAR race, and festivals for wine and craft beer.[17] Although still in the program's technological research phase, DADSS technology is expected to meet "acceptable technology and manufacturing readiness levels" and be integrated into fleets and potentially privately operated vehicles within approximately 5 to 10 years (DADSS, n.d.-a).

---

[17] Ibid.

Implementation Barriers and Considerations

Consumer education and public acceptance are the most critical elements for long-term adoption and successful commercialization of DADSS technology. Installation and use of DADSS devices is currently planned to be voluntary; widespread implementation will depend on public acceptance of addressing alcohol-impaired driving as a society (Griffin, 2017). Many people do not view themselves as part of the problem, as a small minority of drivers is responsible for producing the majority of alcohol-related traffic crashes. The DADSS technology will be made available to consumers as a driver assistance system, similar to lane departure warning systems and automatic emergency braking. Thus, to promote wide acceptance of DADDS, the technology should be seen as a safety feature to make roads safer, rather than a punitive device (Griffin, 2017).

Privacy concerns are another critical consideration for implementation of DADSS technology. The program has prioritized the issue of consumer data privacy since its initiation, with the program's legal authorization and cooperative agreement specifically stating that "security measures and operating procedures must be put in place to protect data from the inadvertent release or disclosure to unauthorized parties" (DADSS, n.d.-a). Additionally, all vehicle manufacturing companies that fund the DADSS program, in partnership with consumer advocacy organizations, have established voluntary privacy principles, standards, and guidance for the use of all vehicle-integrated technology (DADSS, n.d.-a). The industry's voluntary privacy principles were instated in early 2017, with full implementation to take place in early 2018.

Implementation of DADSS devices will be influenced by several technological considerations. For widespread adoption, the technology will need to be completely passive so that it does not impede normal driving activity. Researchers will also need to address the issue of false positives, which may occur in situations where, for example, the driver washed their hands with products that contain alcohol prior to driving, so alcohol is likely to remain on their hands as well as be in the ambient air when they start their vehicle. Additionally, further research is needed to determine the most effective way to convey information to the driver about their BAC (for example, displaying a numeric BAC reading, displaying a red/yellow/green light) and to ensure that the driver's age is not under 21 years. Furthermore, the devices are being tested assuming a BAC limit of 0.08% (ACTS, 2013), so technological development may need to be expanded to account for potentially lower BAC per se laws. Similarly, researchers will need to address how the technology will operate in situations where the driver's BAC changes (for example, a driver's BAC could be under 0.08% when they start their vehicle but increase to above 0.08% after a period of time driving, depending on when alcohol was consumed).

Several financial considerations are also critical for successful implementation of DADSS devices. Although an estimate of the price for the device has not been publicly released, the cost to the consumer should be in line with other electronic vehicle safety features, with the average price of typical electronic vehicle safety features being approximately $200, and that cost would be expected to decrease significantly (to around $50) if the devices became a standard vehicle amenity (Griffin, 2017). Individual automakers will determine consumer prices for DADSS technologies. Insurance discounts, already offered for most other vehicle safety features including airbags and seat belts, and state government incentives such as those already in use for electric cars will need to be considered to help deployment of DADSS. Regarding crash liability, DADSS devices are expected to be treated no differently than antilock braking systems and airbags. In addition to stringent performance specification testing, consumer education on the functions the technology can and cannot perform will be important to understanding and managing expectations of the technology's capabilities.[18]

Potential Effect

The Insurance Institute for Highway Safety (IIHS) conducted a nationally representative phone survey in 2009 and found that about two-thirds of respondents, including nondrinking drivers and drinking drivers, supported DADSS technology (Cicchino, 2017); 40 percent of survey participants indicated they would want DADSS devices in their own cars if the technology was available (IIHS and HLDI, 2009). In addition to public support, the DADSS program is also endorsed by safety and child safety advocacy organizations, insurance companies, state and local government representatives, and alcohol industry stakeholders (DADSS, n.d.-b). IIHS estimates that about 7,000 lives could have been saved in 2015 if DADSS devices set at a BAC limit of 0.08% had been in every vehicle (Cicchino, 2017). Given strong public support and endorsement from various sectors as well as a significant potential reduction of alcohol-impaired driving fatalities, the committee concludes:

> *Conclusion 4-2: If its use becomes widespread, Driver Alcohol Detection System for Safety (DADSS) technology is a passive interlock technology that is very promising for reducing alcohol-impaired driving and related consequences. However, it will require substantial evidence of*

[18] Ibid.

its accuracy in order to be brought to market or become required safety equipment in all new motor vehicles.

Therefore, the committee recommends:

Recommendation 4-3: When the Driver Alcohol Detection System for Safety (DADSS) is accurate and available for public use, auto insurers should provide policy discounts to stimulate the adoption of DADSS. Once the cost is on par with other existing automobile safety features and the technology is demonstrated to be accurate and effective, the National Highway Traffic Safety Administration should make DADSS mandatory in all new vehicles.

DADSS should only be mandated by NHTSA if and when it is deemed safe and effective, in the same manner as other vehicle safety features that are already under mandate. Support from organizations like NHTSA and continued funding from Congress will be needed for DADSS technology to be fully developed, tested, and marketed to the general public. If DADSS is eventually installed in all cars, it would be as effective as having ignition interlock devices installed (see Chapter 5). DADSS as a primary prevention strategy would have the potential to be more effective at the population level than ignition interlock devices because the technology would be in the vehicle indefinitely. In theory, DADSS would also prevent the alcohol-impaired driving crashes that would be caused by drivers without a prior DWI conviction, who would not have an interlock device installed. Potential areas for future research include false positives and negatives from the use of interlock technology, time to peak of BAC from the start of the vehicle, intervention strategies for continuous monitoring systems, and the effect of vehicle interlocks on personal safety.

New Technologies on the Horizon

In-vehicle technologies that aim to improve traffic safety are rapidly being developed and tested. While evidence supporting the effectiveness of these technological interventions will remain limited until they are more widely implemented and adopted, many have the potential to decrease fatalities from alcohol-impaired driving (e.g., smartphone technologies discussed later in this chapter or autonomous vehicles).

Autonomous Vehicles

Vehicles that are autonomous have an automated driving capability that enables them to operate with limited to zero human driver involvement (Hedlund, 2017). Autonomous vehicles use multiple integrated systems, including sensors, GPS, and vehicle-to-vehicle (V2V) and vehicle-to-infrastructure (V2I) technology,[19] to monitor and automatically respond to traffic, road, and weather conditions (Faulks, 2014). The Society of Automotive Engineers and NHTSA categorize autonomous vehicles into five levels ranging from no automation (i.e., the driver maintains full control of the vehicle) (level 0) to full automation (i.e., the vehicle is completely self-driving under all conditions and does not require a human driver) (level 5) (Hedlund, 2017). As of July 2017, 26 states and the District of Columbia have either passed legislation or issued executive orders promoting autonomous vehicle development (NCSL, 2017).[20]

Level 1 features such as cruise control, electronic stability control, and lane departure warning systems have been available since the 1960s, 1990s, and 2000s, respectively (Hedlund, 2017). In October 2015 about 60,000 Tesla cars received a software update for Autopilot, a driver assistance feature that enables the cars to control their speed, stay in and change traffic lanes, and self-park (Hedlund, 2017). Many Tesla cars are also equipped with other level 2 features including automated lane guidance, crash avoidance, and detection of driver fatigue (Litman, 2017). Google has been testing level 3 autonomous vehicles with a fleet that has completed nearly 2 million miles in controlled environments and includes autonomous vehicles without steering wheels and floor pedals (Hedlund, 2017; Litman, 2017). As of October 2016, 15 companies in California are testing autonomous vehicles (Hedlund, 2017). In September 2016 Uber began offering autonomous vehicle rides in Pittsburgh with a human driver present to intervene if needed (Hedlund, 2017). In 2016 a self-driving truck developed by Uber Advanced Technologies Group and Otto, a San Francisco–based autonomous vehicle technology company, successfully drove 120 miles on a Colorado highway carrying a trailer of Budweiser beer (Hedlund, 2017; Uber, n.d.-a).

---

[19] V2V and V2I technologies are intelligent transportation systems that communicate data (such as infrastructure advisories and other environmental factors that may affect traffic safety) wirelessly between vehicles (V2V), which includes trucks and motorcycles, and between vehicles and infrastructure (V2I) (DOT, n.d.-a,b).

[20] Alabama, Arkansas, California, Colorado, Connecticut, Florida, Georgia, Illinois, Louisiana, Michigan, Nevada, New York, North Carolina, North Dakota, Pennsylvania, South Carolina, Tennessee, Texas, Utah, Vermont, and Virginia have passed legislation. Arizona, Delaware, Massachusetts, Washington, and Wisconsin have issued executive orders (NCSL, 2017).

Internationally, Volvo has been testing autonomous vehicles in Gothenburg, Sweden, since September 2016 and plans to begin testing in London in 2017 (Hedlund, 2017). In Australia, autonomous vehicles are expected to share the roads with human-driven vehicles beginning in 2020 to 2025 (Knott, 2017). In 2021, Volvo plans to begin selling autonomous vehicles in Australia, and Ford expects to introduce autonomous vehicles for commercial ridesharing (Knott, 2017). As of August 2016, 33 companies worldwide are involved in autonomous vehicle development (Hedlund, 2017).

Based on the timelines and vehicle fleet turnover rates from implementation of previous vehicle technologies, Litman (2017) predicts that autonomous vehicle capability will not be a standard feature of most new vehicles until the 2050s (see Table 4-2). Litman also estimates that autonomous vehicle use will not improve traffic safety until the 2040s to 2060s, once the majority of vehicle travel is autonomous (Litman, 2017) (see Table 4-3).

Although the research and development of autonomous vehicles shows great promise, the solutions they might provide in the future are not yet feasible. It is important that efforts continue to be made to reduce alcohol-impaired driving and related injuries and fatalities using technological resources. There may come a day when vehicle occupants no longer have to be mindful of their alcohol consumption as it relates to driving and their BAC, but that day is a long time from now and may, in fact, not ever be a reality.

TABLE 4-2 Autonomous Vehicle Implementation Projections

Stage	Decade	Vehicle Sales	Vehicle Fleet	Vehicle Travel
Available with large price premium	2020s	2–5%	1–2%	1–4%
Available with moderate price premium	2030s	20–40%	10–20%	10–30%
Available with minimal price permium	2040s	40–60%	20–40%	30–50%
Standard feature included on most new vehicles	2050s	80–100%	40–60%	50–80%
Saturation (everyone who wants it has it)	2060s	?	?	?
Required for all new and operating vehicles	?	100%	100%	100%

SOURCE: Litman, 2017.

TABLE 4-3 Autonomous Vehicle Planning Impacts by Time Period

Impact	Functional Requirements	Planning Impacts	Time Period
Become legal	Demonstrated functionality and safety	Define performance, testing, and data collection requirements for automated driving on public roads	2015–2025
Increase traffic density by vehicle coordination	Road lanes dedicated to vehicles with coordinated platooning capability	Evaluate impacts; define requirements; identify lanes to be dedicated to vehicles capable of coordinated operation	2020–2040
Independent mobility for nondrivers	Fully autonomous vehicles available for sale	Allows affluent nondrivers to enjoy independent mobility	2020–2030s
Automated car sharing/taxis	Moderate price premium; successful business model	May provide demand and response services in affluent areas; supports car sharing	2030s–2040s
Independent mobility for lower-income driver	Affordable autonomous vehicles for sale	Reduced need for conventional public transit services in some areas	2040–2050s
Reduced parking demand	Major share of vehicles are autonomous	Reduced parking requirements	2040–2050s
Reduced traffic congestion	Major share of urban peak vehicle travel is autonomous	Reduced road supply	2050–2060s
Increased safety	Major share of vehicle travel is autonomous	Reduced traffic risk; possibly increased walking and cycling activity	2040–2060s
Energy conservation and emission reductions	Major share of vehicle travel is autonomous; walking and cycling become safer	Supports energy conservation and emission reduction efforts	2040–2060s

TABLE 4-3 Continued

Impact	Functional Requirements	Planning Impacts	Time Period
Improved vehicle control	Most or all vehicles are autonomous	Allows narrower lanes and interactive traffic controls	2050–2070s
Need to plan for mixed traffic	Major share of vehicles are autonomous	More complex traffic; may justify restrictions on human-driven vehicles	2040–2060s
Mandated autonomous vehicles	Most vehicles are autonomous and large benefits are proven	Allows advanced traffic management	2060–2080s

SOURCE: Litman, 2017.

PHYSICAL ENVIRONMENT AND TRANSPORTATION

Interventions related to the physical environment and transportation are included in the committee's conceptual framework for preventing alcohol-related crash fatalities that was presented in Chapter 1 (see Figure 1-5). This section discusses several interventions—designated drivers, smartphone-enabled transportation network ridesharing, and alternative transportation such as safe ride programs and public transportation.

Designated Driver

Background

A designated driver is commonly understood to be a nondrinking member of a social group who agrees before drinking begins to be the driver for the rest of the group. Definitions for the term vary according to expectations about whether the designated driver should remain abstinent from drinking (or how many drinks are acceptable if abstinence is not required) and whether the designation of the driver should take place prior to drinking.

The designated driver concept originated in Scandinavia (Lange et al., 1998) and was popularized in the United States in the late 1980s and early 1990s by a national media campaign launched by the Harvard Alcohol Project. Begun at the Center for Health Communication at the Harvard T.H. Chan School of Public Health, the project partnered with broadcast television networks and Hollywood studios to produce and air prime time public service announcements that encouraged the use of designated drivers. The announcement featured popular characters from top-rated shows that scripted the designated driver concept into prime time television episodes (Harvard School of Public Health, n.d.; Winsten, 1994, 2017).

The two most common approaches to promoting designated driver use are population-based campaigns and programs that incentivize patrons at drinking establishments to act as designated drivers. Incentives offered to patrons for refraining from drinking alcoholic beverages can include free soft drinks, food, beer or other beverages that do not contain alcohol, or admission to a venue (Ditter et al., 2005). Most research shows that both types of programs have increased awareness and use of the concept (Ditter et al., 2005; Lange et al., 1998; Nielson and Watson, 2009); however, the evidence is insufficient to conclude the effectiveness of either type of program on alcohol-impaired driving (Anderson et al., 2009a,b; Burton et al., 2017; Ditter et al., 2005; Esser et al., 2016; Nielson and Watson, 2009; WHO Regional Office for Europe, 2009).

Evidence

NHTSA's *Countermeasures That Work* rates the effectiveness of designated driver interventions as low (Goodwin et al., 2015). The authors note that although costs are low and implementation time is short, few studies have evaluated the effect of designated driver use on traffic injuries owing to variation in the definition and selection of a designated driver. One relevant study was identified in a systematic review conducted by the Community Preventive Services Task Force (Ditter et al., 2005); the systematic review covered population-based campaigns and incentive programs at drinking establishments and is described below.

Population-based campaigns At the time of the Task Force's review (Ditter et al., 2005), only one study evaluating a population-based campaign was identified. The campaign, known as "Pick-a-Skipper" and targeted at 18- to 35-year-olds in a Western Australian city with a population of about 25,000, consisted of public service announcements and newspaper coverage encouraging drinkers to choose a designated driver before consuming alcohol (Boots and Midford, 1999). Although survey results showed a nearly 13 percent increase in selecting a driver prior to alcohol consumption, the results did not indicate a change in self-reported alcohol-impaired driving or riding with an alcohol-impaired driver. The Task Force concluded that the study did not provide sufficient evidence to determine the effectiveness of population-based designated driver campaigns.

Incentive programs at drinking establishments The task force reviewed eight studies (seven in the United States, one in Australia) evaluating incentive programs at establishments serving alcohol. In the American studies, free nonalcoholic drinks, food, and drink discounts were offered to abstinent designated drivers, with incentives promoted through newspaper advertisements, cable television advertisements, and in-establishment advertising on posters, coasters, and so on. The number of designated drivers each night increased by a median of 0.9, and in two studies the number of designated drivers returned to baseline once the incentives were removed. In the Australian study, three nightclubs in Melbourne suburbs offered free admission and nonalcoholic drinks to designated drivers (who were not required to remain abstinent) of two or more drinkers. Despite contradicting increases in self-reports of both always and never selecting a designated driver before drinking, a 6.5 percent decrease was recorded in the number of drivers or passengers who traveled in a vehicle with a driver whose BAC was estimated to be over the limit set by law. The task force concluded that owing to the small magnitude of observed changes and limitations of measured outcomes, the studies did not provide sufficient evidence to determine whether incentive programs promoting the use of designated drivers were effective.

Evidence regarding the effectiveness of designated driver programs is sparse. The systematic review by Ditter et al. (2005) found inconsistent and insufficient evidence to determine whether designated driver programs are an effective intervention for reducing alcohol-impaired driving or reducing alcohol-impaired driving fatalities. Small increases in the number of designated drivers were seen in studies reviewed by Ditter et al. (2005); however, study participants' responses both for drinking alcoholic versus nonalcoholic drinks during the night and for reports of driving or being a passenger in a vehicle with a driver who had been drinking were collected via self-report. Information was also lacking on prior drinking and driving histories prior to the designated driving incentive programs.

Barriers and Strategies for Improvement

Although the designated driver concept is generally well known, studies have shown that expectations about whether the designated driver should remain abstinent from consuming alcohol differ (Lange et al., 1998). In fact, results from the 1996 National Roadside Survey showed that designated drivers were more likely to have a positive BAC than non-designated drivers when the origin of travel was not limited to drinking establishments (Fell et al., 1997).

In a survey of 937 adults in California, 64.2 percent of respondents indicated that a designated driver should not drink any alcohol within 4 hours of driving; 19.5, 9.6, and 1.7 percent responded that one drink, two drinks, and three or more drinks, respectively, were acceptable within 4 hours of driving (Lange et al., 1998). Notably, 41.3 percent of heavy drinkers (defined as those who consumed four or more drinks on at least 1 day in the past 28 days) found two or more drinks acceptable for a designated driver; men were also more likely to be accepting of this standard than women. In practice, although 80.7 percent of survey respondents who had acted as a designated driver reported that they had abstained from drinking within 4 hours of driving, 12.1 percent reported that they had drank within 4 hours every time they had acted as a designated driver (Lange et al., 1998). More recently, a study of 165 designated drivers found that only 65 percent had remained abstinent while 17 percent had BAC levels between 0.02% and 0.049%, and 18 percent had BAC levels at or greater than 0.05% (Barry et al., 2013).

Expectations of whether the designation of the driver should take place prior to alcohol consumption also vary. In the survey of California adults previously discussed, 55.7 percent of respondents expected a designated driver to be selected prior to drinking and 20.5 percent were ambiguous about when they thought the decision should be made (Lange et al., 1998). In its originally intended and safest version of implementation, a designated driver should be chosen prior to alcohol consumption and remain abstinent; only 39.3 percent of respondents fulfilled both of these criteria (Lange et al., 1998). Ongoing and future efforts to promote designated driver use may be more effective if focused on encouraging designated drivers to remain abstinent and to be selected prior to drinking (Lange et al., 1998). However, as noted in a NHTSA report, prior designation of a driver is often not feasible owing to cultural drinking behavior in the United States where social groups typically change during travel to, between, and from drinking establishments (Decina et al., 2009).

Unintended Consequences and Spillover Effects

Favorable public opinion of the designated driver concept may have helped to reinforce societal norms against alcohol-impaired driving (Ditter et al., 2005). However, the concept may also have contributed to greater alcohol consumption by passengers, as availability of a designated driver may encourage drinking passengers to consume more (DeJong and Wallack, 1992; Ditter et al., 2005; Esser et al., 2016; Harding et al.,

2001; Rivara et al., 2007). A study analyzing data from the 2007 National Roadside Survey found that one-fifth of drinking passengers in vehicles operated by designated drivers reported having consumed five or more drinks (Bergen et al., 2014b). The authors note that the behavior of these intoxicated passengers could distract the driver. Results from a study of 146 drivers ages 18 to 29 in Alberta, Canada, support this concern, as intoxicated passengers driven by peer designated drivers were likely to behave in ways that were distracting to the driver and unsafe to both the driver and passengers (Rothe and Carroll, 2009).

Special Populations

Young and high-risk drinkers, such as college students, may be especially vulnerable to binge drinking or drinking more excessively than they would have in the absence of a designated driver (DeJong and Wallack, 1992; Ditter et al., 2005; Esser et al., 2016; Rivara et al., 2007; Wolburg, 2005). Young drinkers may also be more likely to accept even higher BAC levels for designated drivers. A study of 480 college students found that although BAC levels of designated drivers were lower than for nondesignated drivers, the average BAC of designated drivers was 0.074% for men and 0.022% for women, averaging 0.060% (Timmerman et al., 2003). The authors note that use of male designated drivers may be ineffective at preventing alcohol-impaired driving.

Conclusion

In its finding below, the committee is echoing the conclusion of the Community Preventive Services Task Force by Ditter et al. (2005). At the time of the review, the Task Force found only one study on the effectiveness of designated driver programs (which found no significant change in self-reported alcohol-impaired driving as a result of the program) and eight studies of incentive programs. The Task Force concluded there was insufficient evidence to draw conclusions about the effectiveness of such programs. An evaluation of an Australian program in 2014, and thus after the systematic review was completed, again concluded it was not clear whether the program affected alcohol-impaired driving or involvement in alcohol-related crashes.

> Finding 4-1: The available evidence on designated driver programs is insufficient to determine whether they are effective in reducing alcohol-impaired driving or crashes.

Alternative Transportation

Smartphone-Enabled Transportation Network Ridesharing

Since 2010, smartphone-enabled network ridesharing companies (e.g., Uber, Lyft) have led to a major innovation in on-demand public transportation. For example, in its first 5 years of operation, Uber has provided more than 1 billion rides (Uber, n.d.-b). Because of the added convenience relative to existing public transportation options and often lower costs than traditional taxis, using network ridesharing companies has been widely promoted as an alternative to driving after consuming alcohol.

Empirical evidence is beginning to emerge regarding the association between the uptake of network ridesharing and alcohol-impaired driving crashes, alcohol-related driving fatalities, and potential unintended consequences. The current literature is limited to evaluating data available after the publicly reported start date of Uber's launch in a given local market, given that Uber has had the largest market share to date. There are no publicly available data across jurisdictions regarding rideshare volume in those jurisdictions.

As of September 2017, there had been six independent analyses published, with three of these published in the peer-reviewed literature and three published as online economics working papers. While the study methodologies and specific findings are somewhat heterogeneous, the main findings generally demonstrate either a net positive benefit on addressing alcohol-impaired driving or no difference.

With regard to the primary outcome of alcohol-related fatalities, two of the four papers showed reductions associated with Uber entry (Greenwood and Wattal, 2017; Martin-Buck, 2016) and the other two showed no difference (Brazil and Kirk, 2016; Dills and Mulholland, 2016). The two papers using alcohol-related crashes as the primary outcome measured a reduction in these crashes associated with Uber (Morrison et al., 2017; Peck, 2017). The effects tended to be stronger in the year after the Uber launch (Greenwood and Wattal, 2017; Martin-Buck, 2016). It appears that some of the heterogeneity in effects may be attributable to differences in public transportation availability and usage and other local geographic and market factors (Martin-Buck, 2016; Morrison et al., 2017; Peck, 2017). For example, in a study that explicitly adjusted for public transportation usage, there was a reduction in DWI arrests in cities with low public transportation usage, but no reduction in cities with high public transportation usage (Martin-Buck, 2016). Other reasons for mixed evidence include heterogeneity in methodological risk adjustment approaches and model specifications.

Given the concern of potential unintended consequences, several studies also analyzed the effects of the Uber rideshare launch on other crimes that could theoretically occur if increased ridesharing led to increased alcohol consumption, such as disorderly conduct and sexual assaults. Two studies examined the association with other arrests and found that crimes that could be associated with alcohol consumption actually decreased with Uber entry, with no increase in other "control" crimes (Dills and Mulholland, 2016; Martin-Buck, 2016). However, one study found a marked increase in motor vehicle thefts after Uber entry, theorizing this could be caused by leaving cars behind overnight at drinking establishments (Dills and Mulholland, 2016).

In addition to empirical evaluations on the general effect of rideshare entry on alcohol-impaired driving crashes, there are also emerging news reports on municipal police-reported outcomes after the implementation of public–private partnerships to sponsor free rides home from designated drinking establishment locations during peak drinking times (e.g., 9 p.m. to 2 a.m.). For example, based on 2,000 rides provided in Evesham, New Jersey, the mayor reported a 15 percent decline in DWIs and a 16 percent decline in alcohol-related crashes (New Jersey Opinion, 2016). Costs for this program were supported initially by a U.S. Department of Transportation grant to the state followed by private donations.

While network ridesharing services are operating in most cities in the United States, there are still several cities that have barred these services from operating because of concerns ranging from safety, effect on the taxi industry, and increased congestion (NASEM, 2016). Additional concerns about ridesharing services include questions about the training and screening of drivers and the adequacy of insurance coverage. From the perspective of a broadly scalable, cost-effective intervention to reduce alcohol-impaired driving crash fatalities, it appears that the launch of ridesharing network companies has led to a reduction of these crashes in some cities without documented increases in negative public health consequences.

In this section, the committee reviews the emerging evidence base on the effect of the market entry of smartphone-enabled transportation network ridesharing (e.g., Uber, Lyft) on motor vehicle crashes. The evidence is limited to three peer-reviewed papers and three working papers. The evidence is mixed overall, showing either a positive safety benefit or no effect on crashes, but importantly, no increase in unintended crimes that could be attributed to potentially higher alcohol consumption from forgoing driving. There is some evidence that the effect on reducing alcohol-involved crashes is heterogeneous by geography and that the effect may be strongest in geographies with poor public transportation usage. While the evidence of this novel transportation alternative is still emerging, the committee has recommended that transportation network ridesharing be permitted to operate due to the potential to reduce alcohol-impaired driving crashes as one of many transportation alternatives to driving after drinking (see Recommendation 4-4 in this report).

Safe Ride Programs and Public Transportation

Beyond designated drivers (or letting someone else drive) and smartphone-enabled ridesharing, alternative transportation includes safe ride programs and public transportation. These services provide intoxicated people with additional ways to avoid driving while impaired. Alternative transportation varies considerably in consumer population use, funding sources, modes of transportation, geographical range of service, fee and reservation requirements, and service frequency (e.g., times of day, days of the week, and holidays). Despite these differences, these programs are designed to transport people from residences or other locations to, from, and between drinking establishments. Safe ride programs can include taxis, private cars, limousines, trolleys, tow trucks, and scooters, and these programs usually supplement available public transportation options. Specific college-based programs that commonly use taxi services or shuttles on either a fixed or point-to-point route are also available in many cases. Shuttle buses provide transportation between points on campus, off-campus residences, and sometimes into cities.

Evidence for safe ride programs NHTSA's *Countermeasures That Work* concluded that the effectiveness of safe ride programs has not yet been determined and that different study methods produce different results (Goodwin et al., 2015). Furthermore, most programs have not been studied. Those safe ride programs that have been studied lack robust outcomes, making it difficult to make conclusions regarding the effectiveness of alternative transportation options on reducing alcohol-related driving fatalities (Decina et al., 2009; Huseth, 2012). Two college programs that have been evaluated focused on student attitudes toward drinking and perceptions of the college's alternative transportation option, not on outcomes such as crash reductions (Decina et al., 2009). For example, one assessment of a college late-night bus service found a generally positive view of the program, but the study did not directly survey bus users (Elam et al., 2006).

Two safe ride programs have shown positive outcomes. Tipsy Taxi is a free, year-round service available all day in Pitken County and Aspen, Colorado. It is administered through the sheriff's office with support from the restaurant association; funding for the program, which also covers clients' monetary penalties for leaving vehicles overnight, is mainly provided by grants and fundraising events. Tipsy Taxi provided 20,000 rides between 1984 and 1999 (Decina et al., 2009; Lacey et al., 2000). An interrupted time series analysis found injury crashes reduced significantly, by 15 percent, after the taxi service's implementation (Lacey et al., 2000); however, given the small community, not enough data were available to evaluate changes in fatal crashes (Decina et al., 2009). The atypical resort community may also limit generalizability. Another program with favorable results is the Road Crew safe ride program. Road Crew is based on a social marketing model and was originally aimed at young, primarily blue collar men ages 21 to 34 years. Focus group research found young men wanted to be able to drink while riding and did not want to leave their cars behind at the end of the evening (Rothschild et al., 2006). To that end, Road Crew uses older luxury vehicles and limousines in three rural areas to provide rides from residences to and from bars. The limousine/luxury car is socially acceptable and provides a fun, social environment. Self-reported alcohol consumption did not change after Road Crew's introduction. In an analysis of data from 2002 to 2003, 70 percent of people surveyed were aware of Road Crew, and the program provided almost 20,000 rides (Decina et al., 2009; Rothschild et al., 2006). There was also a 17 percent decline in alcohol-related crashes (Decina et al., 2009; Rothschild et al., 2006).

There are additional benefits of safe ride options. Programs generally do not lead to increased alcohol consumption, and they attract people at higher risk of driving impaired (Huseth, 2012; Rothschild et al., 2006; Sarkar et al., 2005; Sprattler, 2010). The services can be inexpensive and easy for communities to implement. For example, a short-term program offered through existing transportation options and centered on holidays or major sporting events could be implemented in a few weeks and operated by donated rides. Furthermore, community organizations, including restaurants and drinking establishments, as well as the alcohol industry, usually support safe ride programs (Huseth, 2012). For instance, the founders of Road Crew attribute part of the program's success to the variety of partners engaged throughout the service's stages of development and implementation. These groups included groups of bar owners and patrons, law enforcement, Miller Brewing Company, and an advertising agency (Rothschild et al., 2006).

Although safe ride programs can be modified to specific community needs and can play a role in a community's broader strategy to reduce alcohol-impaired driving (Decina et al., 2009; Goodwin et al., 2015), there are several shortcomings to these programs. Some programs can only service people in a limited area (e.g., scooter-based programs or rural versus urban programs) or may not be very discreet (e.g., programs that tow a person's car to their home if they are inebriated). Other safe ride programs require that an individual find their own transportation the following day to reclaim their cars. Depending on the location and target population, some safe ride programs suffer from low ridership when people opt for other methods of transportation, such as using a designated driver, riding with a family member or friend, taking a taxi or other form of alternative transportation, or opting to drive home on their own (Decina et al., 2009; Lavoie et al., 1999; Molof et al., 1995). For example, 44 percent of participants in a program primarily aimed at men ages 21 to 29 years in Sacramento, California, reported they would have driven themselves home if the safe ride service was not available when they were ready to go home (Sarkar et al., 2005). Successful marketing of programs can be problematic; a study of a program in central New York found half of the people surveyed knew about the program but only 15 percent used it (Molof et al., 1995). Similarly, an evaluation of a free holiday ride service in Canada surveyed 544 young drivers and found that while almost everyone was aware of the program, only 17 percent of those who reported drinking to impairment used the service (compared to 63 percent who said they found another way home and 20 percent who drove impaired) (Lavoie et al., 1999).

Evidence for public transportation Mass transit is generally easy to use and can be less expensive than driving.[21] However, there are some disadvantages such as short hours of service, infrequent pickup and drop-off locations, and lack of flexibility that prevent people from using public transportation. Taxis can offer more flexibility when mass transit options are limited, although taxi availability varies considerably in rural areas and may be costly. People may be unfamiliar with mass transit options and may not understand subway or bus systems.

There is a lack of evidence regarding public transportation and impaired driving as it can be difficult to obtain appropriate data and to assess causality. One study of the Phoenix, Arizona, light rail found more frequent light rail use by college students was associated with significantly decreased odds of driving impaired (Broyles, 2014). Additionally, a 2011 study evaluated changes in Washington, DC, metro schedules from 1999 to 2003 that resulted in the system staying open until 3 a.m. on Fridays and Saturdays (Jackson and Owens, 2011). When metro operated until 3 a.m., ridership increased 7 percent per hour. DWIs declined 7 percent per hour of additional service, and alcohol-related arrests increased 8 percent in areas close to a metro station. However, while alcohol-related fatal crashes decreased in areas of DC serviced by metro (including a small

[21] The American Public Transportation Association reports an annual savings of $9,797 if a commuter switches from a car to public transportation (http://www.apta.com/mediacenter/pressreleases/2017/Pages/June-Transit-Savings.aspx) (accessed January 9, 2018).

decrease in Maryland suburbs), there was a small increase in Virginia suburbs not covered by metro (Jackson and Owens, 2011).

Moving Forward

For the reasons above, a NHTSA report on alternative transportation concluded that

> At best, [alternative transportation] programs should be viewed as an adjunct to existing transportation programs and ride services.... But there is hope, and these [alternative transportation] programs can complement other programs and services to offer a range of options for all drinkers in a wide variety of circumstances to enhance opportunities for a safe ride home. (Decina et al., 2009, p. 19)

An ideal alternative transportation program aiming to reduce alcohol-impaired driving fatalities would be consistently available, reliable, accessible and easy to use, and free to users.

There is a need for improved studies of alternative and public transportation options and research into how these forms of transportation can best work in concert (complementarity, substitutability, and synergies). Because it can be difficult to obtain the data necessary to conduct a robust study, many studies of safe ride programs rely on crash data, which can be limited because crashes are rare and data from nonfatal crashes are often subjective (Decina et al., 2009). Ideally studies would develop and use relevant outcome measures and aim to assess how alcohol-impaired driving incidence is affected by the availability and use of alternative transportation (Decina et al., 2009). Studies should also evaluate the effect of ridesharing networks on other alcohol-related consequences (e.g., suicides, assault, and injuries).

Although the limited research into alternative transportation options is mixed, the committee believes that this an area that shows great promise. As technology gains in popularity and becomes accessible and available to more individuals and communities, there is an opportunity to use the alternative transportation options previously discussed—smartphone-enabled network ridesharing, safe ride programs, and public transportation (mass transit, taxis, subways, buses, metro)—more broadly to provide options for drivers who have been drinking. Because the committee sees this as a promising strategy for reducing alcohol-related crashes and alcohol-impaired driving injuries and fatalities, the committee recommends the following:

Recommendation 4-4: Municipalities should support policies and programs that increase the availability, convenience,

affordability, and safety of transportation alternatives for drinkers who might otherwise drive. This includes permitting transportation network company ridesharing, enhancing public transportation options (especially during nighttime and weekend hours), and boosting or incentivizing transportation alternatives in rural areas.

RESEARCH NEEDS

To address the research gaps relevant to alcohol-impaired driving interventions, the committee identified the following research needs:

Policies and laws:

- Research into the effectiveness of BAC criminal sanctions versus administrative laws.
- Monitoring and evaluation of the implementation, compliance, and impact of the Utah 0.05% BAC per se law.
- Research on interventions to stop teen and novice drivers from driving after consuming alcohol.
- Development of strategies to prevent passengers from riding in a vehicle driven by an impaired driver, including vehicles driven by teens or novice drivers.
- Research to identify how new drivers ≥18 years of age fare without GDL restrictions and whether driving restrictions should be compulsory for all novice drivers.

Enforcement and arrest:

- Research examining the effectiveness and impact of child endangerment laws to improve their effectiveness and how to increase public awareness of these laws to reduce child fatalities.
- Research to identify ideal frequency of sobriety checkpoints.
- Update current research on the cost-effectiveness of sobriety checkpoints with studies that have rigorous methods and measurements.
- Research to determine how lowering the BAC limit from 0.08% to 0.05% will affect enforcement of BAC per se laws.

Technology and vehicle factors:

- As more cars are manufactured that contain new technology features, studies to determine their effectiveness for reducing the incidence of alcohol-related crashes or mitigating crash severity will be needed.

- Future DADSS research could include how to address false positives and negatives from the use of interlock technology, BAC time to peak issues after starting of the vehicle, intervention strategies for continuous monitoring systems, and the effect of vehicle interlocks on personal safety.

Physical environment and transportation:

- Research into the effectiveness of designated driver programs and how they could be utilized to reduce the number of alcohol-impaired drivers.
- Further research into the effectiveness and usefulness of alternative rideshare options, including smartphone-enabled network ridesharing, safe ride programs, and public transportation.

REFERENCES

AAA (American Automobile Association). 2017. *Distracted driver and teen driver safety top AAA's state advocacy agenda for 2013.* http://newsroom.aaa.com/tag/aaa-advocacy/ (accessed December 12, 2017).

ABI (American Beverage Institute). 2017a. *American Beverage Institute likens Utah's .05 DUI arrest level to equally silly DWO (driving while older) in full-page ad.* https://abionline.org/press_release/american-beverage-institute-likens-utahs-05-dui-arrest-level-to-equally-silly-dwo-driving-while-older-in-full-page-ad (accessed August 7, 2017).

ABI. 2017b. *American Beverage Institute warns Idaho vacationers of Utah's .05 law in full-page* Idaho Statesman *ad.* https://abionline.org/press_release/american-beverage-institute-warns-idaho-vacationers-of-utahs-05-law-in-full-page-idaho-statesman-ad (accessed August 7, 2017).

ABI. 2017c. *American Beverage Institute cautions Nevada vacationers of Utah's .05 law in full-page* Las Vegas Review-Journal *ad and launches petition opposing .05.* https://abionline.org/press_release/american-beverage-institute-cautions-nevada-vacationers-of-utahs-05-law-in-full-page-las-vegas-review-journal-ad-and-launches-petition-opposing-05 (accessed August 7, 2017).

ABI. 2017d. *American Beverage Institute petition to "Urge the Utah legislature to repeal the .05 BAC legislation."* http://www.responsiblelimits.com/05-petition (accessed August 10, 2017).

ACLU (American Civil Liberties Union). 2016. *Racial disparities in Florida safety belt law enforcement.* New York: American Civil Liberties Union.

ACTS (Automotive Coalition for Traffic Safety). 2013. Statement of the Automotive Coalition for Traffic Safety on the National Transportation Safety Board's (NTSB's) recommendation regarding a 0.05 blood alcohol concentration (BAC) per se limit. *PR Newswire.* http://www.prnewswire.com/news-releases/statement-of-the-automotive-coalition-for-traffic-safety-on-the-national-transportation-safety-boards-ntsbs-recommendation-regarding-a-005-blood-alcohol-concentration-bac-per-se-limit-207398711.html (accessed August 18, 2017).

Advocates for Highway and Auto Safety. 2017. *Have we forgotten what saves lives?: 2017 roadmap of state highway safety laws*. Washington, DC: Advocates for Highway and Auto Safety.

Albalate, D. 2008. Lowering blood alcohol content levels to save lives: The European experience. *Journal of Policy Analysis and Management* 27(1):20–39.

Alcañiz, M., M. Guillén, M. Santolino, D. Sánchez-Moscona, O. Llatje, and L. Ramon. 2014. Prevalence of alcohol-impaired drivers based on random breath tests in a roadside survey in Catalonia (Spain). *Accident Analysis & Prevention* 65:131–141.

Amlung, M. T., D. H. Morris, and D. M. McCarthy. 2014. Effects of acute alcohol tolerance on perceptions of danger and willingness to drive after drinking. *Psychopharmacology* 231(22):4271–4279.

Anderson, P., D. Chisholm, and D. C. Fuhr. 2009a. Effectiveness and cost-effectiveness of policies and programmes to reduce the harm caused by alcohol. *The Lancet* 373(9682): 2234–2246.

Anderson, P., A. de Bruijn, K. Angus, R. Gordon, and G. Hastings. 2009b. Impact of alcohol advertising and media exposure on adolescent alcohol use: A systematic review of longitudinal studies. *Alcohol & Alcoholism* 44(3):229–243.

Andreuccetti, G., H. B. Carvalho, C. J. Cherpitel, Y. Ye, J. C. Ponce, T. Kahn, and V. Leyton. 2011. Reducing the legal blood alcohol concentration limit for driving in developing countries: A time for change? Results and implications derived from a time-series analysis (2001–10) conducted in Brazil. *Addiction* 106(12):2124–2131.

APIS (Alcohol Policy Information System). 2016. *Blood alcohol concentration (BAC) limits: Adult operators of noncommercial motor vehicles*. https://alcoholpolicy.niaaa.nih.gov/Blood_Alcohol_Concentration_Limits_Adult_Operators_of_Noncommercial_Motor_Vehicles.html (accessed March 30, 2017).

APIS. n.d. *Highlight on underage drinking*. https://alcoholpolicy.niaaa.nih.gov/Underage-Drinking.html (accessed March 30, 2017).

Apsler, R., T. M. Klein, W. M. Harding, and A. Char. 1999. *The effects of 0.08 BAC laws*. Washington, DC: National Highway Traffic Safety Administration.

Arthurson, R. M. 1985. *Evaluation of random breath testing*. Sidney, Australia: Traffic Authority of New South Wales.

Ascarelli, B. 2014. *Automatic sobriety checkpoints aim to bar drunk drivers*. http://sverigesradio.se/sida/artikel.aspx?programid=2054&artikel=5963580 (accessed August 18, 2017).

Barry, A. E., B. H. Chaney, and M. L. Stellefson. 2013. Breath alcohol concentrations of designated drivers. *Journal of Studies on Alcohol and Drugs* 74(4):509–513.

Bartl, G., and R. Esberger. 2000. *Effects of lowering the legal BAC limit in Austria*. Paper read at Proceedings of the 15th International Conference on Alcohol, Drugs and Traffic Safety, Stockholm, Sweden.

Beck, K. H., and M. L. Moser. 2004. Exposure to the sobriety "checkpoint strikeforce" campaign in Maryland: Impact on driver perceptions of vulnerability and behavior. *Traffic Injury Prevention* 5(2):101–106.

Bergen, G., A. Pitan, S. Qu, R. A. Shults, S. K. Chattopadhyay, R. W. Elder, D. A. Sleet, H. L. Coleman, R. P. Compton, and J. L. Nichols. 2014a. Publicized sobriety checkpoint programs: A community guide systematic review. *American Journal of Preventive Medicine* 46(5):529–539.

Bergen, G., J. Yao, R. A. Shults, E. Romano, and J. H. Lacey. 2014b. Characteristics of designated drivers and their passengers from the 2007 National Roadside Survey in the United States. *Traffic Injury Prevention* 15(3):273–277.

Bergum, A., B. Catlin, J. Willems Van Dijk, and K. Timberlake. 2016. *What works? Strategies to improve rural health*. Madison, WI: University of Wisconsin Population Health Institute.

Bernat, D. H., W. T. Dunsmuir, and A. C. Wagenaar. 2004. Effects of lowering the legal BAC to 0.08 on single-vehicle-nighttime fatal traffic crashes in 19 jurisdictions. *Accident Analysis & Prevention* 36(6):1089–1097.

Bernhoft, I. M., and I. Behrensdorff. 2003. Effect of lowering the alcohol limit in Denmark. *Accident Analysis & Prevention* 35(4):515–525.

Blais, É., F. Bellavance, A. Marcil, and L. Carnis. 2015. Effects of introducing an administrative .05% blood alcohol concentration limit on law enforcement patterns and alcohol-related collisions in Canada. *Accident Analysis & Prevention* 82:101–111.

Blomberg, R. D. 1992. *Lower BAC limits for youth: Evaluation of the Maryland .02 law.* Washington, DC: National Highway Traffic Safety Administration.

Blomberg, R. D., R. C. Peck, H. Moskowitz, M. Burns, and D. Fiorentino. 2005. *Crash risk of alcohol involved driving: A case-control study.* Stamford, CT: Dunlap and Associates, Inc.

Boots, K., and R. Midford. 1999. "Pick-a-skipper": An evaluation of a designated driver program to prevent alcohol-related injury in a regional Australian city. *Health Promotion International* 14(4):337–345.

Borkenstein, R. F., R. Crowther, R. Shumate, W. B. Ziel, and R. Zylman. 1974. The role of the drinking driver in traffic accidents (the Grand Rapids Study). *Blutalkohol* 11(Suppl): 1–131.

Brazil, N., and D. S. Kirk. 2016. Uber and metropolitan traffic fatalities in the United States. *American Journal of Epidemiology* 184(3):192–198.

Breitmeier, D., I. Seeland-Schulze, H. Hecker, and U. Schneider. 2007. The influence of blood alcohol concentrations of around 0.03% on neuropsychological functions—a double-blind, placebo-controlled investigation. *Addiction Biology* 12(2):183–189.

Brooks, C., and D. Zaal. 1992. Effects of a reduced alcohol limit for driving. Paper read at Proceedings International Council on Alcohol, Drugs and Traffic Safety Conference, Cologne, Germany.

Broyles, J. 2014. Drinking and driving and public transportation: A test of the routine activity framework. Thesis. Tempe: Arizona State University.

Burton, R., C. Henn, D. Lavoie, R. O'Connor, C. Perkins, K. Sweeney, F. Greaves, B. Ferguson, C. Beynon, A. Belloni, V. Musto, J. Marsden, and N. Sheron. 2017. A rapid evidence review of the effectiveness and cost-effectiveness of alcohol control policies: An English perspective. *The Lancet* 389(10078):1558–1580.

Byrne, P. A., T. Ma, R. E. Mann, and Y. Elzohairy. 2016. Evaluation of the general deterrence capacity of recently implemented (2009–2010) low and zero BAC requirements for drivers in Ontario. *Accident Analysis & Prevention* 88(5):56–67.

Calhoun, V. D., J. J. Pekar, and G. D. Pearlson. 2004. Alcohol intoxication effects on simulated driving: Exploring alcohol-dose effects on brain activation using functional MRI. *Neuropsychopharmacology* 29(11):2097–2107.

Cavanaugh, M., P. Lane, and J. C. Frey. 2012. *Escondido police under fire: Many more undocumented Latinos nabbed than drunks at DUI checkpoint.* http://www.kpbs.org/news/2012/mar/12/escondido-police-under-fire (accessed August 18, 2017).

CDC (Centers for Disease Control and Prevention). 2012. Vital signs: Drinking and driving among high school students aged ≥16 years—United States, 1991–2011. *Morbidity and Mortality Weekly Report* 61(39):796–800.

CDC. 2016. *Graduated driver licensing system, planning guide.* https://www.cdc.gov/motorvehiclesafety/pdf/teen/gdl_planning_guide-a.pdf (accessed August 11, 2017).

Chamberlain, E., and R. Solomon. 2002. The case for a 0.05% criminal law blood alcohol concentration limit for driving. *Injury Prevention* 8(Suppl 3):iii–1.

Chang, H. L., and C. K. Shih. 2012. Using a multidimensional Rasch model approach to measure the police's perceived ability to detect, detain and intercept DWI vehicles when conducting sobriety checkpoints. *Accident Analysis & Prevention* 48:505–517.

Cheng, S.-Y., J.-C. Lee, H.-Y. Lee, and S.-Y. Tsai. 2010. Comparing the effects of light alcohol consumption on human response to auditory and visual stimuli. *Perceptual and Motor Skills* 111(2):589–607.

Chuliá, H., M. Guillen, and O. Llatje. 2016. Seasonal and time-trend variation by gender of alcohol-impaired drivers at preventive sobriety checkpoints. *Journal of Studies on Alcohol and Drugs* 77(3):413–420.

Cicchino, J. B. 2017. *Insurance Institute for Highway Safety activities on alcohol-impaired driving.* PowerPoint presentation to the Committee on Accelerating Progress to Reduce Alcohol-Impaired Driving Fatalities in Washington DC, March 22, 2017. http://nationalacademies.org/hmd/~/media/Files/Activity%20Files/AcceleratingProgresstoReduceAlcoholImpairedDrivingFatalities/22%20March%202017/9%20Jessica%20Cicchino.pdf (accessed September 7, 2017).

Cicchino, J. B., and D. S. Zuby. 2017. Prevalence of driver physical factors leading to unintentional lane departure crashes. *Traffic Injury Prevention* 18(5):481–487.

Community Preventive Services Task Force. 2000. *Motor vehicle injury—Alcohol-impaired driving: 0.08% blood alcohol concentration (BAC) laws.* https://www.thecommunityguide.org/findings/motor-vehicle-injury-alcohol-impaired-driving-008-blood-alcohol-concentration-bac-laws (accessed August 7, 2017).

Connor, J., R. Norton, S. Ameratunga, and R. Jackson. 2004. The contribution of alcohol to serious car crash injuries. *Epidemiology* 15(3):337–344.

Creaser, J. I., N. J. Ward, M. E. Rakauskas, C. Shankwitz, and E. R. Boer. 2009. Effects of alcohol impairment on motorcycle riding skills. *Accident Analysis & Prevention* 41(5):906–913.

Cromer, J. R., J. A. Cromer, P. Maruff, and P. J. Snyder. 2010. Perception of alcohol intoxication shows acute tolerance while executive functions remain impaired. *Experimental and Clinical Psychopharmacology* 18(4):329–339.

Curry, A. E., K. B. Metzger, A. F. Williams, and B. C. Tefft. 2017. Comparison of older and younger novice driver crash rates: Informing the need for extended graduated driver licensing restrictions. *Accident Analysis & Prevention* 108:66–73.

DADSS (Driver Alcohol Detection System for Safety). 2016a. *Touch-based technology.* http://www.dadss.org/wp-content/uploads/2015/10/DADSSTouchBasedTechnology.pdf (accessed March 16, 2017).

DADSS. 2016b. *Breath-based technology.* http://www.dadss.org/wp-content/uploads/2015/10/DADSSBreathBasedTechnology.pdf (accessed March 16, 2017).

DADSS. 2016c. *DADSS partners with state of Virginia.* http://www.dadss.org/dadss-program-partners-with-state-of-virginia (accessed May 18, 2017).

DADSS. n.d.-a. *Frequently asked questions.* http://www.dadss.org/faq (accessed July 3, 2017).

DADSS. n.d.-b. *Our supporters.* http://www.dadss.org/our-supporters (accessed July 3, 2017).

De Sanctis, V., N. Soliman, A. T. Soliman, H. Elsedfy, S. Di Maio, M. El Kholy, and B. Fiscina. 2017. Caffeinated energy drink consumption among adolescents and potential health consequences associated with their use: A significant public health hazard. *Acta Biomedica* 88(2):222–231.

Decina, L. E., R. Foss, M. E. Tucker, A. Goodwin, and J. Sohn. 2009. *Alternative transportation programs: A countermeasure for reducing impaired driving.* Washington, DC: National Highway Traffic Safety Administration.

Dee, T. S. 2001. Does setting limits save lives? The case of 0.08 BAC laws. *Journal of Policy Analysis and Management* 20(1):111–128.

DeJong, W., and L. Wallack. 1992. The role of designated driver programs in the prevention of alcohol-impaired driving: A critical reassessment. *Health Education Quarterly* 19(4):429–442.

Desapriya, E., and N. Iwase. 1996. Are lower legal blood alcohol limits and a combination of sanctions desirable in reducing drunken driver-involved traffic fatalities and traffic accidents? *Accident Analysis & Prevention* 28(6):721–731.

Desapriya, E., I. Pike, S. Subzwari, G. Scime, and S. Shimizu. 2007. Impact of lowering the legal blood alcohol concentration limit to 0.03 on male, female and teenage drivers involved in alcohol-related crashes in Japan. *International Journal of Injury Control and Safety Promotion* 14(3):181–187.

Dills, A. K., and S. E. Mulholland. 2016. *Ride-sharing, fatal crashes, and crime.* https://ssrn.com/abstract=2783797 (accessed September 5, 2017).

Ditsuwan, V., J. L. Veerman, M. Bertram, and T. Vos. 2015. Sobriety checkpoints in Thailand: A review of effectiveness and developments over time. *Asia-Pacific Journal of Public Health* 27(2):NP2177–NP2187.

Ditter, S. M., R. W. Elder, R. A. Shults, D. A. Sleet, R. Compton, and J. L. Nichols. 2005. Effectiveness of designated driver programs for reducing alcohol-impaired driving: A systematic review. *American Journal of Preventive Medicine* 28(5S):280–287.

DOT (U.S. Department of Transportation). 1998. *TEA-21: Moving Americans into the 21st century.* https://www.fhwa.dot.gov/tea21 (accessed May 23, 2017).

DOT. n.d.-a. *Vehicle-to-infrastructure (v2i) resources.* https://www.its.dot.gov/v2i (accessed August 21, 2017).

DOT. n.d.-b. *Vehicle-to-vehicle (v2v) communications for safety.* https://www.its.dot.gov/research_archives/safety/v2v_comm_safety.htm (accessed August 21, 2017).

Eby, D. W., L. J. Molnar, L. P. Kostyniuk, R. M. St. Louis, N. Zanier, J. M. Lepkowski, and G. Bergen. 2017. Perceptions of alcohol-impaired driving and the blood alcohol concentration standard in the United States. *Journal of Safety Research* 63:73–81.

Eichelberger, A. H., and A. T. McCartt. 2016. Impaired driving enforcement practices among state and local law enforcement agencies in the United States. *Journal of Safety Research* 58:41–47.

Elam, C., R. N. McKaig, B. Jacobs, M. Whitlow, and K. R. Gros Louis. 2006. Examining a safe ride program: An assessment of the midnight special late night bus service. *NASPA Journal* 43(2):358–376.

Erickson, D. J., K. Farbakhsh, T. L. Toomey, K. M. Lenk, R. Jones-Webb, and T. F. Nelson. 2015. Enforcement of alcohol-impaired driving laws in the United States: A national survey of state and local agencies. *Traffic Injury Prevention* 16(6):533–539.

Erke, A., C. Goldenbeld, and T. Vaa. 2009. The effects of drink-driving checkpoints on crashes—A meta-analysis. *Accident Analysis & Prevention* 41(5):914–923.

Esser, M. B., J. Bao, D. H. Jernigan, and A. A. Hyder. 2016. Evaluation of the evidence base for the alcohol industry's actions to reduce drink driving globally. *American Journal of Public Health* 106(4):707–713.

Factor, R., D. R. Williams, and I. Kawachi. 2013. Social resistance framework for understanding high-risk behavior among nondominant minorities: Preliminary evidence. *American Journal of Public Health* 103(12):2245–2251.

Farmer, C. M., and J. K. Wells. 2010. Effect of enhanced seat belt reminders on driver fatality risk. *Journal of Safety Research* 41(1):53–57.

Farmer, C. M., and A. F. Williams. 2005. Effect on fatality risk of changing from secondary to primary seatbelt enforcement. *Journal of Safety Research* 36(2):189–194.

Faulks, I. J. 2014. Self-driving cars will not help the drinking driver. *The conversation.* http://theconversation.com/self-driving-cars-will-not-help-the-drinking-driver-31747 (accessed August 21, 2017).

Fell, J. C., and C. Compton. 2007. Evaulation of the use and benefit of passive alcohol sensors during routine traffic stops. *Annual Proceedings for the Association for the Advancement of Automotive Research* 51:437–448.

Fell, J. C., and M. Scherer. 2017. Estimation of the potential effectiveness of lowering the blood alcohol concentration (BAC) limit for driving from 0.08 to 0.05 grams per deciliter in the United States. *Alcoholism, Clinical and Experimental Research.* doi: 10.1111/acer.13501. [Epub ahead of print.]

Fell, J. C., and R. B. Voas. 2006. Mothers Against Drunk Driving (MADD): The first 25 years. *Traffic Injury Prevention* 7(3):195–212.

Fell, J. C., R. B. Voas, and J. E. Lange. 1997. Designated driver concept: Extent of use in the USA. *Journal of Traffic Medicine* 25(3-4):109–114.

Fell, J. C., S. A. Ferguson, A. F. Williams, and M. Fields. 2003. Why are sobriety checkpoints not widely adopted as an enforcement strategy in the United States? *Accident Analysis & Prevention* 35(6):897–902.

Fell, J. C., E. A. Langston, and A. S. Tippetts. 2005. Evaluation of four state impaired driving enforcement demonstration programs: Georgia, Tennessee, Pennsylvania and Louisiana. *Annual Proceedings of the Association for the Advancement of Automotive Medicine* 49:311–326.

Fell, J. C., A. S. Tippetts, and M. Levy. 2008. Evaluation of seven publicized enforcement demonstration programs to reduce impaired driving: Georgia, Louisiana, Pennsylvania, Tennessee, Texas, Indiana, and Michigan. *Annals in Advances of Automotive Medicine* 52:23–38.

Fell, J. C., D. A. Fisher, R. B. Voas, K. Blackman, and A. S. Tippetts. 2009. The impact of underage drinking laws on alcohol-related fatal crashes of young drivers. *Alcoholism, Clinical and Experimental Research* 33(7):1208–1219.

Fell, J. C., K. Jones, E. Romano, and R. Voas. 2011. An evaluation of graduated driver licensing effects on fatal crash involvements of young drivers in the United States. *Traffic Injury Prevention* 12(5):423–431.

Fell, J. C., M. Scherer, S. Thomas, and R. B. Voas. 2016. Assessing the impact of twenty underage drinking laws. *Journal of Studies on Alcohol and Drugs* 77(2):249–260.

FHWA (Federal Highway Administration). n.d. *Fixing America's Surface Transportation Act or "Fast Act".* https://www.fhwa.dot.gov/fastact (accessed July 3, 2017).

Fillmore, M. T., C. A. Marczinski, and A. M. Bowman. 2005. Acute tolerance to alcohol effects on inhibitory and activational mechanisms of behavioral control. *Journal of Studies on Alcohol* 66(5):663–672.

Filtness, A. J., C. M. Rudin-Brown, C. Mulvihill, and M. G. Lenné. 2013. Impairment of simulated motorcycle riding performance under low dose alcohol. *Accident Analysis & Prevention* 50:608–615.

FMCSA (Federal Motor Carrier Safety Administration). n.d. *MAP-21—Moving Ahead for Progress in the 21st Century Act.* https://www.fmcsa.dot.gov/mission/policy/map-21-moving-ahead-progress-21st-century-act (accessed July 3, 2017).

Foss, R. D., D. J. Beirness, and K. Sprattler. 1994. Seat belt use among drinking drivers in Minnesota. *American Journal of Public Health* 84(11):1732–1737.

Foss, R. D., J. R. Stewart, and D. W. Reinfurt. 2001. Evaluation of the effects of North Carolina's 0.08% AC law. *Accident Analysis & Prevention* 33(4):507–517.

Freedman, M., S. Lavi, P. Zador, and J. Lopdell. 2007. *The effectiveness of enhanced seat belt reminder systems: Observational field data collection methodology and findings.* DOT HS 810 844. Washington, DC: National Highway Traffic Safety Administration.

Freeman, D. G. 2007. Drunk driving legislation and traffic fatalities: New evidence on BAC 08 laws. *Contemporary Economic Policy* 25(3):293–308.

Freydier, C., C. Berthelon, M. Bastien-Toniazzo, and G. Gineyt. 2014. Divided attention in young drivers under the influence of alcohol. *Journal of Safety Research* 49(13):e11–e18.

Friedman, T. W., S. R. Robinson, and G. W. Yelland. 2011. Impaired perceptual judgment at low blood alcohol concentrations. *Alcohol* 45(7):711–718.

Gabrielson, R. 2010. Car seizures at DUI checkpoints prove profitable for cities, raise legal questions. *California Watch*. https://alethonews.wordpress.com/2010/02/16/car-seizures-at-dui-checkpoints-prove-profitable-for-cities-raise-legal-questions (accessed September 7, 2017).

García Moreno, L. M., A. Capilla, O. García Sánchez, J. Luque, K. Senderek, N. M. Conejo, and J. L. Arias. 2004. Alcohol tolerance in rats submitted to different periods of chronic and acute ethanol intake. *Psicothema* 16(2):211–216.

GHSA (Governors Highway Safety Association). 2011. *2011 winner: No Refusal program*. http://www.ghsa.org/about/safety-awards/2011-winner-no-refusal-program (accessed December 2, 2017).

GHSA. n.d. *Sobriety checkpoints*. http://www.ghsa.org/state-laws/issues/Sobriety-Checkpoints (accessed August 14, 2017).

Goodwin, A., R. Foss, J. Hedlund, J. Sohn, R. Pfefer, T. R. Neuman, K. L. Slack, and K. K. Hardy. 2005. *Guidance for implementation of the AASHTO strategic highway safety plan volume 16: A guide for reducing alcohol-related collisions*. Washington, DC: Transportation Research Board.

Goodwin, A., L. Thomas, B. Kirley, W. Hall, N. O'Brien, and K. Hill. 2015. *Countermeasures that work: A highway safety countermeasure guide for state highway safety offices, eighth edition*. DOT HS 812 202. Washington, DC: National Highway Traffic Safety Administration.

Gorman, D. M., J. C. Huber, and S. E. Carozza. 2006. Evaluation of the Texas 0.08 BAC law. *Alcohol and Alcoholism* 41(2):193–199.

Greenwood, B. N., and S. Wattal. 2017. Show me the way to go home: An empirical investigation of ride-sharing and alcohol related motor vehicle fatalities. *Management Information Systems Quarterly* 41(1):163–187.

Griffin, J. T. 2017. *MADD. Campaign to eliminate drunk driving: Update*. PowerPoint presentation to the Committee on Accelerating Progress to Reduce Alcohol-Impaired Driving Fatalities in Washington DC, March 22, 2017. http://www.nationalacademies.org/hmd/~/media/Files/Activity%20Files/AcceleratingProgresstoReduceAlcoholImpairedDrivingFatalities/22%20March%202017/8%20JT%20Griffin.pdf (accessed July 3, 2017).

Haegerich, T. M., R. A. Shults, R. F. Oman, and S. K. Vesely. 2016. The predictive influence of youth assets on drinking and driving behaviors in adolescence and young adulthood. *Journal of Primary Prevention* 37(3):231–245.

Harding, W. M., B. D. Caudill, and B. A. Moore. 2001. Do companions of designated drivers drink excessively? *Journal of Substance Abuse* 13(4):505–514.

Harvard School of Public Health. n.d. *Harvard alcohol project*. https://www.hsph.harvard.edu/chc/harvard-alcohol-project (accessed June 7, 2017).

Hawaii State Legislature. 2017. *SB18: Relating to the use of intoxicants while operating a vehicle*. https://www.capitol.hawaii.gov/Archives/measure_indiv_Archives.aspx?billtype=SB&billnumber=18&year=2017 (accessed December 12, 2017).

Hedlund, J. 2017. *Autonomous vehicles meet human drivers: Traffic safety issues for states*. Washington, DC: Governors Highway Safety Association.

Henstridge, J., R. Homel, and P. M. Mackay. 1997. *The long-term effects of random breath testing in four Australian states: A time series analysis*. Canberra, Australia: Federal Office of Road Safety.

Hingson, R., T. Heeren, and M. Winter. 1996. Lowering state legal blood alcohol limits to 0.08%: The effect on fatal motor vehicle crashes. *American Journal of Public Health* 86(9):1297–1299.

Høiseth, G., J. P. Bernard, N. Stephanson, P. T. Normann, A. S. Christophersen, J. Mørland, and A. Helander. 2008. Comparison between the urinary alcohol markers EtG, EtS, and GTOL/5-HIAA in a controlled drinking experiment. *Alcohol & Alcoholism* 43(2):187–191.

Høiseth, G., B. Yttredal, R. Karinen, H. Gjerde, J. Mørland, and A. Christophersen. 2010. Ethyl glucuronide concentrations in oral fluid, blood, and urine after volunteers drank 0.5 and 1.0 g/kg doses of ethanol. *Journal of Analytical Toxicology* 34(6):319–324.

Huseth, A. 2012. *Alcohol-impaired driving: Common practices and performance.* Fargo: Rural Transportation Safety and Security Center, Upper Great Plains Transportation Institute, North Dakota State University.

IIHS (Insurance Institute for Highway Safety). 2005. Sobriety checkpoints deter impaired drivers. *Status Report* 40(4). http://www.iihs.org/iihs/sr/statusreport/article/40/4/2 (accessed July 3, 2017).

IIHS. 2017. *Safety belts.* http://www.iihs.org/iihs/topics/t/safety-belts/qanda (accessed December 3, 2017).

IIHS and HLDI (Highway Loss Data Institute). 2009. Alcohol detection devices for all drivers garner widespread support. *Status Report* 44(8). http://www.iihs.org/iihs/sr/statusreport/article/44/8/1 (accessed July 3, 2017).

IIHS and HLDI. 2017. *Impaired driving: Deterrence and enforcement.* http://www.iihs.org/iihs/topics/t/impaired-driving/qanda#alcohol--deterrence-and-enforcement (accessed December 5, 2017).

Irwin, C., E. Iudakhina, B. Desbrow, and D. McCartney. 2017. Effects of acute alcohol consumption on measures of simulated driving: A systematic review and meta-analysis. *Accident Analysis & Prevention* 102:248–266.

Jackson, C. K., and E. G. Owens. 2011. One for the road: Public transportation, alcohol consumption, and intoxicated driving. *Journal of Public Economics* 95(1):106–121.

Jewett, A., R. A. Shults, T. Banerjee, and G. Bergen. 2015. Alcohol-impaired driving among adults—United States, 2012. *Morbidity and Mortality Weekly Report* 64(30):814–817.

Johnson, M. B. 2016. A successful high-visibility enforcement intervention targeting underage drinking drivers. *Addiction* 111(7):1196–1202.

Kahane, C. J. 2015. *Lives saved by vehicle safety technologies and associated federal motor vehicle safety standards, 1960 to 2012-passenger cars and LTVs.* DOT HS 812 069. Washington, DC: U.S. Department of Transportation.

Kelley-Baker, T., and E. Romano. 2014. Child passengers killed in reckless and alcohol-related motor vehicle crashes. *Journal of Safety Research* 48:103–110.

Kelley-Baker, T., and E. Romano. 2016. An examination of the effectiveness of child endangerment laws in preventing child fatalities in alcohol-involved motor vehicle crashes. *Journal of Studies on Alcohol and Drugs* 77(5):828–833.

Kelly, A. T., and A. Mozayani. 2012. An overview of alcohol testing and interpretation in the 21st century. *Journal of Pharmacy Practice* 25(1):30–36.

King, J. Y., and M. Tipperman. 1975. The offense of driving while intoxicated: The development of statutory and case law in New York. *Hofstra Law Review* 3(3):541–604.

Kloeden, C., and A. J. McLean. 1994. *Late night drink driving in Adelaide two years after the introduction of the 0.05 limit.* Walkerville, South Australia: Department of Road Transport, Office of Road Safety.

Knott, M. 2017. "Drunk robots": How driverless cars could leave humans behind within five years. *The Sydney Morning Herald.* http://www.smh.com.au/federal-politics/political-news/drunk-robots-how-driverless-cars-could-leave-humans-behind-within-five-years-20170222-guir7t.html (accessed August 22).

Krüger, H.-P., and M. Vollrath. 2004. The alcohol-related accident risk in Germany: Procedure, methods and results. *Accident Analysis & Prevention* 36(1):125–133.

Krüger, H.-P., E. Schulz, and H. Magerl. 1995. The German Roadside Survey 1992–1994. Saliva analyses from an unselected driver population: Licit and illicit drugs. Paper read at T'95 Proceedings of the 13th International Conference on Alcohol, Drugs and Traffic Safety, Adelaide, Australia.

Kusano, K. D., and H. C. Gabler. 2015. Comparison of expected crash and injury reduction from production forward collision and lane departure warning systems. *Traffic Injury Prevention* 16(Suppl 2):S109–S114.

Kweon, Y.-J., and K. M. Kockelman. 2006. Driver attitudes and choices: Speed limits, seat belt use, and drinking-and-driving. *Journal of the Transportation Research Forum* 45(3):39–56.

Kwo, P. Y., V. A. Ramchandani, S. O'Connor, D. Amann, L. G. Carr, K. Sandrasegaran, K. K. Kopecky, and T.-K. Li. 1998. Gender differences in alcohol metabolism: Relationship to liver volume and effect of adjusting for body mass. *Gastroenterology* 115(6):1552–1557.

Lacey, J. H., R. K. Jones, and E. Anderson. 2000. *Evaluation of a full-time ride service program: Aspen, Colorado's tipsy taxi service.* Washington, DC: National Highway Traffic Safety Administration.

Lacey, J. H., S. A. Ferguson, T. Kelley-Baker, and R. P. Rider. 2006. Low-manpower checkpoints: Can they provide effective DUI enforcement in small communities? *Traffic Injury Prevention* 7(3):213–218.

Lacey, J. H., T. Kelley-Baker, A. Berning, E. Romano, A. Ramirez, J. Yao, C. Moore, K. Brainard, K. Carr, K. Pell, and R. Compton. 2016. *Drug and alcohol crash risk: A case-control study.* Washington, DC: National Highway Traffic Safety Administration.

Lalanne, L., P. E. Lutz, and F. Paille. 2017. Acute impact of caffeinated alcoholic beverages on cognition: A systematic review. *Progress in Neuropsychopharmacology and Biological Psychiatry* 76:188–194.

Lange, J. E., and R. B. Voas. 1998. Nighttime observations of safety belt use: An evaluation of California's primary law. *American Journal of Public Health* 88(11):1718–1720.

Lange, J. E., R. B. Voas, and P. O'Rourke. 1998. What is designated driver anyway?: Results of a California survey on definitions and use of designated drivers. *Journal of Traffic Medicine* 26(3–4):101–108.

Lapham, S. C. 2010. The limits of tolerance: Convicted alcohol-impaired drivers share experiences driving under the influence. *Permanente Journal* 14(2):26.

Lavoie, M., G. Godin, and P. Valois. 1999. Understanding the use of a community-based drive-home service after alcohol consumption among young adults. *Journal of Community Health* 24(3):171–186.

Lenk, K. M., T. F. Nelson, T. L. Toomey, R. Jones-Webb, and D. J. Erickson. 2016. Sobriety checkpoint and open container laws in the United States: Associations with reported drinking-driving. *Traffic Injury Prevention* 17(8):782–787.

Levine, B. 2006. Central nervous system depressants: Miscellaneous. In *Principles of forensic toxicology.* 2nd ed. Washington, DC: American Association for Clinical Psychology. P. 216.

Levitt, M. D., R. Li, E. G. Demaster, M. Elson, J. Furne, and D. G. Levitt. 1997. Use of measurements of ethanol absorption from stomach and intestine to assess human ethanol metabolism. *American Journal of Physiology-Gastrointestinal and Liver Physiology* 273(4):G951–G957.

Li, K., B. G. Simons-Morton, and R. Hingson. 2013. Impaired-driving prevalence among US high school students: Associations with substance use and risky driving behaviors. *American Journal of Public Health* 103(11):e71–e77.

Li, T. K., J. D. Beard, W. E. Orr, P. Y. Kwo, and V. A. Ramchandani. 1998. Gender and ethnic differences in alcohol metabolism. *Alcoholism: Clinical and Experimental Research* 22(3):771–772.

Liang, L., and J. Huang. 2008. Go out or stay in? The effects of zero tolerance laws on alcohol use and drinking and driving patterns among college students. *Health Economics* 17(11):1261–1275.

LII (Legal Information Institute). n.d. *Per se.* https://www.law.cornell.edu/wex/per_se (accessed August 21, 2017).

Litman, T. A. 2017. *Autonomous vehicle implementation predictions: Implications for transport planning*. Paper presented at 2015 Transportation Research Board Annual Meeting, Washington, DC.

Liu, Y.-C., and C. H. Ho. 2010. Effects of different blood alcohol concentrations and post-alcohol impairment on driving behavior and task performance. *Traffic Injury Prevention* 11(4):334–341.

MADD (Mothers Against Drunk Driving). 2017. *MADD website: The Path to 0*. https://www.madd.org/the-solution/drunk-driving/ (accessed December 12, 2017).

Mann, R. E., S. Macdonald, G. Stoduto, S. Bondy, B. Jonah, and A. Shaikh. 2001. The effects of introducing or lowering legal per se blood alcohol limits for driving: An international review. *Accident Analysis & Prevention* 33(5):569–583.

Martin-Buck, F. 2016. *Driving safety: An empirical analysis of ridesharing's impact on drunk driving and alcohol-related crime*. http://www.frankmartinbuck.com/Ridesharing%20and%20Alcohol-Related%20Crime%20by%20Frank%20Martin-Buck.pdf (accessed September 11, 2017).

Masten, S. V., and R. D. Foss. 2010. Long-term effect of the North Carolina graduated driver licensing system on licensed driver crash incidence: A 5-year survival analysis. *Accident Analysis and Prevention* 42(6):1647–1652.

Masten, S. V., R. D. Foss, and S. W. Marshall. 2011. Graduated driver licensing and fatal crashes incolving 16- to 19-year old drivers. *JAMA* 306(10):1098–1103.

McCartt, A. T., and V. S. Northrup. 2004. Factors related to seat belt use among fatally injured teenage drivers. *Journal of Safety Research* 35(1):29–38.

McCartt, A. T., E. R. Teoh, M. Fields, K. A. Braitman, and L. A. Hellinga. 2010. Graduated licensing laws and fatal crashes of teenage drivers: A national study. *Traffic Injury Prevention* 11(3):240–248.

McLean, A., C. N. Kloeden, R. McColl, and R. Laslett. 1995. Reduction in the legal blood alcohol limit from 0.08 to 0.05: Effects on drink driving and alcohol-related crashes in Adelaide. *Alcohol, Drugs and Traffic Safety* 1:373–377.

Mercier-Guyon, C. 1998. *Lowering the BAC limit to 0.05: Results of the French experience*. Paper read at Transportation Research Board 77th Annual Meeting, Washington, DC.

Meskali, M., S. Hirt, I. Aillerie, G. Gineyt, N. Louveton, and C. Berthelon. 2011. Effect of moderated doses of alcohol on behavior of drivers confronted to simulated scenarios of accident. *Advances in Transportation Studies* (25):91–96.

Mets, M. A., E. Kuipers, L. M. Senerpont Domis, M. Leenders, B. Olivier, and J. C. Verster. 2011. Effects of alcohol on highway driving in the STI Sim driving simulator. *Human Psychopharmacology: Clinical and Experimental* 26(6):434–439.

Miller, T. R., M. S. Galbraith, and B. A. Lawrence. 1998. Costs and benefits of a community sobriety checkpoint program. *Journal of Studies on Alcohol* 59(4):462–468.

Miller, T., M. Blewden, and J.-F. Zhang. 2004. Cost savings from a sustained compulsory breath testing and media campaign in New Zealand. *Accident Analysis & Prevention* 36(5):783–794.

Mishra, L., S. Sharma, J. J. Potter, and E. Mezey. 1989. More rapid elimination of alcohol in women as compared to their male siblings. *Alcoholism: Clinical and Experimental Research* 13(6):752–754.

Mitchell, Jr., M. C., E. L. Teigen, and V. A. Ramchandani. 2014. Absorption and peak blood alcohol concentration after drinking beer, wine, or spirits. *Alcoholism: Clinical and Experimental Research* 38(5):1200–1204.

Molnar, L. J., D. W. Eby, L. P. Kostyniuk, R. M. St. Louis, and N. Zanier. 2017. Stakeholder perceptions of lowering the blood alcohol concentration standard in the United States. *Annals of Epidemiology* 27(12):757–762.

Molof, M. J., J. Dresser, S. Ungerleider, C. Kimball, and J. Schaefer. 1995. *Assessment of year-round and holiday ride service programs.* DOT HS 808 203. Washington, DC: National Highway Traffic Safety Administration.

Moore, C., and L. Pierce. 2016. Reactance to transgressors: Why authorities deliver harsher penalties when the social context elicits expectations of leniency. *Frontiers in Psychology* 7(550):1–17.

Morrison, C. N., S. F. Jacoby, B. Dong, M. Delgado, and D. J. Wiebe. 2017. Ridesharing and motor vehicle crashes in four US cities: An interrupted time series analysis. *American Journal of Epidemiology*, June 14.

Moskowitz, H., and D. Fiorentino. 2000. *A review of the literature on the effects of low doses of alcohol on driving-related skills.* Washington, DC: National Highway Traffic Safety Administration.

Moskowitz, H., P. Zador, A. Smiley, D. Fiorentino, and M. Burns. 2000. *Driver characteristics and impairment at various BACs.* Washington, DC: National Highway Traffic Safety Administration.

Mumenthaler, M. S., J. L. Taylor, R. O'Hara, and J. A. Yesavage. 1999. Gender differences in moderate drinking effects. *Alcohol Research and Health* 23(1):55–64.

Nagata, T., D. Hemenway, and M. J. Perry. 2006. The effectiveness of a new law to reduce alcohol-impaired driving in Japan. *Japan Medical Association Journal* 49(11):365–369.

Nagata, T., S. Setoguchi, D. Hemenway, and M. J. Perry. 2008. Effectiveness of a law to reduce alcohol-impaired driving in Japan. *Injury Prevention* 14(1):19–23.

Nagin, D. S. 2013. Deterrence in the 21st century: A review of the evidence. *Crime and Justice: An Annual Review of Research* 42:199–263.

Nakahara, S., K. Katanoda, and M. Ichikawa. 2013. Onset of a declining trend in fatal motor vehicle crashes involving drunk-driving in Japan. *Journal of Epidemiology* 23(3):195–204.

NASEM (National Academies of Sciences, Engineering, and Medicine). 2016. *Between public and private mobility: Examining the rise of technology-enabled transportation services.* Washington, DC: The National Academies Press. https://doi.org/10.17226/21875.

Naz, S., and B. Scott-Parker. 2017. Obstacles to engaging in young driver licensing: Perspectives of parents. *Accident Analysis & Prevention* 99(Pt A):312–320.

NCSA (National Center for Statistical Analysis). 2017. *Occupant protection in passenger vehicles: 2015 data.* DOT HS 812 374. Washington, DC: National Highway Traffic Safety Administration.

NCSL (National Conference of State Legislatures). 2017. *Autonomous vehicles.* http://www.ncsl.org/research/transportation/autonomous-vehicles-self-driving-vehicles-enacted-legislation.aspx (accessed August 21, 2017).

NDAA (National District Attorneys Association). 2015. *Child endangerment statutes and penalties.* Alexandria, VA: Author.

Neil, M. 2006. Low manpower sobriety checkpoints in rural and small communities. *Between the Lines* 15(1):1–2.

New Jersey Opinion. 2016. *Editorial: This town's free ride program to fight DUI should be tested all over N.J.* http://www.nj.com/opinion/index.ssf/2016/09/test_drive_eveshams_dui-fighting_program_all_over.html (accessed January 5, 2018).

NHTSA (National Highway Traffic Safety Administration). 2006. *Low-staffing sobriety checkpoints.* DOT HS 810 590. Washington, DC: U.S. Department of Transportation.

NHTSA. 2013a. *Safety in numbers.* 1(9):1–4. https://www.nhtsa.gov/es/staticfiles/numbers/Safety_In_Numbers_Drive_Sober_811871.pdf (accessed August 24, 2017).

NHTSA. 2013b. *U.S. Department of transportation extends cooperative research program with automotive industry to cut drunk driving on U.S. Roads.* https://www.nhtsa.gov/press-releases/us-department-transportation-extends-cooperative-research-program-automotive-industry (accessed May 19, 2017).

NHTSA. 2015. *Traffic safety facts 2015: A compilation of motor vehicle crash data from the Fatality Analysis Reporting System and the General Estimates System.* DOT HS 812 384. Washington, DC: U.S. Department of Transportation.

NHTSA. 2016a. *Traffic safety facts: Alcohol-impaired driving.* https://crashstats.nhtsa.dot.gov/Api/Public/Publication/812350 (accessed August 28, 2017).

NHTSA. 2016b. *U.S. DOT urges public to "drive sober or get pulled over" and announces funding for innovative technology to end drunk driving.* https://www.nhtsa.gov/press-releases/us-dot-urges-public-%E2%80%98drive-sober-or-get-pulled-over%E2%80%99-and-announces-funding-innovative (accessed May 18, 2017).

NHTSA. 2017a. *Traffic safety facts: Young drivers.* https://crashstats.nhtsa.dot.gov/Api/Public/ViewPublication/812278 (accessed August 28, 2017).

NHTSA. 2017b. *NHTSA's No Refusal toolkit.* https://www.nhtsa.gov/staticfiles/planners/NoRefusalWeekend/index.htm (accessed December 2, 2017).

NHTSA. n.d.-a. *Drunk driving.* https://www.nhtsa.gov/risky-driving/drunk-driving (accessed May 16, 2017).

NHTSA. n.d.-b. *NHTSA No Refusal Weekend toolkit.* https://www.nhtsa.gov/staticfiles/planners/NoRefusalWeekend/index.htm (accessed December 2, 2017).

NIAAA (National Institute on Alcohol Abuse and Alcoholism). 1999. *Alcohol alert: Are women more vulnerable to alcohol's effects?* https://pubs.niaaa.nih.gov/publications/aa46.htm (accessed January 9, 2018).

NIAAA. 2017. *What is a standard drink?* https://www.niaaa.nih.gov/alcohol-health/overview-alcohol-consumption/what-standard-drink (accessed December 6, 2017).

Nielson, A. L., and B. Watson. 2009. The effectiveness of designated driver programs. *Journal of the Australasian College of Road Safety* 20(2):32–37.

Noordzij, P. 1977. The introduction of a statutory BAC limit of 50 mg/100 ml and its effect on drinking and driving habits and traffic accidents. Paper read at Seventh International Conference on Alcohol, Drugs and Traffic Safety, Melbourne, Australia.

Noordzij, P. 1994. *Decline in drinking and driving in the Netherlands.* Washington, DC: Transportation Research Board.

Norstrom, T. 1997. Assessment of the impact of the 0.02 percent BAC-limit in Sweden. *Studies on Crime and Crime Prevention* 6(2):245–258.

NTSB (National Transportation Safety Board). 2013. *Reaching zero: Actions to eliminate alcohol-impaired driving.* https://www.ntsb.gov/safety/safety-studies/Documents/SR1301.pdf (accessed January 9, 2018).

Otero, S., and T. Rau. 2017. The effects of drinking and driving laws on car crashes, injuries, and deaths: Evidence from Chile. *Accident Analysis & Prevention* 106:262–274.

Parks, V., C. Leister, A. Patat, S. Troy, A. Vermeeren, E. Volkerts, and J. Verster. 2002. Effects of ethanol at a blood alcohol concentration of 0.4 g/l on actual driving and memory. *European Neuropsychopharmacology* 12(Suppl 3):432–433.

Peck, J. 2017. *New York City drunk driving after Uber.* New York: City University of New York Graduate Center, Ph.D. Program in Economics.

Peck, R. C., M. A. Gebers, R. B. Voas, and E. Romano. 2008. The relationship between blood alcohol concentration (BAC), age, and crash risk. *Journal of Safety Research* 39(3):311–319.

Peden, M., R. Scurfield, D. Sleet, D. Mohan, A. A. Hyder, E. Jarawan, and C. D. Mathers. 2004. *World report on road traffic injury prevention.* Geneva, Switzerland: World Health Organization.

Phillips, D. P., and K. M. Brewer. 2011. The relationship between serious injury and blood alcohol concentration (BAC) in fatal motor vehicle accidents: BAC = 0.01% is associated with significantly more dangerous accidents than BAC = 0.00%. *Addiction* 106(9):1614–1622.

Pickrell, T. M., and R. Li. 2016. *Seat belt use in 2016—Overall results.* DOT HS 812351. Washington, DC: National Highway Traffic Safety Administration.

Piontkowski, S. R., J. S. Peabody, C. Reede, J. Velascosoltero, G. Tsatoke, T. Shelhamer, and K. R. Hicks. 2015. Reducing motor vehicle-related injuries at an Arizona Indian reservation: Ten years of application of evidence-based strategies. *Global Health: Science and Practice* 3(4):619–629.

Preusser, D. F. 2000. Identification of alcohol-impairment on initial interview. *Transportation Research E-Circular* E1–E7.

Quinlan, K. P., R. D. Brewer, D. A. Sleet, and A. M. Dellinger. 2000. Characteristics of child passenger deaths and injuries involving drunk drivers. *JAMA* 283(17):2249–2252.

Rakauskas, M. E., N. J. Ward, E. R. Boer, E. M. Bernat, M. Cadwallader, and C. J. Patrick. 2008. Combined effects of alcohol and distraction on driving performance. *Accident Analysis & Prevention* 40(5):1742–1749.

Rivara, F. P., A. Relyea-Chew, J. Wang, S. Riley, D. Boisvert, and T. Gomez. 2007. Drinking behaviors in young adults: The potential role of designated driver and safe ride home programs. *Injury Prevention* 13(3):168–172.

Rodriguez-Iglesias, C., C. Wiliszowski, and J. H. Lacey. 2001. *Legislative history of .08 per se laws.* Washington, DC: National Highway Traffic Safety Administration.

Roehrs, T., and T. Roth. n.d. *Sleep, sleepiness, and alcohol use.* https://pubs.niaaa.nih.gov/publications/arh25-2/101-109.htm?utm_source=io9+Newsletter&utm_campaign=6d29bbd775-UA-142218-29&utm_medium=email (accessed August 21, 2017).

Rogers, P. N. 1995. *The general deterrent impact of California's 0.08% blood alcohol concentration limit and administrative per se license suspension laws volume 1 of: An evaluation of the effectiveness of California's 0.08% blood alcohol concentration limit and administrative per se license suspension laws.* Sacramento: California Department of Motor Vehicles.

Rogers, P. N. 1997. *Specific deterrent impact of California's 0.08% blood alcohol concentration limit and administrative per se license suspension laws volume 2 of: An evaluation of the effectiveness of California's 0.08% blood alcohol concentration limit and administrative per se license suspension laws.* Sacramento, CA: Office of Traffic Safety.

Romano E., J. Fell, and R. Voas. 2011. The role of race and ethnicity on the effect of graduated driver licensing laws in the United States. *Annals of Advances in Automotive Medicine* 55:51–61.

Ronen, A., H. S. Chassidim, P. Gershon, Y. Parmet, A. Rabinovich, R. Bar-Hamburger, Y. Cassuto, and D. Shinar. 2010. The effect of alcohol, THC and their combination on perceived effects, willingness to drive and performance of driving and non-driving tasks. *Accident Analysis & Prevention* 42(6):1855–1865.

Rothe, P. J., and L. J. Carroll. 2009. Hazards faced by young designated drivers: In-car risks of driving drunken passengers. *International Journal of Environmental Research and Public Health* 6(6):1760–1777.

Rothschild, M. L., B. Mastin, and T. W. Miller. 2006. Reducing alcohol-impaired driving crashes through the use of social marketing. *Accident Analysis & Prevention* 38(6):1218–1230.

Rudin-Brown, C. M., A. J. Filtness, A. R. Allen, and C. M. Mulvihill. 2013. Performance of a cognitive, but not visual, secondary task interacts with alcohol-induced balance impairment in novice and experienced motorcycle riders. *Accident Analysis & Prevention* 50:895–904.

Rupp, T. L., C. Acebo, R. Seifer, and M. A. Carskadon. 2007. Effects of a moderate evening alcohol dose. II: Performance. *Alcoholism: Clinical and Experimental Research* 31(8): 1365–1371.

Salam, R. A., A. Arshad, J. K. Das, M. N. Khan, W. Mahmood, S. B. Freedman, and Z. A. Bhutta. 2016. Interventions to prevent unintentional injuries among adolescents: A systematic review and meta-analysis. *Journal of Adolescent Health* 59(4 Suppl):S76–S87.

Sanem, J. R., D. J. Erickson, P. C. Rutledge, K. M. Lenk, T. F. Nelson, R. Jones-Webb, and T. L. Toomey. 2015. Association between alcohol-impaired driving enforcement-related strategies and alcohol-impaired driving. *Accident Analysis and Prevention* 78:104–109.

Sarkar, S., M. Andreas, and F. De Faria. 2005. Who uses safe ride programs: An examination of the dynamics of individuals who use a safe ride program instead of driving home while drunk. *American Journal of Drug and Alcohol Abuse* 31(2):305–325.

Schmitt, G., R. Aderjan, T. Keller, and M. Wu. 1995. Ethyl glucuronide: An unusual ethanol metabolite in humans. Synthesis, analytical data, and determination in serum and urine. *Journal of Analytical Toxicology* 19(2):91–94.

Schoettle, B., and M. Sivak. 2013. *The reasons for the recent decline in young driver licensing in the U.S.* 2013. University of Michigan, Transportation Research Institute, Ann Arbor, Michigan.

Schwartz, J., and A. Davaran. 2013. Enforcement following 0.08% BAC law change: Sex-specific consequences of changing arrest practices? *Addictive Behaviors* 38(10):2506–2512.

Schweizer, T. A., and M. Vogel-Sprott. 2008. Alcohol-impaired speed and accuracy of cognitive functions: A review of acute tolerance and recovery of cognitive performance. *Experimental and Clinical Psychopharmacology* 16(3):240.

Shults, R. A., and A. F. Williams. 2016. Graduated driver licensing night driving restrictions and drivers aged 16 or 17 years involved in fatal night crashes—United States, 2009–2014. *Morbidity and Mortality Weekly Report* 65(29):725–730.

Shults, R. A., R. W. Elder, D. A. Sleet, J. L. Nichols, M. O. Alao, V. G. Carande-Kulis, S. Zaza, D. M. Sosin, R. S. Thompson, and Task Force on Community Preventive Services. 2001. Reviews of evidence regarding interventions to reduce alcohol-impaired driving. *American Journal of Preventive Medicine* 21(4):66–88.

Sjöström, L. O., and T. Jonsson. n.d. *Experiences from the trial with automatic sobriety checkpoints ("alco gates") in Frihamnen, Stockholm*. https://auli-yhdistysavain-fi-bin.directo.fi/@Bin/5a556fb5e12fb85959ef290a89d3671f/1503074707/application/pdf/204163/Jonsson_Sjostrom.pdf (accessed August 18, 2017).

Smith, D. I. 1986. Effect of low proscribed blood alcohol levels (BALs) on traffic accidents among newly-licensed drivers. *Medicine, Science and the Law* 26(2):144–148.

Snyder, M. 1992. *Driving under the influence: A report to Congress on alcohol limits*. Washington, DC: National Highway Traffic Safety Administration.

Solomon, D. 2014. *The Court of Criminal Appeals ruled that police can't take blood from DWI suspects without a warrant*. https://www.texasmonthly.com/the-daily-post/the-court-of-criminal-appeals-ruled-that-police-cant-take-blood-from-dwi-suspects-without-a-warrant (accessed December 2, 2017).

Solomon, R., E. Chamberlain, M. Abdoullaeva, and B. Tinholt. 2011. Random breath testing: A Canadian perspective. *Traffic Injury Prevention* 12(2):111–119.

Sommer, K. 2016. *DWI Summit shows "No Refusal" program a success*. http://www.valleymorningstar.com/news/local_news/dwi-summit-shows-no-refusal-program-a-success/article_1678b094-3f05-11e6-88b3-2b11e8c368c5.html (accessed December 2, 2017).

Sprattler, K. 2010. *Minnesota safe ride program report*. Minneapolis: Center for Transportation Studies, University of Minnesota.

Sternlund, S. 2017. The safety potential of lane departure warning systems—A descriptive real-world study of fatal lane departure passenger car crashes in Sweden. *Traffic Injury Prevention* 18(Suppl 1):S18–S23.

Stuster, J. W., and P. A. Blowers. 1995. *Experimental evaluation of sobriety checkpoint programs. Final report*. Washington, DC: National Highway Traffic Safety Administration.

Tefft, B. C., A. F. Williams, and J. G. Grabowski. 2013. *Timing of driver's license acquisition and reasons for delay among young people in the United States, 2012*. AAA Foundation for Traffic Safety, Washington, DC.

Tefft, B. C., A. F. Williams, and J. G. Grabowski. 2014. Driver licensing and reasons for delaying licensure among young adults ages 18–20, United States, 2012. *Injury Epidemiology* 1:4.

Thomas, S., T. Kelley-Baker, E. Romano, R. Treffers, and C. L. Cannon. 2014. Transporting young passengers while impaired: The state of the law. *Health Behavior and Policy Review* 1(4):265–277.

Thomasson, H. 2000. Alcohol elimination: Faster in women? *Alcoholism: Clinical and Experimental Research* 24(4):419–420.

Timmerman, M. A., E. S. Geller, K. E. Glindemann, and A. K. Fournier. 2003. Do the designated drivers of college students stay sober? *Journal of Safety Research* 34(2):127–133.

Tippetts, A. S., R. B. Voas, J. C. Fell, and J. L. Nichols. 2005. A meta-analysis of .08 BAC laws in 19 jurisdictions in the United States. *Accident Analysis & Prevention* 37(1):149–161.

Tison, J., A. F. Williams, and N. K. Chaudhary. 2010. *Daytime and nighttime seat belt use by fatally injured passenger vehicle occupants.* Washington, DC: National Highway Traffic Safety Administration.

Tomblin, E. R., P. Reed, and B. Tipton. 2016. *West Virginia highway safety plan: Federal fiscal year 2017.* Charleston, WV: West Virginia's Governor's Highway Safety Program.

Tremblay, M., F. Gallant, M. Lavallière, M. Chiasson, D. Silvey, D. Behm, W. J. Albert, and M. J. Johnson. 2015. Driving performance on the descending limb of blood alcohol concentration (BAC) in undergraduate students: A pilot study. *PLoS ONE* 10(2):e0118348.

Uber. n.d.-a. *The future of trucking.* https://www.uber.com/info/atg/truck (accessed August 21, 2017).

Uber. n.d.-b. *Uber hits five billion rides milestone.* https://www.uber.com/en-SG/blog/uber-hits-5-billion-rides-milestone (accessed December 4, 2017).

Utah State Legislature. 2017. *H.B. 155 Driving under the influence and public safety revisions.* http://le.utah.gov/~2017/bills/static/HB0155.html (accessed March 30, 2017).

UtahPolicy.com. 2017. *Poll: A majority of Utahns oppose lowering DUI limit.* http://utahpolicy.com/index.php/features/today-at-utah-policy/12806-poll-a-majority-of-utahns-oppose-lowering-dui-limit (accessed August 21, 2017).

Van Ooijen, D. 1977. *The effects of a new DWI law.* Paper read at Seventh International Conference on Alcohol, Drugs and Traffic Safety, Melbourne, Australia.

Verster, J. C., A. E. Wester, M. Goorden, J.-P. Van Wieringen, B. Olivier, and E. R. Volkerts. 2009. Novice drivers' performance after different alcohol dosages and placebo in the divided-attention steering simulator (DASS). *Psychopharmacology* 204(1):127–133.

Vingilis, E., H. Blefgen, H. Lei, K. Sykora, and R. Mann. 1988. An evaluation of the deterrent effects of Ontario BAC law. *Accident Analysis & Prevention* 20:917.

Voas, R. B., and J. C. Fell. 2013. Strengthening impaired-driving enforcement in the United States. *Traffic Injury Prevention* 14(7):661–670.

Voas, R. B., and J. H. Lacey. 1990. Drunk driving enforcement, adjudication, and sanctions in the United States. In *Drinking and driving: Advances in research and prevention*, edited by R. J. Wilson and R. E. Mann. New York: Guilford Press. Pp. 116–158.

Voas, R. B., A. S. Tippetts, and J. Fell. 2000. The relationship of alcohol safety laws to drinking drivers in fatal crashes. *Accident Analysis & Prevention* 32(4):483–492.

Voas, R. B., A. S. Tippetts, and E. P. Taylor. 2002. The Illinois .08 law: An evaluation. *Journal of Safety Research* 33(1):73–80.

Voas, R. B., P. Torres, E. Romano, and J. H. Lacey. 2012. Alcohol-related risk of driver fatalities: An update using 2007 data. *Journal of Studies on Alcohol and Drugs* 73:341–350.

Wagenaar, A. C., M. M. Maldonado-Molina, L. Ma, A. L. Tobler, and K. A. Komro. 2007. Effects of legal BAC limits on fatal crash involvement: Analyses of 28 states from 1976 through 2002. *Journal of Safety Research* 38(5):493–499.

Walker, S., A. J. Treno, J. W. Grube, and J. M. Light. 2003. Ethnic differences in driving after drinking and riding with drinking drivers among adolescents. *Alcoholism: Clinical and Experimental Research* 27(8):1299–1304.

Wall, T. L., S. E. Luczak, and S. Hiller-Sturmhofel. 2016. Biology, genetics, and environment: Underlying factors influencing alcohol metabolism. *Alcohol Research* 38(1):59–68.

Washington State House of Representatives. 2017. *HB1874: Bill analysis.* http://lawfilesext.leg.wa.gov/biennium/2017-18/Pdf/Bill%20Reports/House/1874%20HBA%20PS%2017.pdf (accessed December 6, 2017).

Washington State Legislature. 2017. *HB 1874–201–18: Addressing the blood and breath alcohol concentration of persons operating or in physical control of a vehicle, vessel, or aircraft.* http://app.leg.wa.gov/billsummary?BillNumber=1874&Year=2017 (accessed December 12, 2017).

Weldy, D. L. 2010. Risks of alcoholic energy drinks for youth. *Journal of the American Board of Family Medicine* 23(4):555–558.

Wesemann, P. 1989. Costs and benefits of police enforcement in the Netherlands. Paper read at Alcohol, Drugs, & Traffic Safety: Proceedings of the 11th International Conference on Alcohol, Drugs & Traffic Safety, Chicago, IL.

WHO (World Health Organization). 2014. *Legal BAC limits data by country.* http://apps.who.int/gho/data/node.main.A1147?lang=en (accessed December 21, 2017).

WHO. 2015. *Global status report on road safety 2015.* Geneza, Switzerland: WHO.

WHO Regional Office for Europe. 2009. *Evidence for the effectiveness and cost-effectiveness of interventions to reduce alcohol-related harm.* Copenhagen, Denmark: WHO Regional Office for Europe.

Williams, A. F., A. T. McCartt, and L. B. Sims. 2016. History and current status of state graduated driver licensing (GDL) laws in the United States. *Journal of Safety Research* 56:9–15.

Williams, H., and A. Salamy. 1972. Alcohol and sleep. In *The biology of alcoholism,* edited by B. Kissin and H. Begleiter. New York: Plenum Press. Pp. 435–483.

Winkler, J. 2012. *A DWI offer you can't refuse.* https://www.thefix.com/content/no-refusal-night-austin (accessed December 2, 2017).

Winsten, J. A. 1994. Promoting designated drivers: The Harvard alcohol project. *American Journal of Preventive Medicine* 10(3 Suppl):11–14.

Winsten, J. A. 2017. Developing media messages that save lives. *Stanford Social Innovation Review.* https://ssir.org/transformative_scale/entry/developing_media_messages_that_save_lives (accessed June 26, 2017).

Wolburg, J. M. 2005. How responsible are "responsible" drinking campaigns for preventing alcohol abuse? *Journal of Consumer Marketing* 22(4):176–177.

Wurst, F. M., S. Dresen, J. P. Allen, G. Wiesbeck, M. Graf, and W. Weinmann. 2006. Ethyl sulphate: A direct ethanol metabolite reflecting recent alcohol consumption. *Addiction* 101(2):204–211.

Zador, P. L. 1991. Alcohol-related relative risk of fatal driver injuries in relation to driver age and sex. *Journal of Studies on Alcohol* 52(4):302–310.

Zador, P. L., S. A. Krawchuk, and R. B. Voas. 2000. Alcohol-related relative risk of driver fatalities and driver involvement in fatal crashes in relation to driver age and gender: An update using 1996 data. *Journal of Studies on Alcohol* 61(3):387–395.

Zaouk, A. K., M. Wills, E. Traube, and R. Strassburger. 2015. *Driver alcohol detection system for safety (DADSS)—A status update.* Paper presented at 24th International Technical Conference on the Enhanced Safety of Vehicles, Gothenburg, Sweden.

Zwicker, T., N. K. Chaudhary, S. Maloney, and R. Squeglia. 2007a. *Connecticut's 2003 impaired-driving high-visibility enforcement campaign.* Washington, DC: National Highway Traffic Safety Administration.

Zwicker, T., N. Chaudhary, M. G. Solomon, J. Siegler, and J. Meadows. 2007b. *West Virginia's impaired driving high-visibility enforcement campaign, 2003–2005.* Washington, DC: National Highway and Traffic Safety Administration.

5

Postcrash and Arrest Interventions

INTRODUCTION

While the two previous chapters discuss interventions aimed at influencing behaviors such as drinking to impairment and driving while impaired, this chapter focuses on reducing the likelihood or severity of negative outcomes of these behaviors: motor vehicle crashes and serious injuries and fatalities. As noted throughout the report, alcohol-impaired driving fatalities make up 28 percent of all traffic fatalities, and 10,497 people were killed in alcohol-impaired driving crashes in 2016. Because of data limitations, it can be difficult to obtain accurate arrest data on driving while impaired (DWI), accurate counts of how many offenders reoffend, and estimates of the number of DWI arrests that lead to a conviction (see Chapter 6 and Appendix A for more on data limitations). However, available data show that there were more than 1 million arrests for driving under the influence in 2015 (CDC, 2017; FBI, 2015). About 20 to 28 percent of first-time DWI offenders will repeat the offense (Lapham et al., 2006; Robertson et al., 2016), and recidivists are about 60 percent more likely to be involved in a fatal crash (Fell, 2014; Sloan et al., 2016).

This chapter begins with a section on the interventions (i.e., policies, systems, and programs) in the legal system that focus on deterring the general public (general deterrence) and those who have been previously arrested (specific deterrence) from driving while impaired. According to criminological theories, potential offenders balance risks and benefits when choosing whether to commit a crime (Nagin, 2013); deterrence theory relies on the perception of "swift, certain, and severe" detection and punishment of criminal activity, including alcohol-impaired driving (Goodwin et al., 2015, p. 1-10; NIAAA, 2000; Nichols and Ross, 1989). This perception is built on a system of continued, publicized enforcement (IIHS, 2017a). This section also focuses on treatment of those convicted of alcohol-impaired driving to help modify their behaviors and decrease the likelihood that they will repeat the crime. There are many other points in the legal process that could be improved that are not discussed in this section. The interventions discussed are those the committee determined would have the greatest effect on the population, are feasible, are cost-effective, and target specific high-risk populations. The chapter's second section includes information on how to improve emergency response after a motor vehicle crash, with a focus on rural areas. Although the committee did not focus on emergency response as an intervention, it is a promising area to help reduce fatalities in rural areas. As discussed in Chapter 2, rural areas are an important target population for alcohol-impaired driving because they account for a large proportion of fatal crashes, and many existing interventions are more relevant to urban areas. The interventions in this chapter engage the range of actors required to enforce laws and detect, prosecute, adjudicate, and treat alcohol-impaired drivers as well as respond to alcohol-impaired driving crashes.

LEGAL SYSTEM INTERVENTIONS: ENFORCEMENT

Law enforcement officers are trained to detect and arrest impaired drivers in three phases. The first phase is the law enforcement officer's observation of the driver and any unsafe behaviors that draw the officer's attention to the vehicle, such as lane swerving or failure to obey traffic signs and signals. After pulling over a potentially impaired driver, the second phase of detection involves the officer's personal contact with the driver. Law enforcement officials are trained to use all senses when communicating with the driver. For example, the officer observes how the driver is speaking, any odors coming from the driver or vehicle, and any items visible in the vehicle. If the officer suspects the driver is impaired, he or she can then perform the third phase by requesting the driver to perform the standardized field sobriety tests (SFSTs). The officer will continue to observe the driver as he or she exits the vehicle, looking for additional indicators of impairment such as slurred speech or poor motor control. At this point the officer will also ask the driver if he or she has any medical conditions that would preclude the driver from performing the SFSTs. The SFSTs are made up of three validated parts: the walk and turn; the one-leg stand; and the horizontal gaze nystagmus (although some jurisdictions do not allow admission of testimony regarding the horizontal gaze nystagmus). In this phase, the officer may also administer a preliminary, handheld breath test (PBT) (Voas and Fell, 2011). This device can be used to indicate the presence of alcohol, but the results cannot be used in court in most states. A drug recognition expert could also be summoned if the officer does not think alcohol is the sole cause of the driver's impairment. Taken together, the observations of driving ability, communication with the driver, and performance on the SFSTs can lead an officer to conclude there is probable cause for arrest. Subsequent to arrest, officers will request the driver take a chemical test, such as a blood test, to determine blood alcohol concentration (BAC) (Voas and Fell, 2011). State laws vary with respect to policies criminalizing refusal to take chemical tests and license suspension at the point of arrest.

There are some barriers to the process of successfully detecting and arresting alcohol-impaired drivers. For example, law enforcement officers may not be adequately or consistently trained in the three phases or the agency might be understaffed. Additionally, some states have limited laboratories or personnel to complete tests, and tests are often expensive and resource intensive.

Furthermore, it is important to note that there is evidence of systematic discrimination and disproportionate targeting of people of color by the police in the United States (Aboelata et al., 2017; Ingraham, 2014; NASEM, 2017; President's Task Force on 21st Century Policing, 2015). Implementing a unified approach to reducing alcohol-impaired driving in communities would require intensive officer training and community engagement to foster cooperation and avoid alienating residents as communities and police work toward a common goal of zero lives lost (Aboelata et al., 2017).

Breath and Blood Tests for Detecting Alcohol Impairment

Once an officer arrests a driver, the officer will ask the driver to provide a breath test, which may take place at a roadside location or at a police station (Berning et al., 2008). A driver may decline to provide a breath test. The refusal may significantly affect or hinder subsequent prosecution and sanctions, as the absence of a BAC test result precludes a suspected alcohol-impaired driver from being charged under a per se law (Berning et al., 2008).[1] Driver refusal rates for tests vary greatly among states. In 2011, the range of state breath test refusal rates (of Puerto Rico and 33 states with adequate reporting data) was 1 percent to 82 percent, with a national average of 24 percent. Two states (Florida and New Hampshire) had breath test refusal rates above 70 percent, and two more states had rates above 40 percent. Puerto Rico and 21 states had breath

[1] A per se law means that the act in question is illegal in and of itself.

test refusal rates below 25 percent, and of those, 6 states and Puerto Rico had rates of 10 percent or less (Namuswe et al., 2014).

Toxicologists can use a calculation (retrograde extrapolation) to determine an impaired driver's BAC at the time of an offense using, for example, a later BAC result obtained at the police station after arrest (AAA, 2016). This calculation factors in details such as the driver's weight, height, sex, number and type of drinks consumed, and time passed to establish a metabolism rate and estimated BAC while the person was driving (APRI, 2003). As an estimate based on assumptions, results of retrograde extrapolation are not as accurate as a BAC measured in real time. Results can be used in expert testimony in court; however, they may be challenged or excluded, which can disadvantage a prosecutor's case (APRI, 2003; Robertson and Simpson, 2002).

Testing Alcohol Impairment—Practices and Policies

All 50 states and the District of Columbia have *implied consent* laws, meaning that drivers using state roads (or federally owned park roads) have "consented" to comply with sobriety testing if there is an indication that they are driving while impaired. In an effort to compel drivers to comply with sobriety testing, states have enacted laws that make it a criminal offense to refuse a chemical test (e.g., Minnesota and Nebraska, among 16 other states)[2] (Goodwin et al., 2015). As discussed above, law enforcement officials have few tests at their disposal to identify and detect alcohol-impaired drivers, and each of these tests—the SFSTs, a handheld breath-testing device, and blood or urine tests—come with their own limitations and challenges. While the SFSTs and handheld breath-testing devices can be administered at the point of contact with a driver who is suspected of being alcohol impaired, blood, breath, or urine testing are generally administered by trained technicians at a hospital or police station. Some jurisdictions have introduced enforcement vans with evidentiary equipment, although these can be costly and are not available everywhere (DeMetrick, 2016; Hedlund and McCartt, 2002; NC Health and Human Services, 2017). SFSTs and blood, breath, and urine tests can all be used to facilitate the prosecution of DWI cases, although the extent to which they can be admissible in court varies from state to state.

One challenge that police officers face when it comes to administering alcohol-impairment tests is the possibility that drivers simply refuse to comply with their request for testing. Unless the penalty for refusing a chemical test exceeds the penalty that a driver could incur should they fail the test (e.g., being prosecuted for impaired driving), there is little

[2] Number as of 2013 (Goodwin et al., 2015).

incentive for drivers to comply. See Chapter 4 for more information about no refusal enforcement. Without court-admissible tests results, however, it is difficult for police officers or court officials to prove whether a driver was indeed alcohol impaired at the time he or she was stopped.

In 2016, the Supreme Court ruled on a case involving the admissibility of breath and blood tests in states where drivers were told they were subject to criminal charges if they refused to comply with a police officer's request to take a sobriety test.[3] The defendants argued that their Fourth Amendment rights had been violated because they could not refuse the tests, and were not served a court-ordered warrant for the test, thus constituting an unreasonable search. In their ruling, the court determined that the Fourth Amendment rights of drivers were not violated and no warrant was necessary since the breath tests were not invasive, the tests only measured alcohol in the breath, and no biosamples were stored after the test was administered. In regard to blood tests, however, the court ruled that a warrant would be necessary since the act of drawing blood is invasive, an individual's blood can yield additional information beyond the BAC, and biosamples could be saved or used for other purposes.

One strategy to increase BAC testing at the time of arrest, and to eliminate the need for retrograde extrapolation, is the use of electronic warrants. In many jurisdictions law enforcement officers are able to contact on-call judges remotely at the time of arrest and have an electronic warrant sent directly to their smartphones or computers to avoid a delay in testing. Traditional means of obtaining warrants could take hours. These systems link the officer, prosecutor, and judges and allow for the generation, review, approval, and filing of warrants. Potential challenges related to electronic warrants include the availability of judges to be on call, which could be especially difficult in smaller jurisdictions; organizing the needed services for the blood draws, including during evenings and weekends; training for those who obtain the blood samples (including training to minimize risk to oneself or others); transport of a driver to a hospital or clinic if a trained phlebotomist is not available; and the issue of the chain of evidence for the blood sample, as the assessment of the sample would not be performed by the nurse/practitioner who draws the blood, but would need to be taken or sent to a laboratory for analysis. While hospital laboratories are generally open 24/7, this type of testing is not generally performed on an emergency basis for someone who is not a patient in the emergency department (ED) or hospital. The blood would likely be sent to a state laboratory for processing, thereby not providing an immediate answer to the question related to BAC. In addition, if there are any questions during

[3] *Birchfield v. North Dakota*, 136 S. Ct. 2160 (2016) consolidated with *Bernard v. Minnesota*, 844 N.W.2d 41 (Minn. Ct. App. 2014) and *Beylund v. North Dakota*, 859 N.W.2d 403 (N.D. 2015).

the case about the chain of evidence, the person who draws the blood may need to appear in court to attest to the fact that s/he drew the blood and handed it directly to the police officer who was then responsible for getting it to the next destination. However, many law enforcement agencies need to address these issues regardless of when the blood sample is taken from the defendant. Hedlund (2017) notes that many law enforcement agencies are currently considering transitioning to an electronic warrant system to improve efficiency. While electronic warrants are a promising strategy for obtaining accurate BAC results, more guidance is needed on how to implement them and the required infrastructure and protocols.

A passive test, such as using a flashlight that is equipped with an alcohol sensor, can help police officers screen drivers who they suspect have been drinking. These have been shown to increase the arrest rate for police officers who do not normally make DWI arrests (Fell et al., 2008), but the tests do not aid in charging or prosecuting a driver who may have been driving under the influence of alcohol. A recent survey of law enforcement agencies found infrequent use of passive tests, mainly due to a lack of equipment (Eichelberger and McCartt, 2016), although past research has also documented officer aversion to passive tests because of personal safety concerns (e.g., using the device brings the officer in close contact with the driver and occupies one hand) (Goodwin et al., 2015; Leaf and Preusser, 1996).

LEGAL SYSTEM INTERVENTIONS: ADJUDICATION

The adjudication process begins after an alcohol-impaired driver has been arrested. An offender could be arraigned the same day as the arrest or released to come back to court another time. Before pleading guilty at a court appearance, hearing, or trial, defendants may undergo an alcohol evaluation by a trained, certified individual in some jurisdictions or states; the driver is often referred to a treatment program if he or she meets the criteria for alcohol use disorder (AUD, DSM-5)[4] (SAMHSA, 2005a). Whether or not screening is mandatory and when screening takes place vary by state (Chang et al., 2002), but the results can inform the prosecutor's proposal to the judge, along with other additional information such as performance on the SFSTs, chemical tests, observations of the driver,

[4] Alcohol use disorder, as defined by the *Diagnostic and Statistical Manual of Mental Disorders, Fifth Edition* (DSM-5), is based on the presence of at least two symptoms from a specific set of criteria, with subclassifications of mild, moderate, and severe, whereas the DSM-IV defined two different disorders (alcohol abuse and alcohol dependence) with separate criteria for each. This has implications for how the categories compare across various research studies. In this chapter these disorders will be defined as the study authors defined them in their methodology.

statements made by the offender during the arrest process and/or testing, the offender's driving history, and the effect on the victim if a crash was involved. If the driver is found guilty of alcohol-impaired driving, penalties could include fines, restitution, license suspension or revocation, ignition interlock installation, serving time in a correctional facility, or probation (Goodwin et al., 2015; SAMHSA, 2005a). A driver convicted of DWI could also be sentenced to complete a treatment program, participate in a monitoring program, or attend a victim impact panel (Goodwin et al., 2015; SAMHSA, 2005a). Many states have enacted various vehicle and license plate sanctions, including vehicle immobilization, impoundment, or forfeiture, and license plate impoundment and marked license plates for offenders with revoked or suspended licenses (Goodwin et al., 2015). Implementation of these laws varies by state and the evidence base for individual measures is mixed, but in general these sanctions reduce DWI recidivism (Goodwin et al., 2015; TRB, 2013a). States have varying sanctions for convicted DWI offenders, such as the number of DWIs that raise the charge to a felony, as well as more severe penalties for higher BAC levels or for having a child in the car at the time of arrest or crash (Goodwin et al., 2015).

There are some challenges that can impede the adjudication process for ensuring offenders receive proper sentencing and treatment. For example, because blood test results can take a long time to be processed, a prosecutor may have to proceed to trial without those results and therefore potentially rely on less information when presenting the case. Furthermore, information on past DWI convictions in other states may not be available to inform the decision of whether an offense should be increased to a felony charge (AAA, 2016; Robertson and Simpson, 2002). Additionally, there can be discrepancies between arrest and conviction data since some arrests may lead to a lesser plea, and therefore a driver's conviction may not reflect the initial reason for arrest (see Chapter 6 for more details and information gaps regarding these data sources). For example, someone could be charged with reckless driving in addition to a felony DWI but that driver might plead guilty to the felony and have other charges dropped as a result of a deal with the prosecutor. Moreover, alcohol-impaired driving offenses could be reduced to non-alcohol-impaired driving offenses, or a defendant's record could be sealed.

Prosecution Process

Limits on Diversion and Plea Agreements

After an alcohol-impaired driving arrest, some offenders are given the option of participating in a diversion program or taking a plea agreement.

A diversion program usually takes the form of education or treatment, and if the program is successfully completed, then the defendant may be given the option to plead to a non-alcohol-impaired driving offense such as reckless driving, for example, or in some cases, charges may be dropped and the infraction erased from the offender's record (Goodwin et al., 2015). There is variation in the types of education and treatment used in diversion programs, and as a result, the evidence on whether they are effective is mixed (Voas and Fisher, 2001). A plea agreement is an agreement in which the defendant agrees to plead guilty in return for a concession from the prosecutor. Restrictions on when prosecutors can offer plea agreements have been found to reduce alcohol-impaired driving recidivism (Goodwin et al., 2015; Surla and Koons, 1989). Survey results indicate that up to 75 percent of alcohol-impaired driving cases are resolved with a plea agreement, and the concession offered is most often a reduced penalty (Goodwin et al., 2015; Robertson and Simpson, 2002). Concessions, however, vary by state, and in some states plea agreements result in the elimination of penalties and a clean record (Goodwin et al., 2015). Or, lesser offenses could remain on the record, and at least one state (Washington) maintains a record of completed diversion programs (McCartt et al., 2013).

When the record of an alcohol-impaired driving offense is erased or reduced through participation in a diversion program or a plea agreement, then it becomes impossible to identify recidivist offenders, reducing the severity with which their crime is perceived and in turn, the severity of the consequences associated thereof (Hedlund and McCartt, 2002; NTSB, 2000; Robertson and Simpson, 2002; TRB, 2005a). Grunwald et al. (2001) found that approximately 40 percent of alcohol-impaired driving offenders in Rhode Island that were charged as a first-time offender had previous alcohol-impaired driving arrests that had been erased from their records. As of 2014, 13 states had anti-plea-bargaining statutes limiting when a plea bargain can be offered (NHTSA, 2016). The National Highway Traffic Safety Administration (NHTSA) rates limits on diversion and plea agreements as a four-star intervention (that is, demonstrated to be effective in certain situations) for reducing alcohol-impaired driving (Goodwin et al., 2015). The National Transportation Safety Board (NTSB, 2000), the Transportation Research Board (TRB, 2005a), and the Traffic Injury Research Foundation (Robertson and Simpson, 2002) have also recommended limits on diversion and plea agreements.

Many DWI cases do not proceed to trial and offenders are instead offered participation in diversion programs or plea agreements with reduced charges (AAA, 2016; Robertson and Simpson, 2002; Voas and Fisher, 2001). This section reviews limits on diversion and plea agreements, but notes evidence on diversion program effectiveness is mixed because program components and studies of them vary substantially. The only study directly examining plea agreement restrictions found reduced recidivism in three communities in response to the restrictions (Surla and Koons, 1989). Eliminated offenses because of a diversion program or lessened charges as a result of a plea agreement have implications for the severity of punishment and subsequent offender interactions with the criminal justice system, such as later DWIs, and therefore, general and specific deterrent effects (Robertson and Simpson, 2002). Based on older and mixed evidence on plea agreement restrictions and diversion programs, the committee concludes:

> *Conclusion 5-1: Research is needed on the effects of restrictions on diversion programs that remove alcohol-impaired driving convictions from a driver's record and on the content of plea agreements for alcohol-impaired driving offenders as strategies to reduce DWI recidivism.*

Administrative License Suspension/Administrative License Revocation Laws

Administrative license suspension (ALS) laws permit law enforcement officials to suspend an alcohol-impaired driver's license at the time of arrest for refusing to submit or failing (i.e., the driver's BAC is over the limit set by state law) a chemical test to determine his or her BAC. Administrative license revocation (ALR) laws require driver's license reapplication after a suspension concludes. These pre-conviction laws apply to both first-time and repeat offenders. These measures are separate from criminal convictions; drivers convicted of DWI may also lose their licenses and face additional criminal sanctions. A temporary license, which can be valid from 7 to 90 days, allows time for an administrative hearing and for the driver to obtain alternative transportation (Goodwin et al., 2015; IIHS, 2017a).

ALS laws are enacted in 41 states and the District of Columbia,[5] but they vary in the length of temporary license validity, length of suspension, and whether limited driving privileges can be restored during the suspension period (IIHS, 2017b). For example, Virginia's suspension period is 7 days. Mississippi suspends offenders' licenses for 90 days, and while Arizona's suspension is the same length of time, offenders in that state are allowed limited driving privileges after 30 days. At least 12 states allow driving during the suspension period if the driver agrees to an ignition interlock device (IIHS, 2017b). A recent study found suspension periods of at least 91 days to be more effective than shorter periods (Fell and Scherer,

[5] Nine states do not have ALS/ALR laws: Kentucky, Michigan, Montana, New Jersey, Pennsylvania, Rhode Island, South Carolina, South Dakota, and Tennessee.

2017). NHTSA recommends an initial license suspension for at least 90 days for drivers with a BAC over 0.08% (or, 15 days followed by 75 days with a restricted license if the driver uses an ignition interlock device) and greater penalties for drivers who refuse a BAC test (NHTSA, 2006). Some states also allow a hardship provision, permitting the offender to drive to work or school (Goodwin et al., 2015). Although ALS laws have been challenged, court decisions have upheld these statutes, determining the laws ensure drivers' due process as they provide a timely administrative hearing (IIHS, 2017c).

ALS and ALR laws are swift and certain; the consequences immediately follow the offending behavior, rather than following a conviction (Wagenaar and Maldonado-Molina, 2007). Many studies assessing the effectiveness of ALS and ALR laws were conducted as laws were enacted decades ago (Goodwin et al., 2015). These laws have been shown to affect alcohol-impaired driving crashes and fatalities (IIHS, 2017d; Talpins et al., 2014; Voas et al., 2000a). For example, one study found that alcohol-impaired driving crashes and first-time and repeat DWI convictions significantly declined after California's ALS law was enacted (Rogers, 1997). Voas et al. (2000b) examined about 43,700 records of Ohio DWI offenders from 1990 to 1995. Compared to the time period before Ohio's ALS law was enacted, the authors found reductions in DWI recidivism, moving violations, and crashes for first-time and multiple offenders after the law was implemented, although vehicle sanction legislation was also passed around the same time, which also could have affected driving outcomes. The recidivism rate within 24 months of arrest decreased from 15 to 5 percent for first-time offenders and from 25 to 7 percent among multiple offenders. Furthermore, crash involvement declined from 12 to 5 percent and from 14 to 7 percent among first-time and multiple offenders, respectively, in the 24 months after DWI arrest. Another large study that examined data in 38 states from 1976 to 2002 found a significant 5 percent reduction in alcohol-related fatal crash involvement and estimated the law(s) saved 800 lives per year (Wagenaar and Maldonado-Molina, 2007). This study found no significant effect of post-conviction suspension laws and concluded ALS policies are more effective in deterring alcohol-impaired driving than post-conviction license suspension or revocation (Wagenaar and Maldonado-Molina, 2007). While recent studies on cost-effectiveness of ALS and ALR laws have not been completed, a 1991 analysis of three states concluded that revenues generated from license reinstatement fees compensated for the laws' operating expenses (Lacey et al., 1991).

License suspension or revocation does not, however, stop all DWI offenders from continuing to drive without a valid license (Goodwin et al., 2015; Lenton et al., 2010; McCartt et al., 2002), nor does it affect DWI offenders' alcohol consumption among those with AUD. Approximately half of first-time and repeat DWI offenders in one study delayed license reinstatement for at least 1 year (Voas et al., 2010a); those offenders who postpone license reinstatement are more likely to repeat the DWI offense compared to those drivers who reestablish their licenses (Voas et al., 2010b).

As described earlier in this chapter, the theory of deterrence relies on the perception of immediate, guaranteed, and severe punishment; well-implemented ALS and ALR laws ensure celerity and certainty of punishment (Goodwin et al., 2015; IIHS, 2017d). However, these laws are not in place in all states, and among those that have enacted laws, penalty severity varies among states. Although any suspension period is more effective than having no law, analyses favor ALS laws with longer suspension periods (Fell and Scherer, 2017). While there is a need for additional contemporary research, there is evidence from several studies that ALS and ALR laws have both general and specific deterrence effects, and the laws reduce alcohol-impaired driving crashes and convictions (Rogers, 1997; Voas et al., 2000a,b; Wagenaar and Maldonado-Molina, 2007). These effects can endure past the suspension period as well. In a recent study, Fell and Scherer (2017) found ALR laws had greater general deterrence effects than specific deterrence effects. This is an important finding because some offenders will continue to drive without a license, and these laws are one measure to deter alcohol-impaired driving among the general driving population. Other interventions, such as treatment, counseling, and ignition interlock devices (all discussed in more detail in this chapter), could complement ALS and ALR laws to prevent DWI recidivism (Goodwin et al., 2015; TRB, 2013a).

> *Conclusion 5-2: Nationwide adoption of effective administrative license suspension (ALS) and administrative license revocation (ALR) laws that provide for pre-conviction license suspension/revocation for refusing or failing a BAC test, that include an initial complete suspension, and that are based on updated model legislation would increase the effect of these laws.*

Model legislation on ALS/ALR laws exists (NHTSA, 1986), but should be brought up-to-date. NHTSA could work with organizations that focus on state-level traffic laws and traffic safety to ensure that effective model laws (for example, full suspension for refusal to take a breath test) are in place and disseminated to states.

Treatment Related to the Adjudication Process

Different types of alcohol misuse necessitate the need for different, tailored types of interventions. Figure 5-1 shows a spectrum of problems related to alcohol misuse and the types of interventions that may be most beneficial for individuals suffering from each of these problems. The following sections describe some of these interventions and the individuals who may benefit the most from them, particularly among alcohol-impaired driving offenders. Although alcohol-impaired driving is a crime and law enforcement measures can be very effective, enforcement alone will not fully solve the problem of alcohol-impaired driving.

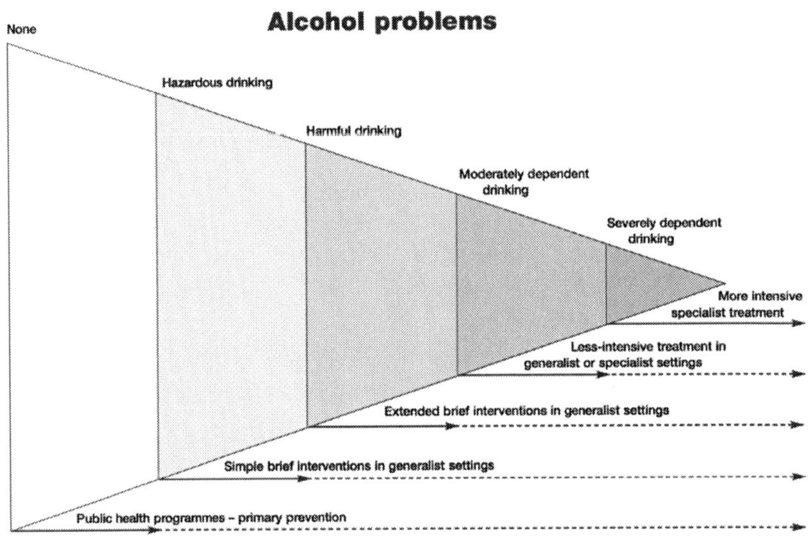

FIGURE 5-1 A spectrum of interventions to treat different types of alcohol misuse.
NOTES: Although the figure is not drawn to scale, the prevalence in the population of each of the categories of alcohol problem is approximated by the area of the triangle occupied; most people have no alcohol problems, a very large number show risky consumption but no current problems, many have risky consumption and less serious alcohol problems, some have moderate dependence and problems, and a few have severe dependence or complicated alcohol problems. In this figure, responses to alcohol problems include public health programs, brief interventions, and treatment. Each of these responses can differ with respect to the setting, duration, and intensity according to the problem.
SOURCE: Raistrick et al., 2006.

Alcohol Use Disorder (AUD) and Convictions for Driving While Impaired

There is a spectrum of reasons individuals drive while alcohol impaired. For those who do not suffer from AUD (DSM-5), swift and appropriate sanctions and penalties, or the use of screening, brief intervention, and referral to treatment (SBIRT) are generally effective. However, apprehension for DWI is an opportunity to identify and provide resources to people with AUD across the entire spectrum. When a convicted individual has AUD, treatment is a key part of the adjudication process to help modify his or her behavior and reduce the likelihood of driving while alcohol impaired again.

More than 15 million adults and 623,000 adolescents had AUD in 2015, according to results from the National Survey on Drug Use and Health (SAMHSA, 2016a). Furthermore, AUD is a highly comorbid condition; 2.7 million adults with AUD in 2015 also had an illicit drug use disorder (SAMHSA, 2016b). Data from the 2012–2013 National Epidemiologic Survey on Alcohol and Related Conditions III showed both 12-month and lifetime AUD were significantly associated with other drug disorders, mood disorders including major depressive and bipolar I disorders, and antisocial and borderline personality disorders (Grant et al., 2015). There is no evidence whether interventions geared toward the general public (e.g., alternative transportation) will be as effective for DWI offenders with AUD. Furthermore, those who drink and drive may also drive while impaired by drugs (Talpins and Rogers, 2017; Talpins et al., 2015). For example, a study of 92 drivers arrested for DWI in Florida found that 41 percent tested positive for at least one of seven drug categories; the most prevalent drugs included cannabinoids, benzodiazepines, and cocaine (Logan et al., 2014).

Among those convicted of DWI, rates of alcoholism appear to increase as the number of DWI convictions increases (Cavaiola et al., 2003). A cohort study found that people with multiple DWIs are five times more likely than the general population to have an alcohol abuse or dependence diagnosis (DSM-IV) (Lapham et al., 2011). Brinkmann et al. (2002) found that more than 80 percent of individuals who drove with a BAC higher than 0.19% were alcoholics in a sample of alcohol-impaired drivers.[6]

Recent national estimates on how many DWI offenders are diagnosed with AUD in the general population are not available in the published literature. Hingson[7] of the National Institute on Alcohol Abuse and Alco-

---

[6] "Alcoholic" is defined in this study by Alc-Indices (calculated using methanol, acetone, 2-propanol, γ-GT, and CDT concentrations).

[7] Personal communication with Ralph Hingson, National Institute on Alcohol Abuse and Alcoholism on April 13, 2017. Available by request from the National Academies of Sciences, Engineering, and Medicine's Public Access Records Office (PARO@nas.edu).

holism (NIAAA) performed a descriptive analysis on data from the 2012 and 2013 National Epidemiology Survey and Related Conditions and found that among the 8 percent (n = 2,091) who reported driving after drinking in the past year, 25 percent met criteria for mild AUD, 21 percent moderate AUD, and 30 percent severe AUD. In the total population, 9 percent met criteria for mild AUD, 5 percent for moderate AUD, and 5 percent for severe AUD.[8] Stasiewicz et al. (2007) found 4.2 and 4.4 percent of convicted DWI offenders from a sample in Erie County, New York, were diagnosed with alcohol abuse and alcohol dependence, respectively (DSM-IV).

Screening DWI offenders for alcohol abuse problems is mandatory in most states, but not all; results can be used to inform treatment recommendations to the court (Chang et al., 2002). Sometimes formal screening methods involving testing and interviewing are used (Chang et al., 2001), but most courts use self-reported information from DWI offenders to screen for AUD, usually by having them complete a simple questionnaire about their alcohol use (NIAAA, 2004/2005). Offenders, however, often underreport their alcohol use for fear of punishment, judgment, or breach in confidentiality, resulting in a missed treatment opportunity for many (Center for Substance Abuse Treatment, 1995; Knight et al., 2002; Lapham et al., 2002, 2004). Although there are effective AUD screening guidelines available (Chang et al., 2002), courts generally cannot hire people specifically trained to screen for AUD because of financial limitations (Knight et al., 2002). The amount it would cost courts to screen and treat these individuals, however, is often much less than the cost of incarceration (Center for Substance Abuse Treatment, 1995; NIAAA, 2004/2005).

Court assessment, referral, intervention, and treatment strategies for DWI offenders vary substantially across the United States (Cavaiola and Wuth, 2014). Some forms of treatment for DWI offenders include motivational interviewing, brief interventions, cognitive behavioral therapy (CBT), and counseling (Robertson et al., 2008; SAMHSA, 2005a). Sentencing practices for driving under the influence of alcohol also vary by state. For example, courts in Washington provide a DWI sentencing grid based on BAC result and number of prior offenses to help judges determine appropriate punishments for DWI offenders. As noted, expanded alcohol assessment and treatment is deemed mandatory in the sentencing grid for any offender with two or three prior offenses (Washington Courts, 2016). A similar sentencing grid created by NHTSA in 2005 recommends alcohol use assessment and treatment for all repeat offenders (NHTSA, 2005).

---

[8] Ibid.

Not all public court sentencing records are available electronically. In most states, court records are available on their website and are searchable by last name or court date, but only by county; they are often unreliable because all data are not routinely entered (see Chapter 6 for more information on data collection). For specific information, such as whether the offender was screened for AUD, one must often contact the court where an individual's action was filed. The number of DWI arrests made per year by state is available through the Federal Bureau of Investigation's Uniform Crime Reporting (UCR) program (FBI, 2010), but these data are neither comprehensive nor timely (Rosenfeld, 2007). The UCR program is made up of crime data reports submitted by police agencies across the country, but these crime rates are often underestimates because of barriers to monitoring and reporting such as financial restrictions, staffing changes, inadequate training, natural disasters, and new computers or crime reporting systems (Maltz and Targonski, 2002). Some states, like California, have been able to overcome these barriers and track not only arrest rates but also types of DWI convictions (Daoud et al., 2015).

DWI Courts

DWI courts are specialized courts aimed at changing DWI offenders' behavior through comprehensive monitoring and substance abuse treatment. As a part of the DWI control system, these post-conviction courts are a systematic mechanism for holding offenders accountable for their actions while treating the underlying cause(s) of their impaired driving. They are a voluntary alternative to traditional probation (Fourth Judicial District Minnesota Judicial Branch, n.d.; Hawaii State Judiciary, n.d.). DWI courts are modeled after the successful drug court system (NADCP, n.d.) and are founded on 10 guiding principles (see Box 5-1).

Some DWI courts are a subset of drug courts; as of August 2014, there were 216 DWI courts across 31 states and 409 hybrid DWI/drug courts (Goodwin et al., 2015). In a 2016 survey, 40 percent of DWI courts reported primarily serving urban areas; more than one-third of programs indicated they mainly serve rural areas, but no respondents described principally serving tribal territory (Block, 2016). DWI courts reported predominantly white, fully employed participants (Block, 2016).

DWI courts are team-based, in which the judge, prosecuting and defense attorneys, probation officer, and treatment staff familiar with DWI laws and addiction issues work together to ensure an effective and individualized sentencing and treatment plan for the offender (Goodwin et al., 2015). Teams meet frequently to report program infractions, offer positive reinforcement, and modify restrictions when deemed appropriate. DWI courts' intensive supervision involves observing the offender in public,

BOX 5-1
10 Guiding Principles of DWI Courts

Identify the population: Clearly define the DWI court's target population based on distinct eligibility criteria in collaboration with the community.

Complete a clinical assessment: Perform an objective evaluation to assess the impaired driver's alcohol use disorder, drug involvement, mental and physical health status, social ties, and self-efficacy to determine the required level of care.

Establish the treatment plan: Based on the clinical assessment, implement an individualized treatment plan made up of multiple, high-quality interventions.

Monitor the offender: The DWI court team, including the probation division and treatment provider, should supervise the offender in his or her home, work, and community environments.

Build partnerships: Develop and use partnerships to foster collaboration between the court, other agencies, and community organizations to reinforce the court's goals.

Encourage a judicial leadership position: Select a DWI court judge who understands alcohol use disorders and who will lead the DWI court team effectively, support the offender, and preserve partnerships.

Use case management methods: Maintain an organized, collaborative, communicative environment for team case management across court, monitoring, and treatment staff; a primary case manager can be designated.

Manage transportation problems: Emphasize offenders should solve transportation issues on their own while acknowledging local contexts and possibly limited transportation alternatives; ensure offenders do not continue to drive without a valid license.

Assess the program: Evaluate the DWI court to analyze operational integrity, identify effective and ineffective program components and interventions, and document successful short- and long-term behavior change attributable to the court.

Plan for a sustainable court: Create a network of support and consider funding, court structure and scale, and organization.

SOURCE: NCDC, n.d.-a.

at home, and at work. This includes adherence to a treatment plan, use of ignition interlocks or car impounds, and alcohol and drug testing (using transdermal or breath test devices). Offender clinical assessments involve screening for alcohol triggers and drug abuse, evaluating physical and mental health, and considering employment and financial status. Motivation for change also plays a role in the treatment plan, which is usually multicomponent and incorporates effective medications (for a discussion of medications, see section on pharmacological treatments), behavioral therapies, peer support groups, and social skills training (NCDC, n.d.-a). Court programs typically last 1 to 3 years, and supervision can be lessened as participants move through a program's different phases (Block, 2016; Goodwin et al., 2015; Hawaii State Judiciary, n.d.; NCDC, n.d.-b). Courts vary in requirements for serving jail time before entering the program; sentences usually do not change after program completion, although some programs reduce sentences (Block, 2016). Participants may be removed from programs for noncompliance or new charges (Block, 2016; Circuit Court of the State of Oregon, n.d.).

Evidence suggests that traditional court processes and sanctions are generally not effective in influencing the behavior of offenders with multiple DWIs (Goodwin et al., 2015; NCDC, n.d.-c). One-third of those arrested annually for driving impaired have a prior DWI conviction (NCDC, n.d.-b). Therefore, most DWI courts are aimed at offenders who have at least one prior DWI and/or who drove with a BAC of 0.15% or higher (NCDC, n.d.-c). DWI courts may disqualify offenders also convicted of felonies or violent crimes (Block, 2016; Hawaii State Judiciary, n.d.; NCDC, n.d.-a). Furthermore, 65 to 80 percent of first-time DWI offenders will not reoffend, and contact with the criminal justice system may offer enough deterrence for first-time offenders to avoid future impaired driving (Goodwin et al., 2015; NCDC, n.d.-b). DWI court resources are best directed toward repeat offenders with whom the treatment program can have the biggest effect. Only about 1 percent of those arrested for DWIs, however, are referred to a specialty court, and approximately half of those referred complete the program (Sloan et al., 2016).

A 2009 systematic review concluded DWI courts are an effective intervention in reducing recidivism, but found many studies were methodologically weak and encouraged additional future research (Marlowe et al., 2009). For example, one of the stronger studies in the review determined participants in an Oregon DWI court were less likely to be convicted of a DWI or other traffic violations (Lapham et al., 2006). Furthermore, 85 percent of studies in a 2012 meta-analysis favored DWI courts over traditional courts (Mitchell et al., 2012). Three of the four randomized studies reviewed in the meta-analysis found DWI courts reduced the odds of recidivism (Mitchell et al., 2012). The fourth experimental study, an evaluation of a DWI court in Los Angeles County, did not find significant differences in drinking behavior or recidivism between the participants assigned to the DWI court and those assigned to a control group (traditional criminal court) during a 24-month follow-up period (MacDonald et al., 2007). The authors note limited jail time in the county for DWI offenders during the study period likely affected incentive to participate in the voluntary DWI court (MacDonald et al., 2007). However, this DWI court was created as an investigational program for a research study, and as such, was not pilot-tested or evaluated for compliance with DWI court guiding principles (Marlowe et al., 2009). Furthermore, aspects of the traditional court (control group) could be considered important elements of a DWI court (such as the number of status hearings in the first 6 months), so the two groups of participants received similar interventions (Marlowe et al., 2009).

Mitchell et al. (2012) found that more DWI court participants graduated from DWI programs compared to adult and juvenile drug court participants (Mitchell et al., 2012). DWI courts characterized by longer program duration and higher quantity of services usually have a higher completion rate, and graduates experience better outcomes, including increased educational fulfilment and enhanced employment status (Robertson et al., 2016; Sloan et al., 2013).

DWI courts have long-term effects on offenders as well. A study of DWI courts in North Carolina found reduced rates of recidivism over 4 years compared to people not referred to the specialty court (Sloan et al., 2016). Similar long-term, positive results were observed in an analysis of three Georgian DWI courts; recidivism rates of comparison groups matched by the number of previous DWI convictions, sex, and age were between 24 and 35 percent, while DWI court graduates' recidivism rate was 9 percent (Fell et al., 2011; Goodwin et al., 2015; NCDC, 2015). Additionally, DWI courts may be more effective than hybrid DWI/drug courts in preventing DWI recidivism because drug courts enroll several types of participants and do not specifically target DWI offenders (Sloan et al., 2016).

Many DWI courts are funded through federal, state, and county grants as well as fees collected from offenders (Block, 2016). Participants often have to pay for program components such as alcohol monitoring and ignition interlocks, substance abuse treatment, and any imposed fines (Carey et al., 2008; Circuit Court of the State of Oregon, n.d.; Fourth Judicial District Minnesota Judicial Branch, n.d.). Although more resources (e.g., time and staff) are needed to provide DWI courts' close monitoring, these courts do not cost more, and sometimes cost less, in up-front costs than traditional probation (Goodwin et al., 2015; NCDC, 2015). Additionally, courts save money by reducing rearrests and total time offenders spend in jail (Carey et al., 2008; NCDC, 2015; NPC Research, 2014).

DWI courts are voluntary programs that couple offender supervision with individualized treatment; courts target high-need offenders who can benefit the most from these components. Characteristics of DWI court programs matter; analyses favor longer program duration and higher intensity contact between the participant and the DWI court (Sloan et al., 2013). Well-done studies by Fell et al. (2011), Lapham et al. (2006), and Sloan et al. (2016) demonstrate that DWI courts have short- and long-term specific deterrent effects. A meta-analysis (Mitchell et al., 2012) generally supports these individual findings, though some methodically weak studies of DWI courts (e.g., inadequately controlling for selection bias) and varying study designs result in different findings. The field could benefit from additional well-designed and executed studies that adhere to established standards. To improve health and safety outcomes and reduce recidivism of repeat offenders and high BAC offenders, the committee recommends:

Recommendation 5-1: Every state should implement DWI courts, guided by the evidence-based standards set by the National Center for DWI Courts, and all DWI courts should include available consultation or referral for evaluation by an addiction-trained clinician.

Screening, Brief Intervention, and Referral to Treatment (SBIRT)

SBIRT may serve to identify hazardous and harmful alcohol intake, as well as provide an opportunity for immediate intervention and referral to treatment, if necessary. DWI offenders are an important population to screen and treat for AUD (DSM-5). As noted earlier, there is not a reliable estimate of AUD among DWI offenders in the criminal justice system (Lapham et al., 2004). However, research suggests recidivists generally exhibit heavier and more frequent drinking behavior (Mullen et al., 2015). Additionally, only about a quarter of impaired drivers treated in EDs are convicted, so many of these offenders do not receive treatment through a court referral (Higgins-Biddle and Dilonardo, 2013). Importantly, many alcohol-impaired driving episodes are caused by binge drinkers, rather than heavy drinkers, so it is equally important to identify these patients and provide treatment before they are involved in an alcohol-impaired driving crash (Flowers et al., 2008; Higgins-Biddle and Dilonardo, 2013). It is clear then that SBIRT plays a role in the other phases of the committee's framework (see Figure 1-5), but it is included in this chapter as it is relevant to many of the treatment options that follow screening and brief intervention.

The main goal of SBIRT is to increase a patient's awareness and understanding of the risks of excessive drinking and to motivate him or her to decrease his or her consumption (Agerwala and McCance-Katz, 2012). A range of health care workers can conduct SBIRT in a variety of settings, including the criminal justice system, EDs, primary care, behavioral health care, and college campuses. Screening, the first component of SBIRT, is usually done using one of several tools (e.g., AUDIT or CAGE) that have been tested and demonstrated to be effective in documenting alcohol consumption as well identifying at-risk alcohol consumption or possible AUD. This may be done in one of several ways: orally, in writing, via computer, or other electronic means (Agerwala and McCance-Katz, 2012; Higgins-Biddle and Dilonardo, 2013). If the screening results indicate at-risk alcohol consumption such as binge drinking or exceeding the recommended limits for low-risk consumption, a brief intervention is performed. In cases in which possible AUD is identified, a more thorough assessment may be done, and the brief intervention may focus on motivating the patient to begin treatment.

A brief intervention is a short, tailored, one-on-one counseling session, usually lasting between 5 and 30 minutes, that uses techniques from motivational interviewing, brief negotiated interviewing, and/or CBT to try to eliminate harmful drinking behaviors such as binge drinking and alcohol-impaired driving (NIAAA, 2005a; SAMHSA, n.d.). During the intervention, practitioners deliver the results of the screening, provide information on low-risk alcohol consumption, assess the patient's motivation to change his or her alcohol consumption, and collaboratively set goals for decreasing consumption (Higgins-Biddle and Dilonardo, 2013). Brief interventions can vary considerably and may consist of one to four sessions depending on the severity of the patient's alcohol problem, the setting, the clinician's expertise, and time constraints (NIAAA, 2005a). Once the brief intervention is completed, the patient may receive follow-up in a primary care or behavioral health setting, or be referred for more extensive treatment if needed (NIAAA, 2005a). Treatment plans can vary in scope and duration, and they are tailored to the patient's specific needs.

Several studies present strong evidence that brief interventions can effectively decrease harmful alcohol consumption (Dunn et al., 2001; Moyer et al., 2002; Vasilaki et al., 2006), especially when conducted in emergency care settings (D'Onofrio and Degutis, 2002; Nilsen et al., 2008), primary care settings (Ballesteros et al., 2004; Bertholet et al., 2005; Kaner et al., 2009; O'Donnell et al., 2014), and college settings (Carey et al., 2007; Larimer and Cronce, 2002). The evidence is inconclusive on whether brief alcohol interventions are effective in general hospital settings (Emmen et al., 2004), among repeat DWI offenders (Brown et al., 2010; Miller et al., 2015; Ouimet et al., 2013), among heavy drinkers or those with alcohol dependence (Saitz, 2010), or among adolescent drivers (Steinka-Fry et al., 2015; Yuma-Guerrero et al., 2012); therefore, more research is needed in these areas. Current studies rely on self-reports of alcohol consumption and include participants who partake in SBIRT and then return for a follow-up assessment. To counteract self-reporting and self-selection bias, future research would benefit from analyzing population health effects in real-world settings. There is also evidence to suggest the positive effects of SBIRT wane over time, and further research is needed to determine the optimum frequency of interventions (O'Donnell et al., 2014). More investigation is also needed into whether brief interventions reduce alcohol-impaired driving (Dill et al., 2004), although at least one study has shown a brief intervention to be effective in decreasing drinking and driving (D'Onofrio et al., 2012).

The U.S. Preventive Services Task Force recommends all adults receive SBIRT at primary care visits (USPSTF, 2013). A recent study from the Centers for Disease Control and Prevention, however, found that only one in three self-reported binge drinkers were screened for alcohol misuse at their last checkup and told that their drinking was risky, and only one in six were screened and advised to reduce their drinking (McKnight-Eily et al., 2017). Primary care physicians have an opportunity to increase their use of SBIRT, allowing them to reach more patients engaging in risky drinking and reduce alcohol-impaired driving injuries. There are barriers, however, that make universal screening difficult. Beich et al. (2003) found approximately 9 percent of patients will screen positive for risky drinking behavior in primary care settings. Madras et al. (2009) found that when EDs and clinics are included, approximately 23 percent of patients screened will self-report risky drinking behavior. These low percentages cause some physicians, who are already strapped for time and resources, to discount SBIRT as an efficient use of their time (Beich et al., 2003). Staff training is also necessary before SBIRT can be effectively administered, which takes additional time and resources (Bernstein et al., 2009; Nilsen et al., 2006).

In addition to busy workloads and financial constraints, other barriers to administering SBIRT include

- underreporting of drinking by patients;
- health care professionals not seeing SBIRT as part of their job;
- more immediate, competing health problems (especially in the ED);
- lack of physician knowledge about alcohol guidelines;
- cultural differences in alcohol consumption; and

- that the topic of alcohol abuse can be a difficult one to discuss (Johnson et al., 2011).

Yokell et al. (2014) found that brief interventions were administered more often in rural EDs and less often in crowded, metropolitan EDs owing to time and financial constraints. In contrast, Colorado initiated a statewide SBIRT initiative over 10 years ago and has documented the strategies necessary for successful implementation of an SBIRT program, including clinical issues, training for health professionals, and reimbursement (Nunes et al., 2017). The Substance Abuse and Mental Health Services Administration (SAMHSA) funded a national initiative to implement SBIRT in general medicine and community settings. Evaluation of 11 of the programs demonstrated that the method used by SAMHSA was an effective way to implement the programs (Bray et al., 2017).

There are also legal reasons why a physician may be hesitant to screen a patient for alcohol misuse. Physicians are required to report "at-risk drivers" to their state Department of Motor Vehicles (DMV) in six states: California, Delaware, Nevada, New Jersey, Oregon, and Pennsylvania (AAA Foundation for Traffic Safety, 2016; State of Nevada, n.d.). The guidelines on which conditions physicians must report, however, are vague and vary by state. All states allow physicians to report medically at-risk patients to the DMV in good faith. Many physicians are more comfortable reporting an impaired driver to the DMV's medical review board rather than to the police (Mello et al., 2003). The reported information is confidential in all states, but most states will release it if they receive a court order (AAA Foundation for Traffic Safety, 2016). Hesitant physicians may be concerned about patient confidentiality and the risk of civil action against the physician (Mello et al., 2003). Furthermore, the implementation of a law in Ontario, Canada, requiring physicians to warn medically at-risk drivers of the consequences of alcohol-impaired driving resulted in a reduced rate of crashes requiring emergency care, but the warning was also associated with increased depression and fewer subsequent doctor visits, suggesting that physicians should decide which patients would benefit most from a warning (Redelmeier et al., 2012). However, warning drivers of consequences without performing interventions to address risky drinking may be part of the difficulty with this approach.

Finally, insurance reimbursement policy may dissuade practitioners from administering SBIRT, although commercial insurance, Medicare, and Medicaid provide reimbursement for SBIRT (SAMHSA, 2017). The Uniform Accident and Sickness Policy Provision Law (UPPL) authorizes health insurance companies to deny claims for injuries sustained while intoxicated, including those that result from driving under the influence (Chezem, 2005). As of 2016, UPPL remains in place in 24 states (APIS,

2016). The National Conference of State Legislators worked to repeal UPPL laws and to ensure that states did not introduce new restrictions on insurance payments. O'Keeffe et al. (2009) assessed the costs associated with caring for patients who are intoxicated compared to those who are not and discussed the implications for costs borne by trauma centers in states with UPPL. The findings showed that alcohol consumption by minimally injured trauma patients is correlated with higher hospital charges, which are exacerbated in UPPL states, and, the authors conclude, are likely to increase with implementation of SBIRT. Gentilello et al. (2005a) analyzed survey data from trauma surgeons and identified UPPL as an important barrier to alcohol screening. The results indicated strong support for alcohol screening and intervention programs, yet the majority (51 percent) of surgeons reported not routinely measuring BAC. Furthermore, almost one-quarter of surgeons reported having a payment denied in the past 6 months based on alcohol screening results. Interestingly, SBIRT does not identify whether the visit at which SBIRT is being performed is for treatment of an alcohol-impaired driving injury, as the screening tool documents patterns of alcohol use, rather than report of use for a single incident. Because of this, SBIRT in itself may not contribute to denial of coverage for an injury.

It is important to note that SBIRT may be performed by a number of members of the health care team who have been trained in its use, which is one way to overcome the limitations of physician time and financial resources (Johnson et al., 2011). This includes nurses, social workers, health educators, and others who interact with patients on a regular basis. Education and training programs have been developed and disseminated through several initiatives by federal agencies, professional organizations such as the American College of Emergency Physicians and the Association for Medical Education and Research in Substance Abuse, and academic centers (ACEP, n.d.; AMERSA, n.d.). Studies have demonstrated that health promotion advocates, who do not have a professional license, can effectively perform SBIRT in the ED (Bernstein et al., 2009; D'Onofrio and Degutis, 2010). Carnegie et al. (1996) found that when provided with proper training, receptionists were open to helping with preventive medicine tasks. Several studies also suggest that SBIRT is cost-effective in the long term because it reduces health care costs by addressing risky alcohol behaviors before they lead to injury (Estee et al., 2010; Fleming et al., 2002; Gentilello et al., 2005b). A redistribution of ED resources that prioritizes SBIRT training and implementation may therefore make financial sense.

As discussed in this section, the evidence on SBIRT's efficacy is strong, but it requires resources, training, and time. Many of the barriers outlined above could also be overcome through new technology that electronically administers screening and brief interventions to patients, such as at computer kiosks, on tablets, or through smartphone applications and text messages. The Community Preventive Services Task Force[9] recommends electronic screening and brief interventions to curtail harmful alcohol consumption (Community Preventive Services Task Force, 2012), and evidence suggests that electronic screening and brief interventions delivered through interactive, online programs and smartphones are effective (Donoghue et al., 2014; White et al., 2010).

Mobile health approaches have emerged as a promising strategy for expanding behavioral alcohol interventions (Kazemi et al., 2017; Muench et al., 2017). Recent studies by Suffoletto et al. (2014, 2015) found that brief interventions delivered by text messages were successful in reducing self-reported binge drinking among young adults discharged from the ED. In fact, findings from Suffoletto et al. (2015) suggested that an intervention consisting of an interactive text message with tailored feedback was more effective than self-monitoring without feedback and no text messaging or feedback (the control condition) in reducing alcohol consumption and related injury. These findings were consistent with a previous study, which also used text messaging to provide feedback to young adults who were identified as hazardous drinkers. The study findings showed that the text message intervention reduced heavy drinking; young adults who received the intervention reported about two fewer drinks per drinking day than they did at baseline and approximately three fewer heavy drinking days in the last month (Suffoletto et al., 2012).

A randomized controlled pilot study tested four types of alcohol-reduction themed text messages for problem drinkers. Participants significantly reduced their weekly drinking in response to loss-framed (i.e., conveys the consequences of harmful drinking) and tailored (i.e., conveys messages tailored to the individual's baseline assessment and goal achievement) messages (Muench et al., 2017). There are many opportunities to reach more patients with alcohol problems as technology continues to develop, but further research is needed to identify which elements of electronic interventions are key to initiating behavioral changes (Bewick et al., 2008). The following sections discuss various treatment and program strategies for people who have AUD or engage in harmful drinking behaviors such as binge drinking.

---

[9] The Community Preventive Services Task Force was formerly known as the Task Force on Community Preventive Services. Task Force publications prior to 2012 are cited as the latter, and those published after 2012 are cited as the former.

Use of Medications for Alcohol Use Disorders

There are four medications approved by the Food and Drug Administration (FDA) for the treatment of alcohol dependence: naltrexone (NTX), extended release naltrexone, acamprosate, and disulfiram (NIAAA, 2005b). NTX is an opioid receptor antagonist approved for the treatment of opioid addiction and AUD (SAMHSA, 2016c). It is taken as a 50 mg pill once per day and has been shown to reduce alcohol consumption and cravings in those with alcohol dependence (Lobmaier et al., 2011; SAMHSA, 2016c). NTX is effective because it blocks the feelings of euphoria associated with alcohol intoxication and has no abuse potential (O'Brien et al., 1996; Roozen et al., 2006). Oral NTX, however, is known for having poor adherence rates (Swift et al., 2011), possibly because of its initial side effects of nausea, vomiting, dizziness, and fatigue, or the patient belief that it is not effective (Carmen et al., 2004; Rohsenow et al., 2000; Srisurapanont and Jarusuraisin, 2005). Research also indicates that family history of alcohol dependence and genetic variations can influence the efficacy of NTX. Most notably, a polymorphism of the μ-opioid receptor gene may be positively associated with the efficacy of NTX (Chamorro et al., 2012; Garbutt et al., 2014; Oslin et al., 2006). Further research is needed to confirm these moderating effects. They have the potential to influence physician decision making by identifying subgroups that are more likely to respond positively to NTX.

Extended-release naltrexone requires intramuscular injection into the gluteus muscle at 380 mg per month (SAMHSA, 2016c). This schedule greatly improves adherence to treatment. The medication has the potential to increase compliance as it requires less frequent administration than NTX. Over 5 percent of users, however, experience complications at the injection site including induration, swelling, nodules, and itching (Walker et al., 2017). Injection site reactions can occur if the injection is made into fat rather than muscle. A recent study by Walker et al. (2017) suggests that a modified injection technique in which the needle is inserted at a 40 degree angle may help decrease injection site complications. Long-acting depot formulations or implants of NTX have also been under development and show promise in terms of increasing treatment efficacy and decreasing noncompliance rates (Goonoo et al., 2014). Although they are not yet approved by FDA, these new delivery systems have the potential to release NTX to the brain for up to 7 months after insertion (Goonoo et al., 2014). More research on the safety and tolerability of these medications is needed before they can be released for use by the general public (Goonoo et al., 2014). All FDA-approved addiction medications are covered by the Patient Protection and Affordable Care Act, and the high cost of naltrexone and extended-release naltrexone to prevent relapse is considered justified by the high cost of alcohol relapse.

Two pilot studies analyzed the specific effects of NTX on alcohol-impaired driving. The first study examined the efficacy of NTX on treating repeat DWI offenders. The researchers found that with NTX, participants' daily drinks decreased by 77 percent and that vehicular failures to start because of an ignition interlock activation decreased from 3.1 to 1.29 percent of tests (Lapham and McMillan, 2011). The second study analyzed the feasibility and effectiveness of using extended-release NTX to treat alcohol dependence (DSM-IV) in three drug court settings. The researchers found that NTX treatment was associated with 57 percent fewer missed court sessions and a reduction in positive drug and alcohol tests (Finigan et al., 2011). An endpoint analysis found that 26 percent of standard-care clients were rearrested compared to 8 percent of clients treated with NTX (Finigan et al., 2011). Randomized, clinically-controlled trials that look specifically at NTX effects on alcohol-impaired driving are needed.

Acamprosate is a glutamate antagonist that is administered in two 333 mg tablets three times per day and is used to maintain abstinence of alcohol after withdrawal has occurred (SAMHSA, 2005b). A recent systematic review and meta-analysis of medications for treating AUD (DSM-5) found that oral NTX and acamprosate are equally effective in reducing rates of drinking relapse (Jonas et al., 2014). NTX has been shown to be more effective in reducing heavy drinking and craving, while acamprosate has been shown to be more effective in maintaining abstinence (Carmen et al., 2004; Maisel et al., 2013; Mann, 2004; Rösner et al., 2008). Research suggests that the combination of NTX and acamprosate is safe and more effective than treatment with either medication alone (Feeney et al., 2006; Kiefer and Wiedemann, 2004). The most common side effect from acamprosate is diarrhea, but this has not been shown to cause any problems in medication adherence (Carmen et al., 2004).

Disulfiram, the first medication approved by the FDA to treat alcohol dependence, is an alcohol-sensitizing agent that causes physical reactions such as sweating, hyperventilation, head and neck throbbing, nausea, vomiting, and weakness when the patient consumes any alcohol (Center for Substance Abuse Treatment, 2009). Once alcohol has been ingested it usually takes 10 to 30 minutes for this reaction to occur; the intensity shows individual variation (Center for Substance Abuse Treatment, 2009). Disulfiram is taken as a pill of 125 to 500 mg once per day (Center for Substance Abuse Treatment, 2009). Evidence on the effectiveness of disulfiram in treating alcohol dependence is mixed. There is compelling evidence to indicate that disulfiram decreases alcohol consumption when the drug is taken in a controlled laboratory setting (Fuller et al., 1986). In real-life settings, however, adherence is very difficult to maintain and ingestion of the medication must be supervised in order to be effective

(Brewer et al., 2000). In addition to compliance issues, high doses of alcohol and disulfiram can be life threatening, leading some physicians to dismiss it as a viable treatment option (Williams, 2005). Disulfiram is most effective and safe when used in substance abuse treatment programs where patients can be closely monitored (Schuckit, 2006).

Topiramate is an antiepileptic drug that was approved by FDA to prevent seizures. It can be used off-label to treat alcohol dependence as well (Kenna et al., 2009). It has been reported to decrease cravings and promote alcohol abstinence by mimicking the presence of alcohol in the brain (Ait-Daoud et al., 2006). Topiramate is taken as a 15 to 200 mg pill twice per day (Kenna et al., 2009). A meta-analysis of pharmacotherapy concluded there is moderate[10] evidence to suggest that topiramate is associated with fewer drink days, fewer heavy drinking days, and fewer drinks per drinking day (Jonas et al., 2014). One review found oral naltrexone and topiramate were equally effective in increasing days of abstinence in those with alcohol dependence (DSM-IV), while acamprosate was only moderately effective (Miller et al., 2011). Topiramate has some side effects that may affect adherence including paresthesia, taste perversion, anorexia, and difficulty concentrating (Johnson et al., 2007). A study conducted on patients taking topiramate for long-term prevention of seizures found that cognitive slowing and dysphasia were the main reasons the medication was discontinued (Bootsma et al., 2004). Topiramate holds promise in producing self-efficacy to resist heavy drinking among a subset of heavy drinkers identified by a specific genotype (Kranzler et al., 2016),[11] but further research is needed to understand how the drug affects alcohol-impaired driving.

Evidence suggests that most antipsychotics are not effective in reducing drinking or craving in patients with alcohol dependence (DSM-IV) (Kishi et al., 2013). While the antipsychotic quetiapine has shown some promising effects in treating alcohol dependence and abuse (DSM-IV) because of its effects on mood, anxiety, and sleep, more research is needed to determine its usefulness and to identify patients most likely to benefit from it (Ray et al., 2010).

Although psychopharmacological approaches to treating AUD have been shown to be cost-effective (Burton et al., 2016; Zarkin et al., 2010) and effective in reducing heavy drinking, medications are underused. In 2016, a survey of DWI courts reported that 31 courts used NTX for alcohol

---

[10] Jonas et al. (2014) based the strength of evidence on published guidance on comparing medical interventions from the Agency for Healthcare Research and Quality (Owens et al., 2008).

[11] Heavy drinking was defined in this study as average weekly consumption of 18 and 24 standard drinks for women and men, respectively (Kranzler et al., 2016).

treatment services and 3 courts used acamprosate (Block, 2016). A 2008 study analyzed state-level policies and their association with the use of NTX in treatment facilities. They found that Medicaid policies that support the use of generic drugs were associated with higher NTX use while policies with preferred drug lists and restricted pharmacy network were not (Heinrich and Hill, 2008).

The quality of the evidence for the efficacy of anti-relapse medications is excellent. For NTX, the first such medication approved by FDA for efficacy in preventing relapse, the evidence is based on placebo-controlled, randomized clinical trials conducted in multiple countries throughout the world. The most reliable finding for success is not total abstinence from drinking, but rather a reduction in the number of heavy drinking days. This translates into fewer opportunities to drive a vehicle in an alcohol-impaired state. While there are reports from drug courts on the benefits of using medication as a means of preventing relapse to alcohol-impaired driving, the published controlled trials were not conducted among drug court participants. The evidence for NTX, acamprosate, and topiramate is mainly based on controlled trials and meta-analyses, while that for disulfiram is poor for efficacy because of high drop-out from treatment. NTX, extended-release NTX, acamprosate, disulfiram, and topiramate all appear to be effective in certain situations, but more research is needed to determine which medications are most beneficial for which patients. Most of the research on the effects of these medications has been done on adults; future research should analyze the effectiveness of pharmacotherapy for younger populations of driving age (Stockings et al., 2016). Although medication is a helpful tool in treating people with AUD, research indicates that psychosocial therapy given in conjunction is beneficial (Miller et al., 2011; Rohsenow, 2004; Roozen et al., 2006; Srisurapanont and Jarusuraisin, 2005).

Conclusion 5-3: Though effect sizes vary, medications in combination with other treatment modalities to treat individuals with alcohol use disorder who have been convicted of alcohol-impaired driving can reduce impaired-driving recidivism.

While a single DWI does not imply an illness, repeat offenders have a high probability of having an AUD. This, like other addictions, is a disease of the brain and requires long-term treatment to prevent relapse. The offender needs to be evaluated by a clinician with addiction training and, if medically indicated, placed in a program that includes relapse prevention medication and the requirement for an extended period of attendance in therapy (see the following section for a discussion of one such therapy—CBT). Because there are barriers to adherence to medication, success in some DWI programs for repeat offenders has involved monthly injections of extended-release naltrexone. As explained above, this medication reduces reward from alcohol drinking, has minimal side effects, and often reduces craving for alcohol. The result reported in most studies is a reduction in heavy drinking, though not total abstinence. There are many barriers to AUD treatment, including stigma, comorbid conditions requiring treatment, lack of perceived need for treatment or motivation for change, lack of adequate training among health care professionals, and decreased access to or increased cost of medications or providers (Knudsen et al., 2011; NIAAA, 2010; Schuler et al., 2015). Furthermore, offenders could refuse to comply with compulsory treatment components of sentences, after which they would face additional punishment; motivational enhancement therapy could be helpful for these offenders (Dill and Wells-Parker, 2006).

Cognitive Behavioral Therapy (CBT)

CBT is a structured behavioral therapy that helps patients solve problems by changing their patterns of thought and therefore their behavior and coping strategies in response to daily situations. There are several effective approaches to CBT in addressing AUD. For example, motivational interventions are relatively brief and focus on readiness to change behavior (Magill and Ray, 2009; Miller and Rollnick, 2002). Contingency management involves the provision of some type of material reinforcement when an individual refrains from drinking alcohol (Petry et al., 2000; Prendergast et al., 2006). The community reinforcement approach is focused on making sobriety more rewarding than alcohol use. Behavioral couples therapy centers around the effects of alcohol use on the relationship (Epstein and McCrady, 1998; Powers et al., 2008). CBT can also be made available online or through other communication technologies, making it more accessible to patients in remote areas. For example, CBT has been adapted to interactive voice response for continuing care after AUD treatment (Rose et al., 2015) and other mobile or Internet-based tools for a variety of conditions (Blankers et al., 2011; Marsch et al., 2014; Vallury et al., 2015).

CBT may also be used in conjunction with other therapies, such as medications that have demonstrated effectiveness in the treatment of AUD. For example, a systematic review found that the community reinforcement approach combined with the medication disulfiram decreased the number of drinking days, but there was conflicting evidence of the impact of a community reinforcement approach on abstinence (Hunt and Azrin, 1973; Roozen et al., 2004). Studies have shown that CBT combined with naltrexone, alone or with acamprosate, is an effective treatment for alcohol dependence (DSM-IV) (Anton et al., 2006; Feeney et al., 2006). However, the COMBINE study did not demonstrate any significant added effectiveness of the combination of naltrexone, acamprosate, and behavioral interventions (Anton et al., 2006). Another study found that while acamprosate was more effective in promoting abstinence, naltrexone had a slight advantage in reducing heavy drinking and craving, but this review did not examine the effect of the medications in conjunction with CBT (Maisel et al., 2013). The degree of effectiveness of CBT in combination with medications warrants further study, given the number of people with AUD and the consequences that can result from the disease for patients and the public.

Cost-Effectiveness of Treatment to Reduce Alcohol-Impaired Driving Crashes

The committee could not identify a study of alcohol treatment that specifically examined the cost-effectiveness related to alcohol-impaired driving crashes and/or fatalities as the single outcome. However, there are multiple studies of the cost-effectiveness of AUD treatment with respect to other outcomes, suggesting that AUD treatment can be cost-effective. Thus, while there are no studies evaluating whether AUD treatment is cost-effective when solely considering reducing alcohol-impaired driving crashes, there would likely be other important effects from AUD treatment to other socially desirable outcomes such that treatment could be cost-effective when considering a broader set of outcomes.

For example, the study by Fleming et al. (2002) included motor vehicle crashes, operating a vehicle while intoxicated, and operating while under the influence as components of the full set of benefits of a brief intervention. However, these were not separate endpoints, but rather they factored into the full benefits (measured as costs averted). The study found that motor vehicle crashes declined with the study's specific brief intervention, which included two in-person physician visits followed up by two nurse calls and other related activities (e.g., a worksheet and an "agreement"). The high-quality study includes randomization to treatment arms, a large sample, and a long follow-up period (48 months). The extent to which the findings can be generalized to other brief interventions or to treatments more generally is not clear. However, a review of multiple screening and counseling studies found that brief intervention was one of the most cost-effective among a number of effective services (Solberg et al., 2008).

Gentilello et al. (2005b) conducted a cost-benefit analysis of alcohol interventions for patients treated in U.S. hospitals and EDs. The authors found that every $1.00 spent on screening and intervention saved $3.81 in health care costs. Net cost savings per patient for screening are $89, and for an intervention the savings are $330. It is important to note that

Gentilello et al. did not take into account societal costs or health care follow-up costs. A similar study by Purshouse et al. (2013) modeled the cost-effectiveness of brief intervention and alcohol screening within primary care in England, using quality-adjusted life years as the outcome. Study researchers found that screening patients upon registering with a general practitioner would be cost-effective, saving £120 million in health care costs over 30 years.

Zarkin et al. (2008) and Dunlap et al. (2010) both examined the cost-effectiveness of several combinations of medications and behavioral therapies for treating alcohol dependence (DSM-IV) that were examined in a large (1,383 patients) randomized clinical trial. However, neither study included alcohol-impaired driving or crashes in their analyses. Instead, the main outcomes of the study were the incremental costs per percentage point increase in percentage of days abstinent, as well as the incremental costs of avoiding heavy drinking and of achieving a good clinical outcome. A recent evidence review on treating alcohol dependence with medication found that it is cost-effective when compared to standard care (Burton et al., 2016). Treatment with medication and psychotherapy has also been found to result in decreased median social costs, such as those associated with motor vehicle crashes, arrests, and health care (Zarkin et al., 2010).

In summary, although cost-effectiveness analyses for alcohol-impaired driving as a primary outcome are not clear at this time, use of medications for AUD to prevent alcohol-impaired driving fatalities should not be discounted.

Conclusion

Assessment, treatment, and monitoring of alcohol-impaired driving offenders remain critical elements in reducing alcohol-impaired driving recidivism and fatal crashes. Therefore, the committee recommends the following:

> **Recommendation 5-2: All health care systems and health insurers should cover and facilitate effective evaluation, prevention, and treatment strategies for binge drinking and alcohol use disorders including screening, brief intervention, and referral to treatment (SBIRT), cognitive behavioral therapy, and medication-assisted therapy.**

Alcoholics Anonymous

Alcoholics Anonymous (AA) is an international, self-help recovery program founded in the 1930s for "alcoholics" (now defined in DSM-5 as a spectrum of alcohol use disorder) to achieve sobriety (AA, 2017). The group frames the disorder as "a progressive illness which can never be 'cured,' but which, like some other illnesses, *can* be arrested" (AA World Services Inc., 1984, p. 9). It is a nonprofessional, nonclinical, peer-to-peer program based on 12 steps, which include an individual admitting a problem with alcohol, asking for help from a higher power, making amends with people who have been harmed by his or her drinking, and providing emotional support for others in the same situation (AA, n.d.). AA and other 12-step programs have become a common part of alcohol and drug treatment and aftercare (Gross, 2010). For example, DWI courts' treatment component includes development of an individual treatment plan that can include participation in a 12-step program to maintain abstinence (NCDC, n.d.-d).

Peer support groups can be an important part of treating those with substance use disorders (Tracy and Wallace, 2016). AA has an estimated 2 million members worldwide and is frequently suggested as an intervention for people with alcohol use disorder (Ferri et al., 2006; Gross, 2010; Tracy and Wallace, 2016). Involvement in AA can be associated with the development of healthy coping mechanisms and increased self-efficacy, which are related to better outcomes (Tracy and Wallace, 2016). However, potential participants may be deterred by the program's lack of treatment or its religious overtones (Tracy and Wallace, 2016).

Research into the effectiveness of AA can be controversial and produces mixed results (Dill and Wells-Parker, 2006; Kaskutas, 2009). For example, mandatory AA attendance as an intervention ranked low in efficacy in a review of 361 controlled trials of various alcohol use disorder treatments (Miller and Wilbourne, 2002). For this reason, the DWI court model compliance checklist cautions DWI courts against assigning AA participation, because forced AA attendance could modify its effectiveness, and because some people in DWI courts are not the target AA population (NCDC, n.d.-d). Additionally, the Cochrane Group reviewed eight trials including mandatory and voluntary participants of AA and other 12-step programs. The authors concluded there was no strong evidence from a number of studies that AA had an effect on therapy acceptance or duration compared to other interventions, nor were there conclusive studies with evidence of AA's effectiveness in reducing alcohol dependence or realizing abstinence (Ferri et al., 2006).

Kaskutas (2009) reviewed additional AA literature and found varied results. Observational research generally associates AA with positive outcomes, but this could be due to self-selection bias (Humphreys et al., 2014;

Kaskutas, 2009). Alcohol abstinence was higher among a large sample of male Veterans Health Administration inpatients who attended AA compared to those who did not attend (Kaskutas, 2009). Sustained and frequent AA attendance was associated with higher alcohol abstinence rates across separate populations and lengths of follow-up, and components of the AA program are aligned with theories of behavioral change (such as adjustments in life outlook, strengthening positive social ties, and improving self-efficacy and relapse prevention skills) (Kaskutas, 2009). However, experimental studies in the sample produced the weakest evidence, and results were similarly wide ranging (indications of positive, negative, or null effects) after adjustment for confounders or flaws in study design (Kaskutas, 2009). Finally, few recent studies explore alcohol-impaired driving outcomes (Dill and Wells-Parker, 2006). One observational study found previously untreated DWI offenders who attended AA and received outpatient treatment were less likely to repeat the offense within 1 and 16 years of follow-up, although results could again be affected by self-selection bias (Timko et al., 2011).

The literature lacks robust, well-designed studies in which AA is compared to interventions where successful elements can be identified. Additional studies are needed to examine AA's effect on alcohol-impaired driving outcomes; the program may be more effective in reducing DWI recidivism if combined with other interventions, although the effects of mandatory versus voluntary participation need further investigation as well (Dill and Wells-Parker, 2006).

Penalties and Sanctions

Offender Monitoring: The 24/7 Program and Continuous Alcohol Monitoring Devices

Close DWI offender monitoring can be accomplished through a variety of approaches, including intensive supervision programs such as DWI courts (discussed earlier in this chapter), staggered sentencing (allows offenders to serve a portion of his or her full sentence in jail followed by 3 to 6 years of additional monitoring and probation in which segments of the full sentence can be stayed), and the 24/7 program. Components of intensive supervision programs can include AUD screening and treatment, supervision (including continuous alcohol monitoring devices), license and/or vehicle sanctions, and punishment for noncompliance, depending on the program, its resources, and community needs (Wiliszowski et al., 2011). Such programs can be offered at state or local levels. There is evidence that close offender monitoring reduces DWI recidivism (AAA, 2016; Goodwin et al., 2015; Wiliszowski et al., 2011).

For example, a Minnesota staggered sentencing program significantly reduced the recidivism rate in program participants for up to 4 years when compared to age- and sex-matched nonparticipants (Wiliszowski et al., 2011).

In 2005, the State of South Dakota enacted the 24/7 Sobriety Program, a statewide program to reduce alcohol- or drug-related incarcerations by eliminating (or limiting) alcohol and drug use by repeat offenders. The 24/7 Program combines thorough alcohol and drug testing and monitoring with immediate and certain punishment for violations, and therefore provides an opportunity for repeat offenders to avoid incarceration and remain active in their communities as long as they abstain from alcohol or drug use. In participating counties, repeat offenders or offenders with BAC levels at or above 0.17% must participate in the 24/7 Program to get a work permit. Participation can also be mandated as a condition of certain court actions—such as sentencing, probation, parole, or court-ordered care or treatment—or may be required in child custody or visitation orders (Loudenburg et al., 2010; Nicosia et al., 2016). In 2009, 59 percent of all 24/7 Program participants were guilty of DWI offenses while the remainder of participants (41 percent) had drug or other alcohol offenses (Loudenburg et al., 2010).

The 24/7 Program's focus on repeated alcohol (and drug) testing and the certainty of immediate consequences for a failed drug- or alcohol-detection test make it unique. Most program participants are subject to twice-daily PBTs, which are typically administered at the local sheriff's office at 12-hour intervals (typically between the hours of 7–9 a.m. and 7–9 p.m.). To pass a test, participants must test negative for alcohol use or be officially excused from taking a test. Missing or failing a PBT (by having alcohol detected) results in immediate but modest jail time, usually lasting overnight or 1 to 2 days. While twice-daily PBTs are the most commonly used monitoring method, transdermal continuous alcohol monitoring and testing can also be conducted electronically through the use of ankle bracelet testing, once-per-day PBT, or urinalysis; occasionally these tests are administered contemporaneously or used in conjunction with ignition interlock devices (Loudenburg et al., 2010). The continuous alcohol monitoring devices use a transdermal sampling method every 30 minutes to detect ethanol vapor at the skin's surface as perspiration evaporates, and wirelessly transmit sampling results from the ankle device to the monitoring agency at predetermined times, one to six times daily (SCRAM Systems, 2017). Continuous alcohol monitoring units are programmed to detect tampering and can also be used to monitor the movement of offenders who are under house arrest.

The use of transdermal devices is seen as an especially promising alternative for offenders who face special challenges securing transportation to and from law enforcement agencies for twice-daily PBT tests, and for populations such as those who live in rural communities (MADD, 2013). 24/7 Sobriety Program participants are responsible for paying testing fees—$1 per PBT test, $10 for a urinalysis, $40 for each drug patch attached, $40 for the activation and deactivation of a mobile testing device, and $4 per day for use, as well as a program participation fee not to exceed $3 per day (South Dakota Legislature, 2017).

Evaluations of South Dakota's 24/7 Sobriety Program have garnered positive results. Loudenburg et al. (2010) reviewed 24/7 Sobriety Program data from 17,874 participants, collected between the program's inception in 2005 through January 2010, to evaluate testing results and recidivism rates for program participants. Researchers found that offenders who had one or two DWI offenses, 24 to 31 percent and 40 to 47 percent, respectively, made up the largest percentage of 24/7 Sobriety Program participants. The majority of offenders participated in the program for at least 31 to 60 days (n = 982) or 91 to 180 days (n = 963). Test results from 802,210 records showed that participants successfully passed 99.4 percent of PBT tests, and of the sample evaluated (n = 4,009), 54.5 percent (2,183 participants) passed all of their tests and only 8.8 percent (351 participants) had failed more than three tests. When compared to controls, participants who entered the program after their second DWI and were tested for at least 30 consecutive days had a statistically significant 74 percent reduction in recidivism for future DWI arrests (from 13.7 percent to 3.6 percent). Participants who had their third DWI when they entered the program and had similar testing had a 44 percent decrease in recidivism (from 15.3 to 8.6 percent) and these results improved when consecutive testing days were increased to 90 days.

Similar results were seen in differences-in-differences analyses conducted by Kilmer et al. (2013) and Nicosia et al. (2016). Using South Dakota county data collected between January 2001 and December 2010, Kilmer et al. (2013) made comparisons using pre- and post-24/7 Sobriety Program implementation data. The authors found a reduction in DWI incidence and reported crashes involving males between 18 and 40 years of age, as well as significant reductions in repeat arrests (12 percent) and domestic violence arrests (9 percent), in counties where the number of participants was at least one-quarter of all DWI arrests in the county. Nicosia et al. (2016) used 24/7 Program data from January 2000 through June 2011 to determine whether the program was associated with a reduction in mortality by evaluating total deaths as well as deaths caused by circulatory or digestive disorders, external injuries, or cancer. Based on 9,108 county-month observations, the authors found a 4.2 percent reduction in all-cause mortality since implementation of the 24/7 Sobriety Program. No deterrent effect for first-time DWI arrests was apparent.

Since being implemented in South Dakota, five other rural states have put the 24/7 Program into place: Alaska, Iowa, Montana, North Dakota, and Wyoming. Several additional states, including Florida, Illinois, New Mexico, Pennsylvania, Tennessee, Virginia, Washington, West Virginia, and Wisconsin, are considering the program as well (Sobering Up, 2016). (See Box 5-2 for how a rural sheriff's department in Tennessee recently used monitoring devices as part of a comprehensive approach to reducing alcohol-impaired driving.) Of the new state programs that have been evaluated, results similar to South Dakota's have been found in the evaluated new state programs. RAND evaluated the Montana program and found "suggestive evidence" that 24/7 participation reduced the probability of DWI rearrest (within 12 months) among second-time offenders by approximately 45 to 70 percent,[12] although many limitations were noted, including missing data or information on the sample participants (Midgette and Kilmer, 2015). The program in North Dakota was found to have more of a deterrent effect on female repeat offenders than males, and the overall deterrent effect was strongest when the program had a mandatory 12-month enrollment period (Kubas et al., 2015).

Although not a 24/7 Sobricty program, a related Sobriety Tags pilot program has been implemented in London, United Kingdom, where ankle monitoring devices are being used for offenders who have committed crimes that can be attributed to the use of alcohol (Greater London Authority, 2016).

In this section, the committee reviews the evidence on the effectiveness of the 24/7 Sobriety Program and continuous alcohol monitoring devices. These are two examples of offender monitoring programs (DWI courts and ignition interlock devices also closely monitor offenders and are discussed elsewhere in this chapter). The 24/7 Program is targeted toward repeat or high-BAC DWI offenders. The PBTs, continuous alcohol monitoring devices, and other tests ensure a high probability of alcohol detection; immediate sanctions are enacted for failed tests. The 24/7 Sobriety Program analysis (Loudenburg et al., 2010) and peer-reviewed differences-in-differences study (Kilmer et al., 2013), both with large sample sizes, consistently found significantly reduced DWI recidivism among 24/7 Program participants; the differences-in-differences analysis by Nicosia et al. (2016) also identified a small reduction in all-cause adult mortality in South Dakota counties. There is also emerging, promising

---

[12] The program was challenged in court for charging program fees to offenders as unconstitutional pretrial punishment, but the Montana Supreme Court upheld the program saying that the associated fees are not unconstitutional, and that judges must consider each case individually (i.e., prior alcohol-related arrests, risk to the community, financial standing) when determining whether to assign an offender to the program (*State v. Spady*, 2015 MT 218, 354 P.3d 590).

BOX 5-2
Grundy County, Tennessee Sheriff's Department

Setting: Grundy County, Tennessee, is a rural county about 50 miles west of Chattanooga with a population of approximately 13,000 people. The sheriff's department is responsible for covering about 300 miles of rural roadways. Since 2014, the county sheriff's department has implemented a number of initiatives aimed at reducing impaired driving and related injuries and damages in the county.

Strategies: In 2014, the county passed Amelia's Law, which mandates that people on probation or parole for impairment-related deaths are monitored as a condition of their release. The personal alcohol monitoring device assigned to offenders detects even small amounts of alcohol in the perpetrator's system. The county also employs an interlock device strategy to keep repeat offenders from being able to start their vehicles while impaired.

The sheriff's department has worked within the court system to change prosecutorial standards to decrease plea deals that would allow DWI charges to be reduced to reckless driving. The courts use a mandatory sentencing system that increases the severity of the sentence with each DWI offense. The sheriff's department has also worked with the courts to help their officers ensure that they are prepared for testimony for DWI cases. Furthermore, the court system provides and encourages education for drug- and alcohol-impaired offenders, as well as cognitive behavioral therapy and recovery support programs.

The Grundy County sheriff's department also uses a system of tracking and trending data to target areas and times for heavier patrols and checkpoints. They now ensure that all officers are trained in field sobriety testing and detection of impaired drivers. The department has a strong presence at community events and local schools to educate the public about the dangers of impaired driving, and to offer suggestions to community members to ensure that they do not put themselves in a potentially dangerous situation.

Initial outcomes: The average number of DWI-related fatalities from 2004 to 2013 was 6.8. Since the program started, the average declined to 3.0 DWI-related fatalities from 2014 to 2016. 2015 marked the first year on record that Grundy County had zero traffic deaths (outcomes as reported by Grundy County).

SOURCE: Shrum, 2017.

evidence from other states with large rural populations that have implemented 24/7 Sobriety Programs and alcohol consumption monitoring. However, the studies in this section report limitations such as failure to account for program fidelity, missing data, and reliance on aggregate analyses rather than individual-level data; additional research is needed using randomization or matched control groups to more completely assess the short- and long-term effects of the program among diverse jurisdictions and offenders.

Finding 5-1: The 24/7 monitoring program for high-risk offenders has been shown to be effective in some rural areas.

Conclusion 5-4: Systems alcohol monitoring programs are a promising intervention for reducing alcohol use and alcohol-impaired driving recidivism among high-risk offenders.

Successful implementation of these monitoring programs requires buy-in from law enforcement agencies and officials. Further investigation is required to see if similar programs could be implemented in other contexts.

Victim Impact Panels

Begun in 1982 by Mothers Against Drunk Driving (MADD), victim impact panels aim to reduce alcohol-impaired driving by exposing DWI offenders to the pain and suffering inflicted on victims of alcohol-impaired driving and their loved ones (Rojek et al., 2003). Victim impact panels follow a restorative justice model in which victims of alcohol-impaired driving and their loved ones are given the opportunity to speak about how the problem has affected their lives. The panels are not intended to condemn or shame audience members, nor are they a replacement for other sanctions (MADD, n.d.). Individuals convicted of alcohol-impaired driving, particularly first-time DWI offenders, are commonly court ordered to attend victim impact panels (AAA, 2016).

Evidence showing the effects of victim impact panels on alcohol-impaired driving and recidivism is mixed. While some studies have indicated that victim impact panels decrease recidivism, others have shown that recidivism rates are not significantly lower for those who attend victim impact panels than for those who do not. Much of the literature examining victim impact panels has not been updated; therefore, the following section presents the available evidence.

In a study measuring rearrest rates of DWI offenders who attended a victim impact panel in a southeastern county of the United States, 15.8 percent of offenders were rearrested over the following 5 years compared to 33.5 percent of the control group (Rojek et al., 2003). The analysis suggested that those who attended victim impact panels were 55.7 percent less likely to be rearrested and that victim impact panels were most effective in the first 2 years following arrest, after which their effectiveness decreased significantly. In an earlier study, rearrest rates during 0 to 6, 7 to 12, and 0 to 12 months after arrest were all found to be lower for those who attended a victim impact panel (Fors and Rojek, 1999). Differences in rearrest rates were most significant for white men, those between the ages of 26 and 35, and those with one previous DWI arrest. The authors suggested that victim impact panels can be cost-effective in reducing rearrest rates of DWI offenders if implemented on a larger scale. An examination of a victim impact panel program in North Dakota demonstrated reduced odds of recidivism among male and female DWI offenders who participated when compared to those who did not. These findings were consistent for multiple DWI offenders (Joyce and Thompson, 2017).

Other studies have shown victim impact panels to be ineffective at reducing recidivism (C'de Baca et al., 2000; Crew and Johnson, 2011; Polacsek et al., 2001; Wheeler et al., 2002, 2004). Results of an unpublished randomized trial of convicted alcohol-impaired drivers in Bernalillo County, New Mexico, showed that victim impact panels potentially increased recidivism among those with multiple previous convictions, as the average number of subsequent convictions for those who attended a victim impact panel (1.81) was significantly higher than for those who did not (1.31) (Woodall et al., 2000). The average number of subsequent convictions for first-time DWI offenders who attended a victim impact panel in addition to DWI classes (0.87) was not significantly lower than for those who only attended DWI classes (1.09).

In a study of more than 2,000 DWI offenders in California and Oregon, recidivism rates following victim impact panel attendance were compared to rates in control groups of offenders matched by age and sex who were convicted of DWIs in the same states and in the same time periods (Shinar and Compton, 1995). Recidivism rates in the group that attended a victim impact panel were also compared with 683 offenders who were ordered to attend a panel but failed to show up. DWI offenders in Oregon who attended a victim impact panel had lower recidivism rates than those in their age-sex matched control group, but they did not have significantly different recidivism rates than those who were ordered to attend but failed to do so. However, DWI offenders in California who attended a victim impact panel did not have lower recidivism rates than those in the control groups and those who were ordered to attend but failed to do so. The authors noted, however, that analysis of more narrow age groups as well as by sex suggested that victim impact panels could be effective for DWI offenders aged 35 years and older.

A modified victim impact panel tailored to represent the local demographics of a community in New Mexico was also found to be ineffective. A randomized trial of first-time DWI offenders in San Juan County found that alcohol consumption, alcohol-impaired driving, and recidivism within 2 years were no different for those who attended a victim impact panel as part of a 28-day treatment program than for those in the treatment program who did not attend the panel (Wheeler et al., 2004). Nevertheless, San Juan County's customized victim impact panel was not found to increase the effectiveness of the treatment program in changing alcohol-impaired driving behavior among first-time DWI offenders.

Although attendees of victim impact panels often recall the experience as highly emotional, the emotional effect only seems to exert a temporary influence and is not influential enough to sustain long-term behavioral change (Lapham and England-Kennedy, 2012). Many court-ordered attendees have also reported that they felt out of place and/or burdened by attending a victim impact panel. Many also discounted the experience because they thought their own impaired driving was not bad enough to be responsible for a serious alcohol-impaired driving crash.

In summary, evidence on the effectiveness of victim impact panels with respect to reducing rearrest recidivism is mixed and needs to be updated. While a number of studies found victim impact panels to be effective at decreasing recidivism rates of DWI offenders (Fors and Rojek, 1999; Joyce and Thompson, 2017), particularly within the first 2 years after arrest (Rojek et al., 2003), several studies produced mixed results (Shinar and Compton, 1995) or found them to be ineffective (C'de Baca et al., 2000; Crew and Johnson, 2011; Polacsek et al., 2001; Wheeler et al., 2002, 2004). Based on its review of the available evidence, the committee offers the following finding:

> Finding 5-2: While victim impact panels may have positive effects for victims and their families, the available evidence is insufficient to determine whether victim impact panels are effective in preventing alcohol-impaired driving recidivism.

Ignition Interlock Devices

An ignition interlock device is a breath alcohol analyzer that is connected to a vehicle's ignition and requires the driver to provide a breath sample in order to start the vehicle's engine (Marques and Voas, 2010; Sprattler, 2009). The device inhibits driving if the driver's breath contains more than a preset alcohol concentration level, which is typically 0.02 g/dL or 0.02% (Goodwin et al., 2015). Interlocks generally have four basic features:

1. breath alcohol sensor in the vehicle and a control unit under the hood;
2. rolling retest system, which requires at least one retest once the trip is under way (for most interlocks, a retest is required every 20 to 30 minutes while driving);[13]

---

[13] This feature can mitigate the potential harm associated with time to peak BAC. For example, if a driver's BAC is ascending, but not yet at or above the limit set by the interlock,

3. tamper-proof system for mounting the engine part of the unit with a system incorporated to detect attempts to bypass the interlock; and
4. data-recording system that logs BAC results, tests compliance, and logs engine operation to determine if the offender is driving the vehicle regularly (Marques and Voas, 2010, p. 1).

Recent models of interlock devices feature an embedded camera, which takes the driver's photograph when a breath sample is required. Facial imaging technology allows for better identification of the driver providing the breath sample (Voas, 2014) and helps prevent circumvention by having someone else provide a sample for an impaired driver. The use of ignition interlocks in the United States is generally managed in programs that are administered at the state level and aim to prevent alcohol-impaired driving recidivism among individuals arrested for alcohol-impaired driving.

History and legislation Interlock devices were first developed in the United States in 1969, and alcohol-detecting interlocks began to gain traction in the 1980s, when the public's attention to the issue of impaired driving demanded solutions (AAMVA, 2015; Marques and Voas, 2010). The first national model standard for interlock devices was not issued until 1992 (Voas, 2014). The devices became more widespread once Congress passed legislation in 1998 that provided financial incentives to states that passed laws requiring interlocks for repeat offenders (AAMVA, 2015). More recently, the 2012 U.S. transportation reauthorization bill, Moving Ahead for Progress in the 21st Century Act, included incentives for states to pass and enforce mandatory interlock laws.[14]

While every state currently has some form of an ignition interlock law, the nature of the law, enforcement, structure, authority, and operational practices of the interlock programs vary (NCSL, 2016; NHTSA, 2013). For example, 30 states, the District of Columbia, and 4 counties in California require interlocks for all alcohol-impaired driving offenders, including first-time offenders (also called "all-offender" ignition interlock laws). Other states have different variations of interlock laws, including only requiring interlocks for repeat offenders and/or offenders with high BAC levels, mandatory interlocks for first-time offenders at the time of

---

then the vehicle may start after the driver provides a breath sample, but a retest would theoretically capture the driver's peak or subsequent increased BAC and not allow further operation of the vehicle if it is above the limit. Best practices for retest requirements vary (see AAMVA, 2015).

[14] Moving Ahead for Progress in the 21st Century Act, Public Law 112-141, 112th Cong. (July 6, 2012).

arrest (Illinois), or no requirements for first-time or repeat offenders (IIHS, 2017c). In some states where offenders are not required by law to install interlocks, there are still incentives for offenders to do so (e.g., avoiding a jail sentence) (Casanova-Powell et al., 2015). In Georgia, for example, first-time offenders are given the option of a limited driving permit if they install an ignition interlock, with the restriction that they can only drive to work, school, treatment, and monthly monitoring meetings (NCSL, 2016). These devices do not stop an offender from driving a car without the device installed. To help avoid this, in states such as Ohio and Oklahoma, the offender is required to obtain a specially marked driver's license indicating that they can only drive a vehicle that is equipped with an interlock.

Additionally, state ignition interlock laws vary in the length of time for which offenders must have an ignition interlock device installed. For example, for a first offense, Arkansas requires 6 months with an ignition interlock, Arizona requires 12 months, and Delaware requires between 4 and 23 months (MADD, 2017). Comparatively, interlocks are not available for first-time offenders in Massachusetts (MADD, 2017). Ignition interlocks can also be purchased by anyone directly from the manufacturer, usually for voluntary personal use, for parents to monitor teen drivers, or for employers to install in company vehicles (Collier, 2013). A recent study conducted discussion groups with parents, teens, and young adults, as well as manufacturing and insurance companies, on the feasibility of using ignition interlocks to monitor young drivers (Kelley-Baker et al., 2017). All groups agreed that in order for ignition interlocks to be seen as a viable vehicle safety addition, they would first have to be destigmatized from their use as a punishment.

State interlock programs also vary in the extent to which compliance is monitored and how sanctions are tied to noncompliance. Evidence from a randomized controlled trial conducted in the state-wide ignition interlock program in Maryland (Zador et al., 2011), combined with evidence from multiple observation studies conducted in Texas (Marques et al., 2004, 2007) and Canada (Marques et al., 1998, 1999, 2000), indicates that dedicated monitoring can increase compliance with the requirements of an interlock program, and that increased compliance is associated with reductions in impaired driving recidivism after completing a period of interlock monitoring. Compliance is an important component of state interlock programs but is one that has received relatively little research attention in comparison to other program components.

Current use Interlock use in the United States has increased dramatically since the early 2000s. Installation of interlocks increased by about 15 percent per year from 2006 to 2012 (Marques and Voas, 2012). Since 2006 the number of interlocks in use has almost tripled, from 101,000 to about 318,714 in 2014 (Casanova-Powell et al., 2015; Roth, 2014). Despite this increase and the prevalence of ignition interlock laws and state monitoring programs throughout the country, research suggests that interlocks are underused relative to the number of eligible offenders. Goodwin et al. (2015) estimate a ratio of one installed interlock to five DWI arrests.

The interlock technology has also evolved over the past few decades, allowing for more accurate, frequent, and in-depth offender monitoring. While data from earlier models of interlocks were only available on a monthly basis, now interlock companies can provide daily and real-time data to monitoring agencies. The availability of GPS data also provides information on the offender's driving patterns and location when a breath sample is being given (Voas, 2014).

Ignition interlocks can be administered through three general types of programs: administrative, judicial, and hybrid. Administrative programs are typically managed by state DMV agencies that require the ignition interlock installation as a condition of both licensing a suspended driver as well as of license reinstatement. These programs do not require a conviction. Judicial programs use the power of the court to mandate an interlock for an offender, either pretrial or post-conviction, and ensure program compliance. While administrative programs are managed uniformly throughout a jurisdiction, judicial programs allow the courts to have discretion and flexibility to tailor sanctions to program participants. Hybrid programs incorporate a combination of administrative and judicial requirements, which demand a great deal of coordination between judicial and administrative operations (AAMVA, 2015).

Fees for ignition interlocks are borne by the DWI offender. Offenders can pay approximately $65 to $90 per month for an interlock device, in addition to installation fees that can vary from $100 to $250 (Marques and Voas, 2010). Indigent funds are provided for low-income offenders based on specific unaffordability criteria in 30 states and Washington, DC (Goodwin et al., 2015; MADD, 2017); providing such funds in the states without them could help increase participation among low-income offenders there (Elder et al., 2011; Marques and Voas, 2010).

In 2013, NHTSA published a *Model Guideline to State Ignition Interlock Programs*, which provides practical strategies on key program features that are critical for effective delivery. These include legislation, education, program administration, and criminal and administrative sanctions (NHTSA, 2013). In 2015 the American Association of Motor Vehicle Administrators (AAMVA) published the *Ignition Interlock Program Best Practices Guide*, which provides recommendations for how ignition interlock programs should be administered, ranging from technical matters including alerts, device calibration, retests, and anti-circumvention measures including cameras, to administrative matters including outlining program rules and the processes individuals must complete to participate (AAMVA, 2015).

Many countries outside the United States also use ignition interlocks including Australia, Belgium, Canada, Denmark, Finland, Ireland, the Netherlands, Sweden, and the United Kingdom (Martino et al., 2014; Schonfeld and Sheehan, 2004). In Sweden, alcohol-impaired driving offenders have the option of choosing between a 12-month license revocation and a 2-year alcohol ignition interlock program. A study found that those who chose the ignition interlock program were more likely to be relicensed 2 and 3 years after the DWI, had lower rates of harmful alcohol consumption, and were less likely to reoffend (Bjerre and Thorsson, 2008). Another study conducted in Québec, Canada, found that participation in their alcohol ignition interlock program reduced recidivism by 80 percent among first-time offenders during the first 12 months and by 74 percent among repeat offenders during the first 24 months (Vézina, 2002).

Evidence of interlocks as related to drinking and driving The benefits of ignition interlocks as they relate to the problem of drinking and driving have been evaluated with respect to several outcomes, including alcohol-impaired driving recidivism while devices are installed, alcohol-impaired motor vehicle crashes and crash fatalities while devices are installed, and alcohol-impaired driving after devices have been removed from drivers' vehicles.

Considerable research has been dedicated to evaluating whether ignition interlocks have an impact on recidivism, defined as arrests for alcohol-impaired driving among individuals who have an ignition interlock device installed on their vehicle. The evidence from these studies is compelling and indicates that interlocks reduce alcohol-impaired driving recidivism by 50 to 90 percent while ignition interlock devices are installed (Beck et al., 1999; Bjerre, 2005; Casanova-Powell et al., 2015; Coben and Larkin, 1999; Fiedler et al., 2012; Roth et al., 2007; Willis et al., 2004). Also compelling, however, is the evidence that this effect is not observed among drivers after interlock devices are removed from drivers' vehicles (Voas et al., 2016; Willis et al., 2004). Most of the studies evaluating how ignition interlocks relate to recidivism used observation designs. Many of those studies were subject to selection bias, as only subsets of offenders were included as interlock users rather than studying the effectiveness of interlocks among all individuals who are eligible for a given program (Willis et al., 2004). Also, based on the findings of their systematic review, Willis et al. (2004) note that some interlock programs are voluntary versus mandatory for offenders in a jurisdiction. Voas et al. (1999) note that interlock programs can only be effective to the extent that offenders participate. Hence, participation has implications both for how research findings are interpreted and for whether interlock programs can be successful.

In 1991, Sweden was the first country to introduce ignition interlocks on commercial vehicles (buses, trucks, and taxis) on a voluntary basis (Bjerre and Kostela, 2008). A study found that the rates of alcohol-impaired driving were similar among professional drivers and general drivers and that although ignition interlocks prevented very few starts in commercial vehicles, the installation increased employer confidence in drivers (Bjerre and Kostela, 2008). A recent report released in Australia called for the universal use of ignition interlocks on commercial fleets and personal vehicles (Fitzharris et al., 2015). Ignition interlocks are not required on U.S. commercial vehicles or fleets, but they are available to interested employers, school districts, and public transportation officials (Intoxalock, n.d.). In 2017, two Rhode Island legislators sponsored a bill that would require ignition interlocks on all state school buses (O'Coin, 2017).

A separate matter is whether ignition interlocks affect alcohol-impaired driving crashes; a small number of studies have considered this outcome (Elder et al., 2011). Of these, a study in Sweden found decreased crashes in the interlock group compared to the control group, but there were low absolute numbers of crashes in both groups, limiting the interpretation of the findings (Bjerre, 2005; Elder et al., 2011). A study in California found that ignition interlocks installed on the vehicles of convicted drivers were effective at preventing alcohol-impaired driving crashes, but they were associated with increases in other types of crashes. However, this study found that interlocks appeared not to prevent alcohol-impaired driving crashes for first-time DWI offenders with high BAC levels (DeYoung et al., 2004). Another study analyzed relocating interlock order issuance to the driver licensing department from courts and expanding the ignition interlock requirement to first-time offenders with BACs below 0.15% in Washington (McCartt et al., 2013). The authors concluded that requiring interlocks for first-time offenders was associated with fewer reconvictions (despite low interlock use rates) and with reduced single-vehicle late-night crashes.

A recent study by Vanlaar et al. (2017) evaluated the ignition interlock program implemented in Nova Scotia to assess its effectiveness in reducing alcohol-impaired driving. The study was conducted by evaluating alcohol-impaired driving charges and convictions and fatal and serious crashes experienced by 929 offenders who had a voluntary or mandatory interlock device and a comparison group of 326 offenders who declined to participate in the interlock program and instead had their drivers' licenses suspended for their revocation period. Over the course of approximately 12 months, the authors observed a conviction recidivism rate of 0.94 and 3.02 percent among the interlock-voluntary and interlock-mandatory groups, respectively, compared to 8.93 percent among the control group, representing a 90 percent reduction in recidivism in the voluntary group and a 66 percent reduction in recidivism in the mandatory group. The recidivism rates increased to 1.89 percent in the voluntary group and 3.73 percent in the mandatory group after devices were removed from vehicles, but these rates were still lower than those observed among the control group. In addition to this evidence of a specific deterrent effect, the authors used an interrupted time series analysis and found evidence of a general deterrent effect among the entire population of Nova Scotia drivers, in the form of a temporary decrease in the number of alcohol-impaired driving charges (13.3 percent within the first month of the program) and the number of alcohol-impaired driving convictions (9.9 percent following the seventh month of program implementation). They also found a small but significant decrease in the number of fatal and serious-injury alcohol-impaired driving crashes. The authors concluded that the interlock program was more effective in preventing harm attributable to alcohol-impaired driving compared to what would have occurred had the interlock program not been implemented.

Barriers to implementing ignition interlock programs include delays to being eligible to install a device in one's vehicle, low installation rates once individuals are eligible, and recidivism after devices are uninstalled. Ma et al. (2016) evaluated the Reduced Suspension with Ignition Interlock Conduct Review Program in Ontario, Canada. The program was implemented to change Ontario's preexisting interlock policy, in which DWI offenders served at least a 12-month license suspension and then completed another 12 months with either an interlock or without driving at all, in an attempt to address these issues. The program shortened the license suspension period to 3 or 6 months if an offender agreed to install an interlock, followed by 9 or 12 months with the device installed. The new program also attempted to shorten the pretrial elapsed time and therefore required an "early" guilty plea within 90 days of the alcohol-impaired driving offense. Finally, the new program also included behavioral feedback and compliance-based removal to affect long-term recidivism rates. The authors analyzed records of first-time offenders (n = 30,200 in both the interlock installation and pretrial elapsed time investigations; n = 9,326 in the post-interlock recidivism assessments) from 2005 to 2014. The authors found positive effects of the incentive program on two outcomes of interest: interlock installation rates improved 54 percent and pretrial elapsed time shortened by 146 days. However, there was no positive effect on reoffense rate after interlocks were removed. The authors concluded ignition interlocks could be incentivized to bolster installation uptake.

Researchers have questioned whether integrating AUD treatment with ignition interlock programs could extend the effectiveness of these devices after their removal. Voas et al. (2016) studied a Florida policy that required AUD treatment for DWI offenders in an ignition interlock program. The program mandated treatment for offenders who committed three violations (a violation was defined as two lockouts within four hours). The authors conducted survival analyses to compare recidivism between offenders with multiple DWIs who received treatment while their vehicles had interlock devices (n = 640) and matched offenders not required to receive treatment while using interlocks (n = 806). In the 48 months after interlock removal, the DWI offenders who benefited from treatment experienced 32 percent lower recidivism compared to the offenders who did not receive treatment. AUD treatment of offenders was estimated to prevent 41 rearrests, 13 crashes, and 9 injuries from crashes among this group after interlock removal.

To the committee's knowledge, no studies had investigated fatalities as outcomes in evaluations of ignition interlock programs or device installation until two such studies were published within the past 2 years. In 2016, Kaufman and Wiebe used a difference-in-differences design to compare U.S. states that introduced an all-offender ignition interlock law versus states that did not introduce such a law between 2004 and 2013. Eighteen states introduced an all-offender ignition interlock law during that period, making interlocks mandatory for all alcohol-impaired driving convictions. Evidence of an effect of the law was apparent 3 years after these laws were implemented, with an average alcohol-related crash death rate of 4.7 per 100,000 people in states with an all-offender interlock requirement, compared to a rate of 5.5 per 100,000 people in states without this requirement, suggesting an absolute reduction of 0.8 deaths per 100,000 people per year. The authors concluded that policies mandating ignition interlocks for all alcohol-impaired driving convictions were associated with 15 percent fewer alcohol-related driving fatalities; they estimated that 915 lives were saved in the universal interlock states during the period of study.

In 2016, McGinty et al. (2017) used a multilevel model to investigate the relationship between state ignition interlock laws and alcohol-impaired fatal crashes in the United States between 1983 and 2013. After accounting for between-state variation and autocorrelation within states over time, the authors found that state laws requiring interlocks for all alcohol-impaired driving convictions had a 7 percent lower rate of fatal crashes with a BAC greater than 0.08% and an 8 percent lower rate of fatal crashes with a BAC of at least 0.15%. The findings of this study, along with those of Kaufman and Wiebe (2016), provide evidence that alcohol-impaired driving crash deaths are prevented through state all-offender ignition interlock laws.

Potential for primary prevention There are opportunities for more widespread implementation of ignition interlocks among offenders and nonoffenders. This has been a subject of discussion since the devices' emergence as a prevention strategy. The use of ignition interlocks to prevent motor vehicle fatalities is not inherently limited to high-risk populations (i.e., people who have already been convicted of DWI). Public support, a major determinant of widespread implementation, has been studied as well. A nationally representative survey of the U.S. population revealed that 84 percent of participants supported mandating ignition interlocks for all convicted DWI offenders. In addition, if affordable, about 42 percent expressed interest in having advanced alcohol test technology in their vehicles (McCartt et al., 2010).[15] See the section on cost-effectiveness data for information on the potential cost savings for interlocks in all new vehicles.

Bjerre (2005) describes a primary prevention pilot conducted in Sweden with three commercial transport companies (buses, trucks, and taxis). Professional drivers of commercial vehicles, as well as their employers and passengers, accepted ignition interlocks; interlocks as a primary prevention measure were reported to be quickly growing in Sweden at the time the 2005 article was written. Ultimately, the authors found the interlock stopped 3 of 1,000 ignition starts after the device detected a BAC above the lock point (and limit set by Swedish law) of 0.02%, providing some evidence of effectiveness.

Ignition interlock devices on motorcycles Opportunities to prevent alcohol-impaired driving crashes might be achieved through the use of ignition interlock devices on motorcycles. Motorcyclist fatalities, as a proportion of all traffic fatalities, increased from 11 percent in 2006 to 14 percent in 2015 (NCSA, 2016); there were 4,976 motorcyclist fatalities in 2015, which is the highest number since 2012 (NCSA, 2016). In 2011, 30 percent of motorcycle riders involved in fatal crashes had a BAC of 0.08% or higher, a proportion higher than for any other type of vehicle (NHTSA, 2017). NHTSA recently examined the feasibility of ignition interlocks for motorcycles by conducting interviews with ignition interlock manufacturers and installers, state officials, and motorcycle riders with interlocks installed on their motorcycles (NHTSA, 2017).

[15] Of the other 58 percent of respondents, about 54 percent would not be interested in having such technology in their vehicles and 4 percent were undecided or refused to answer.

State laws vary on the extent to which motorcycles are addressed in operating standards for interlocks. For example, some states require DWI offenders who are owners of motorcycles to equip them with an interlock, other states disallow interlocks, and other states have laws that require motorcycle owners to install motorcycle interlocks but do not enforce them. Two interlock manufacturing companies currently permit their devices to be installed on motorcycles (NHTSA, 2017). These devices are designed for use on motor vehicles other than motorcycles, but they can be installed to work adequately on a motorcycle. A number of issues pose challenges for this practice, including exposure to weather and vibration, secure storage, power draw on the battery, and circumvention potential (NHTSA, 2017). A particular challenge with implications for safety is the requirement for performing retests while the motorcycle is being operated. These technical challenges can be overcome, however. NHTSA estimates that motorcycle interlocks likely represent less than 0.1 percent of all interlocks in service (NHTSA, 2017). However, interlock manufacturers reported being willing to install interlocks on motorcycles and to work on adapting or developing new technology for this purpose if states require a motorcycle option for interlocks in their laws.

Cost-effectiveness studies for ignition interlock devices Studies on ignition interlock devices can be divided into two types: studies that examine mandatory interlock device policies for high-risk offenders, and those that aim to predict the effect of mandating interlock devices on all new cars. The former typically involves an alcohol-impaired driving crash and a court mandating that the high-risk driver install an interlock device instead of a court-mandated fine and/or jail time. Also, the former can be studied with real-world data as several states have implemented such policies.

Studies on current interlock programs tend to find them to be cost-effective, but care needs to be taken in observing which costs are included. Interlock devices save the public $3 to $7 on every $1 spent on the devices for DWI offenders, and are cost-effective for this population (MADD, 2013). Similarly, a study of mandatory interlocks in New Mexico (Roth et al., 2007) found that the benefits of requiring interlocks for first offense is cost-effective, finding a $3 benefit (cost savings) for $1 spent for this population. First-time offenders are a high-risk population who might more easily be deterred from future offenses, when compared to repeat offenders. Ullman (2016) also focuses on first-time offenders, noting that interlock programs can prevent alcohol-impaired driving and crashes and provide benefits to society, especially when offenders bear the costs of installation and maintenance.

There are several studies that predict a universal ignition interlock policy would be cost-effective. A study by Carter et al. (2015) modeled the cost savings of interlock devices installed in new vehicles in the United States. The study predicted that, over a span of 15 years, 59,554 fatalities would be prevented and approximately 1.25 million injuries averted. The study further predicted that injury-related savings would outweigh the cost of device installation after 3 years, with savings related to fatal and nonfatal injuries estimated to be $342 billion over the 15-year time span. The study concluded that interlock devices are cost-effective in reducing alcohol-impaired driving crashes, most notably among drivers ages 21 to 29.

An Australian study by Lahausse and Fildes (2009) estimated that benefit-cost ratios for interlock devices can range between 0.6:1 and 3.4:1, depending on various factors including discount rates and time horizon. However, because effectiveness rates are not known, the authors assumed several different levels instead. Not surprisingly, the higher assumed level of effectiveness appeared to be cost-effective, while the lower level was not. This means that the results are rather speculative and may not be applicable to U.S. policy, as it was based in Australia and the alternative effectiveness rates were hypothesized and then compared.

In summary, there are relatively few studies examining the cost-effectiveness of interlock devices. The suggestive evidence is that requiring interlock devices for those arrested for alcohol-impaired driving, and specifically first-time offenders, is likely cost-effective. This conclusion is supported by evaluations of cost-effectiveness of implemented programs. However, there is some uncertainty in this conclusion, and more studies are needed.

The findings are less clear for universal ignition interlock devices on all new cars. These studies are necessarily hypothetical; the price of implementing these devices in the future is unknown. It is reasonable to think that requiring interlock devices for those identified as high risk for alcohol-impaired driving (e.g., arrested) would be more cost-beneficial for society when compared to requiring universal interlock devices and their payment even though only some devices would be used to prevent alcohol-impaired driving. The price is an important unknown factor. In contrast, the advantages of universal ignition interlock are that all high-risk individuals would be subject to the interlock whether they have been caught by law enforcement or not. Furthermore, there would be more alcohol-impaired driving prevention, and costs of law enforcement requiring implementation of interlock would be averted.

Conclusions This section provides a considerable body of research from the United States and other countries that have investigated ignition interlock laws and programs and their effects on alcohol-impaired driving recidivism and related harm. There is strong evidence that individuals convicted of alcohol-impaired driving who have an interlock installed on their vehicle are less likely than others to be rearrested for alcohol-impaired driving or to crash while the device is installed. Evidence from a Cochrane systematic review including only randomized controlled trials and controlled trials also suggests that the benefits of an ignition interlock cease once the device is removed from a vehicle; additional randomized controlled trials are needed as nonrandomized studies do not adequately control for selection bias (Willis et al., 2004). Elder et al. (2011) used the Community Guide methodology to synthesize the research from the Cochrane review, in addition to four other studies, and found strong evidence for ignition interlocks' effectiveness to reduce rearrest rates while interlocks are installed. As a result, the Community Preventive Services Task Force concludes that increased and sustained use of interlocks could significantly affect the rate of alcohol-related crashes. However, findings from at least one study suggest a benefit may be gained by pairing an ignition interlock program with a treatment program for AUD (Voas et al., 2016). States that have introduced all-offender ignition interlock laws appear to have experienced reductions in alcohol-related motor vehicle crash deaths (Kaufman and Wiebe, 2016). It is worth noting that there is evidence suggesting ignition interlock laws have general, as well as specific, deterrent effects. Given strong scientific evidence that individuals convicted of alcohol-impaired driving who have an interlock installed on their vehicle are less likely than others to be rearrested for alcohol-impaired driving or to crash while the device is installed, the committee finds ignition interlocks to be a beneficial technological intervention for reducing alcohol-impaired driving. This technology is affordable for many individuals, and made affordable for others through indigent funds for low-income offenders.

Recommendation 5-3: All states should enact all-offender ignition interlock laws to reduce alcohol-impaired driving fatalities. An ignition interlock should be required for all offenders with a blood alcohol concentration (BAC) above the limit set by state law. To increase effectiveness, states should consider increased monitoring periods based on the offender's BAC or past recidivism.

Current monitoring periods vary by state. The monitoring period ranges from a minimum of 6 months (for example, Delaware and South Carolina) for a first offense to 2 to 5 or more years for second, third, and subsequent offenses (for example, Alabama, New Mexico, and Washington) (NCSL, 2016). Evidence indicates that a minimum monitoring period of 2 years is effective for a first offense and 4 years for a second offense, such as the ignition interlock programs administered in Alabama, Illinois, Oklahoma, and Washington. The law should not have a BAC minimum. Furthermore, given the effectiveness of ignition interlock devices in reducing recidivism, additional research and development into the use of these devices for motorcycles is needed because of the high rates of alcohol-impaired driving fatalities for motorcyclists. Based on the limitations of ignition interlocks (e.g., dissipating effects after removal) and in light of the research that indicates most crash fatalities involve drivers who have never been convicted of a DWI, there is a need to integrate alcohol detection technology in all vehicles (see Chapter 4 for a discussion of the Driver Alcohol Detection System for Safety, a passive alcohol detection system for vehicles).

Education and Training of Law Enforcement and Judicial System Experts

For interventions related to law enforcement and the judicial system to be successful, it is important for those on the front lines to have adequate training and education on alcohol impairment, the law, and options during the adjudication process. Prosecutors can regularly be at a disadvantage during DWI cases because retained defense counsel is usually well funded, resource rich, and highly knowledgeable (AAA, 2016), and prosecutors assigned to DWI cases are often newer and less practiced. In fact, almost half of DWI prosecutors in one survey described insufficient training for DWI prosecution before trying cases, and 94 percent reported wanting additional training (Robertson and Simpson, 2002). Inadequate preparation can affect the outcome of a DWI case (Robertson and Simpson, 2002). Therefore, all prosecutors would benefit from training regarding the development of SFSTs, operation and certification procedures for breath-testing devices, toxicology testing and expert testimony, and procedures and protocols for blood and urine testing to determine BAC. State traffic safety resource prosecutors can be used to create and conduct trainings on these issues. Training courses and other educational resources including technical and trial assistance are also available through the National District Attorneys Association's National Traffic Law Center on topics such as alcohol and drug toxicology, the admission of scientific evidence, and cross-examination of expert witnesses (NDAA, n.d.).

Law enforcement officers are the first to interact with impaired drivers as they make observations on roads and highways. As discussed earlier in this chapter, many of the procedures they regularly perform are essential elements in apprehending and processing an alcohol-impaired driver. Administering SFSTs; accurately assessing drivers based on observations of their driving behavior, speech, demeanor, and appearance;

administration of a breath test; collection of urine or blood for analysis; training on alcohol-related laws (Ramirez, 2017); and other evidence collection provide the basis for how DWI cases will move through the criminal justice system (Shrum, 2017; Woodward, 2017). Because of these crucial roles, timely training and education is important. The National Traffic Law Center also has courses and educational materials available to law enforcement officials involved in DWI cases (NDAA, n.d.).

Judges overseeing alcohol-impaired driving cases need to be knowledgeable about how impaired drivers proceed through the justice system and challenges confronting the judiciary in these cases (AAA, 2016; Shrum, 2017). For example, education for judges could include the signs and symptoms of impairment and the history and protocol regarding administration of the SFSTs by law enforcement officers. Additional education needs to center on how the scientific evidence is collected from the driver, on the operation and certification procedures for breath-testing devices, and on the procedures and protocols for blood and urine testing to determine BAC, the results of which may be submitted during a trial. In terms of post-conviction sanctions, judges could also receive education regarding the full range of effective treatment options for repeat offenders and for those with AUD (including the use of SBIRT, therapy, and medications). The National Judicial College offers training to traffic court judges, magistrates, and hearing officers and could be an important partner for expanding and disseminating the needed knowledge to judges (The National Judicial College, n.d.). State and regional judicial outreach liaisons can also be mobilized to create and conduct trainings on these issues.

Clinical staff who provide assessments of offenders and offer treatment suggestions to judges need to be aware of the various effective treatment options. Training for clinicians can include screening for alcohol and/or other drug use, identifying AUD, identifying binge drinking and the relationship of that behavior to alcohol-impaired driving fatalities and injuries, and implementing prevention strategies in the clinical setting.

Given the central role of law enforcement officers and the judicial system experts described above, as well as the Robertson and Simpson (2002) survey, agreement from national organizations (AAA, 2016; Goodwin et al., 2015; The National Judicial College, n.d.; NDAA, n.d.), and in large part based on information gathered during committee meetings (Ramirez, 2017; Shrum, 2017; Woodward, 2017) and committee expertise on this topic, the committee concludes:

> *Conclusion 5-5: To enhance the effectiveness of alcohol-impaired driving interventions, systematic and ongoing training of professionals in law enforcement, prosecution, the judiciary, clinicians, and public health is needed.*

Law Enforcement Activities

As discussed throughout Chapters 3–5, law enforcement and the criminal justice system play a vital role in preventing alcohol-impaired driving fatalities in every phase outlined in the report's conceptual framework (from precrash to postcrash). However, if supportive policies are not in place or data are not available to help target interventions, the effectiveness of enforcement activities and the ability to take a comprehensive approach to addressing alcohol-impaired driving becomes hampered.

Conclusion 5-6: With respect to DWI prevention and enforcement, the criminal justice and legal systems need to have supportive policies and resources at their disposal to do the following: publicize laws or enforcement activities, permit and conduct sobriety checkpoints, conduct other enforcement activities, administer preliminary breath tests, have strong penalties for refusal to take alcohol tests when warranted, conduct investigations, prosecute and adjudicate criminal charges to the fullest extent of the law (i.e., to reduce pleading down to lesser charges), access data monitoring systems to track and report outcomes of DWI-related charges, access place-of-last-drink data to prioritize enforcement activities, and use Alcoholic Beverage Control Commission enforcement agents to assist in conducting enforcement activities and compliance of alcohol licensees.

IMPROVING EMERGENCY MEDICAL AND TRAUMA SYSTEM SERVICES

Surviving injuries and minimizing the harm of crashes from alcohol-impaired driving require receiving definitive trauma care quickly (MacKenzie et al., 2006). Care in a designated level I or level II trauma center can reduce mortality by 25 percent in patients with severe injuries when compared with care in a nontrauma center hospital (MacKenzie et al., 2006). Alcohol-related crashes that occur in rural areas pose a particular concern given that crashes can occur in remote areas with less access to trauma center care. Using data from the 2000 Census and the 2005 American Hospital Association (AHA) annual survey, Hsia and Shen (2011) found two-thirds of Americans in urban areas have easy access to trauma centers (defined in the study as within 10 miles), compared to 24 percent of people living in rural areas. Furthermore, about one-third of Americans in rural areas have difficult access to trauma centers (defined as more than 30 miles away), compared to 12 percent of urban populations. Additionally, increased notification and response times of emergency care (Gonzalez et al., 2009) can lead to more severe disability after injury (Sihler and Hemmila, 2009) and an increased number of fatalities (Muelleman et al., 2007; Zwerling et al., 2005).

As of 2010, the last year data are available, only 5 percent of the U.S. land area and 64 percent of the U.S. population could access a level I or level II trauma center by ground ambulance within 60 minutes of injury (Carr and Branas, n.d.). Increasing geographical access to trauma centers by locating new air medical helicopter services in rural and other under-covered areas could help reduce alcohol-impaired driving crash fatalities (Branas et al., 2013; Brown et al., 2017; Schiller et al., 2009). If existing air medical transport is used, 35 percent of U.S. land area and 90 percent of the U.S. population could access a level I or level II trauma center within 60 minutes of injury (Carr and Branas, n.d.).

Rural Areas

Delays to emergency care in rural areas may be increasing given that over the past several decades rural hospitals have been closing at a rapid rate (Pines and Ernst, 2017). Trauma centers are often safety-net hospitals, treating disproportionately high volumes of patients with Medicaid or no insurance and as a result are often underfunded, owing to poor reimbursement for their provision of lifesaving but expensive care. Because of this, many trauma center closures have occurred over the last 20 years (Hsia and Shen, 2011). As noted earlier, motivation for treatment of problematic drinking is often lacking. Time in the trauma center may be an opportunity for an offender with a history of problematic drinking to receive counseling and connection to a treatment program for AUD.

Emergency medical services (EMS) coverage and response, as well as geographical access to trauma centers, is especially challenging in rural tribal areas (Dernocoeur, 1988). This is likely a contributor to the disparities in fatal crash rates among American Indian/Alaska Native (AI/AN) populations. The AHA Task Force on Ensuring Access in Vulnerable Communities recommends several strategies to improve the capacity of the Indian Health Service (IHS) to provide care to AI/AN communities. These recommendations include ensuring technical expertise so IHS facilities can gain appropriate federal reimbursements, strengthening partnerships among IHS and non-IHS facilities to enhance coordination of care, and increasing IHS funding (AHA, 2017).

Coordinated efforts are needed to improve access to emergency and trauma care for individuals injured in alcohol-impaired driving crashes in rural areas. Some such efforts are described below. The National Cooperative Highway Research Program Guide for Enhancing Rural Emergency Services identifies four objectives (see bullets below) for improving emergency medical services in rural areas. Each objective is linked with a number of strategies that can be pursued by local decision makers based on their level of need and resources.

- Integrate services to enhance emergency medical capabilities.
- Provide or improve management and decision-making tools.
- Provide better education opportunities for rural EMS.
  - Proven strategy: Use technology-based instruction for rural EMS training.[16]
- Reduce time from injury to appropriate definitive care (TRB, 2005b, p. I-1).

Partnering Emergency Medicine and Primary Care

Many rural hospitals and EDs serve as rural patients' source of primary care; these hospitals are often staffed by primary care and emergency medicine practitioners who can provide care in both disciplines. As rurality increases, a patient is seven times more likely to be treated by a primary care practitioner in an ED (versus an emergency physician). Rural health needs can be met by developing a partnership between primary care and emergency medicine in these areas (Greenwood-Ericksen et al., 2017). For example, a hospital leadership team in a rural county in North Carolina recently rebuilt their facility around "a community-focused care model" (Greenwood-Ericksen et al., 2017, p. 641). The new facility includes a primary care clinic, space for specialists, and an ED with a trauma room; there is no separation between components as all patient rooms are grouped in one bay. A physician assistant and ED nurse screen incoming patients so they can best direct them, and the facility employs patient navigators to help with coordinating care. The flexible care delivery supports the community, patients, and providers.

Mueller et al. (2014) conducted a systematic review to assess published tele-emergency models and their associated outcomes. The authors evaluated a large, Midwestern tele-emergency service through a survey sent to all 71 participating hospitals in addition to site visits and telephone interviews. The authors found tele-emergency services effectively enhance clinical quality by broadening and coordinating the clinical care team and amplifying available resources during events, which help reduce time to care. These attributes foster patient-centered care and help maintain rural hospitals' patient bases while increasing family physician recruitment and retention. The study also found regulatory barriers to tele-emergency use such as varying reimbursement policies and cross-state licensure

[16] This strategy is the only one listed in the report that is marked as "proven" (i.e., evidence based).

issues. Payment systems related to outcomes, rather than volume, such as value-based systems, could help alleviate these challenges and expand tele-emergency services.

Freestanding Emergency Centers

Unlike urgent care centers, freestanding emergency centers (either independent or as a hospital satellite of a regional health system) are full-service EDs that may provide a practical solution to the problem of decreasing time to treatment in rural settings in the context of the United States having experienced so many rural hospital closures (Pines and Ernst, 2017). Rural communities may not provide adequate demand for inpatient care and therefore may not be able to sustain a full hospital. Alternatively, freestanding emergency centers have a lower cost structure and higher patient volume, and facilitate sharing of electronic medical records and imaging, as well as faster transfers of those patients who need additional specialty or trauma care. Correctly triaging patients and improving interhospital transfer is important (Haas et al., 2010, 2012), as one study found that patients who were not transferred to trauma centers from nontrauma EDs but should have been were at risk of getting insufficient trauma care (Delgado et al., 2014).

Technological Advances

Automated crash notification (ACN), a vehicle safety technology designed to notify emergency responders of a crash and its location, has been shown to reduce crash to notification times to 1 minute or less, potentially reducing overall response time (Lahausse et al., 2008). It is estimated that a fully implemented ACN system in the United States could save between 400 and 1,600 lives per year by improving EMS response times (Clark and Cushing, 2002).

Advanced automatic crash notification (AACN) builds on the concept of ACN by including more detailed crash data, such as changes in speed, seat belt use, air bag deployment, and direction of impact, to provide an understanding of crash severity; however, data on how AACN affects patient outcomes are not yet available (TRB, 2013b).

Data Linkage

Samra et al. (2014) evaluated the rural transportation system components in South Dakota as they relate to EMS and ultimately recommended linking EMS data with crash data to "predict service delivery more accurately and establish more specific, data-driven, and performance-based measures" (p. 25).

Beyond improving EMS response times, improving the systems of care for seriously injured crash victims would benefit from the development of a national, learning trauma system, as outlined in an NASEM report on the national trauma care system (NASEM, 2016). The report concluded that, despite past recommendations, the United States lacks a governmental civilian health lead agency for prehospital, in-hospital, and post-acute trauma care. Such leadership is needed to support a learning system for trauma care at the national level. The report recommended that

> the White House should lead the integration of military and civilian trauma care to establish a national trauma care system. This initiative would include assigning a locus of accountability and responsibility that would ensure the development of common best practices, data standards, research, and workflow across the continuum of trauma care. (NASEM, 2016, pp. 16–17)

A critical role would be to enable the linking of current data sources (crash, EMS, nontrauma center and trauma center hospital discharge data, and longitudinal postdischarge data such as death certificates) in order to measure and improve system outcomes. Identifying best practices and learning from successes and failures, particularly in rural areas, has the potential to save lives from alcohol-impaired driving crashes as well as other traffic crashes. Trauma centers could be engaged to reduce time to care for rural areas.

This section reviews some of the challenges rural regions face in confronting alcohol-impaired driving fatalities, including longer distances to trauma centers and hospital closures. Several organizations (e.g., the National Cooperative Highway Research Program and the National Academies of Sciences, Engineering, and Medicine) have drawn attention to these issues and made recommendations to integrate services. Emergency response and trauma system improvement is a promising intervention for rural communities, which is particularly important given the large proportion of alcohol-impaired fatalities that occur there and because many other interventions in this report may be more relevant to urban areas. For example, Greenwood-Ericksen et al. (2017) provide a compelling example of how rural hospitals can effectively partner emergency medicine with primary care, and the Mueller et al. (2014) systematic review and survey illustrate ways in which tele-emergency services can positively affect rural health systems. As explained above, the United States lacks a national trauma care system that effectively integrates successful learning system processes from military settings with civilian trauma care; the National Academies report recommended that the White

House lead this effort (NASEM, 2016). Data linkage is a key component in reducing rural alcohol-impaired driving fatalities. Therefore, the committee concludes:

Conclusion 5-7: A coordinated and continuous learning trauma care system is lacking in the United States. Facilitating the linkage of crash, EMS, and hospital data to generate insights on areas for improvement in addition to greater coordination could substantially affect the number of deaths from alcohol-impaired driving, particularly in rural and tribal areas owing to longer response times to crashes and increased distances from trauma care facilities.

REFERENCES

AA (Alcoholics Anonymous). 2017. *What is A.A.?* https://www.aa.org/pages/en_US/what-is-aa (accessed October 3, 2017).

AA. n.d. *The twelve steps of Alcoholics Anonymous.* https://www.aa.org/assets/en_US/smf-121_en.pdf (accessed October 3, 2017).

AA World Services Inc. 1984. *This is A.A.: An introduction to the A.A. recovery program.* New York: Alcoholics Anonymous World Services, Inc.

AAA (American Automobile Association). 2016. *DUI justice link: A resource to help reduce substance-impaired driving.* http://duijusticelink.aaa.com/wp-content/uploads/2016/11/Bench-Book.pdf (accessed December 9, 2017).

AAA Foundation for Traffic Safety. 2016. *Driver licensing policies and practices.* http://lpp.seniordrivers.org/index.cfm?selection=reportingdrs1&orderby= (accessed June 2, 2017).

AAMVA (American Association of Motor Vehicle Administrators). 2015. *Ignition interlock program: Best practices guide.* Arlington, VA: American Association of Motor Vehicle Administrators.

Aboelata, M., E. Yanez, and R. Kharrazi. 2017. *Vision Zero: A health equity road map for getting to zero in every community.* Los Angeles, CA: Prevention Institute.

ACEP (American College of Emergency Physicians). n.d. *Alcohol screening and brief intervention in the ED.* https://www.acep.org/Clinical---Practice-Management/Alcohol-Screening-and-Brief-Intervention-in-the-ED/#sm.0001k2vlbre0odbbru92379zdg78p (accessed November 27, 2017).

Agerwala, S. M., and E. F. McCance-Katz. 2012. Integrating screening, brief intervention, and referral to treatment (SBIRT) into clinical practice settings: A brief review. *Journal of Psychoactive Drugs* 44(4):307–317.

AHA (American Hospital Association). 2017. *Emerging strategies to ensure access to health care services.* http://www.aha.org/content/17/stategies-to-ensure-access.pdf (accessed October 10, 2017).

Ait-Daoud, N., R. J. Malcolm, and B. A. Johnson. 2006. An overview of medications for the treatment of alcohol withdrawal and alcohol dependence with an emphasis on the use of older and newer anticonvulsants. *Addictive Behaviors* 31(9):1628–1649.

AMERSA (Association for Medical Education and Research in Substance Abuse). n.d. *Project Mainstream.* https://amersa.org/resources/educational-resources/project-mainstream (accessed November 27, 2017).

Anton, R. F., S. S. O'Malley, D. A. Ciraulo, R. A. Cisler, D. Couper, D. M. Donovan, D. R. Gastfriend, J. D. Hosking, B. A. Johnson, J. S. LoCastro, R. Longabaugh, B. J. Mason, M. E. Mattson, W. R. Miller, H. M. Pettinati, C. L. Randall, R. Swift, R. D. Weiss, L. D. Williams, and A. Zweben. 2006. Combined pharmacotherapies and behavioral interventions for alcohol dependence: The combine study: A randomized controlled trial. *JAMA* 295(17):2003–2017.

APIS (Alcohol Policy Information System). 2016. *Health care services and financing: Health insurance: Losses due to intoxication ("UPPL").* https://alcoholpolicy.niaaa.nih.gov/Insurers_Liability_for_Losses_Due_to_Intoxication_UPPL.html (accessed June 9, 2017).

APRI (American Prosecutors Research Institute). 2003. *Alcohol toxicology for prosecutors: Targeting hardcore impaired drivers.* Alexandria, VA: American Prosecutors Research Institute.

Ballesteros, J., J. C. Duffy, I. Querejeta, J. Ariño, and A. González-Pinto. 2004. Efficacy of brief interventions for hazardous drinkers in primary care: Systematic review and meta-analyses. *Alcoholism: Clinical and Experimental Research* 28(4):608–618.

Beck, K. H., W. J. Rauch, E. A. Baker, and A. F. Williams. 1999. Effects of ignition interlock license restrictions on drivers with multiple alcohol offenses: A randomized trial in Maryland. *American Journal of Public Health* 89(11):1696–1700.

Beich, A., T. Thorsen, and S. Rollnick. 2003. Screening in brief intervention trials targeting excessive drinkers in general practice: Systematic review and meta-analysis. *BMJ* 327(7414):536–542.

Berning, A., R. Compton, M. Vegega, D. Beirness, J. Hedlund, R. Jones, and J. Nichols. 2008. *Refusal of intoxication testing: A report to Congress.* DOT HS 811 098. Washington, DC: National Highway Traffic Safety Administration.

Bernstein, E., D. Topp, E. Shaw, C. Girard, K. Pressman, E. Woolcock, and J. Bernstein. 2009. A preliminary report of knowledge translation: Lessons from taking screening and brief intervention techniques from the research setting into regional systems of care. *Academic Emergency Medicine* 16(11):1225–1233.

Bertholet, N., J.-B. Daeppen, V. Wietlisbach, M. Fleming, and B. Burnand. 2005. Reduction of alcohol consumption by brief alcohol intervention in primary care: Systematic review and meta-analysis. *Archives of Internal Medicine* 165(9):986–995.

Bewick, B. M., K. Trusler, M. Barkham, A. J. Hill, J. Cahill, and B. Mulhern. 2008. The effectiveness of web-based interventions designed to decrease alcohol consumption—A systematic review. *Preventive Medicine* 47(1):17–26.

Bjerre, B. 2005. Primary and secondary prevention of drink driving by the use of alcolock device and program: Swedish experiences. *Accident Analysis & Prevention* 37(6):1145–1152.

Bjerre, B., and J. Kostela. 2008. Primary prevention of drink driving by the large-scale use of alcolocks in commercial vehicles. *Accident Analysis & Prevention* 40(4):1294–1299.

Bjerre, B., and U. Thorsson. 2008. Is an alcohol ignition interlock programme a useful tool for changing the alcohol and driving habits of drink-drivers? *Accident Analysis & Prevention* 40(1):267–273.

Blankers, M., M. W. Koeter, and G. M. Schippers. 2011. Internet therapy versus Internet self-help versus no treatment for problematic alcohol use: A randomized controlled trial. *Journal of Consulting and Clinical Psychology* 79(3):330–341.

Block, A. 2016. *Survey of DWI courts.* DOT HS 812 283. Washington, DC: National Highway Traffic Safety Administration.

Bootsma, H., F. Coolen, A. Aldenkamp, J. Arends, L. Diepman, J. Hulsman, D. Lambrechts, L. Leenen, M. Majoie, and A. Schellekens. 2004. Topiramate in clinical practice: Long-term experience in patients with refractory epilepsy referred to a tertiary epilepsy center. *Epilepsy & Behavior* 5(3):380–387.

Branas, C. C., C. S. Wolff, J. Williams, G. Margolis, and B. G. Carr. 2013. Simulating changes to emergency care resources to compare system effectiveness. *Journal of Clinical Epidemiology* 66(8 Suppl):S57–S64.

Bray, J. W., F. K. Del Boca, B. G. McRee, S. W. Hayashi, and T. F. Babor. 2017. Screening, brief intervention and referral to treatment (SBIRT): Rationale, program overview, and cross-site evaluation. *Addiction* 112(Suppl 2):3–11.

Brewer, C., R. J. Meyers, and J. Johnsen. 2000. Does disulfiram help to prevent relapse in alcohol abuse? *CNS Drugs* 14(5):329–341.

Brinkmann, B., J. Beike, H. Köhler, A. Heinecke, and T. Bajanowski. 2002. Incidence of alcohol dependence among drunken drivers. *Drug and Alcohol Dependence* 66(1):7–10.

Brown, J. B., M. R. Rosengart, T. R. Billiar, A. B. Peitzman, and J. L. Sperry. 2017. Distance matters: Effect of geographic trauma system resource organization on fatal motor vehicle collisions. *Journal of Trauma and Acute Care Surgery* 83(1):111–118.

Brown, T. G., M. Dongier, M. C. Ouimet, J. Tremblay, F. Chanut, L. Legault, N. Y. Kin, and N. M. Kwong. 2010. Brief motivational interviewing for DWI recidivists who abuse alcohol and are not participating in DWI intervention: A randomized controlled trial. *Alcoholism: Clinical and Experimental Research* 34(2):292–301.

Burton, R., C. Henn, D. Lavoie, R. O'Connor, C. Perkins, K. Sweeney, F. Greaves, B. Ferguson, C. Beynon, A. Belloni, V. Musto, J. Marsden, and N. Sheron. 2016. A rapid evidence review of the effectiveness and cost-effectiveness of alcohol control policies: An English perspective. *The Lancet* 389(10078):15–21.

Carey, K. B., L. A. Scott-Sheldon, M. P. Carey, and K. S. DeMartini. 2007. Individual-level interventions to reduce college student drinking: A meta-analytic review. *Addictive Behaviors* 32(11):2469–2494.

Carey, S. M., B. E. Fuller, K. Kissick, E. Taylor, and P. Zold-Kilbourn. 2008. *Michigan DUI courts outcome evaluation: Final report.* Portland, OR: NPC Research.

Carmen, B., M. Angeles, M. Ana, and A. J. María. 2004. Efficacy and safety of naltrexone and acamprosate in the treatment of alcohol dependence: A systematic review. *Addiction* 99(7):811–828.

Carnegie, M. A., M. K. Gomel, J. B. Saunders, H. Britt, and L. Burns. 1996. General practice receptionists' attitudes and beliefs towards preventive medicine before and after training and support interventions. *Family Practice* 13(6):504–510.

Carr, B. G., and C. C. Branas. n.d. *Traumamaps.org trauma center maps.* http://www.traumamaps.org (accessed October 10, 2017).

Carter, P. M., C. A. C. Flannagan, C. R. Bingham, R. M. Cunningham, and J. D. Rupp. 2015. Modeling the injury prevention impact of mandatory alcohol ignition interlock installation in all new US vehicles. *American Journal of Public Health* 105(5):1028–1035.

Casanova-Powell, T., J. Hedlund, W. Leaf, and J. Tison. 2015. *Evaluation of state ignition interlock programs: Interlock use analyses from 28 states, 2006–2011.* Washington, DC: National Highway Traffic Safety Administration.

Cavaiola, A. A., and C. Wuth. 2014. *Assessment and treatment of the DWI offender*, edited by B. Carruth. New York: Routledge.

Cavaiola, A. A., D. B. Strohmetz, J. M. Wolf, and N. J. Lavender. 2003. Comparison of DWI offenders with non-DWI individuals on the MMPI-2 and the Michigan alcoholism screening test. *Addictive Behaviors* 28(5):971–977.

CDC (Centers for Disease Control and Prevention). 2017. *Impaired driving: Get the facts.* https://www.cdc.gov/motorvehiclesafety/impaired_driving/impaired-drv_factsheet.html (accessed January 30, 2017).

C'de Baca, J., S. C. Lapham, S. Paine, and B. J. Skipper. 2000. Victim impact panels: Who is sentenced to attend? Does attendance affect recidivism of first-time DWI offenders? *Alcoholism: Clinical and Experimental Research* 24(9):1420–1426.

Center for Substance Abuse Treatment. 1995. *Substance abuse treatment for adults in the criminal justice system.* Rockville, MD: Substance Abuse and Mental Health Services Administration.

Center for Substance Abuse Treatment. 2009. Chapter 3 Disulfiram. In *Incorporating alcohol pharmacotherapies into medical practice.* Vol. 49. Rockville, MD: Substance Abuse and Mental Health Services Administration.

Chamorro, A. J., M. Marcos, J. A. Mirón-Canelo, I. Pastor, R. González-Sarmiento, and F. J. Laso. 2012. Association of μ-opioid receptor (OPRM1) gene polymorphism with response to naltrexone in alcohol dependence: A systematic review and meta-analysis. *Addiction Biology* 17(3):505–512.

Chang, I., S. C. Lapham, J. C'de Baca, and J. Davis. 2001. Alcohol use inventory: Screening and assessment of first-time driving-while-impaired offenders. II. Typology and predictive validity. *Alcohol and Alcoholism* 36(2):122–130.

Chang, I., C. Gregory, and S. C. Lapham. 2002. *Review of screening instruments and procedures for evaluating DWI [driving while intoxicated/impaired] offenders.* Washington, DC: AAA Foundation for Traffic Safety.

Chezem, L. 2005. *Legal barriers to alcohol screening in emergency departments and trauma centers.* Lafayette, IN: Purdue University.

Circuit Court of the State of Oregon. n.d. *DISP participant handbook.* Portland, OR: Multnomah County Courthouse.

Clark, D. E., and B. M. Cushing. 2002. Predicted effect of automatic crash notification on traffic mortality. *Accident Analysis & Prevention* 34(4):507–513.

Coben, J., and G. Larkin. 1999. Effectiveness of ignition interlock devices in reducing drunk driving recidivism. *American Journal of Preventive Medicine* 16(Suppl 1):81–87.

Collier, R. 2013. *Ignition interlock devices in California.* http://dmv-defenders.com/ignition-interlock-devices-california (accessed August 25, 2017).

Community Preventive Services Task Force. 2012. *Alcohol—excessive consumption: Electronic screening and brief interventions (E-SBI).* https://www.thecommunityguide.org/findings/alcohol-excessive-consumption-electronic-screening-and-brief-interventions-e-sbi (accessed May 30, 2017).

Crew, B. K., and S. E. Johnson. 2011. Do victim impact programs reduce recidivism for operating a motor vehicle while intoxicated? Findings from an outcomes evaluation. *Criminal Justice Studies* 24(2):153–163.

Daoud, S. O., H. N. Tashima, and R. Grippe. 2015. *2015 annual report of the California DUI management information system.* Sacramento: California Department of Motor Vehicles.

Delgado, M. K., M. A. Yokell, K. L. Staudenmayer, D. A. Spain, T. Hernandez-Boussard, and N. E. Wang. 2014. Factors associated with the disposition of severely injured patients initially seen at non-trauma center emergency departments: Disparities by insurance status. *JAMA Surgery* 149(5):422–430.

DeMetrick, A. 2016. *State police rolling out a mobile breathalyzer truck.* http://baltimore.cbslocal.com/2016/12/15/state-police-rolling-out-a-mobile-breathalyzer-truck (accessed December 5, 2017).

Dernocoeur, K. 1988. The far limits of rural EMS. Challenges on indian reservations. *Journal of Economics and Management Strategy* 13(4):36–39.

DeYoung, D. J., H. N. Tashima, and S. Maston. 2004. *An evaluation of the effectiveness of ignition interlock in California.* Sacramento, CA: Office of Traffic Safety.

Dill, P. L., and E. Wells-Parker. 2006. Court-mandated treatment for convicted drinking drivers. *Alcohol Research and Health* 29(1):41–48.

Dill, P. L., E. Wells-Parker, and C. A. Soderstrom. 2004. The emergency care setting for screening and intervention for alcohol use problems among injured and high-risk drivers: A review. *Traffic Injury Prevention* 5(3):278–291.

D'Onofrio, G., and L. C. Degutis. 2002. Preventive care in the emergency department: Screening and brief intervention for alcohol problems in the emergency department: A systematic review. *Academic Emergency Medicine* 9(6):627–638.

D'Onofrio, G., and L. C. Degutis. 2010. Integrating project assert: A screening, intervention, and referral to treatment program for unhealthy alcohol and drug use into an urban emergency department. *Academic Emergency Medicine* 17(8):903–911.

D'Onofrio, G., D. A. Fiellin, M. V. Pantalon, M. C. Chawarski, P. H. Owens, L. C. Degutis, S. H. Busch, S. L. Bernstein, and P. G. O'Connor. 2012. A brief intervention reduces hazardous and harmful drinking in emergency department patients. *Annals of Emergency Medicine* 60(2):181–192.

Donoghue, K., R. Patton, T. Phillips, P. Deluca, and C. Drummond. 2014. The effectiveness of electronic screening and brief intervention for reducing levels of alcohol consumption: A systematic review and meta-analysis. *Journal of Medical Internet Research* 16(6):e142.

Dunlap, L. J., G. A. Zarkin, J. W. Bray, M. Mills, D. R. Kivlahan, J. R. McKay, P. Latham, and J. S. Tonigan. 2010. Revisiting the cost-effectiveness of the combine study for alcohol-dependent patients. *Medical Care* 48(2):306–313.

Dunn, C., L. Deroo, and F. P. Rivara. 2001. The use of brief interventions adapted from motivational interviewing across behavioral domains: A systematic review. *Addiction* 96(12):1725–1742.

Eichelberger, A. H., and A. T. McCartt. 2016. Impaired driving enforcement practices among state and local law enforcement agencies in the United States. *Journal of Safety Research* 58:41–47.

Elder, R. W., R. Voas, D. Beirness, R. A. Shults, D. A. Sleet, J. L. Nichols, R. Compton, and Task Force on Community Preventive Services. 2011. Effectiveness of ignition interlocks for preventing alcohol-impaired driving and alcohol-related crashes: A community guide systematic review. *American Journal of Preventive Medicine* 40(3):362–376.

Emmen, M. J., G. M. Schippers, G. Bleijenberg, and H. Wollersheim. 2004. Effectiveness of opportunistic brief interventions for problem drinking in a general hospital setting: Systematic review. *BMJ* 328(7435):318.

Epstein, E. E., and B. S. McCrady. 1998. Behavioral couples treatment of alcohol and drug use disorders: Current status and innovations. *Clinical Psychology Review* 18(6):689–711.

Estee, S., T. Wickizer, L. He, M. F. Shah, and D. Mancuso. 2010. Evaluation of the Washington State screening, brief intervention, and referral to treatment project: Cost outcomes for Medicaid patients screened in hospital emergency departments. *Medical Care* 48(1):18–24.

FBI (Federal Bureau of Investigation). 2010. *Crime in the United States table 69: Arrests by state.* https://ucr.fbi.gov/crime-in-the-u.s/2010/crime-in-the-u.s.-2010/tables/10tbl69.xls (accessed April 11, 2017).

FBI. 2015. *Crime in the United States 2015: Table 29, estimated number of arrests.* https://ucr.fbi.gov/crime-in-the-u.s/2015/crime-in-the-u.s.-2015/tables/table-29 (accessed November 15, 2017).

Feeney, G. F., J. P. Connor, R. Young, J. Tucker, and A. McPherson. 2006. Combined acamprosate and naltrexone, with cognitive behavioural therapy is superior to either medication alone for alcohol abstinence: A single centres' experience with pharmacotherapy. *Alcohol and Alcoholism* 41(3):321–327.

Fell, J. C. 2014. Update: Repeat DWI offenders involvement in fatal crashes in 2010. *Traffic Injury Prevention* 15(5):431–433.

Fell, J. C., and M. Scherer. 2017. Administrative license suspension: Does length of suspension matter? *Traffic Injury Prevention* 18(6):577–584.

Fell, J. C., C. Compton, and R. B. Voas. 2008. A note on the use of passive alcohol sensors during routine traffic stops. *Traffic Injury Prevention* 9(6):534–538.

Fell, J. C., A. S. Tippetts, and E. A. Langston. 2011. *An evaluation of the three Georgia DUI courts.* Washington, DC: National Highway Traffic Safety Administration.

Ferri, M., L. Amato, and M. Davoli. 2006. Alcoholics Anonymous and other 12-step programmes for alcohol dependence. *Cochrane Database of Systematic Reviews* (3):CD005032.

Fiedler, K., C. Brittle, and S. Stafford. 2012. *Case studies of ignition interlock programs.* DOT HS 811 594. Washington, DC: National Highway Traffic Safety Administration.

Finigan, M. W., T. Perkins, P. Zold-Kilbourn, J. Parks, and M. Stringer. 2011. Preliminary evaluation of extended-release naltrexone in Michigan and Missouri drug courts. *Journal of Substance Abuse Treatment* 41(3):288–293.

Fitzharris, M., S. Liu, S. Peiris, A. Devlin, K. Young, M. Lenne, D. Bowman, and J. Gatof. 2015. *Options to extend coverage of alcohol interlock programs.* Sydney, Australia: Austroads.

Fleming, M. F., M. P. Mundt, M. T. French, L. B. Manwell, E. A. Stauffacher, and K. L. Barry. 2002. Brief physician advice for problem drinkers: Long-term efficacy and benefit-cost analysis. *Alcoholism: Clinical and Experimental Research* 26(1):36–43.

Flowers, N. T., T. S. Naimi, R. D. Brewer, R. W. Elder, R. A. Shults, and R. Jiles. 2008. Patterns of alcohol consumption and alcohol-impaired driving in the United States. *Alcoholism: Clinical and Experimental Research* 32(4):639–644.

Fors, S. W., and D. G. Rojek. 1999. The effect of victim impact panels on DUI/DWI rearrest rates: A twelve-month follow-up. *Journal of Studies on Alcohol* 60(4):514–520.

Fourth Judicial District Minnesota Judicial Branch. n.d. *Adult DWI court*. Minneapolis, MN: Fourth Judicial District.

Fuller, R. K., L. Branchey, D. R. Brightwell, R. M. Derman, C. D. Emrick, F. L. Iber, K. E. James, R. B. Lacoursiere, K. K. Lee, and I. Lowenstam. 1986. Disulfiram treatment of alcoholism: A Veterans Administration cooperative study. *JAMA* 256(11):1449–1455.

Garbutt, J. C., A. M. Greenblatt, S. L. West, L. C. Morgan, A. Kampov-Polevoy, H. S. Jordan, and G. V. Bobashev. 2014. Clinical and biological moderators of response to naltrexone in alcohol dependence: A systematic review of the evidence. *Addiction* 109(8):1274–1284.

Gentilello, L. M., A. Donato, S. Nolan, R. E. Mackin, F. Liebich, D. B. Hoyt, and R. A. LaBrie. 2005a. Effect of the uniform accident and sickness policy provision law on alcohol screening and intervention in trauma centers. *Journal of Trauma Injury, Infection, and Critical Care* 59(3):629–636.

Gentilello, L. M., B. E. Ebel, T. M. Wickizer, D. S. Salkever, and F. P. Rivara. 2005b. Alcohol interventions for trauma patients treated in emergency departments and hospitals: A cost benefit analysis. *Annals of Surgery* 241(4):541–550.

Gonzalez, R. P., G. R. Cummings, H. A. Phelan, M. S. Mulekar, and C. B. Rodning. 2009. Does increased emergency medical services prehospital time affect patient mortality in rural motor vehicle crashes? A statewide analysis. *American Journal of Surgery* 197(1):30–34.

Goodwin, A., L. Thomas, B. Kirley, W. Hall, N. O'Brien, and K. Hill. 2015. *Countermeasures that work: A highway safety countermeasure guide for state highway safety offices*, 8th ed. DOT HS 812 202. Washington, DC: National Highway Traffic Safety Administration.

Goonoo, N., A. Bhaw-Luximon, R. Ujoodha, A. Jhugroo, G. K. Hulse, and D. Jhurry. 2014. Naltrexone: A review of existing sustained drug delivery systems and emerging nano-based systems. *Journal of Controlled Release* 183:154–166.

Grant, B. F., R. B. Goldstein, T. D. Saha, S. P. Chou, J. Jung, H. Zhang, R. P. Pickering, W. J. Ruan, S. M. Smith, B. Huang, and D. S. Hasin. 2015. Epidemiology of DSM-5 alcohol use disorder: Results from the National Epidemiologic Survey on Alcohol and Related Conditions III. *JAMA Psychiatry* 72(8):757–766.

Greater London Authority. 2016. *"Sobriety tags" rolled out across London.* https://www.london.gov.uk/press-releases/mayoral/crackdown-against-alcohol-related-crime (accessed September 13, 2017).

Greenwood-Ericksen, M. B., R. Tipirneni, and M. Abir. 2017. An emergency medicine-primary care partnership to improve rural population health: Expanding the role of emergency medicine. *Annals of Emergency Medicine* 70(5):640–647.

Gross, M. 2010. Alcoholics Anonymous: Still sober after 75 years. *American Journal of Public Health* 100(12):2361–2363.

Grunwald, D., J. McDonald, and J. Galante. 2001. *Drunk driving in Rhode Island: 1995–1997.* Providence, RI: Brown University.

Haas, B., D. Gomez, B. Zagorski, T. A. Stukel, G. D. Rubenfeld, and A. B. Nathens. 2010. Survival of the fittest: The hidden cost of undertriage of major trauma. *Journal of the American College of Surgeons* 211(6):804–811.

Haas, B., T. A. Stukel, D. Gomez, B. Zagorski, C. De Mestral, S. V. Sharma, G. D. Rubenfeld, and A. B. Nathens. 2012. The mortality benefit of direct trauma center transport in a regional trauma system: A population-based analysis. *Journal of Trauma and Acute Care Surgery* 72(6):1510-1515; discussion 1515–1517.

Hawaii State Judiciary. n.d. *DWI court program overview.* http://www.courts.state.hi.us/docs/special_projects/DWI_Court_Info.pdf (accessed April 19, 2017).

Hedlund, J. 2017. *Drug-impaired driving: A guide for what states can do.* Washington, DC: Governors Highway Safety Association.

Hedlund, J. H., and A. T. McCartt. 2002. *Drunk driving: Seeking additional solutions.* Washington, DC: AAA Foundation for Traffic Safety.

Heinrich, C. J., and C. J. Hill. 2008. Role of state policies in the adoption of naltrexone for substance abuse treatment. *Health Services Research* 43(3):951–970.

Higgins-Biddle, J., and J. Dilonardo. 2013. *Alcohol and highway safety: Screening and brief intervention for alcohol problems as a community approach to improving traffic safety.* DOT HS 811 836. Washington, DC: National Highway Traffic Safety Administration.

Hsia, R., and Y. C. Shen. 2011. Possible geographical barriers to trauma center access for vulnerable patients in the United States: An analysis of urban and rural communities. *Archives of Surgery* 146(1):46–52.

Humphreys, K., J. C. Blodgett, and T. H. Wagner. 2014. Estimating the efficacy of Alcoholics Anonymous without self-selection bias: An instrumental variables re-analysis of randomized clinical trials. *Alcoholism: Clinical and Experimental Research* 38(11):2688–2694.

Hunt, G. M., and N. H. Azrin. 1973. A community-reinforcement approach to alcoholism. *Behavior Research Therapy* 11(1):91–104.

IIHS (Insurance Institute for Highway Safety). 2017a. *Impaired driving: Deterrence and enforcement.* http://www.iihs.org/iihs/topics/t/impaired-driving/qanda#alcohol--deterrence-and-enforcement (accessed November 27, 2017).

IIHS. 2017b. *Impaired driving: DUI/DWI.* http://www.iihs.org/iihs/topics/laws/dui?topicName=impaired-driving (accessed June 28, 2017).

IIHS. 2017c. *Alcohol-impaired driving.* http://www.iihs.org/iihs/topics/t/impaired-driving/qanda#alcohol--general (accessed June 19, 2017).

IIHS. 2017d. *Impaired driving: Administrative license suspension.* http://www.iihs.org/iihs/topics/t/impaired-driving/qanda#alcohol--administrative-license-suspension (accessed November 27, 2017).

Ingraham, C. 2014. You really can get pulled over for driving while black, federal statistics show. *The Washington Post*, September 9.

Intoxalock. n.d. *Alcohol monitoring business solutions.* https://www.intoxalock.com/drunk-driving-prevention/fleets (accessed August 28, 2017).

Johnson, B. A., N. Rosenthal, J. A. Capece, F. Wiegand, L. Mao, K. Beyers, A. McKay, N. Ait-Daoud, R. F. Anton, and D. A. Ciraulo. 2007. Topiramate for treating alcohol dependence: A randomized controlled trial. *JAMA* 298(14):1641–1651.

Johnson, M., R. Jackson, L. Guillaume, P. Meier, and E. Goyder. 2011. Barriers and facilitators to implementing screening and brief intervention for alcohol misuse: A systematic review of qualitative evidence. *Journal of Public Health* 33(3):412–421.

Jonas, D. E., H. R. Amick, C. Feltner, G. Bobashev, K. Thomas, R. Wines, M. M. Kim, E. Shanahan, C. E. Gass, and C. J. Rowe. 2014. Pharmacotherapy for adults with alcohol use disorders in outpatient settings: A systematic review and meta-analysis. *JAMA* 311(18):1889–1900.

Joyce, S., and K. M. Thompson. 2017. Do victim impact panels reduce drunk driving recidivism? *Restorative Justice* 5(2):251–266.

Kaner, E. F., H. O. Dickinson, F. Beyer, E. Pienaar, C. Schlesinger, F. Campbell, J. B. Saunders, B. Burnand, and N. Heather. 2009. The effectiveness of brief alcohol interventions in primary care settings: A systematic review. *Drug and Alcohol Review* 28(3):301–323.

Kaskutas, L. A. 2009. Alcoholics Anonymous effectiveness: Faith meets science. *Journal of Addiction and Disease* 28(2):145–157.

Kaufman, E. J., and D. J. Wiebe. 2016. Impact of state ignition interlock laws on alcohol-involved crash deaths in the United States. *American Journal of Public Health* 106(5):865–871.

Kazemi, D. M., B. Borsari, M. J. Levine, S. Li, K. A. Lamberson, and L. A. Matta. 2017. A systematic review of the mHealth interventions to prevent alcohol and substance abuse. *Journal of Health Communication* 22(5):413–432.

Kelley-Baker, T., E. Taylor, A. Berning, J. Yao, E. Lauer, and D. Watson. 2017. *The feasibility of voluntary ignition interlocks as a prevention strategy for young drivers.* Washington, DC: National Highway Traffic Safety Administration.

Kenna, G. A., T. L. Lomastro, A. Schiesl, L. Leggio, and R. M. Swift. 2009. Review of topiramate: An antiepileptic for the treatment of alcohol dependence. *Current Drug Abuse Reviews* 2(2):135–142.

Kiefer, F., and K. Wiedemann. 2004. Combined therapy: What does acamprosate and naltrexone combination tell us? *Alcohol and Alcoholism* 39(6):542–547.

Kilmer, B., N. Nicosia, P. Heaton, and G. Midgette. 2013. Efficacy of frequent monitoring with swift, certain, and modest sanctions for violations: Insights from South Dakota's 24/7 sobriety project. *American Journal of Public Health* 103(1):e37–e43.

Kishi, T., S. Sevy, R. Chekuri, and C. U. Correll. 2013. Meta-analysis antipsychotics for primary alcohol dependence: A systematic review and meta-analysis. *Journal of Clinical Psychiatry* 74(7):e642–e654.

Knight, K., D. D. Simpson, M. L. Hiller, C. Leukefeld, F. Tims, and D. Farabee. 2002. *Screening and referral for substance-abuse treatment in the criminal justice system.* Washington, DC: Department of Justice.

Knudsen, H. K., A. J. Abraham, and C. B. Oser. 2011. Barriers to the implementation of medication-assisted treatment for substance use disorders: The importance of funding policies and medical infrastructure. *Evaluation and Program Planning* 34(4):375–381.

Kranzler, H. R., S. Armeli, R. Wetherill, R. Feinn, H. Tennen, J. Gelernter, J. Covault, and T. Pond. 2016. Self-efficacy mediates the effects of topiramate and GRIK1 genotype on drinking. *Addiction and Biology* 21(2):450–459.

Kubas, A., P. Kayabas, and K. Vachal. 2015. *Assessment of the 24/7 sobriety program in North Dakota: Participant behavior during enrollment.* Fargo, ND: North Dakota State University.

Lacey, J. H., R. K. Jones, and J. R. Stewart. 1991. *Cost-benefit analysis of administrative license suspensions.* DOT HS 807 689. Washington, DC: National Highway Traffic Safety Administration.

Lahausse, J. A., and B. N. Fildes. 2009. Cost-benefit analysis of an alcohol ignition interlock for installation in all newly registered vehicles. *Traffic Injury Prevention* 10(6):528–537.

Lahausse, J. A., B. N. Fildes, Y. Page, and M. P. Fitzharris. 2008. *The potential for automatic crash notification systems to reduce road fatalities.* Paper presented at Annals of Advances in Automotive Medicine/Annual Scientific Conference, San Diego, CA, October 6–8.

Lapham, S., and E. England-Kennedy. 2012. Convicted driving-while-impaired offenders' views on effectiveness of sanctions and treatment. *Qualitative Health Research* 22(1): 17–30.

Lapham, S. C., and G. P. McMillan. 2011. Open-label pilot study of extended-release naltrexone to reduce drinking and driving among repeat offenders. *Journal of Addiction Medicine* 5(3):163–169.

Lapham, S. C., J. C'de Baca, I. Chang, W. C. Hunt, and L. R. Berger. 2002. Are drunk-driving offenders referred for screening accurately reporting their drug use? *Drug and Alcohol Dependence* 66(3):243–253.

Lapham, S. C., J. C'de Baca, G. McMillan, and W. C. Hunt. 2004. Accuracy of alcohol diagnosis among DWI offenders referred for screening. *Drug and Alcohol Dependence* 76(2):135–141.

Lapham, S. C., L. R. Kapitula, J. C'de Baca, and G. P. McMillan. 2006. Impaired-driving recidivism among repeat offenders following an intensive court-based intervention. *Accident Analysis & Prevention* 38(1):162–169.

Lapham, S. C., R. Stout, G. Laxton, and B. J. Skipper. 2011. Persistence of addictive disorders in a first-offender driving while impaired population. *Archives of General Psychiatry* 68(11):1151–1157.

Larimer, M. E., and J. M. Cronce. 2002. Identification, prevention and treatment: A review of individual-focused strategies to reduce problematic alcohol consumption by college students. *Journal of Studies on Alcohol* (Suppl 14):148–163.

Leaf, W., and D. Preusser. 1996. *Effectiveness of passive alcohol sensors.* DOT HS 808 381. Washington, DC: National Highway Traffic Safety Administration.

Lenton, S., J. Fetherston, and R. Cercarelli. 2010. Recidivist drink drivers' self-reported reasons for driving whilst unlicensed—A qualitative analysis. *Accident Analysis & Prevention* 42(2):637–644.

Lobmaier, P. P., N. Kunøe, M. Gossop, and H. Waal. 2011. Naltrexone depot formulations for opioid and alcohol dependence: A systematic review. *CNS Neuroscience & Therapeutics* 17(6):629–636.

Logan, B. K., A. L. A. Mohr, and S. K. Talpins. 2014. Detection and prevalence of drug use in arrested drivers using the Drager Drug Test 5000 and Affiniton DrugWipe oral fluid drug screening devices. *Journal of Analytical Toxicology* 38(7):444–450.

Loudenburg, R., G. Drube, and G. Leonardson. 2010. *South Dakota 24/7 sobriety program evaluation findings report.* Salem, SD: Mountain Plains Evaluation.

Ma, T., P. A. Byrne, J. A. Bhatti, and Y. Elzohairy. 2016. Program design for incentivizing ignition interlock installation for alcohol-impaired drivers: The Ontario approach. *Accident Analysis & Prevention* 95(Pt A):27–32.

MacDonald, J. M., A. R. Morral, B. Raymond, and C. Eibner. 2007. The efficacy of the Rio Hondo DUI court: A 2-year field experiment. *Evaluation Review* 31(1):4–23.

MacKenzie, E. J., F. P. Rivara, G. J. Jurkovich, A. B. Nathens, K. P. Frey, B. L. Egleston, D. S. Salkever, and D. O. Scharfstein. 2006. A national evaluation of the effect of trauma-center care on mortality. *New England Journal of Medicine* 354(4):366–378.

MADD (Mothers Against Drunk Driving). 2013. *Ignition interlock institutes: Promoting the use of interlocks and improvements to interlock programs.* DOT HS 811 815. Washington, DC: National Highway Traffic Safety Administration.

MADD. 2017. *Ignition interlock laws in the United States of America: A look at how states implement ignition interlock laws.* http://www.madd.org/laws/law-overview/Overview-of-first-offender-interlock-laws.pdf (accessed June 28, 2017).

MADD. n.d. *How it works: Victim impact panel program.* https://www.maddvip.org/how-it-works (accessed July 3, 2017).

Madras, B. K., W. M. Compton, D. Avula, T. Stegbauer, J. B. Stein, and H. W. Clark. 2009. Screening, brief interventions, referral to treatment (SBIRT) for illicit drug and alcohol use at multiple healthcare sites: Comparison at intake and 6 months later. *Drug and Alcohol Dependence* 99(1):280–295.

Magill, M., and L. A. Ray. 2009. Cognitive-behavioral treatment with adult alcohol and illicit drug users: A meta-analysis of randomized controlled trials. *Journal of Studies on Alcohol and Drugs* 70(4):516–527.

Maisel, N. C., J. C. Blodgett, P. L. Wilbourne, K. Humphreys, and J. W. Finney. 2013. Meta-analysis of naltrexone and acamprosate for treating alcohol use disorders: When are these medications most helpful? *Addiction* 108(2):275–293.

Maltz, M. D., and J. Targonski. 2002. A note on the use of county-level UCR data. *Journal of Quantitative Criminology* 18(3):297–318.

Mann, K. 2004. Pharmacotherapy of alcohol dependence: A review of the clinical data. *CNS Drugs* 18(8):485–504.

Marlowe, D. B., D. S. Festinger, P. L. Arabia, J. R. Croft, N. S. Patapis, and K. L. Dugosh. 2009. *A systematic review of DWI court program evaluations.* Alexandria, VA: National Drug Court Institute.

Marques, P. R., and R. B. Voas. 2010. *Key features for ignition interlock programs.* DOT HS 811 262. Washington, DC: National Highway and Traffic Safety Administration.

Marques, P. R., and R. B. Voas. 2012. Are we near a limit or can we get more safety from vehicle alcohol interlocks? *Addiction* 108(4):657–658.

Marques, P. R., R. B. Voas, and D. Hodgins. 1998. Vehicle interlock programs: Protecting the community against the drunk driver. *Journal of Prevention & Intervention in the Community* 17(1):31–44.

Marques, P. R., R. B. Voas, A. S. Tippetts, and D. J. Beirness. 1999. Behavioral monitoring of DUI offenders with the alcohol ignition interlock recorder. *Addiction* 94(12):1861–1870.

Marques, P. R., A. S. Tippets, R. B. Voas, E. R. Danseco, and D. R. Beirness. 2000. Support services provided during interlock usage and post-interlock repeat DUI: Outcomes and processes. In *Proceedings of the 15th International Conference on Alcohol, Drugs and Traffic Safety*, edited by H. Laurell and F. Schlyter. Stockholm, Sweden: X-CD Technologies. Pp. 1127–1132.

Marques, P. R., R. B. Voas, and D. S. Timken. 2004. Preliminary outcomes from a Texas manual-based group motivational intervention supplement for court-stipulated interlock DUI offenders. In *Proceedings of the 17th International Conference on Alcohol, Drugs and Traffic Safety*, edited by J. Oliver, P. Williams, and A. Clayton. Glasgow, Scotland: X-CD Technologies.

Marques, P., R. Voas, S. Tippetts, K. Blackman, D. Timken, and C. Field. 2007. Motivational intervention keyed to interlock use reduces the rate of positive BAC tests. In *Proceedings of the T2007 Joint International Meeting of TIAFT/ICADTS/IIS*, edited by B. K. Logan, D. S. Isenschmid, J. M. Walsh, D. Beirness, and J. Morland. Seattle, WA: ICADTS.

Marsch, L. A., K. M. Carroll, and B. D. Kiluk. 2014. Technology-based interventions for the treatment and recovery management of substance use disorders: A JSAT special issue. *Journal of Substance Abuse and Treatment* 46(1):1–4.

Martino, A., A. Sitran, and C. Rosa. 2014. *Technical development and deployment of alcohol interlocks in road safety policy.* Brussels, Belgium: European Union.

McCartt, A. T., L. L. Geary, and W. J. Nissen. 2002. *Observational study of the extent of driving while suspended for alcohol-impaired driving.* Washington, DC: National Highway Traffic Safety Administration.

McCartt, A. T., J. K. Wells, and E. R. Teoh. 2010. Attitudes toward in-vehicle advanced alcohol detection technology. *Traffic Injury Prevention* 11(2):156–164.

McCartt, A. T., W. A. Leaf, C. M. Farmer, and A. H. Eichelberger. 2013. Washington State's alcohol ignition interlock law: Effects on recidivism among first-time DUI offenders. *Traffic Injury Prevention* 14(3):215–229.

McGinty, E. E., G. Tung, J. Shulman-Laniel, R. Hardy, L. Rutkow, S. Frattaroli, and J. S. Vernick. 2017. Ignition interlock laws: Effects on fatal motor vehicle crashes, 1982–2013. *American Journal of Preventive Medicine* 52(4):417–423.

McKnight-Eily, L. R., C. A. Okoro, R. Mejia, C. H. Denny, J. Higgins-Biddle, D. Hungerford, D. Kanny, and J. E. Sniezek. 2017. Screening for excessive alcohol use and brief counseling of adults—17 states and the District of Columbia, 2014. *Morbidity and Mortality Weekly Report* 66(12):313–319.

Mello, M. J., T. D. Nirenberg, D. Lindquist, H. A. Cullen, and R. Woolard. 2003. Physicians' attitudes regarding reporting alcohol-impaired drivers. *Substance Abuse* 24(4):233–242.

Midgette, G., and B. Kilmer. 2015. *The effect of Montana's 24/7 sobriety program on DUI re-arrest: Insights from a natural experiment with limited administrative data.* Santa Monica, CA: RAND.

Miller, P. G., A. Curtis, A. Sønderlund, A. Day, and N. Droste. 2015. Effectiveness of interventions for convicted DUI offenders in reducing recidivism: A systematic review of the peer-reviewed scientific literature. *The American Journal of Drug and Alcohol Abuse* 41(1):16–29.

Miller, P. M., S. W. Book, and S. H. Stewart. 2011. Medical treatment of alcohol dependence: A systematic review. *International Journal of Psychiatry in Medicine* 42(3):227–266.

Miller, W. R., and S. Rollnick. 2002. *Motivational interviewing: Preparing people for change,* 2nd ed. New York: Guilford Publications.

Miller, W. R., and P. L. Wilbourne. 2002. Mesa Grande: A methodological analysis of clinical trials of treatments for alcohol use disorders. *Addiction* 97(3):265–277.

Mitchell, O., D. B. Wilson, A. Eggers, and D. L. MacKenzie. 2012. Assessing the effectiveness of drug courts on recidivism: A meta-analytic review of traditional and non-traditional drug courts. *Journal of Criminal Justice* 40(1):60–71.

Moyer, A., J. W. Finney, C. E. Swearingen, and P. Vergun. 2002. Brief interventions for alcohol problems: A meta-analytic review of controlled investigations in treatment-seeking and non-treatment-seeking populations. *Addiction* 97(3):279–292.

Muelleman, R. L., M. C. Wadman, T. P. Tran, F. Ullrich, and J. R. Anderson. 2007. Rural motor vehicle crash risk of death is higher after controlling for injury severity. *Journal of Trauma* 62(1):221–225; discussion 225–226.

Mueller, K. J., A. J. Potter, A. C. MacKinney, and M. M. Ward. 2014. Lessons from tele-emergency: Improving care quality and health outcomes by expanding support for rural care systems. *Health Affairs (Millwood)* 33(2):228–234.

Muench, F., K. van Stolk-Cooke, A. Kuerbis, G. Stadler, A. Baumel, S. Shao, J. R. McKay, and J. Morgenstern. 2017. A randomized controlled pilot trial of different mobile messaging interventions for problem drinking compared to weekly drink tracking. *PLoS ONE* 12(2):e0167900.

Mullen, J., S. R. Ryan, C. W. Mathias, and D. M. Dougherty. 2015. Feasibility of a computer-assisted alcohol screening, brief intervention and referral to treatment program for DWI offenders. *Addiction Science and Clinical Practice* 10:25.

NADCP (National Association of Drug Court Professionals). n.d. *What are drug courts?: The most effective justice strategy addressing the drug-addicted and mentally ill.* http://www.nadcp.org/learn/what-are-drug-courts (accessed April 19, 2017).

Nagin, D. 2013. Deterrence in the twenty-first century: A review of the evidence. In *Heniz College Research Showcase.* Pittsburgh, PA: Carnegie Mellon University.

Namuswe, E. S., H. L. Coleman, and A. Berning. 2014. *Breath test refusal rates in the United States—2011 update.* Traffic Safety Facts Report DOT HS 811 881. Washington, DC: National Highway Traffic Safety Administration.

NASEM (National Academies of Sciences, Engineering, and Medicine). 2016. *A national trauma care system: Integrating military and civilian trauma systems to achieve zero preventable deaths after injury.* Washington, DC: The National Academies Press.

NASEM. 2017. *Communities in action: Pathways to health equity.* Washington, DC: The National Academies Press.

The National Judicial College. n.d. *Traffic courses and programs.* http://www.judges.org/courses/courses-by-judge-type/traffic-courses-and-programs (accessed October 10, 2017).

NC (North Carolina) Health and Human Services. 2017. *Forensic tests for alcohol: Breath alcohol testing (BAT) program awareness.* http://publichealth.nc.gov/chronicdiseaseandinjury/fta/bataware.htm (accessed December 5, 2017).

NCDC (National Criminal Defense College). 2015. *The bottom line: Research update on DWI courts.* https://www.dwicourts.org/wp-content/uploads/The%20Bottom%20Line_0.pdf (accessed August 9, 2017).

NCDC. n.d.-a. *The ten guiding principles of DWI courts.* https://www.dwicourts.org/wp-content/uploads/Guiding_Principles_of_DWI_Court_0.pdf (accessed August 16, 2017).

NCDC. n.d.-b. *The bottom line: DWI court: First-time offenders—In or out?* https://www.dwicourts.org/wp-content/uploads/The%20Bottom%20Line_0.pdf (accessed August 9, 2017).

NCDC. n.d.-c. *What is a DWI court?* https://www.dwicourts.org/uncategorized/what-dwi-court (accessed April, 11, 2017).

NCDC. n.d.-d. *DWI court model compliance checklist.* https://www.dwicourts.org/wp-content/uploads/2011%20NCDC%20Checklist%20Final-Form_0.pdf (accessed August 9, 2017).

NCSA (National Center for Statistics and Analysis). 2016. *Traffic safety facts 2015: A compilation of motor vehicle crash data from the Fatality Analysis Reporting System and General Estimates System.* DOT HS 812 384. Washington, DC: National Highway Traffic Safety Administration.

NCSL (National Conference of State Legislators). 2016. *State ignition interlock laws.* http://www.ncsl.org/research/transportation/state-ignition-interlock-laws.aspx (accessed June 16, 2017).

NDAA (National District Attorneys Association). n.d. *National Traffic Law Center: Resources.* http://ndaa.org/ntlc_resources.html (accessed November 28, 2017).

NHTSA (National Highway Traffic Safety Administration). 1986. *Reducing highway crashes through administrative license revocation.* DOT HS 806 921. Washington, DC: National Highway Traffic Safety Administration.

NHTSA. 2005. *A guide to sentencing DUI offenders.* Washington, DC: National Highway Traffic Safety Administration.

NHTSA. 2006. *Uniform guidelines for state highway safety programs: Highway safety program guideline no. 8: Impaired driving.* Washington, DC: National Highway Traffic Safety Administration.

NHTSA. 2013. *Model guideline for state ignition interlock programs.* DOT HS 811 859. Washington, DC: National Highway Traffic Safety Administration.

NHTSA. 2016. *Digest of impaired driving and selected beverage control laws.* Washington, DC: National Highway Traffic Safety Administration.

NHTSA. 2017. *Examining the feasibility of alcohol ignition interlocks for motorcycles.* Traffic Tech Report DOT HS 812 406. Washington, DC: National Highway Traffic Safety Administration.

NIAAA (National Institute on Alcohol Abuse and Alcoholism). 2000. *10th special report to the U.S. Congress on alcohol and health.* Rockville, MD: National Institute on Alcohol Abuse and Alcoholism.

NIAAA. 2004/2005. Screening for alcohol use and alcohol related problems. *Alcohol Alert* 65.

NIAAA. 2005a. *Brief interventions.* Rockville, MD: National Institute on Alcohol Abuse and Alcoholism.

NIAAA. 2005b. *Helping patients who drink too much.* Washington, DC: National Institute on Alcohol Abuse and Alcoholism.

NIAAA. 2010. Exploring treatment options for alcohol use disorders. *Alcohol Alert* 81.

Nichols, J., and H. L. Ross. 1989. The effectiveness of legal sanctions in dealing with drinking drivers. In *Surgeon General's Workshop on Drunk Driving: Background papers.* Rockville, MD: Office of the Surgeon General. Pp. 93–112.

Nicosia, N., B. Kilmer, and P. Heaton. 2016. Can a criminal justice alcohol abstention programme with swift, certain, and modest sanctions (24/7 sobriety) reduce population mortality? A retrospective observational study. *Lancet Psychiatry* 3(3):226–232.

Nilsen, P., M. Aalto, P. Bendtsen, and K. Seppä. 2006. Effectiveness of strategies to implement brief alcohol intervention in primary healthcare: A systematic review. *Scandinavian Journal of Primary Health Care* 24(1):5–15.

Nilsen, P., J. Baird, M. J. Mello, T. Nirenberg, R. Woolard, P. Bendtsen, and R. Longabaugh. 2008. A systematic review of emergency care brief alcohol interventions for injury patients. *Journal of Substance Abuse Treatment* 35(2):184–201.

NPC (Northwest Professional Consortium, Inc.) Research. 2014. *Collection of executive summaries: Evaluation findings in nine DWI court programs.* http://www.mncourts.gov/Documents/0/Public/Drug_Court/DWI_Court_Evaluation_Collection_of_Statewide_and_Program_Summaries.pdf (accessed August 16, 2017).

NTSB (National Transportation Safety Board). 2000. *Actions to reduce fatalities, injuries, and crashes involving the hard core drinking driver.* Washington, DC: National Transportation Safety Board.

Nunes, A. P., M. K. Richmond, K. Marzano, C. Swenson, and J. Lockhart. 2017. Ten years of implementing SBIRT: Lessons learned. *Substance Abuse* 38(4):508–512.

O'Brien, C. P., L. A. Volpicelli, and J. R. Volpicelli. 1996. Naltrexone in the treatment of alcoholism: A clinical review. *Alcohol* 13(1):35–39.

O'Coin, T. 2017. Lawmakers propose ignition locks on school buses. *WPRI*, January 18.

O'Donnell, A., P. Anderson, D. Newbury-Birch, B. Schulte, C. Schmidt, J. Reimer, and E. Kaner. 2014. The impact of brief alcohol interventions in primary healthcare: A systematic review of reviews. *Alcohol and Alcoholism* 49(1):66–78.

O'Keeffe, T., S. Shafi, J. L. Sperry, and L. M. Gentilello. 2009. The implications of alcohol intoxication and the uniform policy provision law on trauma centers; A national trauma data bank analysis of minimally injured patients. *Journal of Trauma* 66(2):495–498.

Oslin, D. W., W. H. Berrettini, and C. P. O'Brien. 2006. Review: Targeting treatments for alcohol dependence: The pharmacogenetics of naltrexone. *Addiction Biology* 11(3–4):397–403.

Ouimet, M. C., M. Dongier, I. Di Leo, L. Legault, J. Tremblay, F. Chanut, and T. G. Brown. 2013. A randomized controlled trial of brief motivational interviewing in impaired driving recidivists: A 5-year follow-up of traffic offenses and crashes. *Alcoholism: Clinical and Experimental Research* 37(11):1979–1985.

Owens, D. K., K. N. Lohr, D. Atkins, J. R. Treadwell, J. T. Reston, E. B. Bass, S. Chang, and M. Helfand. 2008. Grading the strength of a body of evidence when comparing medical interventions. In *Methods guide for effectiveness and comparative effectiveness reviews.* Rockville, MD: Agency for Healthcare Research and Quality.

Petry, N. M., B. Martin, J. L. Cooney, and H. R. Kranzler. 2000. Give them prizes, and they will come: Contingency management for treatment of alcohol dependence. *Journal of Consulting and Clinical Psychology* 68(2):250–257.

Pines, J., and D. Ernst. 2017. *Solving the rural health care access crisis with the freestanding emergency center care model.* http://healthaffairs.org/blog/2017/02/21/solving-the-rural-health-care-access-crisis-with-the-freestanding-emergency-center-care-model (accessed October 10, 2017).

Polacsek, M., E. M. Rogers, W. G. Woodall, H. Delaney, D. Wheeler, and N. Rao. 2001. MADD victim impact panels and stages-of-change in drunk-driving prevention. *Journal of Studies on Alcohol* 62(3):344–350.

Powers, M. B., E. Vedel, and P. M. Emmelkamp. 2008. Behavioral couples therapy (BCT) for alcohol and drug use disorders: A meta-analysis. *Clinical Psychology Review* 28(6): 952–962.

Prendergast, M., D. Podus, J. Finney, L. Greenwell, and J. Roll. 2006. Contingency management for treatment of substance use disorders: A meta-analysis. *Addiction* 101(11): 1546–1560.

President's Task Force on 21st Century Policing. 2015. *Final report of the President's Task Force on 21st Century Policing.* Washington, DC: Office of Community Oriented Policing Services.

Purshouse, R. C., A. Brennan, R. Rafia, N. R. Latimer, R. J. Archer, C. R. Angus, L. R. Preston, and P. S. Meier. 2013. Modelling the cost-effectiveness of alcohol screening and brief interventions in primary care in England. *Alcohol and Alcoholism* 48(2):180–188.

Raistrick, D., N. Heather, and C. Godfrey. 2006. *Review of the effectiveness of treatment for alcohol problems.* London, UK: National Treatment Agency for Substance Misuse.

Ramirez, R. 2017. PowerPoint presentation to the Committee on Accelerating Progress to Reduce Alcohol-Impaired Driving Fatalities in Washington, DC, February 16, 2017. http://nationalacademies.org/hmd/~/media/Files/Activity%20Files/Accelerating ProgresstoReduceAlcoholImpairedDrivingFatalities/16%20FEB%202017/5%20 Ramirez.pdf (accessed December 4, 2017).

Ray, L. A., A. Heydari, and T. Zorick. 2010. Quetiapine for the treatment of alcoholism: Scientific rationale and review of the literature. *Drug and Alcohol Review* 29(5):568–575.

Redelmeier, D. A., C. J. Yarnell, D. Thiruchelvam, and R. J. Tibshirani. 2012. Physicians' warnings for unfit drivers and the risk of trauma from road crashes. *New England Journal of Medicine* 367(13):1228–1236.

Robertson, A., S. Gardner, C. S. Walker, and A. Tatch. 2016. DUI recidivism by intervention adherence: A multiple risk factor approach. *American Journal of Drug and Alcohol Abuse* 42(5):597–605.

Robertson, R. D., and H. M. Simpson. 2002. *DWI system improvements for dealing with hard core drinking drivers: Prosecution. Executive summary.* Ottawa, Canada: Traffic Injury Research Foundation.

Robertson, R., H. Simpson, and P. Parson. 2008. *Screening, assessment and treatment of DWI offenders: A guide for justice professionals and policy makers.* Ottawa, Ontario: Traffic Injury Research Foundation.

Rogers, P. N. 1997. *Specific deterrent impact of California's 0.08% blood alcohol concentration limit and administrative per se license suspension laws.* Sacramento: California Department of Motor Vehicles.

Rohsenow, D. J. 2004. What place does naltrexone have in the treatment of alcoholism? *CNS Drugs* 18(9):547–560.

Rohsenow, D. J., S. M. Colby, P. M. Monti, R. M. Swift, R. A. Martin, T. I. Mueller, A. Gordon, and C. A. Eaton. 2000. Predictors of compliance with naltrexone among alcoholics. *Alcoholism: Clinical and Experimental Research* 24(10):1542–1549.

Rojek, D. G., J. E. Coverdill, and S. W. Fors. 2003. The effect of victim impact panels on DUI rearrest rates: A five-year follow-up. *Criminology* 41(4):1319–1340.

Roozen, H. G., J. J. Boulogne, M. W. van Tulder, W. van den Brink, C. A. De Jong, and A. J. Kerkhof. 2004. A systematic review of the effectiveness of the community reinforcement approach in alcohol, cocaine and opioid addiction. *Drug and Alcohol Dependency* 74(1):1–13.

Roozen, H. G., R. de Waart, D. A. van der Windt, W. van den Brink, C. A. de Jong, and A. J. Kerkhof. 2006. A systematic review of the effectiveness of naltrexone in the maintenance treatment of opioid and alcohol dependence. *European Neuropsychopharmacology* 16(5):311–323.

Rose, G. L., J. M. Skelly, G. J. Badger, T. A. Ferraro, and J. E. Helzer. 2015. Efficacy of automated telephone continuing care following outpatient therapy for alcohol dependence. *Addictive Behavior* 41:223–231.

Rosenfeld, R. 2007. Transfer the uniform crime reporting program from the FBI to the Bureau of Justice Statistics. *Criminology & Public Policy* 6(4):825–833.

Rösner, S., S. Leucht, P. Lehert, and M. Soyka. 2008. Acamprosate supports abstinence, naltrexone prevents excessive drinking: Evidence from a meta-analysis with unreported outcomes. *Journal of Psychopharmacology* 22(1):11–23.

Roth, R. 2014. *2014 survey of currently-installed interlocks in the U.S.* http://www.rothinterlock.org/2014_survey_of_currently_installed_interlocks_in_the_us.pdf (accessed December 20, 2016).

Roth, R., R. Voas, and P. Marques. 2007. Interlocks for first offenders: Effective? *Traffic Injury Prevention* 8(4):346–352.

Saitz, R. 2010. Alcohol screening and brief intervention in primary care: Absence of evidence for efficacy in people with dependence or very heavy drinking. *Drug and Alcohol Review* 29(6):631–640.

SAMHSA (Substance Abuse and Mental Health Services Administration). 2005a. *Substance abuse treatment for adults in the criminal justice system: A treatment improvement protocol.* Rockville, MD: Department of Health and Human Services.

SAMHSA. 2005b. *Acamprosate: A new medication for alcohol use disorder.* Washington, DC: Department of Health and Human Services.

SAMHSA. 2016a. *Results from the 2015 National Survey on Drug Use and Health: Detailed tables.* https://www.samhsa.gov/data/sites/default/files/NSDUH-DetTabs-2015/NSDUH-DetTabs-2015/NSDUH-DetTabs-2015.htm#tab2-41b (accessed March 31, 2017).

SAMHSA. 2016b. *Key substance use and mental health indicators in the United States: Results from the 2015 National Survey on Drug Use and Health.* Washington, DC: Department of Health and Human Services.

SAMHSA. 2016c. *Naltrexone.* https://www.samhsa.gov/medication-assisted-treatment/treatment/naltrexone (accessed June 8, 2017).

SAMHSA. 2017. *Coding for screening and brief intervention reimbursement.* https://www.samhsa.gov/sbirt/coding-reimbursement (accessed November 28, 2017).

SAMHSA. n.d. *SBIRT: Brief intervention.* http://www.integration.samhsa.gov/clinical-practice/sbirt/brief-interventions#Brief_Intervention_Models (accessed June 1, 2017).

Samra, H., X. Qin, and H. Zhaoxiang. 2014. *Improving rural emergency medical services (EMS) through transportation system enhancements.* Brookings: South Dakota State University.

Schiller, J., J. E. McCormack, V. Tarsia, M. J. Shapiro, A. J. Singer, H. C. Thode, Jr., and M. C. Henry. 2009. The effect of adding a second helicopter on trauma-related mortality in a county-based trauma system. *Prehospital Emergency Care* 13(4):437–443.

Schonfeld, C., and M. Sheehan. 2004. *Critical overview of alcohol ignition interlock programs in Australia.* Paper presented at 17th International Conference on Alcohol, Drugs and Traffic Safety, Glasgow, Scotland, August 8–13.

Schuckit, M. A. 2006. Rehabilitation. In *Drug and alcohol abuse: A clinical guide to diagnosis and treatment.* New York: Springer.

Schuler, M. S., S. Puttaiah, R. Mojtabai, and R. M. Crum. 2015. Perceived barriers to treatment for alcohol problems: A latent class analysis. *Psychiatric Services* 66(11):1221–1228.

SCRAM (Secure Continuous Remote Alcohol Monitor) Systems. 2017. *SCRAM continuous alcohol monitoring: Quick facts.* https://www.scramsystems.com/images/uploads/general/media-pdf/media-kits/scram-mediakit-quickFacts.pdf (accessed September 3, 2017).

Shinar, D., and R. P. Compton. 1995. Victim impact panels: Their impact on DWI recidivism. *Alcohol, Drugs and Driving* 11(1):73–87.

Shrum, C. 2017. PowerPoint presentation to the Committee on Accelerating Progress to Reduce Alcohol-Impaired Driving Fatalities in Washington, DC, May 9, 2017. http://nationalacademies.org/hmd/Activities/PublicHealth/ReduceAlcoholImpairedDrivingFatalities/2017-MAY-09.aspx (accessed October 17, 2017).

Sihler, K. C., and M. R. Hemmila. 2009. Injuries in nonurban areas are associated with increased disability at hospital discharge. *Journal of Trauma* 67(5):903–909.

Sloan, F. A., L. M. Chepke, D. V. Davis, K. Acquah, and P. Zold-Kilbourn. 2013. Effects of admission and treatment strategies of DWI courts on offender outcomes. *Accident Analysis & Prevention* 53:112–120.

Sloan, F. A., E. J. Gifford, L. M. Eldred, and S. A. McCutchan. 2016. Does the probability of DWI arrest fall following participation in DWI and hybrid drug treatment court programs? *Accident Analysis & Prevention* 97:197–205.

Sobering Up. 2016. *States make 24/7 sobriety legislation a top priority in 2016.* https://www.scramsystems.com/blog/2016/02/states-make-247-sobriety-legislation-a-top-priority-in-2016 (accessed September 19).

Solberg, L. I., M. V. Maciosek, and N. M. Edwards. 2008. Primary care intervention to reduce alcohol misuse ranking its health impact and cost effectiveness. *American Journal of Preventive Medicine* 34(2):143–152.

South Dakota Legislature. 2017. *24/7 sobriety program, chapter 2:06:03: Fees.* http://sdlegislature.gov/rules/DisplayRule.aspx?Rule=02:06:03 (accessed September 13, 2017).

Sprattler, K. 2009. *Ignition interlocks—what you need to know: A toolkit for policy makers, highway safety professionals, and advocates.* Washington, DC: National Highway Traffic Safety Administration.

Srisurapanont, M., and N. Jarusuraisin. 2005. Naltrexone for the treatment of alcoholism: A meta-analysis of randomized controlled trials. *International Journal of Neuropsychopharmacology* 8(2):267–280.

Stasiewicz, P. R., T. H. Nochajski, and D. L. Homish. 2007. Assessment of alcohol use disorders among court-mandated DWI offenders. *Journal of Addictions & Offender Counseling* 27(2):102–112.

State of Nevada. n.d. *State regulations dementia and driving.* Carson City, NV: Department of Health & Human Services.

Steinka-Fry, K. T., E. E. Tanner-Smith, and E. A. Hennessy. 2015. Effects of brief alcohol interventions on drinking and driving among youth: A systematic review and meta-analysis. *Journal of Addiction & Prevention* 3(1):11.

Stockings, E., W. D. Hall, M. Lynskey, K. I. Morley, N. Reavley, J. Strang, G. Patton, and L. Degenhardt. 2016. Prevention, early intervention, harm reduction, and treatment of substance use in young people. *Lancet Psychiatry* 3(3):280–296.

Suffoletto, B., C. Callaway, J. Kristan, K. Kraemer, and D. B. Clark. 2012. Text-message-based drinking assessments and brief interventions for young adults discharged from the emergency department. *Alcoholism: Clinical and Experimental Research* 36(3):552–560.

Suffoletto, B., J. Kristan, C. Callaway, K. H. Kim, T. Chung, P. M. Monti, and D. B. Clark. 2014. A text message alcohol intervention for young adult emergency department patients: A randomized clinical trial. *Annals of Emergency Medicine* 64(6):664–672.

Suffoletto, B., J. Kristan, T. Chung, K. Jeong, A. Fabio, P. Monti, and D. B. Clark. 2015. An interactive text message intervention to reduce binge drinking in young adults: A randomized controlled trial with 9-month outcomes. *PLoS One* 10(11):e0142877.

Surla, Jr., L., and S. Koons. 1989. *An evaluation of the elimination of plea bargaining for DWI offenders.* Washington, DC: National Highway Traffic Safety Administration.

Swift, R., D. W. Oslin, M. Alexander, and R. Forman. 2011. Adherence monitoring in naltrexone pharmacotherapy trials: A systematic review. *Journal of Studies on Alcohol and Drugs* 72(6):1012–1018.

Talpins, S. K., and P. Rogers. 2017. Overcoming the plateau: Reducing impaired driving by addressing drug-impaired drivers. *Global Journal of Addiciton & Rehabilitation Medicine* 1(4):555–569.

Talpins, S. K., R. DuPont, R. Voas, E. Holmes, K. Sabet, and C. Shea. 2014. License revocation as a tool for combating drugged driving. *Impaired Driving Update* 19(2):29–41.

Talpins, S. K., R. L. DuPont, H. C. Walls, K. Sabet, and D. Wallace. 2015. The Miami-Dade protocol: Making drugged driving enforcement a reality. *Journal of Alcoholism & Drug Dependence* 3(4):212.

Timko, C., A. Desai, D. M. Blonigen, B. S. Moos, and R. H. Moos. 2011. Driving while intoxicated among individuals initially untreated for alcohol use disorders: One- and sixteen-year follow-ups. *Journal of Studies on Alcohol and Drugs* 72(2):173–184.

Tracy, K., and S. P. Wallace. 2016. Benefits of peer support groups in the treatment of addiction. *Substance Abuse and Rehabilitation* 7:143–154.

TRB (Transportation Research Board). 2005a. *Guidance for implementation of the AASHTO strategic highway safety plan. Volume 16: A guide for reducing alcohol-related collisions.* Washington, DC: The National Academies Press.

TRB. 2005b. *Guidance for implementation of the AASHTO strategic highway safety plan. Volume 15: A guide for enhancing rural emergency medical services.* Washington, DC: The National Academies Press.

TRB. 2013a. *Countermeasures to address impaired driving offenders: Toward an integrated model.* Washington, DC: The National Academies Press.

TRB. 2013b. *Emergency medical services response to motor vehicle crashes in rural areas.* Washington, DC: The National Academies Press.

Ullman, D. F. 2016. Locked and not loaded: First time offenders and state ignition interlock programs. *International Review of Law and Economics* 45:1–13.

USPSTF (U.S. Preventive Services Task Force). 2013. *Alcohol misuse: Screening and behavioral counseling interventions in primary care.* https://www.uspreventiveservicestaskforce.org/Page/Document/RecommendationStatementFinal/alcohol-misuse-screening-and-behavioral-counseling-interventions-in-primary-care (accessed June 2, 2017).

Vallury, K. D., M. Jones, and C. Oosterbroek. 2015. Computerized cognitive behavior therapy for anxiety and depression in rural areas: A systematic review. *Journal of Medical Internet Research* 17(6):e139.

Vanlaar, W. G., M. Mainegra Hing, and R. D. Robertson. 2017. An evaluation of Nova Scotia's alcohol ignition interlock program. *Accident Analysis & Prevention* 100:44–52.

Vasilaki, E. I., S. G. Hosier, and W. M. Cox. 2006. The efficacy of motivational interviewing as a brief intervention for excessive drinking: A meta-analytic review. *Alcohol and Alcoholism* 41(3):328–335.

Vézina, L. 2002. The Québec alcohol ignition interlock program: Impact on recidivism and crashes. In *Proceedings of Alcohol, Drugs and Traffic Safety—T2002: 16th International Conference on Alcohol, Drugs and Traffic Safety*, edited by D. Mayhew and C. Dussault. Québec, Canada: Societe de L'assurance automobile du Québec. Pp. 97–104.

Voas, R. B. 2014. Enhancing the use of vehicle alcohol interlocks with emerging technology. *Alcohol Research: Current Reviews* 36(1):81–89.

Voas, R. B., and J. C. Fell. 2011. Preventing impaired driving opportunities and problems. *Alcohol Research & Health* 34(2):225–235.

Voas, R. B., and D. A. Fisher. 2001. Court procedures for handling intoxicated drivers. *Alcohol Research and Health* 25(1):32–42.

Voas, R. B., P. R. Marques, A. S. Tippetts, and D. J. Beirness. 1999. The Alberta interlock program: The evaluation of a province-wide program on DUI recidivism. *Addiction* 94(12):1849–1859.

Voas, R. B., A. S. Tippetts, and J. Fell. 2000a. The relationship of alcohol safety laws to drinking drivers in fatal crashes. *Accident Analysis & Prevention* 32(4):483–492.

Voas, R., A. S. Tippetts, and E. Taylor. 2000b. *Effectiveness of the Ohio vehicle action and administrative license suspension laws.* Washington, DC: National Highway Traffic Safety Administration.

Voas, R. B., A. S. Tippetts, and A. S. McKnight. 2010a. DUI offenders delay license reinstatement: A problem? *Alcoholism: Clinical and Experimental Research* 34(7):1282–1290.

Voas, R. B., S. S. Tippetts, D. Fisher, and M. Grosz. 2010b. Requiring suspended drunk drivers to install alcohol interlocks to reinstate their licenses: Effective? *Addiction* 105(8): 1422–1428.

Voas, R. B., A. S. Tippetts, G. Bergen, M. Grosz, and P. Marques. 2016. Mandating treatment based on interlock performance: Evidence for effectiveness. *Alcoholism: Clinical and Experimental Research* 40(9):1953–1960.

Wagenaar, A. C., and M. M. Maldonado-Molina. 2007. Effects of drivers' license suspension policies on alcohol-related crash involvement: Long-term follow-up in forty-six states. *Alcoholism: Clinical and Experimental Research* 31(8):1399–1406.

Walker, J., D. Santos, C. Rowe, G.-M. Santos, S. Jung, and P. Coffin. 2017. A novel approach to naltrexone injections may reduce complications and increase adherence. *Drug & Alcohol Dependence* 171:e210.

Washington Courts. 2016. *Current DUI sentencing grid.* Olympia, WA: Administrative Office of the Courts.

Wheeler, D. R., G. Woodall, and E. Rogers. 2002. Victim impact panels. Do they impact drinking and driving behavior? Paper presented at 16th International Conference on Alcohol, Drugs and Traffic Safety, Montreal, Canada, August 4–9.

Wheeler, D. R., E. M. Rogers, J. S. Tonigan, and W. G. Woodall. 2004. Effectiveness of customized victim impact panels on first-time DWI offender inmates. *Accident Analysis & Prevention* 36(1):29–35.

White, A., D. Kavanagh, H. Stallman, B. Klein, F. Kay-Lambkin, J. Proudfoot, J. Drennan, J. Connor, A. Baker, and E. Hines. 2010. Online alcohol interventions: A systematic review. *Journal of Medical Internet Research* 12(5):e62.

Wiliszowski, C., J. Fell, S. McKnight, and S. Tippetts. 2011. *An evaluation of intensive supervision programs for serious DWI offenders.* DOT HS 811 446. Washington, DC: National Highway Traffic Safety Administration.

Williams, S. H. 2005. Medications for treating alcohol dependence. *American Family Physician* 72(9):1775–1780.

Willis, C., S. Lybrand, and N. Bellamy. 2004. Alcohol ignition interlock programmes for reducing drink driving recidivism. *The Cochrane Library* 18(4):CD004168.

Woodall, W. G., H. Delaney, E. Rogers, and D. Wheeler. 2000. A randomized trial of victim impact panels' DWI deterrence effectiveness. *Alcoholism: Clinical and Experimental Research* 24(S5):113A.

Woodward, T. 2017. PowerPoint presentation to the Committee on Accelerating Progress to Reduce Alcohol-Impaired Driving Fatalities in Washington, DC, February 16, 2017. http://nationalacademies.org/hmd/~/media/Files/Activity%20Files/Accelerating ProgresstoReduceAlcoholImpairedDrivingFatalities/16%20FEB%202017/4%20 Woodward.pdf (accessed December 4, 2017).

Yokell, M. A., C. A. Camargo, N. E. Wang, and M. K. Delgado. 2014. Characteristics of United States emergency departments that routinely perform alcohol risk screening and counseling for patients presenting with drinking-related complaints. *Western Journal of Emergency Medicine* 15(4):438–445.

Yuma-Guerrero, P. J., K. A. Lawson, M. M. Velasquez, K. von Sternberg, T. Maxson, and N. Garcia. 2012. Screening, brief intervention, and referral for alcohol use in adolescents: A systematic review. *Pediatrics* 130(1):115–122.

Zador, P. L., E. M. Ahlin, W. J. Rauch, J. M. Howard, and G. D. Duncan. 2011. The effects of closer monitoring on driver compliance with interlock restrictions. *Accident Analysis & Prevention* 43(6):1960–1967.

Zarkin, G. A., J. W. Bray, A. Aldridge, D. Mitra, M. J. Mills, D. J. Couper, R. A. Cisler, and COMBINE Cost-Effectiveness Research Group. 2008. Cost and cost-effectiveness of the COMBINE study in alcohol-dependent patients. *Archives of General Psychiatry* 65(10):1214–1221.

Zarkin, G. A., J. W. Bray, A. Aldridge, M. Mills, R. A. Cisler, D. Couper, J. R. McKay, and S. O'Malley. 2010. The impact of alcohol treatment on social costs of alcohol dependence: Results from the COMBINE study. *Medical Care* 48(5):396–401.

Zwerling, C., C. Peek-Asa, P. S. Whitten, S. W. Choi, N. L. Sprince, and M. P. Jones. 2005. Fatal motor vehicle crashes in rural and urban areas: Decomposing rates into contributing factors. *Injury Prevention* 11(1):24–28.

6

Data and Surveillance Needs and Opportunities

INTRODUCTION

There are a variety of datasets and surveillance systems that provide information on alcohol-impaired driving in the United States. Surveys conducted through the mail, over the phone, and at schools provide self-reported behavioral data; on-road data are also collected through passive methods. Information on crash data is available through police reports as well as hospital and emergency medical services (EMS) records. Other related datasets track fatal and nonfatal injuries and road usage. These data systems each have their respective strengths and limitations (see Table 6-2 at the end of the overview section for available data sources on alcohol-impaired driving), but examining them together allows a picture of the state of alcohol-impaired driving in the United States to emerge. Systematic data collection can help to understand causes, determine long-term trends, and identify subpopulations at greater risk; big data and data collected from epidemiological investigations can also improve real-time response rates. Having a comprehensive understanding of alcohol-impaired driving, both in regard to the rates of occurrence, traffic crashes, injuries, fatalities, arrests, and convictions, as well as qualitative data on when and why people drive while impaired, is vital to create targeted interventions to reduce it.

From a public health perspective, understanding the scope and burden of alcohol-impaired driving requires triangulation across multiple sources of data to identify primary, secondary, and tertiary interventions as well as interventions that can be used prior to alcohol consumption, once alcohol has been consumed and driving is likely, and once alcohol-impaired driving has occurred. These interventions may involve policy, vehicle, and road design, as well as human factors.

In the committee's conceptual model (see Figure 1-5) the pathway to an alcohol-related driving fatality includes drinking, driving, crashing, and death. As such, a public health approach to surveillance data includes assessment of burden and trends across all four stages. Public health approaches routinely use collected survey data with reliable and well-validated reports of consumption and high-risk drinking to assess alcohol use. These data sources also provide national and local information on driving after drinking and other driving-related risks. Finally, administrative and hospital records allow for assessment information about crashes and fatalities (for more on public health data sources, see the section in this chapter titled Public Health and Hospital Datasets). No data source is without error and no data source has complete information on all aspects of the impaired driving landscape. As such, harnessing the available resources while being explicit about strengths and limitations enables researchers to sketch the best possible picture of the scope of the problem, risk factors, and potential points of intervention and prevention.

This chapter begins with a short description of relevant datasets; for a more detailed description, see Appendix A. This is followed by sections that summarize the gaps in the data, the barriers to collecting more comprehensive data, and opportunities for enhanced data collection and surveillance. The chapter concludes with a description of the importance of transparency and access in data and the roles that various stakeholders can play in collecting and maintaining data.

OVERVIEW OF AVAILABLE DATA SOURCES ON ALCOHOL-IMPAIRED DRIVING

The datasets described in this section provide behavioral, crash, fatal injury, nonfatal injury, and denominator data related to alcohol-impaired driving and alcohol-related fatalities. They are summarized in Table 6-2 and grouped by the stages of the drinking-to-crash processes in the conceptual framework (see Figure 1-5). This chapter focuses on datasets that specifically track alcohol-impaired driving trends, but other data sources that provide relevant, related data (e.g., Monitoring the Future, a longitudinal survey that collects behavioral information on secondary school and college students as well as young adults) are also available and an opportunity exists for data integration and research expansion.

Alcohol Consumption and Drinking and Driving Data

The Behavioral Risk Factor Surveillance System (BRFSS) is composed of answers from telephone surveys conducted by the Centers for Disease Control and Prevention (CDC) in all 50 states, the District of Columbia, and 3 U.S. territories (CDC, 2017a). It is the largest continuously conducted health survey in the world and includes information from interviews with more than 400,000 adults (age ≥18 years) annually (CDC, 2017a). The data collected cover chronic health conditions, the use of preventive services, and health-related risk behaviors, including a question pertaining to alcohol-impaired driving that has been asked biennially since 2006 (CDC, 2017a; DiMaggio et al., 2018).[1] The core questionnaire has included this alcohol-impaired driving question as an optional module since the survey's inception in 1984 and has included the question every other year (in even years) since 2002. The survey also asks respondents how many alcoholic beverages they consume in a day and how often they wear a seat belt when driving or riding as a passenger (see Appendix A for more information) (DiMaggio et al., 2018). Some limitations of the BRFSS are that it is conducted on the telephone and therefore excludes some populations from participating, it relies on self-reported data that may contain biases, and its results are only valid on national, state, county, and metropolitan and micropolitan statistical area levels (not local) (CDC, 2016; DiMaggio et al., 2018).

The Youth Risk Behavior Surveillance System (YRBSS) is similar to the BRFSS in that it is a health behaviors survey conducted by CDC (CDC, 2017c). Unlike the BRFSS, however, the YRBSS collects information from middle and high school students biennially and is administered in schools (CDC, 2017c). The YRBSS includes a national school-based Youth Risk Behavior Survey (YRBS) conducted by CDC, and state and large urban school district school-based YRBSs conducted by state and local education and health agencies. The YRBSS includes national, state, territorial, tribal government, and local school-based surveys of representative samples of 9th through 12th grade students that are conducted biennially. Questions on the YRBS cover the following topics: behaviors that contribute to unintentional injuries and violence, sexual behaviors related to unintended pregnancy and sexually transmitted infections, diet and exercise, and drug use (including alcohol and tobacco, with two questions that explicitly address behaviors related to alcohol-impaired driving) (CDC, 2017c; DiMaggio et al., 2018). Beginning in 2013, the YRBS alcohol-impaired driving question response categories were modified to include the option

[1] The BRFSS includes the following question that explicitly pertains to alcohol-impaired driving: "During the past 30 days, how many times have you driven when you've had perhaps too much to drink?" Survey respondents may answer with 0 to 76 times.

"I did not drive a car or other vehicle during the past 30 days." Because of this change, the YRBS alcohol-impaired driving estimates now represent prevalence of the behavior among students who drive, and the long-term temporal trend of alcohol-impaired driving among all students is no longer available. Like the BRFSS, the YRBS is limited by self-reported data that may be subject to under- or overreporting biases (Kann et al., 2016). It is also administered in schools, and therefore does not capture the behaviors of youth who do not attend school (Kann et al., 2016). The YRBS is not conducted in every state; in 2015 Minnesota, Oregon, and Washington did not participate (CDC, 2017d). Lastly, there are missing data from states and school districts that do not include all of the standard YRBS questions on their questionnaires (Kann et al., 2016). The National Health Interview Survey (NHIS), conducted by CDC, also collects information on alcohol consumption and injuries from motor vehicle crashes (NCHS, 2015, 2017a). Specifically, the alcohol consumption data collected by the survey include the percentage of adults 18 years and older who had at least one heavy drinking day[2] in the past year, adjusted by age and sex (NCHS, 2017b).

The National Survey on Drug Use and Health (NSDUH)[3] is conducted annually by the Substance Abuse and Mental Health Services Administration (SAMHSA) in the United States and provides prevalence patterns and other information on the consequences of alcohol use (including one question about arrests for alcohol-impaired driving), tobacco, illegal drug use, and mental disorders among noninstitutionalized populations ages 12 years and over (DiMaggio et al., 2018; SAMHSA, 2016). The survey has been in use since 1971 and reaches about 70,000 respondents each year, making it an effective tool for tracking trends over time (DiMaggio et al., 2018). The NSDUH collects information from residents of homes, military bases, and noninstitutional living spaces such as shelters, rooming houses, and dormitories, but excludes homeless individuals who do not use shelters, institutionalized populations, and active duty military personnel (Batts et al., 2014). Other limitations are that the survey relies on self-reported information and does not assess outcomes at a local level (Batts et al., 2014; DiMaggio et al., 2018).

The National Roadside Survey of Alcohol and Drug Use by Drivers was first conducted by the National Highway Traffic Safety Administration (NHTSA) in 1973 and has been repeated four times since (1986, 1996, 2007, and 2013–2014) (NHTSA, n.d.-c). The survey is voluntary and paid, the two most recent surveys recruiting more than 10,000 drivers each at

---

[2] The NHIS defines a heavy drinking day as an occasion on which men consume five or more drinks and women consume four or more drinks (NCHS, 2017a).

[3] The NSDUH was formerly known as the National Household Survey on Drug Abuse.

roadside stops to complete questionnaires and collect breath, oral fluid, and blood samples (Berning et al., 2015; Lacey et al., 2011). Survey data are based on a combination of physical tests and self-reporting, reducing measurement error compared to surveys relying on only self-report (DiMaggio et al., 2018; Lacey et al., 2011). Survey findings have historically been used to estimate the prevalence of alcohol-impaired driving on U.S. roads and can be used to assess injury and fatality risk in relative risk studies (Kelley-Baker, 2017). One limitation to this survey, however, is that participation is voluntary, so those who think or know they are impaired may choose not to participate (Lacey et al., 2011). The use of appropriated funds for NHTSA to conduct roadside surveys was prohibited by Congress (U.S. House of Representatives, 2015),[4] due to the perception that constituents are being unduly coerced to participate (Kelley-Baker, 2017).

The Alcohol Research Group and its National Alcohol Research Center have conducted the National Alcohol Surveys approximately every 5 years since the 1960s. The survey collects detailed information on alcohol use and alcohol-related problems for adults ages 18 years and older and provides information on alcohol-related patterns and trends over the course of eight surveys spanning more than 35 years (ARG, n.d.).

The Alcohol Policy Information System (APIS) collects information on state- and federal-level policies related to alcohol, including detailed information by state on 35 specific policies related to taxation, underage drinking, alcohol beverage pricing, blood alcohol concentration (BAC) limits, transportation, retail sales, alcohol control systems, pregnancy and alcohol, and health care services and financing (APIS, n.d.-b). In addition, the APIS also includes information on regulations related to legalization of recreational cannabis and drug-impaired driving. The APIS is developed and supported by the CDM Group, Inc., the National Institute on Alcohol Abuse and Alcoholism (NIAAA), and the Pacific Institute for Research and Evaluation (APIS, n.d.-a). Many of the NIAAA's recent alcohol policy research program announcements include calls for research on alcohol and drug use and the effect of alcohol and drug policies on outcomes related to alcohol and drug impairment (NIAAA, 2017).

Motor Vehicle Crash Data

NHTSA has been collecting data from police accident reports (PARs) in its State Data System (SDS) since the early 1980s (NHTSA, n.d.-d). The data include information from 34 participating states, and although the information reported in PARs varies by state, the reports usually include information on crashes resulting in injury, death, or vehicle damage

[4] See Section 143.

(DiMaggio et al., 2018; NHTSA, n.d.-d). Most states report if the driver had been drinking alcohol in proximity to the time of the crash, but information about the passengers' alcohol use is usually not included (DiMaggio et al., 2018). Similar to data on arrests for driving while intoxicated (DWI), data from the SDS on property damage only crashes may be useful in determining opportunities for intervention and prevention of more serious crashes. The biggest limitations of the SDS are the variability in data collected by each state and that much of the data are not readily available to the public—access to state data requires permissions from that specific state (DiMaggio et al., 2018). Researchers or others interested in using the data for a specific purpose may apply for access to the data.

From 1992 to 2013, NHTSA oversaw the Crash Outcome Data Evaluation System (CODES), an autonomous system that creates probabilistic data linkages between crash report data, hospital data, and EMS data—some states have opted to also include data from death certificates, trauma registries, driver citations, and motor vehicle licensing (Cook et al., 2015; Kindelberger and Milani, 2015; NHTSA, n.d.-d). The CODES provides a more comprehensive understanding of the medical and financial consequences of a crash and allows for a more accurate analysis of injury diagnosis and crash severity (NHTSA, n.d.-d). There are cases of missing data, data that the CODES cannot access, and instances in which the data that are available fail to link (Kim et al., 2001).

The National Incident-Based Reporting System (NIBRS) is managed by the Federal Bureau of Investigation (FBI) and provides detailed information on crime incidents (including DWI), such as information about location, time of day, the victim, known offenders, arrestees, the relationships between those involved, and any property involved in the crime (DiMaggio et al., 2018; FBI, n.d.-a). The biggest limitation of the NIBRS is that it is only used by about one-third of all U.S. law enforcement agencies. Deterrents to switching to the NIBRS include preliminary startup costs and concerns that initial results can make it appear that the agency has had a spike in crime incidents (FBI, n.d.-a). The Uniform Crime Reporting program is another data reporting system managed by the FBI, but it provides much less qualitative and contextual detail for crimes than the NIBRS (FBI, n.d.-b). The program collects data on violent crime (murder and nonnegligent manslaughter, rape, robbery, and aggravated assault) and property crime (burglary, larceny, theft, and motor vehicle theft) (FBI, n.d.-c).

The National Academies of Sciences, Engineering, and Medicine's (the National Academies') Transportation Research Board manages the second Strategic Highway Research Program (SHRP 2), which collects important information on driver behavior and performance, identifies variables needed to study naturalistic driving behavior, and provides linkages between multiple datasets (TRB, n.d.). One of the research program's primary applied research focus areas is to better understand driver behavior to improve motor vehicle and highway safety (NASEM, 2015). Specifically, the program analyzes how drivers interact with and adapt to vehicles, roadway design and characteristics, and traffic control devices; the program also analyzes changes in crash risk attributed to these variables (TRB, n.d.). The program conducted a naturalistic driving study by collecting data from more than 3,500 volunteer drivers over a 3-year time period, producing a large database that contains important information on driver behavior and interactions (TRB, n.d.).[5] As the drivers self-selected to participate, the study does not claim to be a random sample of drivers in the United States, nor was it designed to study alcohol use. Another limitation relating to the alcohol sensors installed in study participants' vehicles is that they may record false positives from other sources of alcohol; however, data on impairment were also collected through other indicators, including kinematics, driver behavior, and video (NASEM, 2015). The SHRP 2 database provides the largest naturalistic driving study dataset to date; if analyzed appropriately and with data limitations taken into consideration, it offers useful data for examining alcohol use and alcohol-impaired driving issues in new ways. Although alcohol use has not emerged as one of the program's primary research themes, the SHRP 2 provides a promising area of research expansion to gain behavioral insights of alcohol-impaired drivers and their interactions with vehicles and the traffic environment.

Fatal Motor Vehicle Injury Data

The Fatality Analysis Reporting System (FARS) is a census of fatal crashes that occur on public roadways in the United States and Puerto Rico that has been conducted by NHTSA since 1975 (NHTSA, 2014). FARS data are abstracted by trained FARS analysts in each state, and the annually reported dataset provides information on the characteristics of fatal crashes (e.g., location, alcohol involvement, and roadway and atmospheric conditions), the vehicles, and the people involved by collecting data from PARs, state vehicle registration files, state driver licensing files, state highway department data, vital records department data, death certificates, coroner/medical examiner reports, and EMS reports (DiMaggio et al., 2018; NHTSA, 2014).

The FARS dataset has a number of strengths, including a uniform set of data definitions that are used for data submissions. The dataset characterizes the crash, the vehicles, and the people involved, with the

[5] Available at https://insight.shrp2nds.us (accessed October 10, 2017).

primary data source being the PAR. For alcohol-related crashes, when the information is available, the FARS includes data from breath, blood, and urine BAC tests as well as police behavioral assessments, although both types of data are often missing as these tests are not always done (DiMaggio et al., 2018). BAC test results can be submitted to the FARS and are in the dataset, whereas BAC results that are missing from individual records are imputed using a multiple imputation method that has been tested and evaluated. While the imputations may provide estimates that are close to the actual BAC results that fatally injured drivers and pedestrians have, it is not possible to be certain of their accuracy. There is also variability among states with respect to the proportion of fatally injured persons whose BAC results are obtained. The FARS could be improved through more consistent reporting of BAC results across states, which would require increased testing of persons who are suspected of alcohol-impaired driving (see Appendix A for additional discussion of multiple imputation and addressing missing data).

Demographic data are included in the FARS, as is information on survival time from crash to death, but survival data are limited to deaths occurring within 30 days of the crash (i.e., anyone who dies more than 30 days after the crash is not in the dataset as a crash fatality). Injury severity is not scored in a way that is clinically relevant, so it is not possible to determine whether a death is due to a uniformly fatal injury or to factors that are unrelated to the crash itself. Detailed data on injuries that would allow the calculation of an Injury Severity Score, and would also provide information on potential vehicle design modifications to prevent fatal injuries, are not included, as death certificates do not generally contain detailed injury descriptions. Review of autopsy reports as well as details in hospital records would be necessary to obtain this information. In addition, there is not a 100 percent autopsy rate for fatally injured persons, but a death certificate must be completed for each fatality. The FARS collects race and ethnicity information from death certificates, so these data are only known for the fatally injured, with this information missing 14 percent of the time (DiMaggio et al., 2018; NHTSA, 2009).

Drug data are also collected in the FARS, an important inclusion as the scope of the problems of drug-impaired driving as well as drug- and alcohol-impaired driving are not well understood. The percentage of fatally injured drivers tested for drugs is considerably lower than the percentage tested for alcohol, and drug data that are collected by the FARS have several substantial limitations. Although NHTSA has developed an imputation method to predict BACs of fatally injured drivers of alcohol-related crashes, it has not developed a method for impairment from specific drugs such as cannabis,[6] which will likely require greater rates of drug testing of fatally injured drivers. The FARS drug data provide information on if a drug was present in a driver's system but do not differentiate whether the person was impaired by that drug at the time of the crash or the amount of the drug present, although how much of specific drugs, including cannabis, cause impairment is not well understood. This can be an important distinction because some drugs can remain in a person's system weeks after ingestion (Berning and Smither, 2014). In addition, the degree and type of testing, as well as the proportion of tests that are reported to the FARS, vary by state. In addition to reporting variation, states also vary in testing protocols and positive test thresholds. Drivers who die at the scene of a crash are the most likely to be tested, while drivers who survive, regardless of whether they are considered to be responsible for the crash, are least frequently tested. As might be expected, states that have higher BAC testing rates also have higher drug testing rates (Slater et al., 2016).

In some states, hospitals test any drivers who are brought to the emergency department (ED) after a crash, although law enforcement does not uniformly have access to the hospital tests that are performed. There are states that allow law enforcement to obtain a search warrant to search the hospital record to obtain alcohol test results for tests that were obtained for medical purposes. There are various costs that would result from increased testing and reporting, including the costs of the tests and the personnel costs to law enforcement for the time involved in both performing and reporting the tests. In addition, there are multiple challenges to broadening testing for alcohol and other drugs, including resistance on the part of some practitioners and institutions to perform the tests for various reasons. The benefits of testing can be addressed in educational strategies for the range of practitioners and workers who are involved in the testing and reporting process. Enacting and implementing laws that require alcohol and drug testing in serious and fatal crashes, while costly, would aid in understanding alcohol and drug involvement in these crashes. However, testing only in serious and fatal crashes results in missed opportunities to identify alcohol and drug use that contributes to less severe injury, vehicular damage only, and noninjury crashes and decreases the opportunities to intervene when a minor crash that involves alcohol and/or drugs occurs.

Data on driver's license status, i.e., the validity of the driver's license for operating the particular type of vehicle involved in the crash, are reported. Driving record information for the 3 years prior to the fatal

[6] The AAA Foundation for Traffic Safety has developed an imputation method for cannabis (AAA Foundation for Traffic Safety, 2016).

crash is included, but data from the driving record for more than 3 years prior to the crash are not.

Another strength of the FARS is that its data can be downloaded for analysis; there are also options for online queries. The FARS also contains a geographic information system (GIS) mapping system that can be useful for examining data from a particular state or comparing data across states. As with many other datasets that provide a picture of a problem or set of problems at a national level, the FARS has various strengths and weaknesses. Strengths and limitations of the FARS are summarized in Table 6-1. Working to improve the FARS can be a challenge, but there would be benefits to doing so, including a unique opportunity to explore the utility of using the FARS along with other datasets to address specific issues related to alcohol-impaired driving.

Another source of data for fatal motor vehicle crashes is the Web-based Injury Statistics Query and Reporting System (WISQARS), an interactive, electronic database maintained by CDC that provides statistics on all fatal and nonfatal injuries; it is not limited to those resulting from traffic

TABLE 6-1 Strengths and Limitations of the Fatality Analysis Reporting System

Characteristic	Strength	Limitation
BAC imputation	• BACs imputed based on tested method	• Imputed BAC data proportion varies by state
Information on crash, vehicle(s), and persons involved in crash	• Characterizes crash, vehicle(s), and persons involved—beneficial for understanding fatal crashes • Includes some information on survival time from crash to death (instant to 30 days)	• Limited information on injury severity (only death) • No information on autopsy rates • No data on number of survivors and their degree of injury • Does not include data on deaths more than 30 days postcrash
Information on driver's license status and driving record	• Contains data on driver's license status (validity) • Contains data on driving record for 3 years prior to crash	• Does not include data on driving record for more than 3 years prior to crash
Public availability of data	• Data can be downloaded for analyses • Online query system available	• Online query system is somewhat complex

incidents (CDC, 2017b). Cost data are available based on 2010 economic data from CDC reports, but the WISQARS itself does not contain current cost data. The information on fatal injuries reported in the WISQARS is taken from the *International Classification of Diseases* (ICD)-10 codes on death certificates (DiMaggio et al., 2018). There is underreporting of alcohol involvement in injuries and deaths from various causes, including traffic fatalities (Castle et al., 2014). Although a number of efforts have been made to improve the accuracy and completion of death certificates (Dean et al., 2012; Degani et al., 2009; Myers and Farquhar, 1998), the role of the decedent is also routinely left blank on death certificates (Poe et al., 1993), so it can be impossible to determine if the fatality was that of the driver or a passenger.

State-Level Driving and Crash Data

Driving and crash records are available at the state level. Procedures to request them and the variables they contain vary by jurisdiction. Driving records generally consist of identifying and demographic information, current driving status, recorded offenses in the previous 3 to 10 years (depending on state law and the type of offense), and information on all crashes in which the driver was involved. The data elements included in a driving record vary by state but fall under the general domains of court or administrative actions, reports of crashes, moving violations, drug- and alcohol-related offenses, licensure information and issues, and, in some cases, child support and child endangerment violations.

State-level crash data are based primarily on police investigation reports. State law for investigating and reporting traffic crashes differs across states. For example, in New York, police investigate all crashes involving "death, personal injury, or property damage to any one person in excess of $1,000."[7] In Colorado, crashes involving "injury to, serious bodily injury to, or death of any person or any property damage" are investigated.[8] While this kind of heterogeneity introduces difficulties in combining data across jurisdictions, there are similarities that make such analyses possible.

Crash data can be grouped into two general domains: crash characteristics and vehicle/individual characteristics. Crash-level data consist of police-reported data elements related to the environment and circumstances involving the crash. These variables include crash date and time, crash location (sometimes geocoded), and apparent contributing factors such as roadway and weather conditions, apparent involvement

[7] New York State Vehicle and Traffic Law, Sections 600 to 604.

[8] Colorado Uniform Motor Vehicle Law 42-4-1601 to 42-4-1605.

of alcohol, number of lanes, driver actions such as turning, and presence of traffic controls such as stopping signals. In general, police reports of contributing factors, particularly alcohol involvement, are poorly documented for all but the most serious injuries. Additional vehicle/individual-related variables are routinely collected as part of police investigations, including vehicle classifications (e.g., sedan, taxi, light truck, or van), whether pedestrians were involved, degree and type of vehicle damage, and injury severity (often limited to killed or seriously injured [KSI] versus all others).

Nonfatal Motor Vehicle Injury Data

Nonfatal injuries fall into several categories—those that require hospitalization; those that are treated in the ED without hospitalization; those that are treated in a physician's office or clinic; and those that do not require treatment. The range of severity and short-term, long-term, or permanent disability can vary greatly, particularly in the hospitalization group. There are challenges in measuring severity of injury. The Abbreviated Injury Scale (AIS) provides an anatomic severity measurement, and the Injury Severity Score, which is derived from the AIS, is used to classify severity from single or multiple injuries, and has been described as a component of combined measures that can be used to predict likelihood of survival or potentially preventable deaths. Other datasets that can be used to assess injury severity are data from the Healthcare Cost and Utilization Project (HCUP), maintained by the Agency for Healthcare Research and Quality (AHRQ), and the National Hospital Discharge Dataset, which CDC also maintains. The ICD-9 codes can be translated to AIS codes using available software, and, if desired, Injury Severity Score can be calculated. One of the challenges for all of the datasets is that the quality of the coded data is dependent on the data that are recorded in the medical record, as well as the interpretation of the data at the time of coding.

The WISQARS nonfatal injury data are obtained from ED data from the National Electronic Injury Surveillance System (NEISS), which is operated by CDC's National Center for Injury Prevention and Control in collaboration with the Consumer Product Safety Commission (CDC, n.d.-a). The NEISS All Injury Program collects information from a statistical sample of U.S. EDs and provides data on the injured person's characteristics as well as the intent of injury, the principle diagnoses, the body part(s) affected, where the injury occurred, and whether it was an occupational injury (CDC, n.d.-a). A limitation of the nonfatal WISQARS data is that there are large confidence intervals around the estimates they provide, suggesting that they are not a reliable source for tracking trends over a short period of time (SPRC, 2012).

The optimal method of studying nonfatal and fatal crashes requires a combination of clinical (EMS, ED, hospital, and medical examiner/coroner) and law enforcement datasets to obtain a complete picture of the events and their outcomes. For some studies, a single dataset, such as the FARS, may be useful, but it depends on the focus of the report or research question. For example, the FARS data alone may be helpful if one wants to examine which locations (urban versus rural) have the highest incidence of fatal crashes. The discharge dataset alone may be helpful if one is studying a particular type of injury resulting from motor vehicle crashes; however, this is dependent on how the incidents are coded.

Maintained by the American College of Surgeons, the National Trauma Data Bank (NTDB) is the largest aggregation of U.S. trauma registry data, containing nearly 7.5 million records of all types of injuries, including records of injuries specifically related to motor vehicle injury and alcohol use (American College of Surgeons, n.d.). The NTDB data may be used to study particular types of injuries, and while the NTDB is a national dataset, it is not a statistical sample, nor do all hospitals contribute data. Because it is a dataset that is focused on trauma, it does include a great deal of data regarding injury severity and injury treatment. Trauma registry data are submitted by hospitals throughout the country and include injury event information, detailed diagnoses, information on hospital stay, and outcomes.

Developed as part of AHRQ's HCUP, the Nationwide Emergency Department Sample (NEDS) is the largest U.S. database on all-payer ED visits at the national level that includes detailed information on visits related to injury from alcohol misuse and alcohol-impaired driving (DiMaggio et al., 2018; HCUP, n.d.). Among more than 100 variables for which information on each ED visit is collected, patient demographic and payment information is obtained (HCUP, n.d.). The NEDS data, particularly in conjunction with other datasets, can be used to examine trends in underage alcohol misuse and other alcohol-related problems (Naeger, 2017; NIAAA, 2013).

Driver Denominator Data

To determine rates of alcohol-impaired driving and alcohol-related fatalities, absolute numbers of crashes and fatalities need appropriate denominators to calculate and compare rates across time and location (DiMaggio et al., 2018). The following overview describes data sources that provide information for such purposes.

The National Household Travel Survey sponsored by the Federal Highway Administration (FHWA) asks respondents questions about their transportation habits, including the purpose of their trips, how long the trips take, when the trips take place, means of transportation and, if in a private vehicle, the number of vehicle occupants, the driver's characteristics, and the vehicle's attributes (FHWA, n.d.-a). In 2017, more than 129,000 households completed the survey, but the data are limited by low response rates, difficulty reaching demographic subgroups, and because the race and ethnicity of the survey respondent is also applied to the rest of their household (DiMaggio et al., 2018; FHWA, 2015, n.d.-b). The survey is conducted infrequently and irregularly (Garrett, 2014).

The FHWA has also compiled state data on highway vehicle miles traveled (HVMT) since 1945, providing an annual summary of national and state statistics on motor fuel, motor vehicle registration, drivers' licenses, highway miles traveled, highway user taxation, and highway finance (FHWA, 2016). A major limitation of these data is that they are based on vehicle counts, and therefore the demographics of miles traveled are unavailable (DiMaggio et al., 2018). Another limitation is that data are only collected on 4,000 automatic traffic recorders throughout the country, and there are limited corresponding data available on local traffic (DOT, 2016).

Drivers' licensure data are another source of denominator data that may be especially useful at the state level. Public availability of licensure data is governed by the Driver's Privacy Protection Act (DPPA),[9] which mandates all states to protect the privacy of individuals' personal information in their motor vehicle records (Walsh et al., 2011). The DPPA allows the release of licensure data when requests are in compliance with permissible public health research uses (Walsh et al., 2011). In a study conducted in 2009 and 2010 requesting access to licensure data for a hypothetical public health research project, 32 percent of states (16 out of 50) allowed access and 44 percent (22 out of 50) denied access (Walsh et al., 2011). Although accessibility is limited, in some states licensure data can provide information on prior DWI arrests.

In addition to data availability and quality limitations of HVMT for use as a denominator in assessing crash risk, normalizing data across HVMT may obscure the contribution of salient risk factors including, but not limited, to alcohol. There are multiple options for assessing crash risk; measures such as the crash incidence ratio (CIR), for example, provide estimates of the relative risk of crash at various levels of BAC compared with the risk at referent levels of BAC (most commonly, BAC = 0.0%). The addition of such metrics provides an assessment of the contribution of alcohol to crash risk net of other risk factors. Thus, whereas use of HVMT as a denominator provides assessment of absolute alcohol-related crash risk, CIR measures provide assessment of

[9] 18 U.S.C. 2721–2725.

relative alcohol-related crash risk. Voas et al. (2007) demonstrated that underage drivers have a high absolute risk of alcohol-related crash risk compared with older drivers, but a lower relative alcohol-related crash risk. This seeming incongruence is due to the fact that underage drivers who crash do so based on many factors (e.g., inexperience, distraction), including, but not limited to, alcohol, whereas older drivers who crash are more likely to have alcohol involved in the crash. As such, providing evidence across multiple indicators of crash risk is necessary to fully contextualize risk across the myriad of factors that vary across age, other demographics, and the environment (e.g., road conditions). Table 6-2 summarizes the strengths, weaknesses, and biases of the datasets discussed in this section.

GAPS AND BARRIERS

Many data and surveillance needs have been identified throughout Chapters 2–5 regarding alcohol-impaired driving. Below is a discussion of these data gaps and barriers that, if addressed, would help provide a fuller picture of who, where, and when alcohol-impaired fatalities and injuries are taking place to better inform comprehensive interventions at the local, state, and federal levels.

Vehicle miles traveled (VMT) can serve as a meaningful denominator for assessing the effect of interventions to prevent alcohol-impaired driving, as the use of VMT can allow tracking of trends over time, as well as the true proportion of events in specific populations. For example, it is difficult to assess whether the higher proportion of alcohol-impaired driving fatalities in rural areas is related to a higher number of miles traveled in rural areas as compared to urban areas, or some other factors. However, VMTs are not routinely measured, so this method of analysis cannot be used readily.

The lack of availability of data with respect to enforcement of traffic laws makes it difficult to assess the effect of enforcement. There is limited information on the number of people who are arrested for DWI, the outcomes of the arrests, and the long-term effect of arrest on recidivism. In addition, data that are collected and reported are not necessarily collected using standardized or uniform definitions, which is a challenge for traffic safety in general, not just alcohol-impaired driving. One example of the difficulty related to alcohol-impaired driving is the lack of information on drivers convicted of a DWI charge whose licenses are suspended or revoked, but who continue to drive during the suspension or revocation periods. As penalties tend to differ depending upon state policies, as well as the judicial process, data on penalties and how often specific penalties are imposed are lacking. The penalties may be affected by various

TABLE 6-2 Strengths, Weaknesses, and Biases of Datasets That Include Information on Alcohol-Impaired Driving

Conceptual Framework Phase	Data Source	Conducted/Managed by	Data Collection Method and Data Collected	Important Characteristics (Strengths, Weaknesses, Biases, and Limitations)
Alcohol Consumption; Drink to Impairment; Drive Impaired	Behavioral Risk Factor Surveillance System	Centers for Disease Control and Prevention	• Telephone survey that collects information about chronic health conditions, use of preventive services, and health-related risk behaviors	• Health-related risk behavior question on alcohol-impaired driving only asked biennially since 2006 • Conducted via telephone and thus excludes some populations • Nationally representative • Effective tool for tracking trends over time • Relies on self-reported data that may contain biases • Results not available on local level
	Youth Risk Behavior Surveillance System	Centers for Disease Control and Prevention	• In-school survey that collects information on behaviors that contribute to unintentional injuries and violence, sexual behaviors related to unintended pregnancy and sexually transmitted infections, diet and exercise, and drug use (including alcohol and tobacco, with questions related to alcohol-impaired driving)	• Representative of adolescents in school • Effective tool for tracking trends over time • Relies on self-reported data that may contain biases • Administered in schools and thus excludes youth not in school • Not all school districts include all standard Youth Risk Behavior Survey questions on their questionnaires

National Survey on Drug Use and Health	Substance Abuse and Mental Health Services Administration	• Prevalence patterns and other information on consequences of alcohol use (including question about arrests for alcohol-impaired driving), tobacco, illegal drug use, and mental health disorders	• Effective tool for tracking trends over time (in use since 1971 and reaches ~70,000 respondents each year) • Excludes homeless and institutionalized populations and active duty military personnel • Relies on self-reported information • Does not assess outcomes at local level
National Roadside Survey of Alcohol and Drug Use by Drivers	National Highway Traffic Safety Administration	• Drivers complete questionnaires • Breath, oral fluid, and blood samples collected	• Data based on a combination of physical tests and self-report, reducing measurement error compared to surveys relying on self-report only • Survey participation is voluntary, so those who think/know they are impaired may choose not to participate
National Alcohol Surveys	Alcohol Research Group and National Alcohol Research Center	• Conducted ~5 years on alcohol use and alcohol-related problems for adults ages 18 years and older	• Provides information on alcohol-related patterns and trends over time span of 35 years
Alcohol Policy Information System	CDM Group, Inc.; National Institute on Alcohol Abuse and Alcoholism; Pacific Institute for Research and Evaluation	• State- and federal-level policies related to alcohol	• Provides detailed information by state on 35 specific policies related to taxation, underage drinking, alcohol beverage pricing, BAC limits, transportation, retail sales, alcohol control systems, pregnancy and alcohol, and health care services and financing

continued

TABLE 6-2 Continued

Conceptual Framework Phase	Data Source	Conducted/Managed by	Data Collection Method and Data Collected	Important Characteristics (Strengths, Weaknesses, Biases, and Limitations)
Motor Vehicle Crash	State Data System	National Highway Traffic Safety Administration	• Data on crashes resulting in injury, death, or vehicle damage collected from police accident reports • Most states report if driver had been drinking alcohol in proximity to crash; information about passengers' alcohol use usually not included	• Variability in data collected by each state • Data not readily available to the public, as access to state data requires permissions from that specific state
	Crash Outcome Data Evaluation System	National Highway Traffic Safety Administration	• Autonomous system that creates probabilistic data linkages between crash report data, hospital data, and EMS data • Some states also include data from death certificates, trauma registries, driver citations, and motor vehicle licensing	• Provides more comprehensive understanding of medical and financial consequences of a crash • Allows for more accurate analysis of injury diagnosis and crash severity • Cases of missing data, data that Crash Outcome Data Evaluation System cannot access, and instances in which data available fails to link

National Incident-Based Reporting System	Federal Bureau of Investigation	• Information on crime incidents (including DWIs) and location, time of day, victim, known offenders, arrestees, relationships between those involved, property involved in the crime	• Only about one-third of U.S. law enforcement agencies particpate
Uniform Crime Reporting	Federal Bureau of Investigation	• Collects statistics on violent crime (murder and nonnegligent manslaughter, rape, robbery, and aggravated assault) and property crime (burglary, larceny, theft, and motor vehicle theft)	• Provides less qualitative detail than the National Incident-Based Reporting System

continued

TABLE 6-2 Continued

Conceptual Framework Phase	Data Source	Conducted/Managed by	Data Collection Method and Data Collected	Important Characteristics (Strengths, Weaknesses, Biases, and Limitations)
Serious Injuries and Fatalities	Fatality Analysis Reporting System	National Highway Traffic Safety Administration	• Characteristics of fatal crashes (e.g., location, alcohol involvement, roadway and atmospheric conditions), vehicles, and people involved by collecting data from police accident reports, state vehicle registration files, state driver licensing files, state highway department data, vital records department data, death certificates, coroner/medical examiner reports, and EMS reports • Data from breath, blood, and urine BAC tests as well as police behavioral assessments • Information on whether a drug was present in a driver's system	• Information from breath, blood, and urine BAC tests often missing since these tests not always done; therefore, BAC data are imputed • Near complete census of fatal crashes • Well-documented methodology • Only includes information on crashes resulting in at least one fatality within 30 days of a crash • Collects race and ethnicity information from death certificates, so such data only known for those fatally injured • Does not differentiate whether person was impaired by a drug at time of crash

Web-based Injury Statistics Query and Reporting System	Centers for Disease Control and Prevention	• Electronic database providing statistics on all fatal and nonfatal injuries (not limited to those resulting from traffic incidents) • Data on fatal injuries taken from ICD-10 codes on death certificates • Non-fatal injury data obtained through National Electronic Injury Surveillance System (emergency department data)	• Underreporting of alcohol involvement in injuries and deaths from various causes, including traffic fatalities • Role of decedent routinely left blank on death certificate, so it may be impossible to determine if fatality was of driver or passenger • Large confidence intervals for nonfatal injury data (unreliable source for tracking short-term trends)
National Trauma Data Bank	American College of Surgeons	• Trauma registry data submitted by hospitals throughout the country and include injury event information, detailed diagnoses, and information on hospital stay and outcomes	• Does not provide national statistical sample • Not all hospitals contribute data • Focused on trauma, so includes detailed information on injury severity and injury treatment

continued

TABLE 6-2 Continued

Conceptual Framework Phase	Data Source	Conducted/Managed by	Data Collection Method and Data Collected	Important Characteristics (Strengths, Weaknesses, Biases, and Limitations)
	Nationwide Emergency Department Sample	Agency for Healthcare Research and Quality's Healthcare Cost and Utilization Project	• Largest U.S. database on all-payer emergency department visits at the national level that includes detailed information on visits related to injury from alcohol misuse and alcohol-impaired driving	• Collects data for more than 100 variables, including patient demographic and payment information
Denominator Data	National Household Travel Survey	Federal Highway Administration	• Transportation habits including purpose of trips, how long trips take, when trips take place, means of transportation; if in a private vehicle, number of vehicle occupants, driver's characteristics, and vehicle's attributes	• Low response rates • Difficulty reaching demographic subgroups • Race and ethnicity of survey respondent applied to rest of his or her household
	Highway Vehicle Miles Travel	Federal Highway Administration	• Statistics on motor fuel, motor vehicle registration, driver licenses, highway miles traveled, highway user taxation, and highway finance	• Based on vehicle counts, therefore demographics of miles traveled unavailable • Only collected on 4,000 automatic traffic recorders nationwide • Limited data available on local traffic

factors in addition to the specific charge, including legal defense strategies, courtroom advocates, local standards, and biases. One of the difficulties across the data collection spectrum is the time and financial burden of data collection and submission. Incentives can be used to increase the reliability of and routine approach to data collection. Another limitation is that for all but serious injuries, law enforcement reporting of contributing factors (such as alcohol) is often poorly documented (DiMaggio et al., 2018). Apparent alcohol involvement does not necessarily involve the results of testing for alcohol or obtaining a BAC result and may be based on the judgment of the officer at the scene, which is a subjective rather than objective assessment. Data collected on injury severity may suffer from similar limitations, as injury severity in many cases is a subjective measure with broad categories of severity and differs from anatomic and physiological measures of severity. For crash report documentation, injury severity may be limited to KSI or killed, severe injury, minor injury, no injury (KABCO).

An additional gap is data on the involvement of alcohol in motor vehicle crashes resulting in hospital admissions, as BAC testing is not always performed for fatally injured drivers and infrequently performed for hospitalized persons. The NTDB contains information on alcohol involvement but lacks data from many hospitals with low rates of BAC testing, particularly as state laws vary on whether law enforcement has access to the results of BAC tests that are obtained for clinical purposes (Meisel, 2006). In addition, drawing a patient's blood without a medical reason to do so may be interpreted as a violation of the Hippocratic oath and presents a bioethical dilemma for physicians (Meisel, 2006). This may be an issue with respect to expecting practitioners to obtain a BAC result purely for legal reasons, although in some EDs, there are existing policies that allow practitioners to obtain a serum BAC from noninjured drivers suspected of DWI for legal evidence with the consent of the person from whom the BAC is being drawn (once drawn, the serum is placed in an evidence container and given to law enforcement to submit to a laboratory for testing). However, there are clinical reasons why BAC testing may be helpful, including the potential effect of alcohol consumption on treatment as well as the potential for alcohol withdrawal that may occur during hospitalization of a person who is alcohol dependent. The BAC itself may provide some indication of alcohol dependence, as tolerance to higher BACs may be a sign of chronic alcohol use and tolerance (Lapham, 2010). In addition, knowledge of a patient's BAC at the time of a crash or shortly thereafter can provide an indication of the need for intervention or treatment for alcohol use disorders. Although there are several clinical reasons for BAC testing, evidence that mandatory BAC testing in hospitals decreases reported rates of alcohol-impaired driving does not currently exist (Meisel, 2006). However, uniform BAC testing in hospitals could provide stronger evidence for law enforcement officials to pursue legal sanctions and/or prosecution more swiftly and is an increasingly important data need as greater numbers of drivers survive serious crashes due to improved motor vehicle safety features.

While alternative transportation options are growing across the country, data on the options, their availability, and the challenges in implementing and maintaining these options are not readily available. This is particularly true in rural areas, which may have more limited access to transportation options, including public transportation, than urban and suburban areas.

There are numerous data gaps related to the alcohol industry and policy. While proprietary data may exist on consumption patterns and sales of alcohol in both on-premise and off-premise environments, public access to these data is limited. Data on marketing and marketing policy are not readily available and could affect regulatory approaches to marketing and advertising. The APIS has detailed data on some major policies at the state and federal level based on information provided by NHTSA, but it lacks data on other policies that may be influential in decreasing alcohol-impaired driving, including data on administrative license revocation (detailed data for each state are not available), sobriety checkpoints, saturation patrols, and ignition interlock devices. In addition, the APIS does not provide data on laws that might affect alcohol-impaired driving or be affected by it, such as laws on speeding, occupant restraints, distracted driving, and impairment due to drugs other than cannabis. On the policy level, data on innovative policies that are in place in some states to increase the availability of evidence of DWI, such as allowing the use of hospital-obtained BAC levels that are part of routine ED/trauma care, are not readily available. Other policy information such as medical examiner/coroner standards for testing for BAC in a person who dies as a result of a traffic crash, even if an autopsy is not performed, is limited. More information on the impact and effectiveness of reporting of at-risk drivers to the DMV is needed, as is detailed information about the effectiveness of various methods of reviewing the reports and acting on them.

There are examples of data collection methods and datasets that might be helpful in designing optimal data collection methods (CDC, n.d.-b). The National Violent Death Reporting System (NVDRS), which exists in the majority of states, may have some lessons to be learned about standardized data collection, as well as data linkages, as the lack of standardized and coordinated data jeopardizes public health activities in addition to law enforcement and policy development. One of the potential difficulties with NVDRS is that the same data elements may be entered from multiple sources (Crosby et al., 2016) and may differ among the sources. A system has been set up within NVDRS to select the most authoritative source for specific data elements. While NVDRS has some potential issues with data quality, timeliness, and consistency, it does provide a comprehensive picture of violent deaths. However, there is difficulty in agreement on data definitions, legal access to data, data system gaps, and data quality concerns. The accuracy and completeness of NVDRS data depend on coding, completeness, and accuracy in the data systems that contribute to it. One issue is the number of deaths for which an intent is listed as "undetermined;" this means that it is not possible to determine whether these deaths are due to suicide or some other factor (Breiding and Wiersema, 2006; Rockett et al., 2014). Much like the FARS, NVDRS has a bias in that it only focuses on fatalities and does not provide a comprehensive picture of violence, just as the FARS does not provide a comprehensive picture of motor vehicle crash-related injuries and vehicular damage.

There are a number of issues with documenting the presence of alcohol in crash injuries or fatalities. When BAC and/or field sobriety testing are not performed, the assessment of whether alcohol was a factor in a crash is far less reliable, as studies have shown. Use of law enforcement estimates of severity are less specific than identifying the actual severity of injury using diagnoses made in a health care setting. Limiting attribution of a death that occurs later than 30 days after a crash may result in an underestimate of the number of fatalities caused by alcohol-impaired driving crashes. While a late death may be affected by other factors, a review of late deaths would be critical to determining this.

PUBLIC HEALTH AND HOSPITAL DATASETS

While public health datasets may not contain all of the traffic information that is present in a dataset focused on transportation, they often include information on the use of occupant restraints, motorcycle or bicycle helmets, and sometimes the circumstances of a crash. In hospital and ED datasets, coding is performed based on documentation in the medical record about the event that led to injury. This may also include the type of crash (head-on, rear-end, side impact, pedestrian struck by a car, bus, or other vehicle). In addition, clinical datasets that are used by public health researchers have more sensitive measures of injury severity, such as the Injury Severity Score, primarily on a continuous numeric scale using a standardized scoring system that accounts for injuries to various organ systems.

Data on BAC alone may be helpful in estimating degree of alcohol consumption by persons who have been injured or killed in a traffic-related event. BAC information that is obtained as part of routine trauma care in an ED may be used as the basis for providing an intervention to decrease the risk of future events in a person who exhibits at-risk drinking. In other words, the knowledge of how frequently an opportunity to intervene in order to prevent future alcohol-impaired driving events exists in the ED, or in a hospital ward, and can aid in decreasing future events. In health care settings, practitioners can use the window of opportunity provided by detecting an elevated BAC to address problematic alcohol consumption and its potential consequences (see Chapter 5 for more information). BAC information that may be available in a hospital setting may also affect the care that is provided as well as survival of the person who is injured.

Information obtained from various datasets that have different data points can aid researchers and evaluators in identifying unique risk factors that are associated with the consequences of alcohol impairment. A dataset that focuses on reported alcohol consumption across various age groups in a population provides the patterns of alcohol use that are most common in various age groups. For example, it could be found that young adults are more likely to have a higher rate of binge drinking than older adults, or that college students are more likely to engage in the practice of "pre-gaming" (consuming alcohol prior to going out to a party or social event). The data may also provide researchers with information about where alcohol is obtained, as well as what type of alcohol is consumed by various age, sex, and racial and ethnic groups. These data can then be used to identify and evaluate interventions targeted at the provision of alcohol to youth under the minimum legal drinking age or to promoting sales of excessive numbers of drinks in on-premise settings. Combining various datasets can give a comprehensive picture of risks for, and associated with, alcohol consumption and subsequent alcohol-impaired driving. Researchers may find that there are differing risks for older adults due to the combination of alcohol with medications for chronic conditions, that there are differences in consumption patterns in different communities, and/or that states differ in the proportions of various groups reporting driving after drinking. When combined with data on DWI arrests and prosecutions, these data can provide a more comprehensive picture of how enforcement affects drinking practices or the use of alternative transportation. Leveraging and, when possible, combining available datasets with awareness of their strengths and limitations enables researchers to obtain a more comprehensive understanding of alcohol-impaired driving and determine more effective intervention and prevention strategies.

OPPORTUNITIES FOR DATA COLLECTION AND SURVEILLANCE

Applying an Epidemiological Investigation Approach

There are strategies and insights that could be extracted from epidemiological approaches and translated to efforts to prevent alcohol-impaired driving fatalities by identifying high-impact targets (e.g., bars that overserve patrons or specific locations where a high proportion of crashes occur). These kinds of investigative approaches have been highly effective for public health agencies that are facing an infectious disease outbreak or that want to identify populations at high risk of specific diseases or conditions. Epidemic-assistance investigations (Epi-Aids) conducted by CDC are one example of public health data-driven approaches that have provided rapid and pertinent information to guide targeted interventions for over 70 years (Brachman and Thacker, 2011). The Crash Injury Research and Engineering Network (CIREN) project provides multisector data that can be used to research alcohol-related crashes and fatalities (NHTSA, n.d.-a).[10] The CIREN process combines prospective data collection with professional multidisciplinary analysis of medical and engineering evidence to determine injury causation in every crash investigation conducted. Analyses might involve multiple agencies, and might use an approach similar to the CIREN strategy.

The Epi-Aid strategy is often used when there are a number of illnesses or deaths occurring in a particular state or region and the investigative team is sent out to explore the incidents and gather data, then document findings. It is labor intensive, and there are limitations on the number of teams potentially available at any given time and costs incurred to send them to a location. Ideally public health, law enforcement, health care, traffic safety engineers, and researchers would all be involved in such an approach for studying alcohol-impaired driving. Departments of transportation also need to be engaged in funding an organization to serve as a repository for the reports.

One related strategy that is already being implemented among certain law enforcement agencies is source investigations following an alcohol-related crash. Source investigations use criminal and administrative techniques to determine where alcohol was purchased and/or consumed (Ramirez, 2017). These investigations have been identified as promising strategies for holding irresponsible licensed entities and sellers accountable for selling to intoxicated or underage persons (Curtis and Ramirez,

---

[10] CIREN was established as a result of a recommendation in the report *Injury in America: A Continuing Public Health Problem* that injury should be studied with a multidisciplinary approach involving experts from engineering, medicine, and other relevant fields (NHTSA, n.d.-a; NRC and IOM, 1985).

2011). The information could also be used to better target education efforts on overserving. However, the investigations can be very resource intensive. Curtis and Ramirez (2011) offer recommendations to improve source investigations through interagency collaboration, training for enforcement officials, and media coverage of the investigations. To enhance the implementation of source investigations, the National Liquor Law Enforcement Association created a toolkit as an online resource for local enforcement agencies.[11]

Another approach that could effectively identify areas in need of intervention is the spatial mapping of motor vehicle crashes. This allows for the visual identification of high-impact locations, trends (e.g., times, days, traffic flow), and outliers. For example, Schneider et al. (2017) conducted a spatiotemporal analysis of alcohol-related crashes in Cuyahoga County, Ohio, which enabled the authors to identify the movement of hotspots through the time of day and day of the week. This kind of data would be valuable to a local law enforcement agency as it could, for example, help identify optimal times and locations for deploying resources for publicized sobriety checkpoints. Researchers have already begun to use spatial analyses to assess the relationships between alcohol-related crashes and specific environmental factors, such as retail alcohol density (see Li et al., 2013, and Morrison et al., 2016), but more small-area analyses are needed. Finally, this tactic would align well with the NHTSA's Data-Driven Approaches to Crime and Traffic Safety framework (NHTSA, n.d.-b). The following section on big data opportunities expands this discussion to include the role of geographic information systems in tracking motor vehicle crashes.

Big Data Opportunities

Modern technological advances have enabled passive collection of enormous quantities of "big data" and created an increasingly data-driven society. Big data, as described by IBM, is characterized by four attributes: volume (increasingly large quantities of data), velocity (increasingly more capabilities to generate data), variety (increasingly diverse sources of data), and veracity (increasingly greater chances of inaccurate and/or poor quality data) (IBM, n.d.-a). Big data collection has had significant implications for the health and transportation sectors, and data collected on drinking and driving are important for determining effective interventions and strategies to reduce alcohol-related driving fatalities. As noted earlier, data related to drinking and driving have the potential to inform

[11] For more information, see http://www.nllea.org/SIT/sit.asp (accessed September 6, 2017).

place-based interventions, improve enforcement efforts, and guide more efficient allocation of resources. The following section describes sources, uses, and limitations of big data and ways in which various public- and private-sector stakeholders have leveraged big data to improve traffic safety. Barriers and challenges to using big data, such as difficulty merging different sources, privacy concerns, and lack of state-level resources for data dissemination, are important considerations as potential sources and uses of big data continue to grow.

Big Data from Smartphone Apps

New generations of smartphones are equipped with increasingly sophisticated sensors that have the ability to passively collect data relevant to alcohol-impaired driving. Mobile phone apps have been developed to estimate an individual's alcohol consumption level by their gait; these apps also record geographical location and time to help identify patterns of unsafe drinking (Arnold et al., 2015; Kao et al., 2012).

Smartphone sensors can also be used to detect unsafe driving behavior, including unsafe behavior specifically related to alcohol impairment. Uber, for example, has begun using GPS and gyroscopes on both driver and passenger smartphones to identify and track unsafe drivers (Brian, 2016). Mobile apps have been developed to detect alcohol-impaired driving behavior through data collected from built-in sensors that are compared with data collected from alcohol-impaired driving tests (Dai et al., 2010). More recently, researchers in China developed and tested a smartphone autocalibration algorithm that uses a smartphone's accelerometer, gyroscope, GPS, and microphone to collect and process data related to unsafe driving behavior (Ma et al., 2017). Known as DrivingSense, the algorithm is designed to specifically identify speeding, unusual changes in direction, and abnormal control of speed. If unsafe driving behavior is detected, the tool can alert the driver to potentially decrease the risk of crash. Published results indicate that the algorithm detects unusual changes in direction and abnormal control of speed with about 94 percent precision and 91 percent recall; the tool also estimated speed with less than 2 meters per second of error (Ma et al., 2017).

Big Data from the Private Sector

The beverage, health care, and insurance industries routinely collect massive quantities of data related to alcohol-impaired driving. Such data may have the potential to be immensely useful for identifying patterns of beverage service and alcohol consumption and pinpointing locations at which these behaviors take place. The alcohol industry would have consumption data, including data, for example, on how frequently laws that allow restaurant patrons to have an unfinished bottle of wine resealed for them to take home are used, and whether these laws have resulted in increased sales. It is likely that the alcohol industry would also have data on the time of day and day of the week for both on-premise and off-premise sales.

Auto insurance companies have collected vast amounts of data related to their customers' driving behavior. Progressive Corporation began offering devices that track driving behavior in 1998, becoming the first auto insurance company to offer telematics devices (for more information on telematics, see the Telematics and Usage-Based Insurance section in this chapter) (Rainie and Duggan, 2016; Threewitt, 2016). Since 2008 the company has used an optional tracking device known as Snapshot (used to track driving behavior to more accurately assess risk and price premiums) to collect 10 billion miles of time, speed, and GPS data (Gagliordi, 2014).

Sources and Opportunities for Big Data Linkages

The Crash Injury Research and Engineering Network As mentioned earlier in this chapter, CIREN, which began in 1996, is a research program that links level I trauma centers through a computer network, enabling each center to add discrete crash and medical data on motor vehicle crashes to a single database (NHTSA, n.d.-a). CIREN's data collection process includes initial detection of environmental, technical, or human factors related to injury causation; routine collection of more than 1,000 data points on each crash; and detailed information on occupant injury, vehicle damage, restraint technology, and crash environment. Each case is reviewed by a team of medical and engineering professionals (such as trauma surgeons, emergency physicians, mechanical engineers trained in biomechanics, epidemiologists, and nurses), as well as a crash investigator.

Crash Outcome Data Evaluation System As discussed earlier in the chapter, CODES is a state-based program that links motor vehicle crash report data and hospital record data using probabilistic linkage methodology designed to combine information from different databases into a single dataset for analysis (Kindelberger and Milani, 2015). Initially, CODES consisted of cooperative agreements between NHTSA and participating states that allowed NHTSA to provide technical assistance and funding. After NHTSA transitioned the program to the state level in 2013, many states ceased to continue the program (Kindelberger and Milani, 2015; Milani et al., 2015).

While neither CIREN nor CODES were specifically designed to study alcohol-impaired driving, both programs can add to the information on the effects of alcohol-impaired driving. For example, injury data are helpful in understanding how many people are seriously injured by an impaired driver. CIREN in particular may not be intended for the study of alcohol-impaired driving, but nonetheless provides valuable information about vehicles and crash circumstances that can help to understand vehicular protective factors that help prevent injuries and fatalities when a driver is alcohol impaired.

Predictive Crash Analytics

Many new approaches and software to leverage big data (e.g., machine learning) are emerging. In the past few years several states have begun initiatives to leverage big data to predict high-risk crash areas and more effectively and efficiently allocate resources to improve traffic safety. Recently, the Tennessee Highway Patrol partnered with IBM to create predictive crash software that the agency began using in late 2013 (Bergal, 2017; IBM, 2015). In 2016, Indiana's state police agency and Management Performance Hub (a state office tasked with improving government operations via enterprise-wide data sharing and transparency efforts) developed an interactive daily crash prediction map that is not only used by law enforcement but is also accessible to the public (Carmen, 2016).[12] Boxes 6-1 and 6-2 provide more information on the funding, implementation, and available outcomes of these two states' efforts.

The initial success of Tennessee and Indiana's efforts has prompted other states to invest in predictive crash analytics initiatives as well. The Missouri State Highway Patrol received a 3-year $148,000 federal grant to collect data, purchase software, and run computer model testing (Bergal, 2017). The agency plans for the tool to be implemented in early 2018. The Wisconsin State Patrol and University of Wisconsin are collecting the time, day, and location of crashes in Wisconsin and factors that contributed to the crashes to develop a program that will assist in dispatching law enforcement personnel to areas where crashes with fatalities or serious injuries have occurred (Bergal, 2017). The program is expected to launch in late 2017.

Some cities are also using predictive crash analytics to improve traffic and road safety. DataKind and Microsoft began a partnership in 2015 to support Vision Zero efforts in New York (expanding to New Orleans, San Jose, and Seattle in 2016) by using public and private data to better understand the most effective engineering and enforcement interventions to improve traffic safety and inform local policy making (DataKind,

---

[12] See https://in.gov/isp/ispCrashApp/main.html (accessed July 17, 2017). See also Box 6-2 and Figure 6-1.

BOX 6-1
Using Predictive Crash Analytics in Tennessee

Using state crash reports, weather conditions, information about special events, and traffic enforcement citations, the Tennessee Highway Patrol's predictive analytics software maps the risk of a serious crash or fatality taking place every 4 hours within 6 × 7 mile areas. Maps generated by the software are used to create monthly enforcement plans, which include locations for seat belt and sobriety checkpoints. They can be checked inside vehicles so troopers can prioritize which areas to patrol. Initial funding from federal grants was $263,000 through what was then called the Governor's Highway Safety Office (Bergal, 2017); staffing and maintenance cost about $125,000 per year.

From 2013 to 2015 traffic fatalities in Tennessee decreased by 3 percent from 995 to 962; in the same time period traffic fatalities increased by 7 percent nationally (Bergal, 2017). In the first year of the initiative, traffic fatalities in the state fell to their second lowest level since 1963 (IBM, 2015). Other outcomes include an 8.9 percent reduction in alcohol-related crashes (IBM, n.d.-b) and a 34 percent increase in DWI arrests (IBM, 2015). Additionally, from 2012 to 2016 average crash response time decreased by almost 33 percent from 37 to 25 minutes (Bergal, 2017).

In 2016 traffic fatalities in Tennessee increased by 8 percent to 1,042, a similar increase to the national rate over the same time period, and it is unclear whether the predictive model's shortcomings were related to increased road traffic or other factors (Bergal, 2017). The program's crash probability predictions have an accuracy rate of 72 percent, and accuracy is expected to improve as the system continues to evolve (Buckley, 2017; Freeze, n.d.).

2016). Each municipality began by sharing a traffic safety challenge specific to their city, around which city-specific data were used to build and train machine learning models to assess effects of and potential sites for local interventions (Grossman, 2017). Figure 6-2 shows locations of street improvement projects in New York and subsequent changes in crashes. Researchers have built models using open data and internal data (used by government departments) that have enabled estimates of the citywide number of motor vehicles on individual streets, which street and signal designs at intersections contribute to bicycle and pedestrian collisions and their severity (i.e., high-risk areas between intersections), and so on (Shueh, 2017).

Predictive analytics may also be an important data source. Milliman, an actuarial and consulting firm, used crash descriptions from NHTSA data on 7,000 automobile crashes to collect narrative data on the involvement of medications, prescriptions, drugs, and illegal narcotics in automobile crashes (Borba, 2013). Narrative descriptions were broken into

BOX 6-2
Using Predictive Crash Analytics in Indiana

Using daily historical crash data from the Indiana Department of Transportation, historical weather trends, and census data, software rates and maps crash risk by using color-coding to indicate crash probability within 1-square-kilometer areas. A portion of the map, with 1-square-kilometer areas color-coded by probable crash risk, is depicted in Figure 6-1. The map displays crash risk within the current 3-hour time window, and users can also select an alternate time period for that day. The map also includes locations of past crashes that were fatal or where EMS responded (red dots) and past traffic crashes that resulted in property damage (grey dots). The primary factor that led to each crash, such as failure to yield or distracted driving, is also included. This kind of analysis could be applied to alcohol-impaired driving.

Law enforcement officers can refer to the map to locate areas with increased crash likelihood and strategically dispatch officers to these locations. The map is also available to the public to use as an "accident forecast," similar to using weather forecasts to prepare for and plan around potentially hazardous weather conditions. Data from the Indiana Department of Transportation suggest that a 1 percent reduction in all crashes in the state could generate $35 million in annual savings (Carmen, 2016).

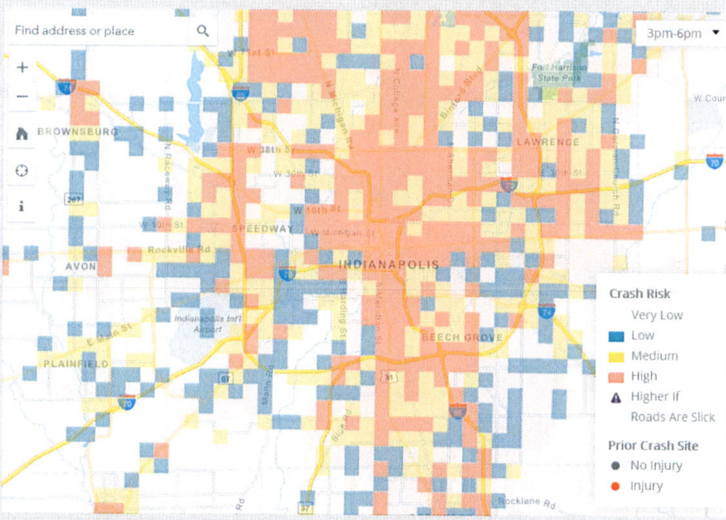

FIGURE 6-1 Indiana daily crash prediction map.
SOURCE: Indiana State Police and Indiana Management Performance Hub, 2017.

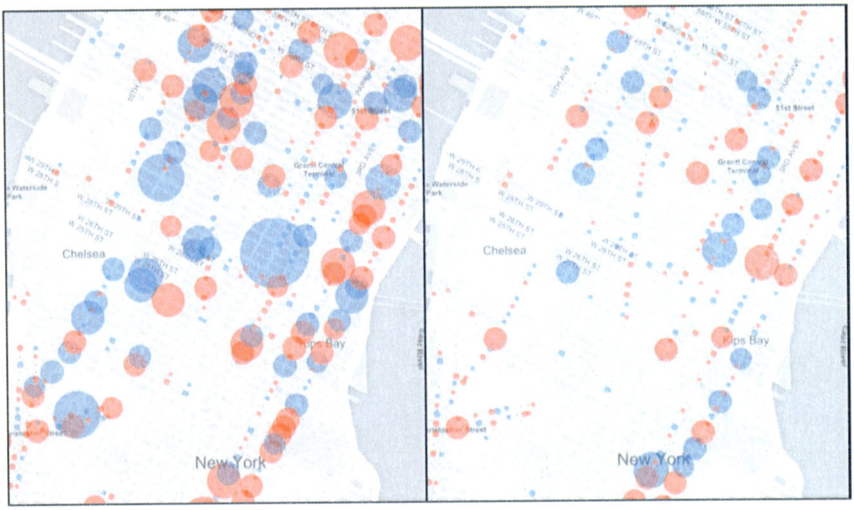

FIGURE 6-2 Locations of street improvement projects in New York and changes in crashes.
SOURCE: DataKind, 2017.

phrases, with more than 13 million unique phrases generated. A statistically significant relationship was found between drug-impaired driving descriptions and crash severity (i.e., whether an injury occurred), indicating that narrative data obtained from crash descriptions, claim adjuster notes, and so on can be beneficial for increasing the accuracy of risk calculation (Borba, 2013).

Government, nonprofit, and private-sector (e.g., IBM and Microsoft) collaboration has enabled state and municipal agencies to leverage various public and private data sources to locate traffic crash hotspots and implement proven and promising safety interventions in these areas with consideration of local circumstances.

Telematics and Usage-Based Insurance

Usage-based insurance involves real-time monitoring of driver behavior (vehicle miles driven, time of day, location of driving activity, speed and acceleration, and braking) to assess and price auto insurance premiums (National Association of Insurance Commissioners, 2017). Driver behavior, including behaviors related to alcohol-impaired driving, can be monitored through GPS sensors, odometers, and in-vehicle telecommunication devices (telematics) that can be self-installed or installed by car manufacturers, subscription-based car connectivity services, and mobile apps (Marquand, 2016; National Association of Insurance Commissioners, 2017). In addition, many cars have internal real-time communication devices that relate crash information, including vehicle condition and crash location, to call centers (e.g., GM's OnStar) and/or that transmit warnings for lane deviation, excessive braking, and other driving-related behaviors (e.g., Toyota's Safety Sense), many of which may indicate and can be used to detect alcohol impairment on the part of the driver (OnStar, n.d.; Toyota, n.d.).

Soleymanian et al. (2016) examined the effect of usage-based insurance on changing customers' driving behavior and found improvements in driving behavior after adoption of usage-based insurance. Daily average frequency of hard braking decreased 21 percent after adopting usage-based insurance for 6 months; however, no significant effect on mileage driven was found. Relative to older drivers, younger drivers adopted usage-based insurance at higher rates and improved their driving scores more quickly. Significant differences were recorded in individual driving scores, suggesting that auto insurance companies can benefit with more accurate risk assessment calculated from usage-based insurance. Soleymanian et al. (2016) concluded that usage-based insurance can be beneficial for both drivers and insurance companies.

Using GIS to Study Motor Vehicle Crashes

Evidence suggests that GIS can be an effective tool for collecting geolocation data to analyze motor vehicle crashes. GIS data can be used to identify and examine a range of factors that contribute to alcohol-impaired driving fatalities, including spatial relationships between motor vehicle crashes and alcohol outlets as well as areas with high risk for crashes owing to poor roadway design and adverse weather conditions.

Stevenson et al. (1998) analyzed whether alcohol-related crashes occur more frequently and/or cluster near on-premises drinking establishments. GIS was used to determine distances between crash locations and on-premises drinking establishments. The authors did not find a statistically significant correlation but concluded that "GIS technology can be useful for assessing potential environmental risk factors for alcohol-related motor vehicle crashes, such as retail alcohol outlets, and for planning public health interventions that promote traffic safety" (Stevenson et al., 1998, p. 197). Similarly, Meliker et al. (2004) conducted a cross-sectional study to examine geographic patterns between alcohol-impaired driving crashes and retail alcohol outlet locations. Using spatial analysis, distance analysis (using ArcGIS), and other statistical methods to analyze BAC levels, traffic and roadway information, census data, and distribution of retail alcohol outlets, the authors found that areas with low population density had more alcohol-impaired driving crashes; no significant relationship between retail alcohol outlets and alcohol-impaired driving crashes was found (Meliker et al., 2004).

Li et al. (2007) analyzed motor vehicle crashes in Harris County (primarily Houston), Texas, to identify roadway segments with potentially high crash risk. Using a GIS-based mapping approach, the authors identified spatial-temporal patterns of relative crash risks and used these data to rank risky roadway segments. Similarly, Saha et al. (2016) analyzed spatial relationships between driving fatalities by state and adverse weather conditions. ArcGIS was used to create state-level maps for total fatality rates by state and fatality rates by vehicle miles traveled related to adverse weather conditions.

Data Integration

The opportunities for short- and long-term data integration continue to increase as new technologies emerge and information systems become more powerful and accessible. There are opportunities for exploring the options of connecting and linking existing data systems to obtain a more complete picture of alcohol-related crashes, as projects such as the CODES project have demonstrated.

A current injury-related project that is linking health care, law enforcement, and medical examiner/coroner data is the NVDRS, which is overseen by CDC (CDC, n.d.-b). As with the CODES project, the NVDRS provides a more detailed picture of an event, and the factors possibly leading up to it, as well as circumstances surrounding the event (Crosby et al., 2016). NVDRS requires no additional data collection; all data are collected by other existing data systems. NVDRS can provide information on linked homicide/suicide, details about types of homicides and suicides, and information that might highlight risk factors for violent death. As data are obtained from medical examiner/coroner offices, there may be both primary and secondary data sources that contribute information to NVDRS. In addition, data are obtained from hospital records, as well as law enforcement. Because NVDRS is based on state-based data systems, each state's violent death reporting system may look different as states may decide to collect data in addition to the data that are submitted to NVDRS.

Data from technologies such as ignition interlock devices, smartphones, and vehicle telematics can contribute to an understanding of crash-related factors and can be combined with EMS, law enforcement, hospital, and medical examiner/coroner data to add to the information about a crash. Drivers' license data can be added to provide a perspective on prior DWI arrests. These various existing datasets could be used in conjunction with one another, even if not linked, to provide a more complete picture of alcohol-impaired driving and related fatalities.

With any data, there is a concern about confidentiality and protection of an individual's protected information. Aggregate data reporting can aid in addressing this, but individual data are clearly needed for enforcement and prosecution in an alcohol-impaired driving crash. Data that are used for public health purposes have protections and exemptions in place, but other data sources may not have these protections. However, research projects generally require review by an institutional review board to ensure compliance with privacy protections and access to identifiable data.

DATA TRANSPARENCY, ACCESS, AND STAKEHOLDERS

Data transparency and access are crucial in understanding the context and patterns of alcohol purchase and consumption, risks and factors associated with alcohol-impaired driving and its consequences, and the effect of policies in place to prevent alcohol-impaired driving crashes. Data are the building blocks of interventions that are effective and lasting.

There are challenges to data access, cost of data access, and transparency, but these barriers can be mitigated and overcome through thoughtful and collaborative initiatives to provide access to the data that are needed. One of the keys to developing these strategies is the identification of the desired outcomes of data collection and analysis. For some outcomes studied, data on individual cases may not be needed, while aggregate data can be helpful. For example, in looking at alternative transportation as a prevention method, aggregate data on the numbers and locations of alternative transportation options, combined with information on the trends in alcohol-impaired driving crashes in the areas where alternative transportation options are available as compared to areas with limited alternative transportation options, may provide valuable information on the effect of such transports on decreasing alcohol-impaired driving crashes. This is an example of combining information from multiple datasets that illustrates the potential for combining publicly available data with private or proprietary data in a way that allows for the use of summary data rather than detailed data that a private entity might be reluctant to release. A similar kind of strategy might examine the relationship between alcohol advertising and alcohol-impaired driving crashes in a specific locale, particularly after an event at which alcohol is heavily marketed and/or consumed. Monitoring of new product development and marketing and the effect on alcohol-related crashes is also needed so when such products as premixed alcoholic energy drinks come on the market, there is some early assessment of their effect on public safety and welfare. Such data collection could be done, for instance, in the ED if persons admitted for injury who had been drinking prior to that injury were asked what alcoholic beverage they drank prior to injury (Jernigan et al., 2013). Looking at the effect of the transport use on insurance companies may highlight a benefit to health insurance companies and auto insurance companies, which could also be studied using aggregate data.

There are multiple stakeholders for the data initiatives, even if the stakeholder groups are not necessarily aware of their stake in having accurate data. Consumers, who may not necessarily use the data or access it, can benefit from policies and practices that are based on data and decrease their risk of injury and death caused by alcohol-impaired driving. Health care systems benefit from decreased needs for treatment of critical and life-threatening injuries, as this care places financial, personnel, and facility/space burdens on a system. The beverage and hospitality industries can benefit from consumers remaining active and healthy and able to consume their products and services. Public health benefits from the contribution of decreased alcohol-impaired driving fatality deaths, which affect community and family health.

FUTURE DATA AND SURVEILLANCE NEEDS

Efforts toward surveillance of alcohol-impaired driving, crashes, fatalities, arrests, and outcomes are hampered by the lack of available, high-quality, consistent data across states and local jurisdictions. To accelerate progress toward the goal of achieving zero motor vehicle fatalities, strong data collection and analysis of transportation safety and hospital data are critically important (Shahum and Vanderkooy, 2017). Current data collection and surveillance systems need to be strengthened, and harmonization of existing sources and definitions are needed to perform more targeted analyses of the data and to get interpretation to those who can take action, such as law enforcement, policy makers, auto makers, and public health agencies. Ultimately this will result in a better use of resources and provide more targeted and effective solutions. Data from multiple sources (insurers, transportation sector, law enforcement, automobiles, payment systems, and so on) can be combined and used in real time for research. Public–private partnerships exist for data mining and analysis to identify high-risk areas and populations, and can be useful for alcohol-impaired driving research.

Having a comprehensive understanding of alcohol-impaired driving, both in regard to the rates of occurrence, traffic crashes, injuries, fatalities, arrests, and convictions, as well as qualitative data on when and why people drive impaired, is vital to creating specific and targeted interventions to reduce it. However, there are several barriers to gaining a comprehensive picture and identifying needs at the federal, state, and local levels. There are data gaps (such as lack of data on place of last drink), methodological issues (such as inconsistent data collection), and a lack of integration of datasets (e.g., how many people are arrested, outcomes of arrest, and long-term outcomes in terms of recidivism). Therefore, the committee concludes:

Conclusion 6-1: Data collection and reporting of high-risk intersections, outlets, drinking behaviors before driving, risk factors, and demographic trends are needed to measure, evaluate, and accelerate progress in reducing risk of fatalities. This evaluation would be facilitated by regular, systematic data collection on geocoded crash locations linked to data systems that monitor injury and fatality information, as well as criminal justice outcomes.

While data quality, timeliness, completeness, and data element definitions and coding can be challenging with respect to the development and maintenance of datasets that provide information on alcohol-impaired driving, advances in technology and means of accessing data can aid in improving datasets so that they are more readily accessible and useful. There is a range of stakeholders who are interested in the data for various uses, including tracking changes in crash rates, injury rates and fatality rates, and identifying risks for crashing. Data are also used to inform the development of new interventions and policies and need to be accessible and usable for evaluating the impact of interventions of various types. While data may come from multiple sources, methods of data linkages have been tested in other datasets and the success of the linkages has been demonstrated. Strategies that involve migrating and transforming variables have been used in large datasets. Standardizing data definitions so that the data can be used to answer the questions posed by stakeholders may involve bringing together stakeholders, agencies, and organizations that collect the data to develop consensus on critical variables. This is not to say that all variables in every dataset will need to be brought into a larger dataset, as various agencies may have needs for specific variables that other agencies do not. Critical issues include timeliness as well as some degree of uniformity in the reporting of variables. The committee recommends:

Recommendation 6-1: The National Highway Traffic Safety Administration should ensure that timely standardized data on alcohol-impaired driving, crashes, serious injuries, and fatalities are collected and accessible for evaluation, research, and strategic public dissemination; should ensure that data

from other government agencies and private organizations are included as needed; and should explore the usefulness of big data for inclusion in alcohol-impaired driving information strategies.

Reducing alcohol-impaired driving requires diligent and accurate collection of surveillance data. Examples of improvements necessary for advancing the science include

- Standardized data definitions across multiple sectors regarding assessment of crash occurrence, severity, and alcohol involvement;
- Harmonization of reported data regarding assessment of alcohol involvement, including use of imputation models for assessment of alcohol-related crashes;
- Universal assessment of drug involvement among fatally injured drivers across states; and
- Increased capacity and resources for data linkages (e.g., state data systems that feed into national databanks) for research purposes across multiple systems including EMS, hospital and other care facilities, law enforcement, and medical examiners/coroners.

While it can be difficult to develop a consensus on data definitions, reporting strategies, and dataset linkages, bringing stakeholders together to resolve the issues that exist due to a lack of data and/or difficulties with access to datasets is a method that has been used successfully in developing datasets that can be used by multiple stakeholders. CODES projects highlight the impact of combined datasets that provide information that multiple stakeholders use for their own, as well as combined, purposes. Another example of a dataset that has been developed and is used by a large group of stakeholders, who sometimes have different needs for the data, is the NTDB, which has been implemented in trauma centers across the United States and whose design and data definitions have formed the basis for discussion of trauma datasets on an international level. While it may seem as though the stakeholders who are engaged in the care and treatment of trauma patients lack diverse needs for data, the stakeholders include trauma surgeons, emergency physicians, hospital administrators, public health practitioners, epidemiologists, and emergency medical services (American College of Surgeons, n.d.).

Another example of a multistakeholder group that has successfully formulated action plans and strategies is the Interagency Coordinating Committee on the Prevention of Underage Drinking (ICCPUD), which was mandated by the Sober Truth on Preventing Underage Drinking (STOP) Act passed by Congress in 2006 (SAMHSA, 2017b). ICCPUD members are representatives from 15 federal agencies, with SAMHSA taking on the role of lead agency, tasked with coordinating federal efforts to address underage drinking issues. ICCPUD's formation carried out a recommendation from the 2004 National Research Council and Institute of Medicine report *Reducing Underage Drinking: A Collective Responsibility*, namely the establishment of "a federal interagency coordinating committee on prevention of underage drinking" (Dowdall, 2013; NRC and IOM, 2004). ICCPUD continues to be active in efforts to reduce and prevent underage drinking by producing mandated annual reports to Congress and generating other initiatives involving all member federal agencies (SAMHSA, 2017a,b). Efforts to reduce alcohol-impaired driving through improved surveillance and data have potential to benefit by following a similar model of streamlining federal efforts with a multistakeholder coordinating entity. The committee recommends:

> **Recommendation 6-2: To facilitate surveillance of alcohol-impaired driving that is timely, ongoing, concise, and actionable, the National Highway Traffic Safety Administration should convene a diverse group of stakeholders that includes academic researchers, law enforcement, city and state public health, transportation sector, and other federal agency representation to create and maintain a metrics dashboard, and publish brief, visually appealing quarterly and annual national and state-by-state reports that analyze and interpret progress in reducing alcohol-impaired driving.**

This recommendation entails identifying the data elements and data sources that are needed to monitor changes in rates of alcohol-impaired driving risk factors (including place of last drink), arrests, crashes, injuries, and fatalities, as well as data elements needed to inform quarterly metrics and reports designed for dissemination to the public, public and private stakeholders, and local, state, and national policy makers through various communication strategies. In addition, it involves ensuring that data for research on the effect of interventions to reduce alcohol-impaired driving are accessible and available using techniques that reflect contemporary standards for data acquisition and downloading. To be impactful and to raise awareness of the problem of alcohol-impaired driving, the data should be strategically released to inculcate action. The dashboard (a user-friendly interface) should contain analyzed data, including longitudinal data linking crash data with licensing data, hospital data that includes costs for care, arrest data, and the results of arrest.

REFERENCES

AAA (American Automobile Association) Foundation for Traffic Safety. 2016. *Prevalence of marijuana involvement in fatal crashes: Washington, 2010-2014*. Washington, DC: AAA Foundation for Traffic Safety.

American College of Surgeons. n.d. *National Trauma Data Bank*. https://www.facs.org/quality-programs/trauma/ntdb (accessed August 7, 2017).

APIS (Alcohol Policy Information System). n.d.-a. *About the Alcohol Policy Information System (APIS)*. https://alcoholpolicy.niaaa.nih.gov/About_APIS.html (accessed November 7, 2017).

APIS. n.d.-b. *Welcome to the Alcohol Policy Information System*. https://alcoholpolicy.niaaa.nih.gov (accessed October 10, 2017).

ARG (Alcohol Research Group). n.d. *National Alcohol Surveys*. http://arg.org/center/national-alcohol-surveys (accessed October 10, 2017).

Arnold, Z., D. Larose, and E. Agu. 2015. *Smartphone inference of alcohol consumption levels from gait*. Paper presented at 2015 International Conference on Healthcare Informatics, Dallas, TX.

Batts, K., M. Pemberton, J. Bose, B. Weimer, L. Henderson, M. Penne, J. Gfoerer, D. Trunzo, and A. Strashny. 2014. *Comparing and evaluating substance use treatment utilization estimates from the National Survey on Drug Use and Health and other data sources*. Rockville, MD: Center for Behavioral Health Statistics and Quality.

Bergal, J. 2017. *Troopers use "big data" to predict crash sites*. http://www.pewtrusts.org/en/research-and-analysis/blogs/stateline/2017/02/09/troopers-use-big-data-to-predict-crash-sites (accessed July 17, 2017).

Berning, A., and D. D. Smither. 2014. *Understanding the limitations of drug test information, reporting, and testing practices in fatal crashes*. Washington, DC: National Highway Traffic Safety Administration.

Berning, A., R. Compton, and K. Wochinger. 2015. *Results of the 2013-2014 National Roadside Survey of alcohol and drug use by drivers*. DOT HS 812 118. Washington, DC: National Highway Traffic Safety Administration.

Borba, P. S. 2013. *Predictive analytics, text mining, and drug-impaired driving in automobile accidents*. http://www.milliman.com/insight/pc/Predictive-analytics--text-mining--and-drug-impaired-driving-in-automobile-accidents/ (accessed August 1, 2017).

Brachman, P. S., and S. B. Thacker. 2011. Evolution of epidemic investigations and field epidemiology during the MMWR era at CDC—1961–2011. *Morbidity and Mortality Weekly Report* 60(4):22–26.

Breiding, M. J., and B. Wiersema. 2006. Variability of undetermined manner of death classification in the US. *Injury Prevention* 12(Suppl 2):ii49–ii54.

Brian, M. 2016. *Uber is using smartphone data to alert it to bad drivers*. https://www.engadget.com/2016/01/26/uber-gyroscopes-data-bad-driving-safety (accessed September 6, 2017).

Buckley, J. 2017. *Preventing car crashes with big data analytics*. https://datafloq.com/read/preventing-car-crashes-with-big-data-analytics/1117 (accessed July 17, 2017).

Carmen, M. 2016. *Indiana state police unveil daily crash prediction map*. http://statescoop.com/indiana-state-police-unveil-car-crash-forecast-map-to-help-reduce-traffic-accidents-in-indiana (accessed July 17, 2017).

Castle, I. J., H. Y. Yi, R. W. Hingson, and A. M. White. 2014. State variation in underreporting of alcohol involvement on death certificates: Motor vehicle traffic crash fatalities as an example. *Journal of Studies on Alcohol and Drugs* 75(2):299–312.

CDC (Centers for Disease Control and Prevention). 2016. *Behavioral Risk Factor Surveillance System: Comparability of data BRFSS 2015.* Version 1—Revised: June 2016. https://www.cdc.gov/brfss/annual_data/2015/pdf/compare_2015.pdf (accessed December 12, 2017).

CDC. 2017a. *Behavioral Risk Factor Surveillance System.* https://www.cdc.gov/brfss/index.html (accessed August 31, 2017).

CDC. 2017b. *Welcome to WISQARS.* https://www.cdc.gov/injury/wisqars/index.html (accessed September 1, 2017).

CDC. 2017c. *Youth Risk Behavior Surveillance System (YRBSS) overview.* https://www.cdc.gov/healthyyouth/data/yrbs/overview.htm (accessed August 31, 2017).

CDC. 2017d. *YRBSS participation maps and history.* https://www.cdc.gov/healthyyouth/data/yrbs/participation.htm (accessed October 4, 2017).

CDC. n.d.-a. *5.0 Data sources for WISQARS nonfatal.* https://www.cdc.gov/ncipc/wisqars/nonfatal/datasources.htm (accessed September 1, 2017).

CDC. n.d.-b. *National Violent Death Reporting System.* https://www.cdc.gov/injury/wisqars/nvdrs.html (accessed November 15, 2017).

Cook, L. J., A. Thomas, C. Olson, T. Funai, and T. Simmons. 2015. *Crash Outcome Data Evaluation System (CODES): An examination of methodologies and multi-state traffic safety applications.* DOT HS 812 179. Washington, DC: National Highway Traffic Safety Administration.

Crosby, A. E., J. A. Mercy, and D. Houry. 2016. The National Violent Death Reporting System: Past, present, and future. *American Journal of Preventive Medicine* 51(5 Suppl 3):S169–S172.

Curtis, S. C., and R. L. Ramirez. 2011. *Source investigations: A tool to combat impaired driving.* DOT HS 811 519. Washington, DC: National Highway Traffic Safety Administration.

Dai, J., J. Teng, X. Bai, Z. Shen, and D. Xuan. 2010. *Mobile phone based drunk driving detection.* Paper read at 2010 4th International Conference on Pervasive Computing Technologies for Healthcare, March 22–25, 2010.

DataKind. 2016. *Data science supporting Vision Zero in three new cities.* http://www.datakind.org/blog/data-science-supporting-vision-zero-in-three-new-cities (accessed August 3, 2017).

DataKind. 2017. *Creating safer streets through data science.* http://www.datakind.org/projects/creating-safer-streets-through-data-science (accessed August 4, 2017).

Dean, S., L. Litzky, B. Fuchs, and C. Cambor. 2012. Assessing the accuracy of death certificate completion by physicians using the "Death Module": An academic institution's experience with an electronic death registration program. *American Journal of Clinical Pathology* 138(Suppl 2):A130.

Degani, A. T., R. M. Patel, B. E. Smith, and E. Grimsley. 2009. The effect of student training on accuracy of completion of death certificates. *Medical Education Online* 14:17.

DiMaggio, C., K. Wheeler-Martin, and J. Oliver. 2018. *Alcohol-impaired driving in the United States: Overview, review of data sources and analyses.* Paper commissioned by the Committee on Accelerating Progress to Reduce Alcohol-Impaired Driving Fatalities (see Appendix A).

DOT (U.S. Department of Transportation). 2016. *VMT per capita.* https://www.transportation.gov/mission/health/vmt-capita (accessed September 1, 2017).

Dowdall, G. W. 2013. *College drinking: Reframing a social problem/changing the culture.* Sterling, VA: Stylus Pub.

FBI (Federal Bureau of Investigation). n.d.-a. *NIBRS overview.* https://ucr.fbi.gov/nibrs-overview (accessed August 31, 2017).

FBI. n.d.-b. *Uniform Crime Reporting.* https://ucr.fbi.gov/crime-in-the-u.s (accessed August 4, 2017).

FBI. n.d.-c. *Welcome to a new way to access UCR statistics.* https://www.ucrdatatool.gov (accessed October 5, 2017).

FHWA (Federal Highway Administration). 2015. *Expert panel review of the 2016 National Household Travel Survey—April 28, 2015.* Washington, DC: U.S. Department of Transportation.

FHWA. 2016. *Highway statistics series.* https://www.fhwa.dot.gov/policyinformation/statistics.cfm (accessed September 1, 2017).

FHWA. n.d.-a. *Introduction to the 2009 NHTS.* http://nhts.ornl.gov/introduction.shtml (accessed September 1, 2017).

FHWA. n.d.-b. *National Household Travel Survey.* http://nhts.ornl.gov (accessed September 1, 2017).

Freeze, B. n.d. *Traffic Incident Management Decision Support System Project.* https://www.pcb.its.dot.gov/t3/s170607/s170607_Traffic_Incident_Management_Whats_New_presentation_Freeze.ppt (accessed October 9, 2017).

Gagliordi, N. 2014. *How auto insurer Progressive collected 10 billion miles of driving data from its customers.* http://www.zdnet.com/article/how-auto-insurer-progressive-collected-10-billion-miles-of-driving-data-from-its-customers (accessed September 6, 2017).

Garrett, M. E. 2014. *Encyclopedia of transportation: Social science and policy.* Thousand Oaks, CA: SAGE Publications, Inc.

Grossman, E. L. 2017. *A street-level look at an innovative data-driven partnership.* https://blogs.microsoft.com/on-the-issues/2017/04/19/street-level-look-innovative-data-driven-partnership (accessed August 4, 2017).

HCUP (Healthcare Cost and Utilization Project). n.d. *Overview of the National Emergency Department Sample (NEDS).* https://www.hcup-us.ahrq.gov/nedsoverview.jsp#about (accessed October 10, 2017).

IBM (International Business Machines). 2015. *Tennessee Highway Patrol.* http://www-03.ibm.com/software/businesscasestudies/nz/en/corp?synkey=G711453G16461R35 (accessed July 14, 2017).

IBM. n.d.-a. *Ingographics & animations. The four v's of big data.* http://www.ibmbigdatahub.com/infographic/four-vs-big-data (accessed December 6, 2017).

IBM. n.d.-b. *Tennessee Highway Patrol.* https://www-01.ibm.com/common/ssi/cgi-bin/ssialias?subtype=ST&infotype=SA&htmlfid=GVJ03030USEN&attachment=GVJ03030USEN.PDF (accessed July 14, 2017).

Indiana State Police and Indiana Management Performance Hub. 2017. *Indiana crash risk map.* https://in.gov/isp/3268.htm (accessed Decemeber 11, 2017).

Jernigan, D. H., S. Cukier, C. Ross, S. R. Ahmed, and A. Stolbach. 2013. Alcohol brand use and injury in the emergency department: A pilot study. *Substance Use & Misuse* 49(1–2):59–65.

Kann, L., T. McManus, W. A. Harris, S. L. Shanklin, K. H. Flint, J. Hawkins, B. Queen, R. Lowry, E. O. M. Olsen, D. Chyen, L. Whittle, J. Thornton, C. Lim, Y. Yamakawa, N. Brener, and S. Zaza. 2016. Youth risk behavior surveillance—United States, 2015. *Morbidity and Mortality Weekly* 65(6):1–174.

Kao, H.-L., B.-J. Ho, A. C. Lin, and H.-H. Chu. 2012. *Phone-based gait analysis to detect alcohol usage.* Paper presented at 2012 ACM Conference on Ubiquitous Computing, Pittsburgh, PA.

Kelley-Baker, T. 2017. PowerPoint presentation to the Committee on Accelerating Progress to Reduce Alcohol-Impaired Driving Fatalities, Washington, DC, March 22, 2017. http://nationalacademies.org/hmd/~/media/Files/Activity%20Files/AcceleratingProgresstoReduceAlcoholImpairedDrivingFatalities/22%20March%202017/11%20Tara%20KelleyBaker.pdf (accessed September 7, 2017).

Kim, K., D. Harmon, M. Singleton, K. Finison, T. Kerns, M. Qu, G. Thaxton, T. Hettinger, S. Brynildsen, A. Lunde, R. Clarke, M. Allen, M. Pease, K. Dougherty, M. Dean, and W. Bigelow. 2001. *Problems, solutions and recommendations for implementing CODES (Crash Outcome Data Evaluation System)*. Washington, DC: National Highway Traffic Safety Administration.

Kindelberger, J., and J. A. Milani. 2015. *Crash Outcome Data Evaluation System (CODES): Program transition and promising practices*. Washington, DC: National Highway Traffic Safety Administration.

Lacey, J. H., T. Kelley-Baker, R. B. Voas, E. Romano, C. D. Furr-Holden, P. Torres, and A. Berning. 2011. Alcohol- and drug-involved driving in the United States: Methodology for the 2007 National Roadside Survey. *Evaluation Review* 35(4):319–353.

Lapham, S. C. 2010. The limits of tolerance: Convicted alcohol-impaired drivers share experiences driving under the influence. *The Permanente Journal* 14(2):26–30.

Li, L., L. Zhu, and D. Z. Sui. 2007. A GIS-based Bayesian approach for analyzing spatial-temporal patterns of intra-city motor vehicle crashes. *Journal of Transport Geography* 15(4):274–285.

Li, Y., N.-N. Sze, and S. Wong. 2013. Spatial–temporal analysis of drink-driving patterns in Hong Kong. *Accident Analysis & Prevention* 59:415–424.

Ma, C., X. Dai, J. Zhu, N. Liu, H. Sun, and M. Liu. 2017. DrivingSense: Dangerous driving behavior identification based on smartphone autocalibration. *Mobile Information Systems* 2017:1–15.

Marquand, B. 2016. *Comparing Drivewise, Snapshot and other usage-based insurance plans.* https://www.nerdwallet.com/blog/insurance/comparing-drivewise-snapshot-usage-based-insurance (accessed July 14, 2017).

Meisel, Z. 2006. *Spare the needle. Doctors shouldn't have to draw blood on behalf of cops.* http://www.slate.com/articles/health_and_science/medical_examiner/2006/09/spare_the_needle.html (accessed November 27, 2017).

Meliker, J. R., R. F. Maio, M. A. Zimmerman, H. M. Kim, S. C. Smith, and M. L. Wilson. 2004. Spatial analysis of alcohol-related motor vehicle crash injuries in southeastern Michigan. *Accident Analysis & Prevention* 36(6):1129–1135.

Milani, J., J. Kindelberger, G. Bergen, E. J. Novicki, C. Burch, S. M. Ho, and B. A. West. 2015. *Assessment of characteristics of state data linkage systems*. DOT HS 812 180. Washington, DC and Atlanta, GA: National Highway Traffic Safety Administration and Centers for Disease Control and Prevention.

Morrison, C., W. R. Ponicki, P. J. Gruenewald, D. J. Wiebe, and K. Smith. 2016. Spatial relationships between alcohol-related road crashes and retail alcohol availability. *Drug and Alcohol Dependence* 162:241–244.

Myers, K. A., and D. R. Farquhar. 1998. Improving the accuracy of death certification. *Canadian Medical Association Journal* 158(10):1317–1323.

Naeger, S. 2017. *Emergency department visits involving underage alcohol misuse: 2010 to 2013.* https://www.samhsa.gov/data/sites/default/files/report_3061/ShortReport-3061.html (accessed October 10, 2017).

NASEM (National Academies of Sciences, Engineering, and Medicine). 2015. *Naturalistic driving study: Alcohol sensor performance*. Washington, DC: The National Academies Press.

National Association of Insurance Commissioners. 2017. *Usage-based insurance and telematics.* http://www.naic.org/cipr_topics/topic_usage_based_insurance.htm (accessed July 31, 2017).

NCHS (National Center for Health Statistics). 2015. *Injury and poisoning questions on the National Health Interview survey: 1997–present.* https://www.cdc.gov/nchs/nhis/injury_poisoning/ip_questions_1997_present.htm (accessed December 6, 2017).

NCHS. 2017a. *Alcohol use.* https://www.cdc.gov/nchs/fastats/alcohol.htm (accessed December 6, 2017).

NCHS. 2017b. *Early release of selected estimates based on data from the 2016 National Health Interview Survey.* Washington, DC: National Center for Health Statistics.

NHTSA (National Highway Traffic Safety Administration). 2009. *Race and ethnicity: 2006 data. Traffic Safety Facts.* DOT HS 810 995. Washington, DC: National Highway Traffic Safety Administration.

NHTSA. 2014. *Fatality Analysis Reporting System.* Washington, DC: U.S. Department of Transportation.

NHTSA. n.d.-a. *Crash Injury Research (CIREN).* https://one.nhtsa.gov/Research/Crash-Injury-Research-(CIREN) (accessed October 5, 2017).

NHTSA. n.d.-b. *Data-Driven Approaches to Crime and Traffic Safety (DDACTS).* https://one.nhtsa.gov/Driving-Safety/Enforcement-&-Justice-Services/Data%E2%80%93Driven-Approaches-to-Crime-and-Traffic-Safety-(DDACTS) (accessed December 13, 2017).

NHTSA. n.d.-c. *Fact sheet: National Roadside Survey of Alcohol and Drug Use by Drivers.* Washington, DC: U.S. Department of Transportation.

NHTSA. n.d.-d. *State data programs.* https://www.nhtsa.gov/research-data/state-data-programs (accessed October 5, 2017).

NIAAA (National Institute on Alcohol Abuse and Alcoholism). 2013. *Alcohol-related emergency department visits and hospitalizations and their co-occurring drug-related, mental health, and injury conditions in the United States: Findings from the 2006-2010 Natiowide Emergency Department Sample (NEDS) and Nationwide Inpatient sample (NIS).* NIH Publication No. 13-8000. Bethesda, MD: National Institute on Alcohol Abuse and Alcoholism.

NIAAA. 2017. *Division of Epidemiology and Prevention Research (DEPR). Funding opportunities.* https://www.niaaa.nih.gov/research/extramural-research/depr#FOA (accessed December 6, 2017).

NRC and IOM (National Research Council and Institute of Medicine). 1985. *Injury in America: A continuing public health problem.* Washington, DC: National Academy Press.

NRC and IOM. 2004. *Reducing underage drinking: A collective responsibility.* Washington, DC: The National Academies Press.

OnStar. n.d. *OnStar.* https://www.onstar.com/us/en/home.html (accessed December 21, 2017).

Poe, G. S., E. Powell-Griner, and J. K. McLaughlin. 1993. *Comparability of the death certificate and the 1986 National Mortality Followback Survey. Vital and Health Statistics.* DHHS Publication No. (PHS) 94-1392. Hyattsville, MD: National Center for Health Statistics.

Rainie, L., and M. Duggan. 2016. *5. Scenario: Auto insurance discounts and monitoring.* http://www.pewinternet.org/2016/01/14/scenario-auto-insurance-discounts-and-monitoring (accessed December 20, 2017).

Ramirez, R. 2017. PowerPoint presentation to the Committee on Accelerating Progress to Reduce Alcohol-Impaired Driving Fatalities, Washington, DC, February 16, 2017. http://nationalacademies.org/hmd/~/media/Files/Activity%20Files/AcceleratingProgresstoReduceAlcoholImpairedDrivingFatalities/16%20FEB%202017/5%20Ramirez.pdf (accessed April 24, 2017).

Rockett, I. R., N. D. Kapusta, and J. H. Coben. 2014. Beyond suicide: Action needed to improve self-injury mortality accounting. *JAMA Psychiatry* 71(3):231–232.

Saha, S., P. Schramm, A. Nolan, and J. Hess. 2016. Adverse weather conditions and fatal motor vehicle crashes in the United States, 1994-2012. *Environmental Health* 15(1):104.

SAMHSA (Substance Abuse and Mental Health Services Administration). 2016. *Population data/NSDUH.* https://www.samhsa.gov/data/population-data-nsduh (accessed August 31, 2017).

SAMHSA. 2017a. *SAMHSA's efforts related to prevention and early intervention.* https://www.samhsa.gov/prevention/samhsas-efforts (accessed November 30, 2017).

SAMHSA. 2017b. *STOP Act legislation*. https://www.samhsa.gov/underage-drinking-topic/stop-act-legislation (accessed November 30, 2017).

Schneider, W. H., B. Stakleff, and L. Buser. 2017. *Alcohol-related hot-spot analysis and prediction*. Minneapolis, MN: Center for Transportation Studies, University of Minnesota.

Shahum, L., and Z. Vanderkooy. 2017. *Moving from vision to action: Fundamental principles, policies & practices to advance Vision Zero in the U.S.* Vision Zero Network.

Shueh, J. 2017. *Mapping collision-prone intersections in Seattle, New York and New Orleans*. http://statescoop.com/mapping-collision-prone-intersections-in-seattle-new-york-and-new-orleans (accessed August 3, 2017).

Slater, M. E., I. J. Castle, B. K. Logan, and R. W. Hingson. 2016. Differences in state drug testing and reporting by driver type in U.S. fatal traffic crashes. *Accident Analysis & Prevention* 92:122–129.

Soleymanian, M., C. Weinberg, and T. Zhu. 2016. *The value of usage-based insurance beyond better targeting: Better driving*. https://research.chicagobooth.edu/~/media/8aeee2a8af83412c954d331dc412cc55.pdf (accessed July 31, 2017).

SPRC (Suicide Prevention Resource Center). 2012. *Data source: WISQARS nonfatal injury data*. Waltham, MA: SPRC.

Stevenson, M., R. D. Brewer, and V. Lee. 1998. The spatial relationship between licensed alcohol outlets and alcohol-related motor vehicle crashes in Gwinnett County, Georgia. *Journal of Safety Research* 29(3):197–203.

Threewitt, C. 2016. *How do those car insurance tracking devices work?* https://cars.usnews.com/cars-trucks/best-cars-blog/2016/10/how-do-those-car-insurance-tracking-devices-work (accessed December 20, 2017).

Toyota. n.d. *Safety Sense™*. https://www.toyota.com/safety-sense (accessed December 21, 2017).

TRB (Transportation Research Board). n.d. *What is the SHRP 2 safety data?* http://www.trb.org/StrategicHighwayResearchProgram2SHRP2/SHRP2DataSafetyAbout.aspx (accessed October 10, 2017).

U.S. House of Representatives. 2015. *Departments of Transportation, and Housing and Urban Development, and related agencies appropriations bill, 2016. Report 114–129*. https://www.congress.gov/114/crpt/hrpt129/CRPT-114hrpt129.pdf (accessed December 6, 2017).

Voas, R. B., A. S. Tippetts, E. Romano, D. A. Fisher, and T. Kelley-Baker. 2007. Alcohol involvement in fatal crashes under three crash exposure measures. *Traffic Injury Prevention* 8(2):107–114.

Walsh, M. C., A. Trentham-Dietz, and M. Palta. 2011. Availability of driver's license master lists for use in government-sponsored public health research. *American Journal of Epidemiology* 173(12):1414–1418.

7

Generating Action

INTRODUCTION

To initiate and sustain action that will bolster progress to reduce alcohol-impaired driving fatalities, the United States needs a strategic and comprehensive national effort. Such an effort requires the engagement of stakeholders across multiple sectors such as transportation, law enforcement, public health, the private sector, philanthropy, and others. Furthermore, it will entail garnering public will to address alcohol-impaired driving and allocating the resources needed to do so by creating and sustaining public discourse to underscore the magnitude of the problem and outline strategies to move these efforts forward. A multilevel ecological approach that targets individual beliefs and attitudes, community-level collaboration, institutional partnerships, and social norms (see Figure 1-6 for an illustration of these levels in the socioecological model) will be needed to catalyze a movement to achieve reductions in alcohol-impaired driving fatalities once again. This chapter highlights the key elements, approaches, innovations, and partnerships that could generate such action and overcome existing barriers. The chapter begins with a discussion of the role of historic and current social movements. This is followed by sections that explore the role of community-based approaches, the media environment and media advocacy, and discussions of stakeholder accountability and recommendations for action to reduce alcohol-impaired driving fatalities.

THE ROLE OF SOCIAL MOVEMENTS

Mothers Against Drunk Driving: A Historical Perspective

There is a significant and understandable tendency to look back at Mothers Against Drunk Driving (MADD) and credit that organization with much of the progress that has been made in reducing alcohol-impaired driving in the United States. Indeed, Fell and Voas (2006) do so, concluding that MADD made such a difference by contributing to the public view that alcohol-impaired driving is socially unacceptable, encouraging state legislatures and Congress to adopt laws and policies, and creating an unparalleled network of victims' services.

MADD has a compelling history. Founded in 1980, it received early on more seed money from the federal government (National Highway Traffic Safety Administration [NHTSA]) than any other source (including alcohol manufacturers, who ultimately donated $50,000 but were no longer involved with MADD by the mid-1980s) (Fell and Voas, 2006). By 1985, MADD had 377 chapters, with at least one in every state except Montana (Wolfson, 1995), and a budget approaching $10 million (Reinarman, 1988). By 1990, it had annual revenues of almost $50 million (Fell and Voas, 2006).

Although not solely attributable to MADD, from 1981 to 1986 states passed 729 laws concerning drinking and driving, with an accompanying dramatic drop in deaths from alcohol-impaired driving (Fell and Voas, 2006). One analysis of MADD's state-level activism concluded that MADD did this without reliance on conventional resources (Wolfson, 1995). Wolfson found that legitimacy, based in the fact that state chapter presidents were generally personally affected by alcohol-impaired driving and there were high levels of victim membership in state chapters, combined with lobbying and legislative activity were more important in explaining significant policy change at the state level (i.e., passage of 21 as the minimum purchase age for alcohol) than the age of members, the overall size of the membership, the revenues of the chapter, network cohesiveness, or the level of organization—all of which are more usual measures of a social movement's magnitude and likely success (Wolfson, 1995).

The salience of alcohol-impaired driving in the media, and particularly the role of the Ad Council and NHTSA's "Friends don't let friends drive drunk" campaign, is worth noting during this time period as well. The campaign is often regarded as an integral contributing factor to the shifting social norms around alcohol-impaired driving (Ad Council, n.d.; Glascoff et al., 2013). While this campaign lacks rigorous evaluative studies, its airing being coincident with MADD's activities could suggest the importance of coordinating media approaches with grassroots efforts to maximize impact. (For more on media approaches, see the section in this chapter on The Media Environment and Media Advocacy.)

In historical review, MADD meets the five "core practices" Ganz posits for the development of a successful social movement in a 2013 Institute of Medicine (IOM) workshop (2014). In putting victims first—and particularly, as Reinarman (1988) points out, unequivocally innocent victims, such as the parents and relatives of children (nondrivers) who were in car crashes—MADD built a "people," a *network of relationships* based in common experience and commitments. From these people, MADD built *a narrative*, a meta-story that every MADD president can tell of the progression from happy family to unjust tragedy to righteous and sympathetic activist. MADD then *developed strategy*, which for Ganz translates to "figuring out how to turn what people have—that is, resources—into what they need—power—in order to get what they want" (IOM, 2014, p. 12). Ganz also encourages viewing resources as political, economic, and cultural or moral. MADD used a moral stance, along with its compelling narrative, to attract significant media attention and create collective outrage, which in turn generated political pressure for change. It did this through *action*, from marching around the White House in 1980 to organizing a national summit of 435 youth from every congressional district in 2000 to encourage Congress to adopt a law requiring all states to set the maximum permissible blood alcohol concentration at 0.08%. Finally, MADD organized a national *structure*, which has endured, with a symbolic presidency rotating among victim members who can carry the organizational narrative with legitimacy, matched by a professional CEO and permanent staff that ensure continuity and focus.

This valuable historical perspective does not provide insights into why MADD arose when it did, what conditions facilitated its emergence, and if those conditions can be replicated today. Currently, a new or renewed social movement to end deaths from alcohol-impaired driving could emerge and carry the work forward. Sociologists generally view social movements as oppositional to the existing order. Thus, Polletta defines a social movement as "an organized effort to change laws, policies, or practices by people who do not have the power to effect change through conventional channels" (IOM, 2014, p. 6). To this extent, the conditions in which MADD arose certainly no longer exist. Alcohol-impaired driving is no longer seen as an acceptable behavior; it has already been stigmatized and more uniformly criminalized (Greenfield and Room, 1997). While Ross feared that it would become "a normal consequence of a society that accepts alcohol in recreation and provides no means of transportation other than private vehicles," the fact that politicians arrested for driving while impaired (DWI) can expect news stories pillorying their behavior suggests otherwise (1997, p. 13). A 2017 content analysis of print and television news media found that about 15 percent of news stories regarding an alcohol-impaired driving incident featured a local person of prominence in the community (e.g., local politician) as the perpetrator (Fisher, 2018).

Building on its success from the 1980s, MADD officially added "and prevent underage drinking" to its mission statement in the late 1990s (Fell and Voas, 2006). It has since worked in coalition with other organizations to implement the much broader public policy agenda foreshadowed in the 1989 report of the *Surgeon General's Workshop on Drunk Driving* and laid out in the National Research Council and the IOM report *Reducing Underage Drinking: A Collective Responsibility* (NRC and IOM, 2004). This agenda includes increasing alcohol taxes and enhancing voluntary restrictions on alcohol advertising, an issue MADD did not address in its earlier history. The broadened mission has not led to the levels of success earlier achieved by MADD.

More recently, MADD's activities have focused on advancing promising technological solutions to address alcohol-impaired driving. This includes advocating and lobbying for all-offender ignition interlock laws in every state (see Recommendation 5-3 in this report) as part of its Campaign to Eliminate Drunk Driving, which launched in 2006 (MADD, 2017). MADD was also instrumental in establishing the Driver Alcohol Detection System for Safety (DADSS) initiative (see Chapter 4 for more on DADSS) and testifies to legislative committees on the promise of new technologies such as autonomous vehicles (Sheehey-Church, 2017).

Creating a Social Movement in the Current Environment

It is worth examining the differences in the current environment and the environment during the era when MADD emerged. In addition to alcohol-impaired driving no longer being normative, media attention to the issue has waned. MADD's competitor, Remove Intoxicated Drivers, received differential treatment for its advocacy of advertising restrictions, while MADD's avoidance of that issue was key to the organization's success in the news media, particularly television news, in the 1980s (Mosher and Jernigan, 1989). Reinarman (1988, p. 112) argued that "MADD did in some senses suit the interests of the alcohol, advertising, and broadcasting industries who were facing what they saw as a broader threat, and the movement both aided and was aided by broader conservative currents." Yanovitzky found that media attention to alcohol-impaired driving, instigated largely by MADD's efforts, played a key role in influencing state and federal legislative action, which in turn stimulated population-level behavior changes around alcohol-impaired driving (Yanovitzky, 2002a).

If MADD is to recover its earlier influence, or if some other organization or emerging movement is to pick up the torch of alcohol-impaired driving as a social issue, it will likely need to be able to capture media attention as MADD did in its early years. The role of funding from NHTSA in getting MADD off the ground and the lesson it offers as to the ability of well-aimed seed funding to sprout results need to be taken into consideration. As described below, support for media advocacy training, and updating that training to encompass social media, would also be a key ingredient for success (Dorfman et al., 2005). This is a critical role that foundations can play in the support of social movements (for guidance to philanthropy on how to support movement building, see Masters and Osborn, 2010).

The sociological literature on social movements has long focused on resource mobilization, meaning the "ability to organize, recruit adherents, deploy strategy, gain strength, and achieve their aims—within the limits of existing political opportunities" (Walder, 2009, pp. 397–398), as key to the success of those movements. What this focus neglects, however, as Walder points out, is the relationship between prevailing social structures and the political orientations taken by social movements. At the height of its success in the 1980s, MADD matched the political climate of the Reagan–George H. W. Bush years, charting a course in line with conservative values at the same time that it took an oppositional stance to the normative nature of drinking and driving. In his analysis of MADD, Reinarman (1988, p. 92) argues that MADD's "foci and tactics succeeded when they did largely (although not merely) because they were in harmony with the morality, policy ideologies, and social-control strategies of the Reagan administration." For example, MADD's individualistic focus, lack of attention to structural factors, and limited retributive solutions could be thought of as aligning with the conservatism at the time (Reinarman, 1988). While multiple authors have pointed to protecting the public's health as the frame most likely to succeed MADD in movements to reduce alcohol-impaired driving (Reinarman, 1988; Ross, 1997), that frame, even as it has been espoused by MADD itself, has yet to capture the public imagination or the media attention so critical to MADD's earlier success.

Efforts to rekindle interest in these issues by stimulating action in other sectors are also currently at their historical nadir. The Enforcing Underage Drinking Laws program in the U.S. Department of Justice sent tens of millions of dollars to local law enforcement each year for more than a decade. As discussed in Chapter 2, while still authorized, that program's funding fell from $25 million in 2009–2010 to $10 million in fiscal year 2013 and subsequently disappeared from the federal budget. Meanwhile, there has been a dramatic drop in federal funding for more

TABLE 7-1 Funding for Federal Substance Abuse Prevention Programs, 2009–2014

	2009	2010	2011	2012	2013*	2014	2015	2016	2017
Drug-Free Communities Program	$90	$95	$95	$92	$87.4	$92	$93.5	$95	$97
Comprehensive Addiction and Recovery Act Enhancement Grants	N/A	N/A	N/A	N/A	N/A	N/A	N/A	N/A	$3
Center for Substance Abuse Prevention	$201	$201.2	$201.2	$186.4	$177.1	$175.6	$175.2	$211.2	$223.2
20% Set-Aside within Substance Abuse Prevention and Treatment Block Grant	$355.8	$355.8	$355.8	$360	$342	$363.9	$363.9	$371.6	$371.6
State Grants Portion of the Safe and Drug Free Schools and Communities Program	$294.8	—	—	—	—	—	—	—	—
National Youth Anti-Drug Media Campaign	$70	$45	$35	—	—	—	—	—	—
Enforcing Underage Drinking Laws	$25	$25	$20.8	$5	$4.8	$2.5	—	—	—
Total	$1.04 billion	$723	$708.8	$643.4	$611.3	$634	$632.6	$677.8	$694.8

NOTES: Dollar amounts are presented in the millions unless otherwise noted and are not adjusted for inflation; *with sequester.
SOURCE: Personal communication with Sue Thau, December 12, 2017, Community Anti-Drug Coalitions of America. Available by request from the National Academies of Sciences, Engineering, and Medicine's Public Access Records Office (PARO@nas.edu).

general work on substance abuse (see Table 7-1 for data on funding of federal substance abuse prevention programs from 2009 to 2014).

Meanwhile, led by craft brewers and their congressional representatives, efforts to roll back federal excise taxes on alcohol have achieved traction and may well succeed, with 218 cosponsors in the House as of June 2017.[1] This stands in stark contrast to the Reagan–Bush era, when (in 1991) federal beer and wine taxes were increased for the first time since 1951.

Polletta describes social movements as having three "essential ingredients": political opportunities, mobilizing structures, and resonant frames (IOM, 2014). MADD's frame on alcohol-impaired driving, while novel in 1981, is no longer capturing media attention and as such it is less resonant, at least in the media environment. MADD continues, largely because of its victim services, to possess a substantial mobilizing structure, matched in the alcohol and other drug space only by Community Anti-Drug Coalitions of America (CADCA), the other major national organizing effort with alcohol explicitly in its mission. Federal funding for the efforts of CADCA's approximately 3,000 member coalitions has also shrunken substantially, while language added in Section 503 of the 2012 federal appropriations bill further restricted what federally funded coalitions can do regarding public policy. Political opportunities, unpredictable as they are, may present themselves in the future, providing an opening for alcohol-impaired driving to regain its place in the national agenda.

RECENT COMMUNITY-BASED APPROACHES

Community Coalitions

While the concept of coalitions has evolved over time, coalitions can be broadly defined as formal, long-term alliances among organizations that collaborate toward a common goal (Butterfoss, 2007). Community-based coalitions are a widely accepted tool for public health promotion and prevention efforts. They have also been identified as important elements of multicomponent initiatives to promote motor vehicle safety (Goodwin et al., 2015; Shults et al., 2009) and to prevent alcohol-related harms (D'Onofrio et al., 2005). Butterfoss et al. (1993) identify six attributes of coalitions that make them instrumental in generating action. The authors assert that coalitions:

[1] At the time this report was being finalized in December 2017, Congress passed a tax bill (Tax Cuts and Jobs Act of 2017, H.R.1, 115th Cong., 1st sess.) that would decrease federal alcohol excise taxes by about 16 percent.

1. Allow organizations to confront new and broader issues without having to take on sole responsibility;
2. Develop and demonstrate public support for a particular issue;
3. Maximize the effect of individuals and groups through joint action;
4. Minimize duplication of efforts;
5. Mobilize more resources and strategies than any one actor could garner alone; and
6. Provide an opportunity to engage participants from various constituencies.

The characteristics of an effective coalition can be measured by the capacity of organizations to be effective coalition members,[2] the capacity of the coalition, and the outcomes and effects of the coalition activities (Raynor, 2011). Chavis argues that although community coalitions can be powerful catalysts for mobilizing and focusing resources, they have not traditionally been successful at developing and managing services and activities in the community. He also suggests that it may behoove coalitions to delegate those tasks to community organizations with the necessary capacity (Chavis, 2001). Cramer et al. (2006) offer a conceptual model for understanding effective coalitions in health promotion, titled the "Internal Coalition Outcome Hierarchy." The authors posit that effective coalitions have two important features. The first is a diverse membership that collaborates well to achieve objectives within the following seven constructs: shared social vision, efficient practices, knowledge and training, relationships, participation, activities, and resources. The second is leadership that fosters a learning environment that is conducive to achieving the collectively desired outcomes (Cramer et al., 2006).

Lessons from Previous Community-Based Funding Efforts

There is a significant history of federal funding of community-based efforts in tobacco control from which efforts to reduce alcohol-impaired driving deaths can benefit. Two major community-level funding initiatives—the Community Intervention Trial for Smoking Cessation (COMMIT) and the American Stop Smoking Intervention Study for Cancer Prevention (ASSIST)—made significant contributions to national capacity

[2] Raynor (2011) details the capacities of effective coalition members, which include but are not limited to skills/knowledge to work collaboratively; commitment to the coalition in action as well as its name; ability to articulate what they bring to the table; willingness to share resources; willingness to share power/credit; and strategic use of coalitions to fill critical gaps and leverage resources toward achieving the mission.

and success in reducing tobacco-related disease and death. Both have been carefully evaluated. COMMIT was a 4-year effort in 11 intervention communities; ASSIST was more policy focused, and ultimately sent $114 million to 17 states over 8 years—an average of $1.14 million per state per year. ASSIST benefited from the COMMIT experience, and focused on building state capacity to deliver comprehensive tobacco use prevention and control. ASSIST showed that implementation of effective policies would lead to concrete reductions in the problem "on the ground." It demonstrated that states with greater capacity, such as high-functioning tobacco control staff and structures in the health department, staff with experience in tobacco use control and prevention, and strong collaboration between agencies and across the state, had better outcomes. It also showed that such an intervention was comparable in its cost-effectiveness to other public health preventive interventions (NCI, 2006).

The Robert Wood Johnson Foundation in the 1990s also made a significant investment in community-based prevention in alcohol control. In particular, its A Matter of Degree program that funded colleges to reduce excess drinking and related problems confirmed the finding from ASSIST that community-based efforts could produce policy and environmental change, and that those sites that focused more on environmental and policy change were the most likely to affect the problem (Weitzman et al., 2004).

The abovementioned and other previous efforts demonstrate that a substantial investment in community-level policy and environmental change can be a cost-effective approach to the improvement of health and safety in that community. Applying such an approach to alcohol-impaired driving at the community level would require a willingness to invest significant government and/or private philanthropic dollars in the effort. This willingness in and of itself may be a measure of the degree to which there is a general commitment to addressing and reducing alcohol-impaired driving fatalities.

Community Coalitions and Alcohol-Impaired Driving

Community coalitions with the goal of addressing alcohol-impaired driving exist around the country. For example, the Texas Impaired Driving Task Force began with an informal meeting of stakeholders and evolved into a coalition that meets to discuss progress to eliminate alcohol- and drug-related crashes through stakeholder work projects and to provide guidance and technical assistance to the Texas Department of Transportation. The coalition is a multisector group, including representatives from law enforcement, media development/communications, treatment, research, alcohol service, driver licensing, public health, and more (Texas

BOX 7-1
The Safe Communities Coalition's Southeast Louisiana DWI Taskforce

The Safe Communities Coalition (SCC) is an initiative of the National Highway Traffic Safety Administration (NHTSA), formed in 1997 with the goal of identifying the major causes of unintentional injury in the greater New Orleans area. The Southeast Louisiana DWI Taskforce (SELA) is a subcommittee of the coalition, which was established in response to a high incidence of alcohol-related crashes and fatalities in metropolitan New Orleans. Also of concern were the perceived lack of emphasis on DWI enforcement and prosecutions by state agencies and the recognition that the DWI issue was a specialized problem requiring expertise not found in SCC. Thus, SELA was created to change the permissive culture around alcohol-impaired driving. According to its mission statement, SELA's mission is to "form a partnership between law enforcement, judiciary, communities, businesses, leaders, civic organizations, and individuals in an effort to reduce the incidence of DWI/DUI through awareness, education, and legislative change."

As described in its mission statement, SELA engages stakeholders across multiple sectors. Participating members include the American Automobile Association, Charity Hospital Trauma Program, the Council on Alcohol and Drug Abuse for Greater New Orleans, the Federal Highway Administration, Jefferson Parish Safe and Drug Free, the Louisiana Property and Casualty Commission, Medical Center of Louisiana in New Orleans, Mothers Against Drunk Driving, Progressive Insurance Company, law enforcement agencies, prosecutors, and schools.

SELA has been a catalyst for important legislative and enforcement changes in the New Orleans area. For example, three parishes—Jefferson, Orleans, and St. Tammany—adopted aggressive DWI enforcement policies within 3 years of the task force's creation. Additionally, SELA was part of the impetus for legislative reform regarding refusal for chemical testing and DWI suspension. Other important activities include hosting conferences to convene law enforcement actors, helping establish the first DWI court in Louisiana, and providing trainings for drug recognition experts in the area.

SOURCE: Fell et al., 2011.

A&M Transportation Institute, 2016). Many states are forming coalitions to advance Vision Zero efforts to eliminate all traffic fatalities and serious injuries, including California, Colorado, and Massachusetts (see Chapter 1 for more information on Vision Zero). Box 7-1 describes a community coalition that developed a DWI taskforce in Louisiana.

Community-level collaboration has been identified as a key element of efforts to reduce alcohol-impaired driving fatalities. The Community Preventive Services Task Force conducted a systematic review of multicomponent interventions with community mobilization for reducing alcohol-impaired driving,[3] and found strong evidence that "carefully planned, well-executed multicomponent programs with community mobilization can reduce alcohol-related crashes" and produce cost savings (Shults et al., 2009, p. 368). One of the positive spillover effects of community mobilization identified in the review was the promotion of individual and community empowerment, as well as the development of problem-solving capacity. In addition, a synthesis of lessons learned from demonstration site projects to reduce impaired driving in rural communities cited the importance of allocating time and resources to build community support through a variety of strategies including coalition building (Cox and Fisher, 2009).

Aguilar and Delehanty (2009) documented the implementation and evaluation of a community-based social marketing initiative in Wisconsin that aimed to reduce alcohol-impaired driving among motorcyclists, a group that has high rates of impaired driving fatalities. One key aspect of the initiative was a coalition made up of tavern and restaurant owners, law enforcement officers, local business owners, members of the motorcycling community, and community activists. The authors reported encouraging outcomes, which included the assembly of a coalition of nontraditional partners and a reduction in the number of motorcycle crashes in which alcohol was a reported factor by 35 percent in the experimental counties, compared to 2 percent in other urban Wisconsin counties, but the reduction did not reach statistical significance ($p = 0.07$) (Aguilar and Delehanty, 2009).

Shults et al. (2009) identified some of the barriers faced by community coalitions in their review of multicomponent interventions to reduce alcohol-impaired driving. Among these challenges, the authors express particular concern for the tendency to engage in less effective interventions (e.g., public education) because they may be more palatable based on the community's social and economic interests. Other challenges include gaining and sustaining consensus among group members, inefficiency in implementing decisions and interventions, ideological differences between member organizations, competition over resources, power imbalances, and existing sociocultural tensions among the various actors.

Alcohol tax coalitions Coalitions can also facilitate progress on alcohol-impaired driving fatalities by focusing their efforts on population-based preventive interventions such as increasing alcohol taxes

[3] Multicomponent programs here are defined as the implementation of interventions or policies in multiple settings (e.g., responsible beverage service in bars and sobriety checkpoints), or that modify the community environment to reduce alcohol-impaired driving (Shults et al., 2009).

(see Recommendation 3-1 in this report). As referenced in Chapter 3, one barrier to the implementation of alcohol tax increases is the lack of awareness of the efficacy of taxes to reduce harmful drinking and related consequences such as alcohol-impaired driving fatalities (Jernigan and Waters, 2009). Policy makers tend to view alcohol taxes primarily as revenue-raising measures, and to be unaware of the positive public health effects related to tax increases. Inserting a public health "voice" into public debates over alcohol taxes can be challenging (Ramirez and Jernigan, 2017). Broad-based coalitions are an important and promising tool for communities to employ to educate the public and policy makers about alcohol taxes.

Ramirez and Jernigan (2017) analyzed the ability of diverse coalitions in three states to pass laws increasing alcohol excise taxes. They found that strategic use of polling data, leveraging existing political champions, broad-based coalition building (beyond the alcohol and drug fields), past experience with legislative initiatives, allocating tax revenues strategically to build political and coalition support, and generating media coverage through intentional media advocacy were key elements of successful campaigns. The most successful grassroots effort occurred in Maryland, where the statewide coalition of more than 1,200 organizations generated 239 media articles mentioning the state sales tax increase on alcohol by 3 percent in significant print media outlets, and succeeded without a leading politician as champion in increasing the tax and generating more than $70 million in revenues, leading to a significant drop in alcohol-impaired drivers on Maryland roadways (Ramirez and Jernigan, 2017). One study found that the tax increase led to a 3.8 percent drop in alcohol consumption relative to what would have been expected given prior sales trends (Esser et al., 2016), while another found that the tax increase was associated with a decline in crashes involving drivers with alcohol in their system (12 percent for drivers 15–34 years old and 6 percent for all drivers) (Lavoie et al., 2017). The formation of such coalitions is an important tool to advance evidence and catalyze action on interventions that can be challenging to implement in the policy-making arena.

Effective Community-Based Approaches for Alcohol-Related Issues

Multicomponent, community-based approaches are a viable way to reduce alcohol-related harms at the local level, as they address the social and environmental conditions that shape the problems at hand (Aguirre-Molina and Gorman, 1996; Shults et al., 2009). In their review of the literature on community-based programs, Aguirre-Molina and Gorman (1994) found that the most promising community prevention efforts:

- Are grounded in models of community action for social change;
- Value community empowerment and have origins in community development;[4]
- Target multiple systems and employ multiple strategies;
- Recognize the importance of social policy;
- Use tools from a public health model (e.g., addressing social and environmental factors beyond individual behaviors); and
- Use the best available evidence to inform the interventions.

The authors also cite two examples of comprehensive community-based alcohol prevention programs, the Prevention Research Center and Communities Mobilizing for Change on Alcohol (CMCA), both of which targeted community-level policies, practices, and the alcohol environment to reduce alcohol-related harm.

CMCA was a 15-community randomized trial in which the intervention was a community organizing project that targeted policies, practices, and social norms to reduce underage persons' access to alcohol. The project involved community organizers working with stakeholders such as public officials, enforcement agencies, alcohol merchants, the media, and schools to change community policies regarding youth drinking. The organizing effort led to institutional policy changes in all seven intervention communities including changes in retailer policies, media coverage, and law enforcement practices (Wagenaar et al., 1999). Wagenaar et al. (2000) evaluated the intervention's effect on youth drinking and driving using arrest and crash data from state departments of public safety and transportation. The findings demonstrated a reduction in arrest and traffic crashes for 15- to 20-year-olds and a statistically significant reduction in DWI arrests among 18- to 20-year-olds.

Another effective community prevention model is Communities That Care (CTC),[5] a coalition-based system that seeks to prevent adolescent problem behaviors (e.g., alcohol use, substance use, delinquency, and violence). A community-randomized trial assessing the system's effects on adolescents 8 years after implementation found that students in the CTC communities were more likely than students in the control communities to have abstained from drinking alcohol (relative risk = 1.31; 95% confidence interval 1.09–1.58) (Hawkins et al., 2014). It is important to note that the program also showed sustained effects on tobacco use,

---

[4] Community empowerment is defined by Wallerstein and Bernstein as a "social-action process in which individuals and groups act to gain mastery over their lives in the context of changing their social and political environment" (1994, p. 142).

[5] For more information, see http://www.communitiesthatcare.net (accessed September 5, 2017).

delinquency, and violence. The CTC model is unique in that it does not focus solely on alcohol use; it also addresses shared risk factors and trains local communities to select the evidence-based intervention(s) that best suit that community's needs and assets.

Tools for Communities to Generate Action

There are a variety of publicly available tools and resources for communities that seek to take action on alcohol-impaired driving. For example, CADCA developed an Impaired Driving Prevention Toolkit for communities that seek to develop a comprehensive plan to address alcohol-impaired driving.[6] The toolkit provides guidance on how to:

- Conduct a community assessment;
- Use a logic model to guide the planning process;
- Examine the research and evidence-based interventions that target the problem; and
- Design an intervention map for a defined local condition (CADCA, n.d.).

In 2011 NHTSA published *A Guide for Local Impaired-Driving Task Forces*, which features case studies of task forces around the country and discusses their histories, structures, and approaches (Fell et al., 2011). Other community resources exist to provide guidance on starting and maintaining coalitions for a broad range of issues, such as the Community Tool Box from the Center for Community Health and Development at the University of Kansas.[7] In addition, the Pan American Health Organization offers a free online course in alcohol policy advocacy that walks through the elements of an alcohol policy change campaign.[8]

THE MEDIA ENVIRONMENT AND MEDIA ADVOCACY

Media discussions and framing of a problem are important influences on what is actually done about that problem (Iyengar, 1991). Content analyses of the current news media environment are essential to inform media advocacy efforts to reframe coverage of health-related issues in ways that advance public health goals (Dorfman, 2003). Fisher (2018) noted that

---

[6] For more information, see http://www.preventimpaireddriving.org (accessed August 21, 2017).

[7] For more information, see http://ctb.ku.edu/en/table-of-contents/assessment/promotion-strategies/start-a-coaltion/main (accessed August 24, 2017).

[8] For more information, see https://mooc.campusvirtualsp.org/enrol/index.php?id=40 (accessed August 24, 2017).

in the U.S. news media, alcohol-impaired driving stories mainly focus on victimization and punishment and show it as an individual problem and an individual responsibility. The stories overwhelmingly focus on the perpetrators. The most common voices in the stories are law enforcement, traffic safety advocates, prosecutors, and other attorneys. Strikingly missing from this list are victims themselves—the focus and key strength of MADD as a social movement in an earlier era and generally a voice often perceived as authentic in advocacy approaches. The presence of traffic safety advocates points to a potential for presenting broader solutions such as those described in this report; however, Fisher found little mention of such solutions, even among thematically framed stories which placed the problem in a broader societal context. These findings are indicative of a greater need for training and capacity in the use of mass media in support of community-based policy and environmental interventions—in other words, of a need for greater use of media advocacy. (See Appendix B for Fisher's media content analysis.)

Media Advocacy

Definition and Theory

Decades of theory and research on agenda setting and framing emphasize that the news media both shape what the public and policy makers think about (see McCombs and Reynolds, 2009; McCombs and Shaw, 1972) and invite certain perspectives about how to think about them (see Iyengar, 1991, 1996). The default news media frame for social problems, including most health issues, is one that focuses on portrayals of people as villains and victims (termed "episodic" coverage, in contrast to "systemic" coverage of underlying causes and population-level consequences and solutions) and thus emphasizes individual responsibility for causing and solving social problems (Dorfman and Krasnow, 2014; Iyengar, 1991).

Media advocacy seeks to reframe public health issues in terms of broader, upstream causes that are best addressed through collective action (community mobilization) and local, state, or federal policy changes to create healthier physical, built, social, and economic environments (see Wallack et al., 1999). Media advocacy involves the strategic use of the news media in support of community organizing to increase public and policy-maker awareness of public health problems, identify effective systems and policy changes to address them, and support progress toward their passage and implementation (Wallack et al., 1993). The theory and practice of media advocacy combine insights from the fields of communication, political science, public health, and sociology, resting on the assumptions that strategic efforts can influence the volume and nature of media coverage to emphasize upstream policy solutions to complex health problems, and that media coverage, in turn, influences the likelihood of policy debate, passage, and successful implementation (Chapman and Lupton, 1994; Dorfman and Krasnow, 2014).

Case Studies of Policy Success Involving Media Advocacy

Much like paid media campaigns, media advocacy interventions face major challenges in evaluation (see Stead et al., 2002). Media advocacy interventions are often conducted concurrently and intertwined with a variety of other intervention strategies, including paid media, community mobilization, and more direct forms of policy advocacy, such as direct contact with policy makers. In addition, the desired outcome for media advocacy is the passage of a particular policy; in a particular community, this amounts to a sample size of a single observation, making broader generalizations very difficult. As a result, many media advocacy evaluations have employed a case study approach, describing media advocacy efforts (along with other activities) and detailing the timeline of political action (or inaction) related to these efforts.

A variety of case studies have described the probable role of media advocacy in shaping policy debates and outcomes surrounding a variety of issues, including violence prevention (Wallack and Dorfman, 1996), tobacco (Jernigan and Wright, 1996; Lane and Carter, 2012; Wakefield et al., 2005), and health disparities and food insecurity (Rock et al., 2011). Several media advocacy case studies have also examined policy debates in the context of alcohol control and policy to limit alcohol-impaired driving. Various authors have credited media advocacy efforts with helping to shape policy debates surrounding a variety of policies to reduce violence against women via changes in messages conveyed in alcohol advertising (Woodruff, 1996), reduce the volume of alcohol-related marketing (Jernigan and Wright, 1996), and reduce rates of alcohol-impaired driving (Russell et al., 1995).

Evidence of Media Advocacy Effects in Shaping Favorable News Coverage

A few studies have moved beyond case study reports to describe systematic changes in the volume and nature of news media coverage in response to media advocacy intervention featuring multiple communities. These studies provide mixed evidence for the success of multisite media advocacy in shaping favorable news coverage. Schooler et al. (1996) compared tobacco-related media coverage between two intervention communities and two comparison sites as part of the Stanford Five-City Project to reduce risk factors for cardiovascular disease. Schooler et al. (1996, p. 346) concluded that media advocacy efforts were highly successful in one treatment community but not the other. They attributed success in the successful intervention community to "frequent, regular, systematic contact with media professionals and provision of materials." Stillman et al. (2001) evaluated changes in news coverage of tobacco control policy in response to ASSIST, a multistate intervention that featured media advocacy efforts as part of broader efforts to change policy and increase rates of smoking cessation. While the authors found that rates of tobacco control policy-related news coverage were greater in intervention states compared to nonintervention states, there were no differences in the rates of change between these groups. This indicates that preexisting differences in the states could account for the observed differences. The authors recommended caution in interpreting group differences as evidence of media advocacy effects.

The strongest evidence in support of media advocacy effects in promoting favorable news coverage comes from a community trial to reduce alcohol-related injury (largely focused on alcohol-impaired driving fatalities). The Community Trials Project sought to inform and mobilize three communities (compared to three matched control communities) to take individual and policy action to reduce alcohol-related injury and death through a variety of intervention strategies, including the strategic use of news media to promote alcohol control policy. Two evaluation studies concluded that media advocacy efforts as a part of this trial, over and above other trial activities, succeeded at increasing the volume of alcohol policy-related coverage, relative to both the comparison communities and larger state and national trends (Treno et al., 1996), and community awareness of alcohol control policies (Holder and Treno, 1997).

Combined, this work provides additional evidence that media advocacy can, under the right conditions, increase the volume and framing of news media coverage in ways that support proposed health policy changes, but more work is needed to parse out factors (at the community level) that shape the likelihood of success in promoting favorable coverage.

Evidence of Media Advocacy Effects on Policy Change

A few studies have used time series analysis and event history models to provide evidence that news coverage of health policy topics can increase policy debate and enactment in local communities. Asbridge (2004) concluded that print media coverage of the health effects of secondhand smoke, combined with direct advocacy efforts, contributed to an increase in the adoption of laws restricting public areas where people could smoke in Canadian communities. Niederdeppe et al. (2007) argued that local newspaper coverage of youth antismoking advocacy activities contributed to increases in the passage of tobacco product placement ordinances targeting retail establishments. Yanovitzky (2002b) found that increased news media coverage of alcohol-impaired driving was associated with increased policy attention (measured by the number of congressional hearings about alcohol-impaired driving and the number of anti-alcohol-impaired driving bills introduced to Congress in a particular month) and policy action (measured by the number of anti-alcohol-impaired driving laws passed by U.S. states over time). These studies offer consistent evidence that strategic efforts to increase news coverage relevant to policy goals can generate policy debate and action favorable to improving public health.

Challenges for Media Advocacy in the New Media Environment

Despite some available evidence supporting media advocacy as an effective strategy to advance public health goals, a variety of caveats and cautions are in order. Several authors have identified a variety of potential unintended consequences and limitations of media advocacy. DeJong (1996) cautions that media advocacy can be a high-risk as well as a high-reward strategy for community coalitions. He cites a case in Massachusetts in which media advocacy brought to light significant internal debates about MADD's mission, rendering it less effective thereafter than it might otherwise have been. Harwood et al. (2005) further warn that media advocacy efforts need to take into account the local political culture. They describe how while media advocacy regarding efforts at alcohol control policy change in Louisiana succeeded in placing the issue on the public agenda, continued attention once policy campaigns entered sensitive periods of negotiation and compromise in the state legislature inadvertently catalyzed the attention and opposition of powerful interests in that state. Gibson (2010) notes that media advocacy's typical reliance on commercial, mainstream media may fundamentally constrain its ability to shape policy debates owing to inherent limitations of journalistic norms and practice. This concern is particularly noteworthy in light of recent changes in the news media landscape, including widespread declines in the number of local newspapers, newspaper circulation, and advertising revenues. This has contributed to smaller newsroom staff, limiting resources for nuanced coverage of health policy topics (Pew Research Center, 2017).

In response to these challenges, media advocacy efforts have increasingly moved toward the use of interactive, participatory, and social media. Clark and Marchi (2017) coined the term "connective journalism" to describe the user-centric practices of information sharing that have emerged over the past decade among youth. Clark and Marchi (2017) assert that youth who engage in connective journalism use "social media to communicate their concerns to one another and to mobilize community members in response" (p. 13). Several studies describe cases where advocacy organizations have effectively used hashtags and other social network tactics to generate public discussion about health and social policy topics (Bail, 2016; Saxton et al., 2015). The Truth Initiative, a nonprofit formerly known as the American Legacy Foundation, extended its anti-tobacco countermarketing campaign to reach youth on social networking sites. This targeting of social networking sites was associated with prompting more than 800,000 visitors to the campaign's website (Duke, 2007). There are reasons for caution in an overreliance on social media approaches, however. Tufekci (2017) studied use of social media to galvanize social protest movements in venues as disparate as the Arab Spring and the Occupy Movement, and concludes that while social media may make mobilization of large numbers of people easier, they may also make movements vulnerable to failure owing to "a lack of organizational depth and experience, of tools or culture for collective decision making, and strategic, long-term action" (p. xxvii).

Media advocacy efforts in the future will need to monitor and adapt to the changing media environment in an effort to shape the nature of public and policy-maker discussions of policy approaches to reduce alcohol-impaired driving fatalities, and exclusive reliance on traditional news media will likely be insufficient to change the national conversation on this issue. Community organizing and media advocacy, along with the use of paid media when feasible, are best viewed as complementary strategies to shape the broader media environment and help to accelerate progress toward further reductions in alcohol-related fatal crashes (Slater et al., 2000). The following sections will explore the roles of a number of stakeholders to take action on reducing alcohol-impaired driving fatalities.

STAKEHOLDER ACTION

Thus far, this chapter has discussed various strategies and tools to create awareness and capacity in addition to garnering support for activities to reduce alcohol-impaired driving. Much of this entails a grassroots approach that engages many stakeholders across sectors. Likewise, efforts to ensure that a sustainable infrastructure is in place to address this problem require a comprehensive, multisector approach that will create opportunities for action. There are a number of stakeholders that need to be engaged—some are traditional, and others are novel for the field of alcohol-impaired driving. Some important stakeholders include, but are not limited to,

- Federal, state, and local governments (e.g., departments of health, transportation, and law enforcement);
- Legal sector (e.g., judges and attorneys);
- Health care sector (e.g., clinicians, hospitals, addiction treatment providers, and insurers);
- Alcohol industry (e.g., producers, wholesalers, and retailers);
- Hospitality sector;
- Automobile industry;
- News media/advertising (television, print, radio, and social media);
- General public;
- Community coalitions; and
- Alcohol consumers.

See Table 8-1 for a summary of stakeholders who are needed to ensure implementation of the evidence-based and promising interventions discussed throughout this report.

To begin, a revised approach to renew and further progress on alcohol-impaired driving would require a change in the status quo and the setting of ambitious goals, such as zero alcohol-impaired driving fatalities. One stakeholder that could spearhead such an effort would be the U.S. Department of Health and Human Services' Healthy People decadal initiative. Healthy People has provided evidence-based benchmarks and monitored progress for improving the health of the nation for three decades.[9] This includes objectives for reducing substance abuse and specifically alcohol-related driving fatalities. The Healthy People 2020 baseline and target objectives for alcohol-related deaths per 100 million vehicle miles traveled were 0.39 and 0.38, respectively (Healthy People, 2017). Based on the stagnation in progress to reduce alcohol-impaired driving fatalities and the growing movement toward zero deaths in the traffic safety community, the committee concludes:

> *Conclusion 7-1: In the development of Healthy People 2030 objectives, a more ambitious target for alcohol-related deaths per 100 million vehicle miles traveled would better align with "zero deaths" initiatives across the country.*

[9] For more information, see https://www.healthypeople.gov (accessed October 3, 2017).

However, the most important factor in reducing deaths, injuries, and adverse socioeconomic effects of impaired driving is actually taking action to achieve stated targets.

Accountability

To achieve a more ambitious goal for reducing alcohol-impaired driving fatalities, it is important to have specific roles and accountabilities identified for each actor. When multiple sectors have a role to play to address a pressing and multifaceted problem, accountability can be difficult to operationalize. Accountability refers to "the principle that individuals, organizations, and the community are responsible for their actions and may be required to explain them to others" (Benjamin et al., 2006, p. 30) and can have different meanings to various fields (IOM, 2011). The U.S. Department of Transportation and law enforcement agencies are not the only actors accountable for or involved in accelerating progress toward zero deaths from alcohol-impaired driving. However, sharing accountability across sectors can be challenging. A 2011 IOM report provided a framework for accountability for improving health. That framework is applicable to alcohol-impaired driving as well. The report notes that the following four elements need to be in place to measure accountability:

1. An identified body with a clear charge to accomplish particular steps toward health goals;
2. Ensuring that the body has the capacity to undertake the required activities;
3. Measurement of what is accomplished against the identified body's clear charge; and
4. The availability of tools to assess and improve effectiveness and quality (such as a feedback loop as part of a learning system, incentives, and technical assistance).

The following sections discuss the roles and accountabilities of stakeholders who play a role in reducing alcohol-impaired driving fatalities. In some cases, the committee makes recommendations to specific stakeholders to accelerate progress.

The Role of the Health Sector

The health sector (i.e., health care delivery systems and governmental public health agencies) is one of many that could take on an expanded role in preventing alcohol-impaired driving fatalities.

The Role of Health Care

Chapter 5 discusses a number of opportunities for the health sector to screen individuals for hazardous drinking, provide timely and adequate care for injured persons, and evaluate and treat those who engage in hazardous drinking. (For example, see Recommendation 5-2 to health care systems and health insurers regarding their role in facilitating effective evaluation and treatment strategies for those who need it.) This section will highlight the changing nature of the health care system and opportunities to leverage those changes.

The health care system is changing dramatically, transitioning from small independent hospitals into large complex health systems that encompass greater geographical areas to serve larger populations. New partnerships and access points such as urgent care and retail clinics are often integrated into a health system network to support provision of care across a spectrum of needs. These new health care systems are often incentivized not only to provide care but also to improve the health of the population they serve and to ensure that the system also provides community health benefits.[10] This has created greater awareness of the diverse needs of the population, the effect of socioeconomic status on health, the need for accessible transportation, the effects of the built environment and local policies on health outcomes, and the locations of businesses such as grocery stores and pharmacies (Howard and Norris, 2015; NASEM, 2017). Health care systems are encouraged to collect more information about these varied determinants of health on patients and link data to identify high-risk and vulnerable populations and patients (Alley et al., 2016; Wyatt et al., 2016). Health care delivery systems can also do the following:

- Ensure that patients who are admitted for an alcohol-related injury are screened and treatment is offered.
- Share and link injury data with public health agencies to identify high-risk or vulnerable groups.
- Work with communities to identify sources of alcohol that contribute to alcohol impairment.
- Provide information on alcohol impairment for civic entities such as schools, employers, and churches so that they can increase awareness of community risks and take steps to intervene.

These are also opportunities for demonstrating community health benefits. Redelmeier and Detsky (2017) offer specific guidance for the role

[10] 26 CFR § 1.501 (r)-3.

BOX 7-2
Physician Strategies to Prevent Alcohol-Impaired Driving

- Alcohol screening and brief interventions for patients with alcohol problems
- Treatment of patients diagnosed with alcohol use disorder
- Counseling of patients not to ride with impaired drivers
- Supporting enforcement of laws against alcohol-impaired driving
- Promoting sobriety checkpoints in local communities
- Lending voice to mass media campaigns against alcohol-impaired driving
- Joining multicomponent interventions in coalitions of community group members

SOURCE: Adapted from Redelmeier and Detsky, 2017.

of clinical providers to take action against alcohol-impaired driving. The authors assert that physicians are positioned to identify high-risk patients and to provide advice that will be taken seriously. See Box 7-2 for an adapted list of Redelmeier and Detsky's physician strategies to prevent alcohol-impaired driving.

The Role of Public Health

Local and state public health departments could also engage in efforts to inform and facilitate initiatives to reduce alcohol-impaired driving. As discussed in Chapter 6, applying an epidemiological investigative approach to identify high-risk establishments (e.g., on-premise outlets that overserve patrons) and areas where crashes occur would be an activity for which local public health agencies could offer their technical expertise. Such an approach would require collaboration and sharing data with local departments of transportation and planning, law enforcement, researchers, the hospitality sector, and health care providers such as hospitals and emergency medical technicians. Public health agencies are also effective conveners for local issues that may necessitate the engagement of multiple stakeholders, often because of their use of population-based data and existing relationships in a given community (NASEM, 2017). As this report underscores the need for a comprehensive, public health (i.e., preventive) approach to alcohol-impaired driving, it is important to note that local and state public health agencies do not generally receive much funding to address alcohol-related harms in contrast to other health issues such as tobacco, which often has several dedicated funding streams.

Chapter 1 discusses the importance of applying a health equity lens to the issue of alcohol-impaired driving. With many local and state public health agencies already adopting a health equity focus in their activities, ensuring that inequities are not perpetuated is a natural role for public health agencies (NASEM, 2017). This is particularly relevant for the implementation of alcohol-impaired driving interventions that have the potential to exacerbate inequities in the criminal justice system, such as enforcement efforts (Horn et al., 2014) or plea bargains for DWI offenders (Rousseau and Pezzullo, 2013). Another strategy to ensure that equity issues are addressed at the local level is to engage community residents in the development of solutions (NASEM, 2017). As discussed earlier in the chapter, community coalitions are a powerful tool to ensure the needs of a community are being met.

In terms of national public health actors, the Surgeon General is particularly well positioned to highlight alcohol-impaired driving and evidence-based solutions as a public health priority. Creating high visibility for the topic in the public health arena can lead to sustained action among the public and policy makers. For example, the Surgeon General's 1964 report on smoking and health had enormous impact on how the country moved forward with tobacco policy (CDC, 2006). With respect to alcohol-impaired driving specifically, the 1989 *Surgeon General's Workshop Proceedings on Drunk Driving* very clearly outlines the interventions that are supported by the available research base. This included increasing alcohol taxes, which were a centerpiece of the Surgeon General's recommendations on impaired driving (HHS, 1989). In summary, leveraging the influence of a public health figure such as the Surgeon General could raise awareness and support for proven and sometimes neglected interventions that could reduce alcohol-impaired driving injuries and fatalities.

The Role of the Alcohol Industry

As Babor et al. (2018) have summarized, alcohol companies have taken on an active role in traffic safety and alcohol-impaired driving. As alcoholic beverage producers are becoming increasingly concentrated in terms of ownership, both in the United States and globally, they have amassed significant resources with which to influence alcohol policies and problems (Jernigan, 2009; Jernigan and Babor, 2015). Some of this influence may be negative. Commercial activities that may contribute to alcohol-impaired driving include

- Increasing the overall availability or decreasing the real price of alcohol;

- Developing products that mix or marketing that encourages the mixing of alcohol and energy drinks, which may facilitate heavier drinking and risk taking (McKetin et al., 2015; Striley and Kahn, 2014);
- Juxtaposing alcohol marketing with motor vehicle speed through auto racing sponsorships (Babor et al., 2018; EuroCare Institute of Alcohol Studies and Monash University, 2015); and
- Heavy exposure of youth to alcohol marketing during a period in life when young people are particularly vulnerable to marketing regarding risky behaviors like alcohol-impaired driving (Pechmann et al., 2005).

Corporate political activities seek to create a favorable regulatory environment for their products through influencing decision makers, promoting ineffective over effective policies, and building partnerships with civil society and governmental organizations that weaken the ability of those organizations to pursue or implement effective policies (Getz, 1997; Hillman et al., 1999; Schuler, 1996). These are normal activities for corporations seeking to maximize revenues and profits; however, in the case of alcohol and alcohol-impaired driving, these activities can function as barriers to progress. A content analysis of 97 industry actions on alcohol-impaired driving concluded that nearly all (97.9 percent)[11] were either ineffective or of unknown effectiveness (Babor et al., 2018). See Appendix C for a content analysis by Babor and colleagues.

The pattern of alcohol companies or their corporate social responsibility organizations is to express concern about the problem of impaired driving and alcohol-related crashes and their resulting deaths, injuries, and economic costs. However, they generally promote ineffective or non-evidence-based policies and generally oppose effective population-based strategies to reduce binge drinking and impaired driving (Babor et al., 2018).

Guidance on the role of the alcohol industry in reducing the burden of harmful drinking is provided in the World Health Organization's (2010) *Global Strategy to Reduce the Harmful Use of Alcohol*. This strategy, endorsed by the 63rd World Health Assembly, provides the following conclusion and recommendations to the industry:

> Economic operators in alcohol production and trade are important players in their role as developers, producers, distributors, marketers and sellers of alcoholic beverages. They are especially encouraged to consider effective ways to prevent and reduce harmful use of alcohol within their

[11] This information was updated after the prepublication release.

> core roles mentioned above, including self-regulatory actions and initiatives. They could also contribute by making available data on sales and consumption of alcohol beverages. (p. 20)

To that end, based on the literature, documented practices of the alcohol industry, and the committee's expertise, the committee concludes:

> *Conclusion 7-2: Alcohol companies and alcohol-related businesses could assist efforts to reduce alcohol-impaired driving fatalities by reducing the alcohol content of existing products, refraining from marketing including sponsorships that are likely to influence excessive alcohol use, and supporting or at least not opposing effective alcohol-impaired driving countermeasures.*

Actions by the alcohol industry to support efforts to reduce alcohol-impaired driving could also include

- At a minimum, adhering to and strengthening self-regulatory standards;
- Submitting needed data on alcohol sales and consumption (WHO, 2010); and
- Subjecting industry activities to reduce harmful use of alcohol to rigorous independent evaluations, free of conflict of interest (i.e., employing evaluation design methods as robust as those used to evaluate public health interventions) (Anderson and Rehm, 2016).

Model Legislation

As discussed throughout this report, policies that address alcohol and impaired driving vary substantially from state to state. In part, this is attributable to the decision to delegate alcohol control and regulation to the states after Prohibition. Many of the strategies outlined in this report require new legislation to be passed at the state level. Stakeholder groups such as community coalitions often lack the technical expertise to develop such legislation. While each state could design and implement the policies and laws that are tailored to its respective population, benchmarks for the states would provide guidance on which evidence-based strategies to adopt. As technology and practice at the state level move forward, there is a constant need to be able to learn from state experiences and not continually be faced with "reinventing the wheel" of model state legislation. To that end, and in an effort to improve uniformity and the adoption of effective policies nationwide, the committee recommends:

Recommendation 7-1: The National Conference of State Legislatures should draft model legislation to provide benchmarks for states that seek to reduce alcohol-impaired driving fatalities.

This would allow states that choose to adopt various policies or laws to reduce alcohol-impaired driving to do so based on the best available evidence, or to update policies or laws currently in place to ensure they are as effective as possible. States often adapt model laws to ensure they are consistent with state laws and community needs and resources and such model legislation has been developed for alcohol-impaired driving policies in the past. For example, model legislation published in 1984 was developed for administrative license suspension (NHTSA, 1986). The National Conference of State Legislatures could provide updated legislation for this law and new model legislation for a number of other laws, including policies regarding DWI look-back periods, limits on plea agreements and diversion programs, child endangerment laws, open container laws, and use of electronic warrants, among others.

Multisector Collaboration

Alcohol policy, and by extension policy approaches for reducing alcohol-impaired driving, is often not housed in one particular place in state or federal government because the responsibility for regulating alcohol is spread across government agencies. To address this, Congress mandated in the Sober Truth on Preventing Underage Drinking Act of 2006[12] the creation of an Interagency Coordinating Committee on the Prevention of Underage Drinking (ICCPUD), composed of the heads of 15 government agencies and others as needed. In the past, the creation of federally appointed committees to address alcohol-impaired driving has been a catalyst for action. For example, the Presidential Commission on Drunk Driving, convened in 1982, and its successor, the National Commission Against Drunk Driving, both contributed to public policy development around impaired driving (Fell and Voas, 2006) in the 1980s. A new, multisector group is needed to coordinate and reinvigorate progress to reduce alcohol-impaired driving fatalities. A comprehensive approach will require the cooperation and expertise of the U.S. Departments of the Treasury, Transportation, Health and Human Services, and Justice, and other federal agencies. In the case of underage drinking, Congress mandated in legislation the creation of the ICCPUD. Ideally, such a coordinating body on alcohol-impaired driving can be created without a congressional mandate. To this end, the committee recommends:

[12] Public Law 109-422.

Recommendation 7-2: The National Highway Traffic Safety Administration should create a federal interagency coordinating committee to develop and oversee an integrated strategy for reducing alcohol-impaired driving, ensure collaboration, maintain accountability, and share information among organizations committed to reducing alcohol-impaired driving.

A federal interagency coordinating committee could include

- U.S. Department of Health and Human Services—Centers for Disease Control and Prevention, Substance Abuse and Mental Health Services Administration, Indian Health Service, National Institutes of Health;
- Alcohol and Tobacco Tax and Trade Bureau;
- U.S. Department of Transportation—National Highway Traffic Safety Administration, Federal Highway Administration;
- U.S. Department of Homeland Security (emergency services sector);
- U.S. Department of Justice;
- U.S. Department of Defense; and
- U.S. Department of Veterans Affairs.

The interagency committee could convene other stakeholders such as private philanthropy, schools, hospitals, public health, health care, the hospitality/restaurant industry, payers, medical insurers, and trial lawyers to further maintain accountability and transparency by sharing information.

Funding and Organizational Commitment

The majority of this chapter focuses on community action and the need for a renewed social movement. The history of MADD included critical investment by NHTSA early on in what at the time likely appeared as a promising but unproven community-based strategy. The history of tobacco control has demonstrated the importance of a demonstration project approach to build capacity within the field, establish the feasibility of effective approaches, and contribute to a paradigm shift both in social norms and in policy environments far beyond where the demonstration projects initially occurred. Based on extensive evidence and experience in the use of community coalitions both in the alcohol field and in other areas of public health, the committee recommends:

Recommendation 7-3: The National Highway Traffic Safety Administration, other federal partners, and private funding

sources free of conflicts of interest should support training, technical assistance, and demonstration projects in the implementation of effective strategies, including policy changes, for reducing alcohol-impaired driving.

Such an approach should create an infrastructure for change. At a minimum, it would combine one or more coordinating centers providing training, technical assistance, and ongoing coaching with demonstration project sites in a diverse array of states and settings situated, for example, within state health or transportation departments with existing infrastructures that can promote sustainability when the funding expires. As was the case with the ASSIST project, there should also be funding for careful scientific evaluation of this effort, so lessons learned may be captured and translated into health and safety policies and practices across the country. Beyond this minimal approach, there is a great need for the funding of stronger advocacy organizations and of media infrastructures that can support the kind of countermarketing that has been so effective in promoting effective tobacco control. Dedicated funding streams for some of these activities could come from earmarked taxes on alcohol itself. However, the need for funding for effective advocacy and education of policy makers points to the importance of complementing public funding with initiatives from private philanthropy that are commensurate in size with the scale of the problem of alcohol-impaired driving in the United States.

Social movements can be powerful catalysts for change. MADD changed the landscape regarding alcohol-impaired driving in the 1980s. Their efforts led to decades of reductions in deaths on the nation's roadways. The end of that decline should be a powerful motivation to generate a social movement that can "finish the job" that MADD so ably began. Such a movement should bring together an unprecedentedly broad array of stakeholders, build on the lessons of past efforts, integrate and take advantage of emerging technologies and practices, and engage states and the federal government in a new "race to the bottom": a race to zero alcohol-related fatalities on our roadways by the year 2030.

CONCLUDING OBSERVATIONS

This chapter largely explores strategies and approaches that address the overarching social, economic, political, legal, and physical context that is identified in the committee's conceptual framework (see Figure 1-5). As emphasized throughout the report, generating sustained action requires comprehensive approaches that target multiple levels, including communities and the media environment. Furthermore, traditional and novel stakeholders need to be engaged in efforts to reduce alcohol-impaired driving fatalities to fulfill their various accountabilities. With support for and creation of innovative projects, multisector collaboration, benchmarks to guide states, and stakeholder engagement, the vision of zero deaths from alcohol-impaired driving fatalities will be attainable.

REFERENCES

Ad Council. n.d. *Drunk driving prevention.* https://www.adcouncil.org/Our-Campaigns/The-Classics/Drunk-Driving-Prevention (accessed November 27, 2017).

Aguilar, M., and H. Delehanty. 2009. *A social marketing initiative to reduce impaired motorcycle operation.* DOT HS 811 095. Washington, DC: National Highway Traffic Safety Administration.

Aguirre-Molina, M., and D. M. Gorman. 1996. Community-based approaches for the prevention of alcohol, tobacco, and other drug use. *Annual Review of Public Health* 17:337–358.

Alley, D. E., C. N. Asomugha, P. H. Conway, and D. M. Sanghavi. 2016. Accountable health communities—addressing social needs through Medicare and Medicaid. *New England Journal of Medicine* 374:8–11.

Anderson, P., and J. Rehm. 2016. Evaluating alcohol industry action to reduce the harmful use of alcohol. *Alcohol and Alcoholism* 51(4):383–387.

Asbridge, M. 2004. Public place restrictions on smoking in Canada: Assessing the role of the state, media, science and public health advocacy. *Social Science & Medicine* 58(1):13–24.

Babor, T., K. Robaina, and J. Noel. 2018. *The role of the alcohol industry in policy interventions for alcohol-impaired driving.* Paper commissioned by the Committee on Accelerating Progress to Reduce Alcohol-Impaired Driving Fatalities (see Appendix C).

Bail, C. A. 2016. Combining natural language processing and network analysis to examine how advocacy organizations stimulate conversation on social media. *Proceedings of the National Academy of Sciences of the United States of America* 113(42):11823–11828.

Benjamin, G., M. Fallon, P. E. Jarris, and P. Libbey. 2006. *Final recommendations for a voluntary national accreditation program for state and local public health departments.* Alexandria, VA: Public Health Accreditation Board.

Butterfoss, F. D. 2007. *Coalitions and partnerships in community health.* San Francisco, CA: Jossey-Bass.

Butterfoss, F. D., R. M. Goodman, and A. Wandersman. 1993. Community coalitions for prevention and health promotion. *Health Education Research* 8(3):315–330.

CADCA (Community Anti-Drug Coalitions of America). n.d. *Prevent impaired driving: A CADCA toolkit: About the toolkit.* http://www.preventimpaireddriving.org/about-the-tool-kit/about-the-toolkit (accessed August 22, 2017).

CDC (Centers for Disease Control and Prevention). 2006. *History of the Surgeon General's reports on smoking and health.* https://www.cdc.gov/tobacco/data_statistics/sgr/history/index.htm (accessed December 5, 2017).

Chapman, S., and D. Lupton. 1994. *Fight for public health: Principles and practice of media advocacy.* London: BMJ Books.

Chavis, D. M. 2001. The paradoxes and promise of community coalitions. *American Journal of Community Psychology* 29(2):309–320.

Clark, L. S., and R. Marchi. 2017. *Young people and the future of news: Social media and the rise of connective journalism.* Cambridge, UK: Cambridge University Press.

Cox, E., and S. Fisher. 2009. Drinking on the dirt roads of America: NACCHO's impaired driving prevention in rural communities demonstration site project. *Journal of Public Health Management Practice* 15(3):278–280.

Cramer, M. E., J. R. Atwood, and J. A. Stoner. 2006. A conceptual model for understanding effective coalitions involved in health promotion programing. *Public Health Nursing* 23(1):67–73.

DeJong, W. 1996. MADD Massachusetts versus Senator Burke: A media advocacy case study. *Health Education Quarterly* 23(3):318–329.
D'Onofrio, G., L. C. Degutis, J. S. Ahluwalia, and J. H. Samet. 2005. Physician involvement in community coalitions to prevent substance abuse. *Substance Abuse* 25(2):1–4.
Dorfman, L. 2003. Studying the news on public health: How content analysis supports media advocacy. *American Journal of Health Behavior* 27(1):217–226.
Dorfman, L., and I. D. Krasnow. 2014. Public health and media advocacy. *Annual Review of Public Health* 35:293–306.
Dorfman, L., L. Wallack, and K. Woodruff. 2005. More than a message: Framing public health advocacy to change corporate practices. *Health Education and Behavior* 32(3):320–336.
Duke, J. D. 2007. *Truth®: Spreading the infections.* Paper read at NCI/NIDA Sponsored Conference on Adolescent Tobacco Use at National Institutes of Health, Bethesda, MD.
Esser, M. B., H. Waters, M. Smart, and D. H. Jernigan. 2016. Impact of Maryland's 2011 alcohol sales tax increase on alcoholic beverage sales. *American Journal of Drug and Alcohol Abuse* 42(4):404–411.
EuroCare Institute of Alcohol Studies and Monash University. 2015. *Alcohol advertising and sponsorship in formula one: A dangerous cocktail.* http://eurocare.org/resources/eurocare_papers_and_publications/2015/alcohol_advertising_and_sponsorship_in_formula_one_a_dangerous_cocktail (accessed October 10, 2017).
Fell, J. C., and R. B. Voas. 2006. Mothers Against Drunk Driving (MADD): The first 25 years. *Traffic Injury Prevention* 7(3):195–212.
Fell, J. C., D. A. Fisher, and S. McKnight. 2011. *A guide for local impaired driving task forces,* Vol. I: Final report. DOT HS 811 460a. Washington, DC: National Highway Traffic Safety Administration.
Fisher, D. A. 2018. *Content analysis of alcohol-impaired driving stories in the news.* Paper commissioned by the Committee on Accelerating Progress to Reduce Alcohol-Impaired Driving Fatalities (see Appendix B).
Getz, K. 1997. Research in corporate political activity: Integration and assessment. *Business and Society* 36:32–77.
Gibson, T. A. 2010. The limits of media advocacy. *Communication, Culture & Critique* 3(1):44–65.
Glascoff, M. A., J. S. Shrader, and R. K. Haddock. 2013. Friends don't let friends drive drunk, but do they let friends drive high? *Journal of Alcohol and Drug Education* 57(1):66–84.
Goodwin, A., L. Thomas, B. Kirley, W. Hall, N. O'Brien, and K. Hill. 2015. *Countermeasures that work: A highway safety countermeasure guide for state highway safety offices*, 8th ed. DOT HS 812 202. Washington, DC: National Highway Traffic Safety Administration.
Greenfield, T. K., and R. Room. 1997. Situational norms for drinking and drunkeness: Trends in the US adult population, 1979–1990. *Addiction* 92(1):33–47.
Harwood, E. M., J. C. Witson, D. P. Fan, and A. C. Wagenaar. 2005. Media advocacy and underage drinking policies: A study of Louisiana news media from 1994 through 2003. *Health Promotion Practice* 6(3):246–257.
Hawkins, J. D., S. Oesterle, E. C. Brown, R. D. Abbott, and R. F. Catalano. 2014. Youth problem behaviors 8 years after implementing the communities that care prevention system: A community-randomized trial. *JAMA Pediatrics* 168(2):122–129.
Healthy People. 2017. *Healthy People 2020: Substance abuse objectives.* https://www.healthypeople.gov/2020/topics-objectives/topic/substance-abuse/objectives (accessed October 2, 2017).
HHS (U.S. Department of Health and Human Services). 1989. *Surgeon General's workshop on drunk driving: Proceedings.* Rockville, MD: Office of the Surgeon General.
Hillman, A., A. Zardkoohi, and L. Bierman. 1999. Corporate political strategies and firm performance: Indications of firm-specific benefits from personal service in the U.S. government. *Strategic Management Journal* 20(1):67–81.

Holder, H. D., and A. J. Treno. 1997. Media advocacy in community prevention: News as a means to advance policy change. *Addiction* 92(Suppl 2):S189–S199.

Horn, B. P., J. J. McCluskey, and R. C. Mittelhammer. 2014. Quantifying bias in driving-under-the-influence enforcement. *Economic Inquiry* 52(1):269–284.

Howard, T., and T. Norris. 2015. *Can hospitals heal America's communities? All in mission is the emerging model impact.* Takoma Park, MD: The Democracy Collaborative.

IOM (Institute of Medicine). 2011. *For the public's health: The role of measurement in action and accountability.* Washington, DC: The National Academies Press.

IOM. 2014. *Supporting a movement for health and health equity: Lessons from social movements: Workshop summary.* Washington, DC: The National Academies Press.

Iyengar, S. 1991. *Is anyone responsible? How television frames political issues.* Chicago, IL: University of Chicago Press.

Iyengar, S. 1996. Framing responsibility for political issues. *Annals of the American Academy of Political and Social Science* 546:59–70.

Jernigan, D. 2009. The global alcohol industry: An overview. *Addiction* 104(Suppl 1):6–12.

Jernigan, D., and T. Babor. 2015. The concentration of the global alcohol industry and its penetration in the African region. *Addiction* 110(4):551–560.

Jernigan, D., and H. Waters. 2009. *The potential benefits of alcohol excise tax increases in Maryland.* Baltimore, MD: Johns Hopkins Bloomberg School of Public Health.

Jernigan, D. H., and P. A. Wright. 1996. Media advocacy: Lessons from community experiences. *Journal of Public Health Policy* 17(3):281–288.

Lane, C. H., and M. I. Carter. 2012. The role of evidence-based media advocacy in the promotion of tobacco control policies. *Salud Publica de Mexico* 54(3):281–288.

Lavoie, M.-C., P. Langenberg, A. Villaveces, P. C. Dischinger, L. Simoni-Wastila, K. Hoke, and G. S. Smith. 2017. Effect of Maryland's 2011 alcohol sales tax increase on alcohol-positive driving. *American Journal of Preventive Medicine* 53(1):17–24.

MADD (Mothers Against Drunk Driving). 2017. *Increase in traffic fatalities highlights need for strong ignition interlock laws: Safety council recommendations support MADD's push for all-offender laws in every state.* https://www.madd.org/blog/press-release/increase-in-traffic-fatalities-highlights-need-for-strong-ignition-interlock-laws (accessed December 4, 2017).

Masters, B., and T. Osborn. 2010. Social movements and philanthropy: How foundations can support movement building. *The Foundation Review* 2(2):12–27.

McCombs, M., and A. Reynolds. 2009. How the news shapes our civic agenda. In *Media effects: Advances in theory and research,* edited by J. Bryant and M. Oliver. New York: Taylor and Francis.

McCombs, M., and D. L. Shaw. 1972. The agenda-setting function of mass media. *Public Opinion Quarterly* 36(2):176–187.

McKetin, R., A. Coen, and S. Kaye. 2015. A comprehensive review of the effects of mixing caffeinated energy drinks with alcohol. *Drug and Alcohol Dependence* 151:15–30.

Mosher, J. F., and D. H. Jernigan. 1989. New directions in alcohol policy. *Annual Review of Public Health* 10:245–279.

NASEM (National Academies of Sciences, Engineering, and Medicine). 2017. *Communities in action: Pathways to health equity.* Washington, DC: The National Academies Press.

NCI (National Cancer Institute). 2006. *Evaluating ASSIST: A blueprint for understanding state-level tobacco control.* NIH publication 06–6058. Bethesda, MD: National Cancer Institute.

NHTSA (National Highway Traffic Safety Administration). 1986. *Reducing highway crashes through administrative license revocation.* Washington, DC: U.S. Department of Transportation.

Niederdeppe, J., M. C. Farrelly, and D. Wenter. 2007. Media advocacy, tobacco control policy change and teen smoking in Florida. *Tobacco Control* 16:47–52.

NRC (National Research Council) and IOM. 2004. *Reducing underage drinking: A collective responsibility.* Washington, DC: The National Academies Press.
Pechmann, C., L. Levine, S. Loughlin, and F. Leslie. 2005. Impulsive and self-conscious: Adolescents' vulnerability to advertising and promotion. *Journal of Public Policy and Marketing* 24(2):202–221.
Pew Research Center. 2017. *Newspapers fact sheet.* http://www.journalism.org/fact-sheet/newspapers (accessed October 12, 2017).
Ramirez, R. L., and D. H. Jernigan. 2017. Increasing alcohol taxes: Analysis of case studies from Illinois, Maryland, and Massachusetts. *Journal of Studies on Alcohol and Drugs* 78(5):763–770.
Raynor, J. 2011. *What makes an effective coalition: Evidence-based indicators of success.* Los Angeles: The California Endowment.
Redelmeier, D. A., and A. S. Detsky. 2017. Clinical action against drunk driving. *PLoS Medicine* 14(2):e1002231.
Reinarman, C. 1988. The social construction of an alcohol problem. *Theory and Society* 17(1):91–120.
Rock, M. J., L. McIntyre, S. A. Persaud, and K. L. Thomas. 2011. A media advocacy intervention linking health disparities and food insecurity. *Health Education Research* 26(6):948–960.
Ross, H. L. 1997. The rise and fall of drunk driving as a social problem in the USA. Paper read at 14th International Conference on Alcohol, Drugs, and Traffic Safety, September 21–26, 1997, Annecy, France.
Rousseau, D. M., and G. P. Pezzullo. 2013. Race and context in the criminal labeling of drunk driving offenders: A multilevel examination of extralegal variables on discretionary plea decisions. *Criminal Justice Policy Review* 25(6):683–702.
Russell, A., R. B. Voas, W. DeJong, and M. Chaloupka. 1995. MADD rates the states: A media advocacy event to advance the agenda against alcohol-impaired driving. *Public Health Reports* 110(3):240–245.
Saxton, G. D., J. N. Niyirora, C. Guo, and R. D. Waters. 2015. #advocatingforchange: The strategic use of hashtags in social media advocacy. *Advances in Social Work* 16(1):154–169.
Schooler, C., S. S. Sundar, and J. Flora. 1996. Effects of the Stanford five-city project media advocacy program. *Health Education Quarterly* 23(3):346–364.
Schuler, D. 1996. Corporate political strategy and foreign competition: The case of the steel industry. *Academy of Management Journal* 39(3):720–737.
Sheehey-Church, C. 2017. *Testimony of Colleen Sheehey-Church, national president, Mothers Against Drunk Driving, to United States Senate Committee on Commerce, Science, and Transportation. Paving the way for self-driving vehicles.* https://www.commerce.senate.gov/public/_cache/files/d1c28b83-2dca-42e8-aabc-b2755718c1d3/BC6FD6634C9510727ECFECCAE30EE620.colleen-sheehey-church---testimony.pdf (accessed December 4, 2017).
Shults, R. A., R. W. Elder, J. L. Nichols, D. A. Sleet, R. Compton, S. K. Chattopadhyay, and Community Preventive Services Task Force. 2009. Effectiveness of multicomponent programs with community mobilization for reducing alcohol-impaired driving. *American Journal of Preventive Medicine* 37(4):360–371.
Slater, M. D., K. Kelly, and R. Edwards. 2000. Integrating social marketing, community readiness and media advocacy in community-based prevention efforts. *Social Marketing Quarterly* 6(3):124–137.
Stead, M., G. Hastings, and D. Eadie. 2002. The challenge of evaluating complex interventions: A framework for evaluating media advocacy. *Health Education Research* 17(3): 351–364.

Stillman, F. A., K. A. Cronin, W. D. Evans, and A. Ulasevich. 2001. Can media advocacy influence newspaper coverage of tobacco: Measuring the effectiveness of the American Stop Smoking Intervention Study's (ASSIST) media advocacy strategies. *Tobacco Control* 10:137–144.

Striley, C. W., and S. R. Kahn. 2014. Review of the energy drink literature from 2013: Findings continue to support most risk from mixing with alcohol. *Current Opinions in Psychiatry* 27(4):263–268.

Texas A&M Transportation Institute. 2016. *Texas Impaired Driving Task Force*. https://www.dyingtodrink.org/about/texas-impaired-driving-task-force (accessed August 24, 2017).

Treno, A. J., L. Breed, H. H. D., P. Roeper, B. A. Thomas, and P. D. Gruenewald. 1996. Evaluation of media advocacy efforts within a community trial to reduce alcohol-involved injury. *Evaluation Review* 20(4):404–423.

Tufekci, Z. 2017. How social media changed protest forever. In *Twitter and tear gas: The power and fragility of networked protest*. New Haven, CT: Yale University Press.

Wagenaar, A. C., J. P. Gehan, R. Jones-Webb, T. Toomey, J. L. Forster, M. Wolfson, and D. M. Murray. 1999. Communities mobilizing for change on alcohol: Lessons and results from a 15-community randomized trial. *Journal of Community Psychology* 27(3):315–326.

Wagenaar, A. C., D. M. Murray, and T. L. Toomey. 2000. Communities mobilizing for change on alcohol (CMCA): Effects of a randomized trial on arrests and traffic crashes. *Addiction* 95(2):209–217.

Wakefield, M., K. Clegg Smith, and S. Chapman. 2005. Framing of Australian newspaper coverage of a secondhand smoke injury claim: Lessons for media advocacy. *Critical Public Health* 15(1):53–63.

Walder, A. G. 2009. Political sociology and social movements. *Annual Review of Sociology* 35(1):393–412.

Wallack, L., and L. Dorfman. 1996. Media advocacy: A strategy for advancing policy and promoting health. *Health Education Quarterly* 23(3):293–317.

Wallack, L., L. Dorfman, D. Jernigan, and M. Themba-Nixon. 1993. *Media advocacy and public health: Power for prevention*. Newbury Park, CA: Sage.

Wallack, L., K. Woodruff, L. Dorfman, and I. Diaz. 1999. *News for a change: An advocate's guide to working with the media*. Newbury Park, CA: Sage.

Wallerstein, N., and E. Bernstein. 1994. Introduction to community empowerment, participatory education, and health. *Health Education Quarterly* 21(2):141–148.

Weitzman, E. R., T. F. Nelson, H. Lee, and H. Wechsler. 2004. Reducing drinking and related harms in college: Evaluation of the "a matter of degree" program. *American Journal of Preventive Medicine* 27(3):187–196.

WHO (World Health Organization). 2010. *Global strategy to reduce the harmful use of alcohol*. Geneva, Switzerland: World Health Organization.

Wolfson, M. 1995. The legislative impact of social movement organizations: The anti-drunken-driving movement and the 21-year-old drinking age. *Social Science Quarterly* 76(2):311–327.

Woodruff, K. 1996. Alcohol advertising and violence against women: A media advocacy case study. *Health Education Quarterly* 23(3):330–345.

Wyatt, R., M. Laderman, L. Botwinick, K. Mate, and J. Whittington. 2016. *Achieving health equity: A guide for health care organizations*. Cambridge, MA: Institute for Healthcare Improvement.

Yanovitzky, I. 2002a. Effect of news coverage on the prevalence of drunk-driving behavior: Evidence from a longitudinal study. *Journal of Studies on Alcohol* 63(3):342–351.

Yanovitzky, I. 2002b. Effects of news coverage on policy attention and actions: A closer look into the media-policy connection. *Communication Research* 29(4):422–451.

8

Conclusion

Despite years of progress in the United States, alcohol-impaired driving remains a major preventable public health and safety issue. Over the past 10 years progress has stalled, and for the past 2 years the number of alcohol-impaired fatalities has increased. Alcohol-impaired driving crashes cost the nation billions of dollars in terms of loss of life, injury and disability, lost productivity, and social and economic consequences, and it needs to become a priority issue across stakeholders and sectors. Changes in the social, economic, technological, and clinical arenas have opened up new opportunities to take action on this multifaceted problem. A renewed and comprehensive approach is needed to successfully reduce serious injuries and fatalities. Furthermore, a one-size-fits-all approach will not suffice, as U.S. states make up a patchwork of different existing policies, needs, and resources. Vision Zero, a philosophy that is grounded in the belief that no death caused by a motor vehicle crash is acceptable, provides a framework to engage novel stakeholders and a system with the goal of eliminating alcohol-impaired traffic fatalities. With this philosophy, each alcohol-impaired driver represents a system failure.

With this vision in mind, the committee examined the causes and consequences of alcohol-impaired driving and delineated the most promising and evidence-based solutions to employ. This report begins with an update on the burden of alcohol-impaired driving crashes (see Chapters 1 and 2) and delves into the complex factors that shape alcohol-impaired driving including the current alcohol and driving environments (see Chapter 2). Using the committee's conceptual framework (see Figure 8-1) as a guiding schema, the report then discusses interventions (i.e., programs, policies,

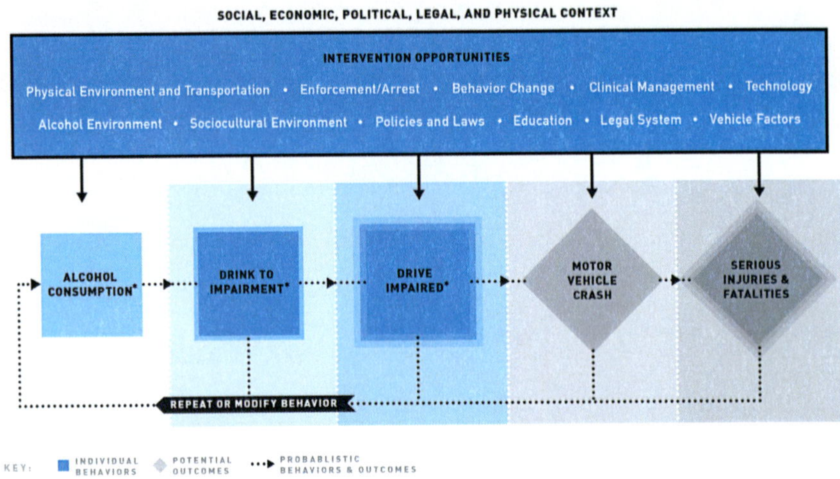

FIGURE 8-1 Preventing alcohol-impaired driving crash fatalities conceptual framework.
NOTES: Each of the phases in this figure represents an opportunity to intervene and prevent alcohol-impaired driving fatalities. A square denotes a behavior, a diamond denotes an outcome, and dotted lines denote potential progression to an outcome. Extra layers around a square or a diamond denote increased likelihood or increased severity, respectively. The asterisks signify that there are alternative behaviors not represented in the three first phases that would preclude an alcohol-impaired driving fatality (e.g., not drinking or not drinking to the level of impairment).

and systems) to be used at the various phases of an alcohol-impaired driving crash: alcohol consumption and drinking to the point of impairment (see Chapter 3); driving while impaired (see Chapter 4); and postcrash and/or arrest (see Chapter 5). These interventions target multiple levels identified in the socioecological model (see Figure 1-6). The report then examines the current state of data and surveillance systems for alcohol-impaired driving and makes recommendations on how to improve the comprehensiveness and accessibility of data (see Chapter 6). Finally, the report explores the strategies and tools needed to generate action and discusses the roles of a few important stakeholders (see Chapter 7).

As illustrated in the committee's conceptual framework, there are intervention opportunities across multiple sectors and disciplines. When interventions are implemented collectively, they can achieve the vision of zero alcohol-impaired driving fatalities. These cross-cutting relationships are visible in the synergies of the interventions that the committee recommends throughout the report. For example, some of the drinking-oriented policies discussed in Chapter 3 that address illegal sales require public support and enhanced enforcement efforts to be most effective. Other strategies, including those related to taxation, outlet density, or hours of sale, do not depend on law enforcement and have population-level impact and therefore the potential for a large impact if prioritized. A systematic approach to addressing the alcohol environment would engage policy makers, alcoholic beverage control agencies, public health agencies, local law enforcement agencies, alcohol retailers, the legal community, and potentially other local institutions such as schools, health care systems, small businesses, local development agencies, and faith-based institutions.

Chapter 4 also illustrates the interdependent nature of interventions to reduce alcohol-impaired driving in the discussion of sobriety checkpoints. These enforcement activities are effective when the public is aware of them and the perceived risk of apprehension while driving impaired is significant. For example, the implementation of a lower blood alcohol concentration (BAC) limit set by state law will require publicity through media campaigns and visible enforcement to change norms. In addition, if the Driver Alcohol Detection System for Safety (DADSS) comes to market, it is unique in that it is a prevention technology that once in place will not require enforcement; however, it will require a successful media campaign to inform the public on what it is and why it is important. Furthermore, readily available data on high-risk areas and intersections or place-of-last-drink for driving while impaired (DWI) offenders would inform targeted enforcement interventions such as sobriety checkpoints.

Other recommendations would have an increased effect among specific populations when implemented in conjunction with each other. For example, for alcohol-impaired drivers with alcohol use disorder (AUD), a system such as DWI courts to engage high-rate recidivists or high BAC offenders could address the underlying causes of their behaviors. Moreover, if court-appointed practitioners use evidence-based evaluation and treatment practices, this would increase the likelihood that the individual will not repeat the offense. Importantly, many of the alcohol-impaired driving interventions in the report would also address drug-impaired driving, a growing public health and safety issue. For example, enhanced resources for law enforcement—trained to identify general impairment in drivers—to conduct frequent and publicized sobriety checkpoints and proper treatment of AUD would likely improve apprehension, deterrence, and treatment of individuals who drive under the influence of drugs. In summary, the synergies of the interventions discussed throughout the report need to be taken into account by policy and decision makers as they create a comprehensive plan for their state or locality. Implementing these interventions in combination would also permit the development of improved evidence to inform the optimal mix of policies and interventions in the long term.

Rural areas are at particularly high risk, as interventions applicable in urban areas may be less practical in rural settings. A comprehensive approach that involves multiple sectors will be important to address the disproportionate number of fatalities in rural areas. For example, primary seat belt laws and enforcement, improved road design, improved emergency response, lower BAC limits set by state law, increased alcohol taxes, and use of ignition interlocks (and eventually DADSS), among other interventions, have the potential to be effective in rural areas when used together.

Applying a Vision Zero approach wherein every stakeholder has an opportunity and responsibility to take action and hold others accountable will help sustain comprehensive solutions for alcohol-impaired driving. Throughout the report, the roles of specific stakeholders are identified. For instance, Chapter 3 highlights the role of alcohol law enforcement agencies in monitoring and enforcing violations to reduce illegal sales to already-intoxicated adults and underage persons. Chapter 4 discusses the role of local departments of transportation in promoting the availability and affordability of alternative transportation options for individuals who drink alcohol. Chapter 7 outlines the role of the health sector, including public health, in providing care to individuals at risk for impaired driving, supplying data, and convening important stakeholders. Table 8-1 categorizes the interventions that are discussed in this report as evidence based or promising and identifies the important stakeholders and time frame for implementation.[1] Collectively, the committee's conclusions and recommendations offer a blueprint for stakeholders across many sectors to take part in reducing alcohol-impaired driving fatalities.

Conclusion 8-1: To achieve the goal of zero alcohol-related crash fatalities, a systematic multipronged approach with clear roles and accountabilities across sectors (including public health, transportation, law enforcement, and health care providers, among others) is needed.

This comprehensive multisector approach has the potential to renew progress and save lives from alcohol-impaired driving crashes.

[1] Time frame (approximations of when these interventions could be in place): short term is 0–2 years, midterm is 3–10 years; long term is 10 years or more.

TABLE 8-1 Tools and Stakeholders to Accelerate Progress to Reduce Alcohol-Impaired Driving Fatalities

Alcohol Consumption and Drinking to Impairment		
Evidence-based	Increase alcohol taxes	**Stakeholders:** *State and federal governments; alcohol producers; consumers; community coalitions **Time frame:** short term
	Implement policies to address physical availability of alcohol	**Stakeholders:** *Local and state governments; alcohol producers; hospitality and retail sectors; community coalitions **Time frame:** short term
	Implement policies to reduce illegal sales of alcohol	**Stakeholders:** *Local, state, and federal governments; alcohol producers; hospitality and retail sectors; community coalitions **Time frame:** short term
	Regulate alcohol marketing	**Stakeholders:** *Local, state, and federal governments; alcohol producers; hospitality and retail sectors; media (television, radio, print, social media); community coalitions **Time frame:** short term
Driving While Impaired		
Evidence-based	Lower BAC per se laws to 0.05%	**Stakeholders:** *State and federal governments; law enforcement; news media/advertising (television, radio, print, social media); alcohol producers; hospitality and retail sectors; public/consumers; community coalitions **Time frame:** short term
	Conduct frequent, publicized sobriety checkpoints	**Stakeholders:** *Local and state governments; law enforcement, news media/advertising (television, radio, print, social media) **Time frame:** short term
	Universal primary seat belt laws	**Stakeholders:** *Local and state governments; law enforcement; public/consumers **Time frame:** short term

continued

TABLE 8-1 Continued

Promising	Future use of DADSS	**Stakeholders:** *NHTSA; automobile industry; automobile insurance industry; Congress; health insurers **Time frame:** long term
	Increase availability of transportation alternatives	**Stakeholders:** *Local government; transportation sector; hospitality and retail sectors; news media/advertising (television, radio, print, social media); public/consumers; private sector **Time frame:** short term
	Postcrash and/or Arrest	
Evidence-based	Evaluation and treatment of binge drinking and AUD (e.g., SBIRT, CBT, medication-assisted therapy)	**Stakeholders:** *Health care sector; *health insurers; *state government; law enforcement; legal sector **Time frame:** short term to midterm
	Implement DWI courts using standards set by National Center for DWI Courts	**Stakeholders:** *Legal sector; law enforcement; National Center for DWI Courts; victims' rights organizations (e.g., MADD) **Time frame:** short term to midterm
	Increased use of ignition interlocks and extended monitoring periods	**Stakeholders:** *State governments; legal sector; law enforcement **Time frame:** short term
Promising	Improving administrative license suspension/revocation laws	**Stakeholders:** *Local, state, and federal governments; law enforcement; legal sector **Time frame:** short term
	Coordinated and continuous learning trauma care system	**Stakeholders:** *Health care sector; law enforcement **Time frame:** short term to midterm
	Professional education and training (judiciary, law enforcement, health professionals)	**Stakeholders:** *Law enforcement; *legal sector; *health care sector; state and local public health **Time frame:** short term to midterm
	Limits on diversion programs and plea agreements	**Stakeholders:** *Research sector; legal sector; law enforcement **Time frame:** short term
	Use of systems alcohol monitoring programs	**Stakeholders:** *Law enforcement; legal sector; local and state government **Time frame:** short term to midterm

TABLE 8-1 Continued

Tools for Addressing the Social, Economic, Political, Legal, and Physical Context		
System-level interventions	Systematic approach to alcohol law enforcement	**Stakeholders:** *Law enforcement; health care sector, local and state government **Time frame:** short term
	Ensure timely, standardized, and accessible data on alcohol-impaired driving with strategic dissemination to the public, and explore big data opportunities	**Stakeholders:** *NHTSA **Time frame:** short term
	Convening of diverse stakeholders to create and maintain a metrics dashboard for alcohol-impaired driving	**Stakeholders:** *NHTSA; academia/research; law enforcement; state and local public health; transportation sector; other federal agencies as needed **Time frame:** short term
	Publish brief, visually appealing quarterly and annual reports that analyze and interpret progress in reducing alcohol-impaired driving	**Stakeholders:** *NHTSA; academia/research; law enforcement; state and local public health; transportation sector; other federal agencies as needed; news media/advertising (television, radio, print, social media) **Time frame:** short term
	Funding and support for community-level demonstration projects	**Stakeholders:** *NHTSA; other federal agencies as needed; private funders **Time frame:** short term
	Create interagency coordinating committee on alcohol-impaired driving	**Stakeholders:** *NHTSA; other DOT agencies as needed; HHS; TTB; DHS; DOJ; NIH; IHS; other federal agencies as needed; state and local governments **Time frame:** short term
	Development of model legislation from NCSL	**Stakeholders:** *National Conference of State Legislatures; NHTSA; state governments **Time frame:** short term to midterm
	Update Healthy People 2030 objectives for alcohol-impaired driving fatalities	**Stakeholders:** *HHS; other federal agencies as needed **Time frame:** short term

continued

TABLE 8-1 Continued

NOTES: Stakeholders marked with an asterisk are the primary actor(s) responsible for initiating action for the intervention. The rows shaded in gray are report conclusions and those in white are recommendations. The committee applied the Healthy People 2020 typology to inform the classification of evidence-based, promising, and emerging tools in this table. Time frame (approximations of when these interventions could be in place): short term is 0–2 years, midterm is 3–10 years; long term is 10 years or more. In some cases, the time horizon may be longer depending on the length of time it takes for a bill to be passed and signed into law. AUD = alcohol use disorder; CBT = cognitive behavioral therapy; DADSS = Driver Alcohol Detection System for Safety; DHS = U.S. Department of Homeland Security; DOJ = U.S. Department of Justice; DOT = U.S. Department of Transportation; DWI = driving while impaired; HHS = U.S. Department of Health and Human Services; IHS = Indian Health Service; NCSL = National Conference of State Legislators; NHTSA = National Highway Traffic Safety Administration; NIH = National Institutes of Health; SBIRT = screening, brief intervention, and referral to treatment; TTB = Alcohol and Tobacco Tax and Trade Bureau.

REFERENCE

Secretary's Advisory Committee on National Health Promotion and Disease Prevention Objectives for 2020. 2010. *Evidence-based clinical and public health: Generating and applying the evidence.* http://www.healthypeople.gov/2010/hp2020/advisory/pdfs/EvidenceBasedClinicalPH2010.pdf (accessed October 5, 2017).

A

Alcohol-Impaired Driving in the United States: Review of Data Sources and Analyses[1]

Charles DiMaggio, Ph.D., M.P.H.,
Katherine Wheeler-Martin, M.P.H., and Jamie Oliver

SUMMARY[2]

The consequences of alcohol-impaired driving continue to affect the United States. A review of the current literature and analyses of recent data indicate a need for renewed surveillance across the spectrum of potential interventions, including law enforcement, engineering and technology, education and behavioral change, built environment, enactment and evaluation of policies, and emergency trauma care. Among these so-called *E*s of motor vehicle crash injury prevention, alcohol itself (ethanol) remains critically important. There has been considerable success in addressing the role alcohol plays in motor vehicle crash injury risk in the United States, but alcohol has been persistently present in nearly a quarter of fatal crashes for the past two decades. Initial decreases of

[1] This background paper was commissioned at the direction of the Committee on Accelerating Progress to Reduce Alcohol-Impaired Driving Fatalities to offer insight into the data and surveillance systems that could inform alcohol-impaired driving interventions in the United States. In addition, this paper provides the descriptive epidemiology of fatal and nonfatal alcohol-involved crashes in the United States over time, describes trends in patterns of alcohol consumption and alcohol-impaired driving over time, and identifies the strengths and weaknesses of existing data sources that inform this epidemiology.

[2] This is an abridged version of the paper. A full version including all tables and figures can be found in the public access file for the Committee on Accelerating Progress to Reduce Alcohol-Impaired Driving Fatalities. Available by request from the National Academies of Sciences, Engineering, and Medicine's Public Access Records Office (PARO@nas.edu).

30 to 40 percent dating from the 1990s have slowed to 5 to 10 percent or leveled off entirely.

Law enforcement has been, and remains, a cornerstone of alcohol-impaired driving control and prevention, but enforcement activity varies widely across states, and there is evidence of an overall decline in alcohol-impaired arrest rates across the nation. While alcohol-impaired driving accounts for over 10 percent of all arrests reported to the Federal Bureau of Investigation's (FBI's) National Incident-Based Reporting System (NIBRS), arrest rates and enforcement activity vary as much as 32-fold across states. The population-based rate of alcohol-impaired driving arrests reported to the NIBRS in 2014 decreased by 13 percent from a high in 2003.

Educational and behavioral interventions have been a foundational feature of the public health approach to alcohol-impaired driving since the earliest days of community-level activism that led to the formation of such groups as Mothers Against Drunk Driving. Identifying what behaviors are associated with which groups is essential to this effort. Some features of alcohol-impaired driving behavior remain unchanged. Men are still three to four times as likely to report recent incidents of alcohol-impaired driving, and the highest population-based rates continue to be among younger drivers. But there have been notable recent changes in behaviors among some groups, indicating an evolution in risks posed by alcohol-impaired driving.

Teens and young adults are driving less, which is reflected in decreases in alcohol-impaired driving arrests, crashes, and fatalities. However, this group may now be at increasing risk of injury as passengers, and behaviors leading to decisions to ride as a passenger with alcohol-impaired drivers deserve increasing attention. The rate of women in the United States reporting a recent arrest for alcohol-impaired driving increased 40 percent between 2002 and 2014. Statistics reported to the FBI over the same time period show a similar increase. This increase may reflect, in part, an increase in marketing of alcohol to women. Motorcyclists, particularly those 55 to 64 years old, have experienced a notable increase in alcohol-related crash fatalities in the United States. In Florida, between 2011 and 2013, the fatality rate for motorcyclist crashes in which alcohol was not involved was 5 percent; when alcohol was involved, the fatality rate was 21 percent. In Nebraska, between 2002 and 2013, all crashes with a driver suspected of using alcohol or with a positive blood alcohol concentration (BAC) report decreased 25 percent, but rates among motorcyclists remained stubbornly persistent. Surveys consistently indicate that alcohol-impaired driving is associated with other risky behaviors such as binge drinking and not using seat belts. Investigating and addressing these interactions may help better tailor interventions that result in decreased morbidity and mortality.

Much of what we know about alcohol-impaired driving behavior comes from national surveys, such as the Centers for Disease Control and Prevention's (CDC's) Behavioral Risk Factor Surveillance System (BRFSS), which is among the most well-accepted and reliable sources of data on health-related behavior in the United States. Surveys can be enhanced to include questions, on alcohol-impaired driving on an annual basis. Additional survey questions. such as whether a person has been stopped at a sobriety checkpoint or been assigned to use an ignition interlock system, can provide information that may help track interventions. But there is a need for objective data to balance survey results. The FBI's NIBRS has the potential to provide important information on alcohol-impaired driving behavior and enforcement in the United States. It is limited in that it is not yet fully implemented across all states or representative of the entire United States. Roadside surveys conducted by the National Highway Traffic Safety Administration (NHTSA) provide perhaps the most valid and reliable estimates of alcohol-impaired driving behavior in the United States, but they are only conducted sporadically.

There is a need for additional, updated research addressing environmental factors associated with alcohol-impaired driving. Approximately 60 percent of alcohol-related motor vehicle crash deaths in the United States occur in rural areas. Adjusting for vehicle miles traveled indicates a risk three times greater than that of urban areas. Possible explanations for the rural–urban difference may include differences in access to alcohol on a per capita basis, and limited access to low-cost public transportation in rural areas. The availability of large data sources, which can be linked, and advances in small-area analyses can allow for better characterization of that risk and targeting of interventions. The NHTSA Fatality Analysis Reporting System (FARS), the premier and most successful source of alcohol-impaired driving fatality statistics in the United States, can contribute to that effort by consistently including geolocations. Most states participating in the NHTSA's State Data System (SDS) already collect and provide information about alcohol involvement in motor vehicle crashes. However, there is substantial variation in how this information has been collected over time and from state to state. Beginning in 2006, NHTSA began standardizing data elements across several of its data systems. Increased state participation in that system using consistent definitions will contribute to a better understanding of the actual incidence of alcohol-related motor vehicle crash fatalities in the United States.

There have been few studies looking explicitly at ethnic and racial patterns of alcohol-impaired driving behavior. More information is needed to better inform and target control efforts. Similarly, studies of the effectiveness of engineering and technological interventions for alcohol-impaired driving have been largely limited to ignition interlock systems. Despite the tremendous potential of self-driving and assisted driving technologies to affect alcohol-impaired driving outcomes, the research literature on the topic is virtually nonexistent. Lastly, while most analyses of alcohol-impaired driving in the United States rightly address the overall public health impact through absolute numbers of fatalities, additional analyses attempting to capture risk, as measured through rates of both crashes and fatalities, can better inform prevention and control through the use of estimates of vehicle miles driven to serve as denominators for analyses.

In summary, much has been achieved in controlling and preventing the consequences of alcohol-impaired driving in the United States, but much remains to be done. Recent evidence and analyses can help point the way to opportunities for additional advancements. Further success will require a renewed commitment to the prevention and control of alcohol-impaired driving in the United States with resources targeted at those individuals and areas most at risk.

ABOUT DATA SOURCES

This paper reviews administrative secondary data sources with information relevant to alcohol-impaired driving. CDC's BRFSS is among the most well-accepted and reliable sources of health-related behavior in the United States, and it should be enhanced to include a question on alcohol-impaired driving on an annual basis. Summary information about key data sources is listed below.

- Behavioral data characterized by self-reports may be biased.
- The NIBRS has the potential to provide important information on alcohol-impaired driving behavior and enforcement in the United States. It is limited in that it is not yet fully implemented by all states nor representative of the entire United States.
- Most states participating in the NHTSA's SDS collect and provide information about alcohol involvement in motor vehicle crashes. However, there is substantial variation in how this information has been collected over time and from state to state. Consistent definitions and greater participation among states can provide valuable surveillance information.
- The NHTSA's FARS is the premier source of alcohol-impaired driving fatality statistics in the United States. Data have been collected in the FARS from all 50 states since 1975.

- Data on alcohol involvement in the FARS are often missing, resulting in likely undercounts of the actual incidence of alcohol-related motor vehicle crash fatalities.
- The U.S. Department of Transportation's National Household Travel Survey provides reasonable estimates of vehicle miles driven to serve as denominators for analyses.

Behavioral Data

The Behavioral Risk Factor Surveillance System

The BRFSS is an annual nationwide survey conducted by CDC and is perhaps the most important, reliable, and long-standing source of information on health behavior in the United States. Since 2006, every other year, the BRFSS has included an explicit question on alcohol-impaired driving that asks, "During the past 30 days, how many times have you driven when you've had perhaps too much to drink?" Respondents answer with the number of times, from 0 to 76. There is an annual question on the number of alcoholic beverages a person consumes each day, which is used to calculate the total number of alcoholic beverages consumed in a month, and determine whether an individual can be considered a binge or heavy drinker. There is an annual question on seatbelt use ("How often do you use seat belts when you drive or ride in a car?"), which can be evaluated in relation to alcohol use.

Among the strengths of the BRFSS is the well-accepted reliability and validity of the results over a long period of time. Among the weaknesses are (1) because it is a phone-based survey, some of that strength is challenged by changes in phone use patterns, (2) self-report of what might be considered deviant behavior is likely to result in bias, (3) questions pertaining to alcohol-impaired driving are only present every other year and therefore provide data for 6 years, making it difficult to establish trends, and (4) results are only valid at the national and state levels, making local behavior patterns difficult to assess. The usefulness of the BRFSS to track alcohol-impaired driving in the United States can be enhanced by including a related question every year. Potential biases in self-reports can be at least partially addressed through the inclusion of such methods as randomized response or item count techniques (Miller et al., 1986; Warner, 1965).

Similar to the BRFSS is the Youth Risk Behavior Surveillance System (YRBSS), which monitors health behaviors among U.S. youth and young adults. The survey is conducted every other year and dates to 1991. Separate versions of the survey are administered to high school and middle school students. Among the six specific health behaviors monitored are alcohol and other drug use, and there are two specific questions relating to alcohol-impaired driving:

1. Have you ever ridden in a car driven by someone who had been drinking alcohol?
2. During the past 30 days, how many times did you ride in a car or other vehicle driven by someone who had been drinking alcohol?

Among the strengths of the YRBSS are that it has consistently included questions on alcohol-impaired driving that allow for reliable estimates of trends and addresses risk among a vulnerable population. Weaknesses of the YRBSS include (1) data may not be available for all states, (2) limited geographic specificity similar to the BRFSS, and (3) biases associated with self-reported behavior likely similar to the BRFSS, although there may be some added level of anonymity in the way the YRBSS is administered.

National Survey on Drug Use and Health

The National Survey on Drug Use and Health is a yearly survey of "national and state-level estimates on the use of tobacco products, alcohol, illicit drugs (including nonmedical use of prescription drugs) and mental health in the United States" conducted by the Substance Abuse and Mental Health Services Administration. Included among the questions is "In the past 12 months, were you arrested and booked for driving under the influence of alcohol or drugs?" A strength of this data source is that it is a large survey of approximately 70,000 individuals conducted yearly since 1971, making it an effective resource to validly track trends at the state and national levels. Unlike the BRFSS, the survey includes individuals in institutional settings such as shelters, rooming houses, and dormitories. Like the BRFSS, the survey is subject to bias in that it relies on self-reported data and is not powered to assess outcomes at smaller geographic levels.

National Incident-Based Reporting System

The FBI maintains the NIBRS as a means of quantifying criminal activity in the United States. In contrast to the FBI's longer-standing traditional Uniform Crime Reporting (UCR) statistics, the NIBRS collects data on a wider array of crimes and goes into greater detail on the circumstances surrounding offenses. Unlike the UCR, and among its weaknesses, the NIBRS is not yet nationally representative. As of June 2012, 32 states were participating. According to the U.S. Department of Justice, "In 2015, 6,648 law enforcement agencies, representing coverage of more than 96 million U.S. inhabitants, submitted NIBRS data. While not yet nationally representative (there are no estimates for agencies that did not submit NIBRS data), this coverage represents 36.1 percent of all law enforcement agencies that participate in the UCR program" (FBI, 2016). The target date for full national representation is 2021.

Among the strengths of these data are that they are (for the states represented) essentially a census of crimes, rather than a survey, and are less sensitive to statistical heterogeneity. Driving while impaired (DWI) has been a reportable offense since the inception of the NIBRS. It is classified as a so-called Group B offense for which only arrestee data are reported. Among the weaknesses of these data as a source of surveillance information on alcohol-impaired driving is that they are as much a reflection of enforcement activity and availability of resources as they are an estimate of actual behavior.

National Roadside Survey of Alcohol and Drugged Driving

NHTSA has conducted the National Roadside Survey of Alcohol and Drugged Driving five times since 1973. The most recent iteration was conducted in 2013 and 2014 and consisted of a sample size of approximately 9,000 persons in 60 U.S. cities. The major strength of this survey is that results are based on breath, saliva, and blood testing rather than self-reporting, increasing the validity of the conclusions. Among the weaknesses is the intermittent nature of the survey, making it difficult to assess trends.

Crash Data

The State Data System

The primary source of alcohol-related motor vehicle crash injury data is the NHTSA SDS. The SDS is based on data from police crash reports submitted by participating states. Police crash reports are completed by police officers at the scene of motor vehicle crashes and contain information about the crash, the vehicles involved, and the motorists and nonmotorists (e.g., pedestrians, cyclists) involved in the crash. Each state determines its own reporting criteria. Generally, crashes are reportable if they involve injuries or deaths. Other common reporting criteria include damages in excess of a designated cost or damages requiring a vehicle to be towed away from the scene. While the specific nature and quantity of information collected at the crash site varies from state to state (and over time within each state), the SDS applies a common nomenclature to field names when processing and storing state datasets to aid in research efforts across states.

As of June 15, 2017, there were 34 states participating in the SDS. Access to state data requires special permission from each individual state data owner. Not all states allow NHTSA to rerelease their data.

Most states participating in the SDS collect and provide information about alcohol involvement in motor vehicle crashes. However, there is substantial variation in how this information has been collected over time and from state to state. The range of language and specific indicators used to identify alcohol use include

- Individual had been drinking.
- Individual was/appeared to be under the influence of alcohol.
- Individual was/appeared to be intoxicated.
- Individual received an alcohol test.
- Individual BAC percentage ranging from 0.00% (0%) to 0.99% (9%).
- Alcohol was a contributing factor, circumstance, or cause of the crash.
- Alcohol was present in the vehicle/at the scene.
- Individual was issued a violation for alcohol use, being under the influence, etc.

Alcohol information is almost always available for drivers. Very few states collect or report alcohol information for passengers. Some states provide indicators at the crash level that may be used to readily identify crashes that involved alcohol on some level. Alcohol indicators are more commonly reported at the individual level, which can allow for analysis by role (driver, pedestrian/cyclist), age, and gender.

The strengths and weaknesses of alcohol-related motor vehicle crash data in the SDS vary considerably by state. For example, before 2011, Florida SDS datasets included alcohol information for individuals using the language "under the influence." Beginning in 2011, Florida began including information about alcohol testing and test results, and added a flag for "alcohol use suspected," which captures a wider range of crashes with alcohol involvement. By contrast, Nebraska data are based on "officer deemed alcohol related to crash," with additional fields available for whether an alcohol test was performed and whether results are known.

By contrast, New York State SDS datasets identify alcohol information only in the context of violations issued, which essentially pertain to drivers only. Violation data files were added to New York's SDS files beginning as early as 2002. There are a number of different types of violations with language ranging from *alcohol use, impairment, intoxication, BAC above 0.08% (CDL)* or *0.1% (private vehicle)*, and *open container of alcohol*.

Because SDS data include injuries as well as fatalities, an additional strength of this data source is that fatality rates can be calculated and compared across crash characteristics. Additionally, the number of participating states has grown over time and now covers the majority of the continental United States. Most states provide a substantial array of variables related to crash circumstances, vehicles involved, and some information about persons involved.

While the SDS provides a common naming structure and language, as noted, a limitation is that there are many differences in how variables are defined and how information is collected and reported from state to state. Also, states have also changed their coding and reporting practices over time, requiring careful attention to the coding manuals. In particular, as noted above, alcohol involvement is recorded in numerous ways and makes state-to-state comparisons problematic. Finally, geographical information in the SDS is limited to city and county.

National Automotive Sampling System General Estimates System

NHTSA's National Automotive Sampling System General Estimates System (NASS GES) is based on a sample of police crash reports. The data are used to track trends and identify emerging issues. Starting in 2006, NHTSA began standardizing data elements across the FARS and the NASS GES, increasing the usefulness of the system.

Fatality Data

Fatality Analysis Reporting System

The primary data source available in the United States for traffic-related mortality is the NHTSA's FARS. When combined with U.S. Census population estimates, or person-miles traveled estimates such as those available from the National Household Travel Survey, and vehicle miles traveled estimates from the Federal Highway Administration, reliable motor vehicle mortality-related rates can be calculated.

The FARS is a national census of fatal motor vehicle crashes (MVCs) and is maintained by the National Center for Statistics and Analysis, a component of NHTSA. Initially established in 1975, the FARS contains detailed information on all crashes that occur on U.S. public roadways that result in the death of one or more motorists or nonmotorists within 30 days. FARS data are acquired from police reports, state administrative files, and medical records from all 50 states and are analyzed by data analysts using standardized protocols. As a result, FARS data elements generally have relatively little missing data and are well documented and maintained.

For each fatal crash, the FARS provides detailed information related to the crash circumstances as well as the people and vehicles involved in that crash. The FARS lists the county, city, state, and longitude and latitude of each crash and also includes roadway information (road surface type, number of lanes, speed limit, traffic control device), and light and atmospheric conditions. The time of the crash and emergency medical services transportation information (arrival at the scene and to the hospital) are also included. In addition, driving maneuvers avoiding and contributing to each crash are documented. Data on each vehicle involved include the make, model, and model year as well as less detailed variables to aggregate and compare crashes by vehicle type.

Data on all motorists and nonmotorists involved in each crash, including age, sex, seating position, vehicle occupant restraint use, and injury severity, are provided. For drivers, information on prior crashes, license suspensions, and other driving violations within 3–5 years preceding the crash is available. Of note, certain information such as race and ethnicity, which is collected from death certificates, is only available for fatally injured individuals.

The FARS also has data on alcohol and drug intoxication that are gathered from breath, blood, and urine tests, as well as police behavioral assessments. Since these data are based on the extent of testing performed by law enforcement, alcohol involvement data are often missing. As a result, the FARS may undercount the actual incidence of alcohol-related motor vehicle crashes, and testing rates are a potential confounding variable for regional comparisons of alcohol-related crashes.

Strengths of the FARS The various strong points of the FARS are listed below.

- Data have been collected in the FARS from all 50 states since 1975, allowing for long-term trend analysis.
- Significant data are available to analyze crashes at the crash level, vehicle level, and person level, and these data are quite detailed at every level.
- For drivers, detailed information is available on a driver's previous traffic and driving violations prior to the crash.
- Data elements are well documented and maintained.
- The majority of FARS variables have very little missing data.

Weaknesses of the FARS The various weak points of the FARS are listed below.

- The FARS only has information on crashes resulting in at least one fatality within 30 days of the crash.
- Data on alcohol involvement are often missing, meaning the FARS may undercount the actual incidence of alcohol-related motor vehicle crashes.
- Police testing for illicit substances may vary between different states and regions and is a confounding variable for state-level comparisons.
- Data on race and ethnicity are collected from death certificates, meaning that it is only available for individuals fatally injured in crashes. Even among deceased individuals in alcohol-related crashes, race and ethnicity information is missing for 14 percent of persons.
- The FARS occasionally has errors in data element coding, but these errors are well documented and can be worked around.

Multiple imputation of alcohol data in FARS Missing data are an issue in most rigorous data analyses and are particularly problematic in alcohol-related crash analyses. While it is the standard for such analyses, more than half of FARS records are missing BAC data (Subramanian and Utter, 2003). Over the years, NHTSA has taken several approaches to estimating missing BAC values in the FARS. Prior to 2001, a linear discriminant method was used to estimate the probability that a driver or nondriver (pedestrian or cyclist) had a BAC of 0.0, 0.01–0.09, or >0.10 g/dl. Starting in 2001, NHTSA moved to multiple imputation methods (Subramanian, 2002). The algorithm generates 10 estimates for BAC values for each missing BAC observation. The models used to estimate missing values include variables such as age, sex, injury severity, and day and time of crash that are likely to be associated with BAC. The final imputed value is a combination of the 10 estimates and includes a measure of the uncertainty, which is added to variances for overall point prevalence. Multiple imputation methods are superior to some other missing data methods, and the methods pioneered by NHTSA have been applied to missing drug testing data in truck crashes (Brady et al., 2009). However, they cannot substitute for actual testing results. Data imputation is least biased when values are missing at random, which is unlikely in the case of alcohol-related fatalities. It is important to evaluate results based on imputed values in comparison to complete-case analyses and explain any discrepancies (Sterne et al., 2009).

Clinical Data

Nationwide Emergency Department Sample

The Agency for Healthcare Research and Quality (AHRQ) Healthcare Cost and Utilization Project (HCUP) maintains the Nationwide Emergency Department Sample (NEDS) (AHRQ, 2015). The HCUP is a group of inpatient and outpatient files created by AHRQ. NEDS is the largest single publicly available emergency department (ED) database in the United States. It is based on a 20 percent stratified single-cluster sample of all U.S. hospital-based EDs. As of 2012, 30 states participated in NEDS, accounting for 66 percent of all national ED visits. Each year's core file contains 100 percent of visits from sampled hospitals. The most recent NEDS database contains about 30 million ED records. Hospitals are defined as nonfederal general and specialty hospitals, including public hospitals and academic medical centers. Additional stratification variables include geographical area, urban/rural, ownership, trauma center and teaching status, and bed size.

Motor vehicle crashes can be identified using external cause of injury e-codes. Alcohol intoxication can be determined using *International Classification of Diseases* (ICD)-9 diagnostic codes. Combining the two variables can allow for the identification of alcohol-related motor vehicle crashes. Among the strengths of the NEDS is the large, comprehensively representative sample with few missing data that can allow for the analysis of rare outcomes. Among the weaknesses is the difficulty in working with the large datasets required for multiyear analyses. An important bias common to clinical datasets based on administrative diagnostic codes is that diagnoses of alcohol intoxication are almost invariably limited to the most intoxicated individuals, resulting in important selection bias.

Web-Based Injury Statistics Query and Reporting System

CDC's Web-based Injury Statistics Query and Reporting System (WISQARS) is an online, publicly available resource for both fatal and nonfatal injury-related statistics. Fatality data are drawn from CDC's National Center for Health Statistics, National Vital Statistics System Mortality Data, which are themselves based on death certificate ICD-10 assignments. The ICD-10 coding system allows for inclusion of alcohol as an attributable cause (Codes X45, Y15, T51.0, T51.1, T51.9) of motor vehicle crashes (Codes E820–E825), but this combination is not routinely reported as part of the WISQARS. Injury data are drawn from the National Electronic Injury Surveillance System All Injury Program (NEISS-AIP) operated by the Consumer Protection Safety Commission. The NEISS is a national probability sample of approximately 100 hospitals in the United

States and its territories drawn from a commercially purchased sampling frame (Schroeder and Ault, 2001).

Data Linkage: Crash Outcome Data Evaluation System

NHTSA developed the Crash Outcome Data Evaluation System (CODES) to help researchers link crash records with clinical records. The CODES uses a match weight test statistic and has been used in a number of motor vehicle crash injury studies (see, for example, Clark et al., 2004; Loo and Tsui, 2007; Lopez et al., 2000). Advances in probabilistic and fuzzy matching methods offer additional approaches to matching datasets (Lujic et al., 2008).

The CODES was created by NHTSA in the early 1990s to inform motor vehicle safety legislation. NHTSA initially funded 16 states to develop and implement the probabilistic data linkage algorithms for motor vehicle crash data sources. Some states expanded their efforts to link crash data with hospital discharge records, emergency medical transport call reports, and trauma registry records. Many of these efforts rely on deterministic linkage using identifiers not generally available to nongovernment researchers. Commercial software that replicates the CODES methodology is also available.

Denominator Data

Among the more challenging aspects of measuring alcohol-related motor vehicle crashes in the United States is determining an appropriate denominator to use to calculate comparable rates across time and place. While absolute numbers of fatalities, crashes, and incidents provide important information on the effect of alcohol-impaired driving in the United States, additional attention to normalizing such numerators by appropriate denominators can help better define risk at a time when resources need to be most efficiently deployed. A common approach is to use census data for population denominators, but other approaches based on travel patterns are possible.

National Household Travel Survey

The U.S. Department of Transportation conducts periodic national surveys about how people travel across the United States in their daily lives; the most relevant to alcohol-impaired driving is the National Household Travel Survey (NHTS). Data are available online for the years 1995, 2001, and 2009. The 2016 survey was recently administered and should be available in the near future. Data collected include

- Purpose of the trip (work, shopping, etc.);
- Means of transportation used (car, bus, subway, walk, etc.);
- How long the trip took (i.e., travel time);
- Time of day when the trip took place;
- Day of the week when the trip took place;
- If a private vehicle trip, number of people in the vehicle (i.e., vehicle occupancy);
- Driver characteristics (age, sex, worker status, education level, etc.); and
- Vehicle attributes (make, model, model year, amount of miles driven in 1 year).

The 1995 and 2001 surveys provide national estimates, and the 2009 survey provides both national- and state-level estimates, as it included a larger sample size. A full description of the NHTS methods and data use considerations may be found online.

To account for intervening years one can apply linear regression to NHTS point estimates from 1995, 2001, and 2009 to create annual estimates of drivers, vehicle miles driven, and person-miles traveled (total and subdivided miles traveled in privately owned vehicles, walking, and biking). Each estimate was stratified by age and sex and by race and ethnicity, and linear interpolation was conducted separately for each stratum.

Among the strengths of the NHTS is that it allows analysis of driver counts, miles driven, and person-miles traveled across a range of household and person characteristics as well as vehicle and trip characteristics, and that it is a large sample—a nationally representative survey.

Among its limitations are that race and ethnicity are applied to driver and household persons based on the primary household respondent. In one stratum, the linear regression produced a negative value for the first observation. In this case (bicycling miles traveled by men ages 75 and older), the intercept was manually adjusted such that the first value was the actual 1995 estimated value.

While 2009 survey estimates are valid at the state level and may be further stratified by demographic characteristics within state, some strata may contain small numbers and aggregation may be required. Because state-level data are not available before 2009, linear interpolation was only conducted at the national level to produce annual estimates.

Federal Highway Administration Highway Vehicle Miles Traveled

The Federal Highway Administration (FHWA) highway vehicle miles traveled (HVMT) provides annual summary statistics at the national and state level on registered vehicles, drivers' licenses, highway miles traveled, and highway user taxation. FHWA compiles the data as submitted by individual states. The data have been collected annually since 1945.

This paper uses annual highway miles traveled by state for SDS analyses at the state level. Urban and rural highway miles traveled were also used with FARS data on urban and rural fatal alcohol-related crashes.

Among the strengths of FHWA highway statistics is that the survey provides a nationally consistent measure of vehicle miles traveled. Among its limitations are that data are based on vehicle counts and therefore demographics of miles traveled are unavailable. A full description of FHWA highway statistics data use considerations may be found online.

Issues and Limitations of Denominator Data

While vehicle miles traveled (VMT) provides a valid approach to estimating risk based on a direct measurement of exposure, there are some methodological challenges in its use (see Table A-1). The NHTS and the FHWA measures are structured differently and cannot be easily or reliably combined. The NHTS, for example, may allow for age stratification, while the FHWA estimates can be broken down by urban or rural geography. More granular stratifications, such as combining age groups and urban versus rural status, are not a trivial problem and require careful use of one dataset or the other. Measuring change over time will generally require interpolation over a limited number of measurements (in some cases just two), with an underlying assumption of linearity that may not be supported.

TABLE A-1 Strengths and Limitations of Denominator Data

Data Type	Strengths	Potential Weakness/Bias
1. Count data	Commonly reported Estimates absolute public health impact Allows for stratification	Cannot estimate risk
2. Census population	Easy to obtain Estimate risk Age stratification Geographic stratification Estimates over time Race/ethnicity data Economic data	May not accurately represent population at risk
3. Vehicle miles traveled	Accurately represents exposure	Limited stratification variables Limited local geography Limited years of observation

ANALYSES

BRFSS Data Analysis

- The number of adults in the United States reporting an instance of alcohol-impaired driving over the previous 30 days decreased about 38 percent from 2006 to 2014. There was an approximate 10 percent decrease between 2010 and 2014.
- Men were three times more likely to report recent alcohol-impaired driving.
- The youngest age groups were more likely to experience a decline in recent alcohol-impaired driving.
- Much of the decrease in reported rates of alcohol-impaired driving in the past 30 days for all age groups (≥18 years) occurred between 2006 and 2008.

The mean number of times an adult (≥18 years of age) reported alcohol-impaired driving over the past 30 days for all the data years and all states was 0.09 (standard error [s.e.] = 0.02, 95% confidence interval [CI] 0.09, 0.10). This represented 189.9 persons (≥18 years old), per 10,000 surveyed U.S. adult population members (s.e. = 2.0, 95% CI 185.6, 194.1), reporting that they drove while alcohol impaired during the previous 30 days. This population-based count decreased 38.4 percent (s.e. = 0.07) from 251.4 per 10,000 in 2006 (95% CI 238.3, 264.4) to 154.9 per 10,000 in 2014 (95% CI 147.5, 162.3). There was a 10.5 percent (s.e. = 0.5) decline from 2010 to 2014.

The overall rate of respondents reporting at least one incident of DWI in the previous month varied by U.S. state and territory, with the highest rate of 414.1 per 10,000 (95% CI 334.6, 493.6) in Guam and the lowest of 62.7 per 10,000 in Utah (95% CI 51.9, 73.6) (see Figure A-1). There was some graphical indication of clustering of higher rates in the northern United States (see Figure A-2). There was some variation, but the general geographic patterns prevailed over time.

More than three times more male (293.9 per 10,000; 95% CI 286.0, 301.7) than female (91.5 per 10,000; 95% CI 87.8, 95.2) respondents reported at least one incident of DWI in the previous 30 days. There was a decline during the study period in the number of both male and female respondents reporting at least one incident of DWI. The rate per 10,000 of respondents reporting at least one incident of DWI in the previous 30 days was inversely related to age group. All age groups experienced a decline from 2006 to 2014 in the rate per 10,000 of respondents reporting at least one incident of DWI in the previous 30 days, with the steepest declines among the youngest age groups (see Figure A-3).

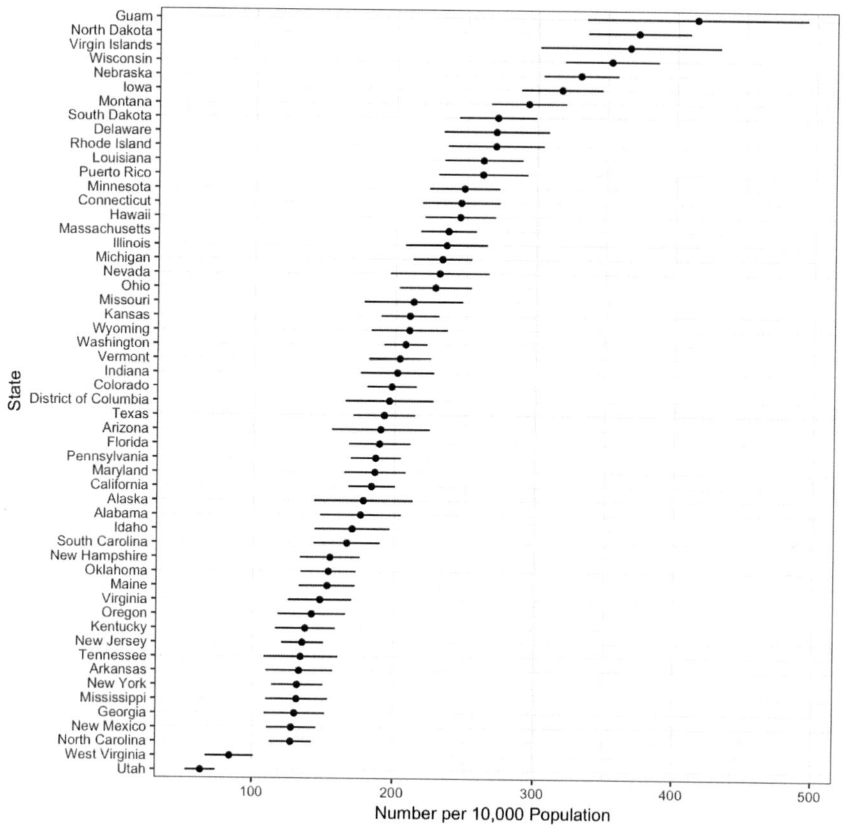

FIGURE A-1 Number of respondents reporting at least one instance of alcohol-impaired driving in the past 30 days per 10,000 target adult survey population by state or territory.
SOURCE: BRFSS data, 2006–2014.

National Survey on Drug Use and Health Data Analysis

- There was a 27 percent decrease from 2002 to 2014 in the rate of persons reporting an arrest for alcohol-impaired driving in the past month, with a more modest and more variable decline of approximately 10 percent since 2011.
- Men were four times more likely to report a recent arrest for alcohol-impaired driving.
- The rate of women reporting a recent arrest for alcohol-impaired driving increased 40 percent between 2002 and 2014.

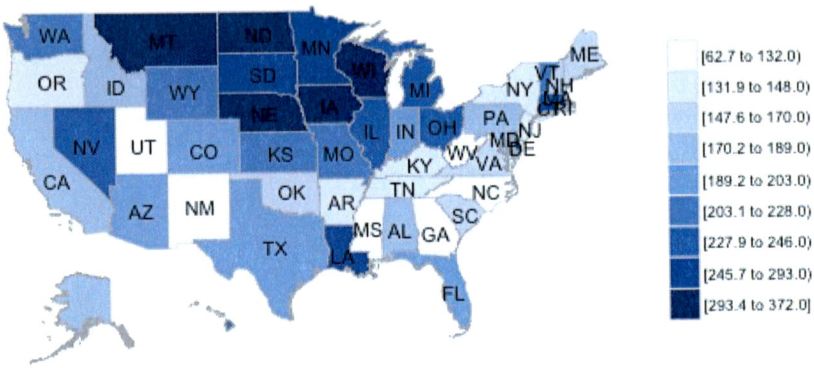

FIGURE A-2 Choropleth number of respondents reporting alcohol-impaired driving in the past 30 days per 10,000 target adult survey population by state.
SOURCE: BRFSS data, 2006–2014.

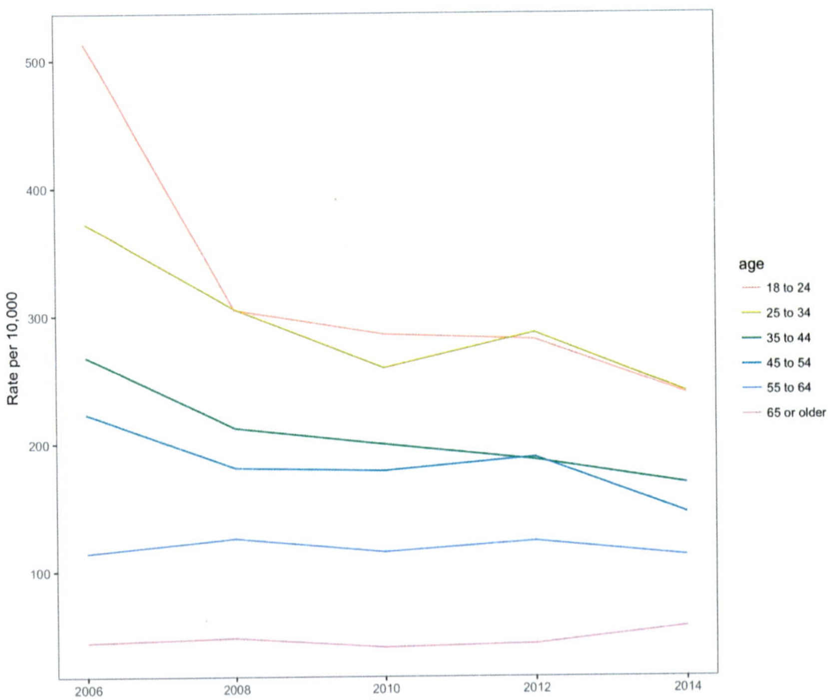

FIGURE A-3 Number of respondents reporting alcohol-impaired driving in the past 30 days per 10,000 target adult survey population by age group over time.
SOURCE: BRFSS data, 2006–2014.

There were 723,283 entries in the National Survey on Drug Use and Health for the years 2002 to 2014, representing a survey-adjusted total of 3,250,847,536 (s.e. = 9,889,020) observations. The yearly survey count mirrored the total U.S. population for the years 2002 to 2014.

The overall rate of persons responding yes to questions regarding whether they had been arrested for DWI in the preceding 12 months was 57.8 per 10,000 survey-adjusted target population (s.e. = 0.0001). The rate per 10,000 of responses of yes to questions regarding arrest for DWI showed a fairly steady pattern from 2002 to 2010, after which there was evidence of a decline. The rate declined 26.7 percent (s.e. = 8.9) from 65.9 per 10,000 in 2002 to 47.9 per 10,000 in 2014. The decline between 2011 and 2014 was more modest (9.4 percent) and more subject to chance (s.e. = 12.4). The rates for 19- to 29-year-olds were nearly three times those for other age groups, although there was graphical evidence of a decrease among 19- to 21-year-olds.

The rate for men answering yes to questions regarding recent DWI arrests was nearly four times that of women, 94.0 per 10,000 target population men (95% CI 88.7, 99.3) versus 23.9 per 10,000 women (95% CI 21.8, 26.0). There was graphical evidence that the rates for men responding yes to questions regarding DWI declined over the study period, while rates among women appeared to be increasing. The rate for male respondents declined 38.6 percent (s.e. = 10.6) from 118.2 per 10,000 in 2002 to 73.1 per 10,000 in 2014, while the rate for female respondents increased 43.7 percent (s.e. = 28.9), from 17.1 per 10,000 target population in 2002 to 24.4 per 10,000 in 2014.

The age-gender category with the highest overall rate of responding yes to questions regarding DWI in the previous year was men aged 18–25, which at 213.8 per 10,000 target population (95% CI 200.3, 227.2) was over three times that of the next highest category. It was also the age category with the steepest decline in rates over the study period, decreasing 43.3 percent (s.e. = 11.6) from 296.1 per 10,000 in 2002 to 169.6 per 10,000 in 2014.

Rates of positive responses to questions regarding DWI were higher in less population-dense core-based statistical areas (CBSAs). These differences were statistically significant ($p = 0.0001$) in a survey-adjusted analysis of variance comparing CBSAs for a positive response to DWI questions. CBSAs of greater and less than 1 million people both experienced declines between 2002 and 2014 in the rates of individuals responding yes to questions about DWI. Although non-CBSA geographic segments had a 38.8 percent (s.e. = 44.2) increase in the rate of positive responses to questions regarding DWI from 2002 to 2014, there was considerable variability in the yearly data.

NIBRS Data Analysis

- There were more than 4.5 million arrests for alcohol-impaired driving reported to the FBI between 1995 and 2014, accounting for more than 10 percent of all reported arrests.
- Alcohol-impaired driving arrest rates varied 32-fold across states.
- The population-based rate of alcohol-impaired driving arrests reported to the FBI in 2014 decreased 13 percent from a high in 2003.
- There has been a decrease in alcohol-impaired driving arrests as a proportion of all arrest activity in the United States.
- There has been a notable and sustained increase in the percentage of female alcohol-impaired driving arrestees over the past 20 years.

There were 4,681,475 recorded DWI arrests reported to the NIBRS over the years 1995 to 2014, which accounted for 10.2 percent of all 45,978,155 reported arrests during that period. The overall population-based rate of DWI arrests for the entire 20-year period was 526.5 arrests per 100,000 persons covered by the reporting agencies. The average age of an arrestee was 34.4 years old (95% CI 34.3, 34.4), and listed ages ranged from 7 to 99 years old. Approximately 78.0 percent (95% CI 78.0, 78.1) of arrestees were male.

The median annual arrest rate for alcohol-impaired driving was 503.4 per 100,000 covered population. While a linear increasing trend line could be fit to the annual arrest rates, the data were more consistent with a period of increased enforcement from a low of 458.1 arrests per 100,000 covered population in 2003 to a high of 563.6 in 2009, followed by a 12.7 percent decline (95% CI 10.2, 15.8) to 491.9 in 2014.

When examined as the percentage of all arrests, there was an apparent decline in alcohol-impaired driving arrests as a proportion of all enforcement activity from 10 percent in 1995 to 9 percent in 2005, with evidence of some recovery in activity to approximately 10 percent of all arrests in 2014. The overall trend, though, indicated a significant decrease in alcohol-impaired driving arrests as a proportion of all arrest activity in the United States.

There was a slight increase in the mean age of arrestees for alcohol-impaired driving from approximately 34 years old in 1995 to 35.8 years old in 2014, with much of the increase occurring after 2010. Women were a rapidly increasing proportion of persons arrested for alcohol-impaired driving during the study period, increasing 40.0 percent (95% CI 22.0, 60.1) from 15.32 percent of all arrestees in 1995 to 25.56 percent in 2014 (see Figure A-4). There was a significant linear increase in the percentage of female arrestees of approximately 0.6 percent each year.

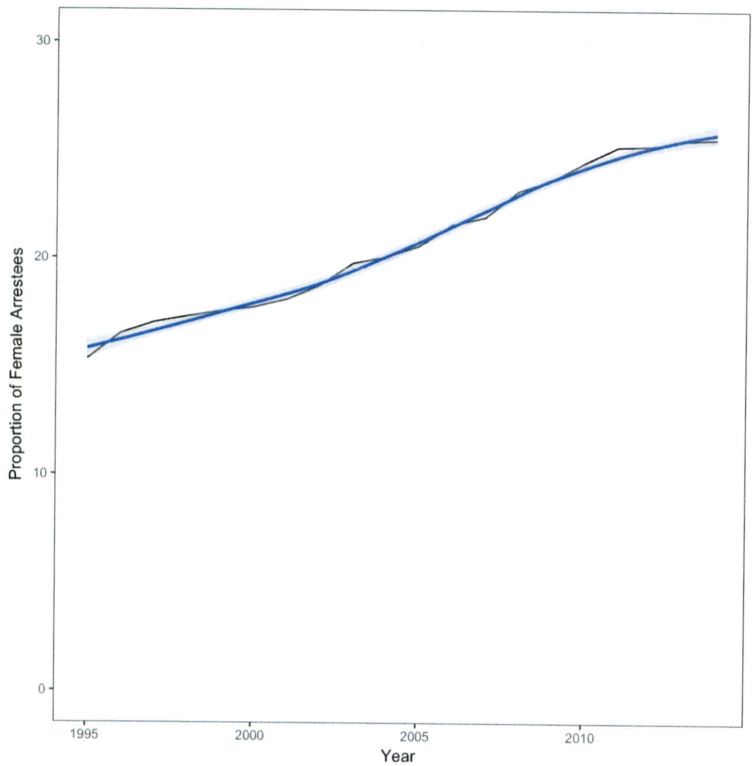

FIGURE A-4 Proportion of women arrestees with overlying LOESS line, incidents of driving under the influence of alcohol.
SOURCE: NIBRS data, 1995–2014.

Rates of reported arrests for alcohol-impaired driving varied considerably by state from a low of 30.9 per 100,000 covered population in Delaware to a high of 960.8 in Kansas, with most states clustered around a median of approximately 490 arrests per 100,000 covered population and some evidence of regional variation. The percentage of all arrests represented by alcohol-impaired driving also varied across states, ranging from a low of 0.43 per 100,000 covered population in the District of Columbia to 21.87 in Vermont but with less overall heterogeneity. Persons arrested for alcohol-impaired driving were on average 5 years younger than the state median for every state except Delaware and Utah, where they were 2 to 3 years older. States also varied considerably in the percentage of women among alcohol-impaired driving arrestees, from a low of 6.98 percent of all arrestees in Georgia to 29.37 percent in Maine.

NHTS Analysis

The NHTS estimates that the overall number of drivers increased 20 percent from 176,331,000 in 1995 to 212,309,000 in 2009, although growth was slower between 2001 and 2009 than between 1995 and 2001. The overall rate of growth varied by age group, and in fact there was an estimated decline in drivers in the 21- to 25-year-old and 26- to 35-year-old age groups (both men and women) between 1995 and 2009. By race and ethnicity, Hispanic drivers experienced the largest rate of growth, approximately 75 percent over the time period, followed by Asian drivers (66 percent), non-Hispanic blacks (33 percent), other non-Hispanic drivers (21 percent), and non-Hispanic whites (11 percent).

Estimates of total vehicle miles driven increased between 1995 and 2001 and decreased from 2001 to 2009, for a net change of +8.8 percent overall from 2.063 trillion in 1995 to 2.245 trillion in 2009. Patterns by age corresponded with driver trends; that is, there were declines in vehicle miles driven for adults 21 to 35 years of age. Vehicle miles driven by race and ethnicity mirrored the aforementioned rates of growth among drivers by race and ethnicity.

Estimated total miles per person of travel across all modalities (private vehicle, walking, biking, transit, air, and other) likewise increased between 1995 and 2001 and decreased between 2001 and 2009, with a net increase of 9 percent from 3.411 trillion to 3.732 trillion. By modality, private vehicle miles accounted for the majority of travel, increasing 6 percent from 3.110 trillion in 1995 to 3.298 trillion in 2009. A decline in overall vehicular travel was observed among 25- to 34-year-olds, similar to the observations above for drivers and vehicle miles driven. Men 16 to 24 years of age also experienced less overall vehicular travel from 1995 to 2009. While a smaller fraction of total travel, walking and biking estimates meanwhile increased both between 1995 and 2001 and between 2001 and 2009. Walking miles increased remarkably by 160 percent from 10.821 billion in 1995 to 27.943 billion in 2009. Estimated total biking miles likewise grew sharply by 95 percent from 4.585 billion in 1995 to 8.956 billion in 2009. Increases in miles walked were observed across all categories of age and gender. Biking trends by age and gender had some fluctuations likely as a result of smaller numbers.

Based on our review of the FHWA HVMT, across the United States, vehicle miles traveled increased between 1995 and 2008, declined somewhat between 2007 and 2009, and then increased again between 2010 and 2015.

FARS Data Analysis

- From 1995 to 2015 there was a 30 percent decrease in the absolute number of alcohol-related motor vehicle crash deaths in the United States, while there was a population increase of 40 percent and a 35 percent increase in VMT.
- The greatest declines in alcohol-related motor vehicle crash mortality occurred among the youngest drivers and passengers.
- Men accounted for 77 percent of all alcohol-related motor vehicle crash deaths in the United States.
- Approximately 60 percent of alcohol-related motor vehicle crash deaths in the United States occur in rural areas.
- Adjusted for VMT, the risk of an alcohol-related motor vehicle crash fatality in rural areas is nearly three times that of urban areas.
- Non-Hispanic Asians had population-adjusted alcohol-related motor vehicle crash fatality rates more than three times lower than any other racial and ethnic group.
- Motorcyclists, particularly those 55 to 64 years old, experienced a marked increase in alcohol-related crash fatalities.

This paper analyzes the FARS data from the years 1995 to 2015, acquired online from NHTSA. The FARS is a nationwide U.S. census providing annual data on all fatalities suffered from MVCs. Specifically, this study examines MVC fatalities with documented alcohol use. Fatal car crashes were considered alcohol related if any motor vehicle driver had police-reported alcohol intoxication or a positive laboratory BAC (BAC = 0.01 g/dL). Alcohol use by passengers, pedestrians, and cyclists did not classify a crash as an alcohol-related MVC.

Analyses focused on persons fatally injured from these crashes. Data were analyzed over this 21-year interval in terms of age, sex, race, and ethnicity. In addition, analyses compared urban and rural crash rates as well as crash rates between different states. Subanalyses were also performed on fatally injured cyclists, pedestrians, and motor vehicle occupants. Crash and fatality rates were adjusted in terms of census population counts obtained from the HCUP website as well as estimates of person-miles traveled obtained from the NHTS website. Results are presented as tables and time series plots.[3] Analyses were completed using *R*.

[3] Available by request from the National Academies of Sciences, Engineering, and Medicine's Public Access Records Office (PARO@nas.edu).

Throughout the 1995–2015 study period, deaths from alcohol-related MVCs decreased by 29 percent. This decline was even greater after adjusting for population increases (41 percent) and person-miles traveled (37 percent). The greatest reductions were observed in younger persons, with 16- to 20-year-olds and children under 16 experiencing 56 and 66 percent decreases in alcohol-related MVC fatalities, respectively. The age group most frequently fatally injured in alcohol-related MVCs, 21- to 24-year-olds, experienced a 34 percent decrease in fatalities from 2,118 deaths in 1995 to 1,393 in 2015. Interestingly, individuals from 45 to 64 years of age experienced a 30 percent increase in alcohol-related MVC fatalities over the study period, but after adjusting for population increases this group also experienced a modest decline (15 percent).

Men accounted for 77 percent of all alcohol-related MVC fatalities. Despite this, both men and women experienced a decline in alcohol-related MVC fatalities of similar proportion, with male fatalities decreasing 29 percent from 10,667 deaths in 1995 to 7,545 in 2015, and female fatalities also decreasing 29 percent from 3,270 in 1995 to 2,312 in 2015. Non-Hispanic whites accounted for 68 percent of alcohol-related MVC fatalities from 2000 to 2015. However, after accounting for population size, non-Hispanic whites had approximately equal alcohol-related MVC fatalities per 100,000 population (3.52) as Hispanics (3.41) and non-Hispanic blacks (3.44) from 2000 to 2015. Non-Hispanic Asians, on the other hand, had population-adjusted fatality rates more than three times lower than all other racial and ethnic groups (1.08). During this period, non-Hispanic whites experienced a 24 percent decline in population-adjusted, alcohol-related MVC fatalities, compared to declines of 10, 56, and 41 percent in non-Hispanic blacks, non-Hispanic Asians, and Hispanics, respectively.

From 1995 to 2014, 60 percent of alcohol-related MVC fatalities occurred in rural areas. After adjusting for VMT, rural areas had a fatality rate of 7.24 deaths per billion VMT, 2.67 times greater than that of urban areas (2.71 deaths per billion VMT). This was relatively constant over the study period (see Figure A-5). During this period rural areas also experienced a greater decline in alcohol-related MVC fatalities (41 percent) compared to urban areas. However, after adjusting for VMT, the declines in MVC fatalities of urban areas (38 percent) and rural areas (40 percent) were similar. Of note, declines in rural fatalities were disproportionately reduced in individuals under 45 years of age (52 percent decrease), with the largest decreases in those under 21 years of age (64 percent). Rural individuals 45 and older had a slight increase in fatalities (4 percent). Changes in urban fatalities had less variance by age between individuals under 45 years of age (22 percent decline) and 45 years of age or older (22 percent increase).

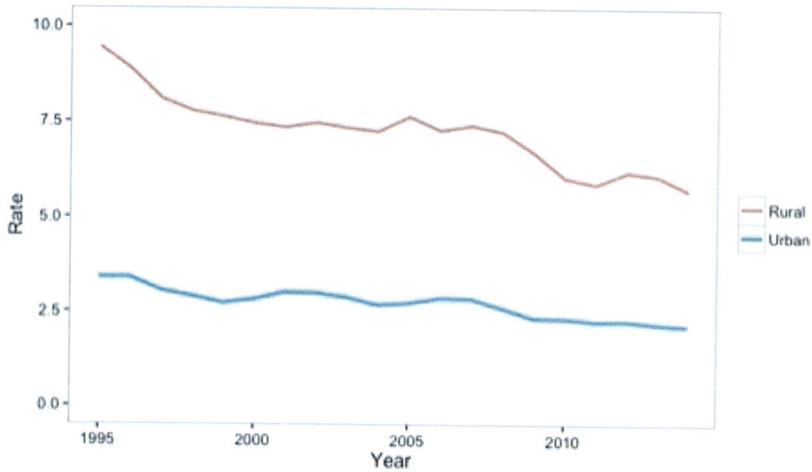

FIGURE A-5 Deaths from alcohol-related crashes by year per billion vehicle miles traveled—urban versus rural.
SOURCE: FARS data, 1995–2014.

Of all those fatally injured in alcohol-related motor vehicle crashes, 95.4 percent were occupants of motor vehicles, 4.0 percent were pedestrians, and 0.6 percent were cyclists. After adjusting for person-miles traveled, pedestrians had the highest fatality rate (22.2 fatalities per billion person-miles traveled), followed by cyclists (11.2) and then motorists (5.2). Over the study period, pedestrians had the greatest reduction in fatalities (36 percent) compared to motor vehicle occupants (29 percent) and cyclists (22 percent). Motorcyclists, particularly those 55 to 64 years old, experienced a marked increase in both number and rate of alcohol-impaired fatalities, with a specific increase following 2010.

From 1995 to 2015 the yearly rate of alcohol-related MVC fatalities was 4.44 persons per 100,000 population. Fatality rates differed substantially between states with the highest population-adjusted fatality rates in Montana, New Mexico, North Dakota, South Carolina, and Wyoming (8.13–11.38 yearly deaths per 100,000 population) and the lowest fatality rates in the District of Columbia, Massachusetts, New Jersey, New York, and Utah (1.73–2.38). Four states, Maine, North Dakota, Rhode Island, and South Dakota, experienced increases in population-adjusted fatalities from 1995 to 2015 (from 1 to 28 percent), while the District of Columbia, Hawaii, Kansas, New Mexico, and Vermont had the greatest declines in population-adjusted fatality rates, with reductions ranging from 58 to 69 percent.

Limitations

In this FARS database analysis, MVCs were considered alcohol related if a motor vehicle driver had police-reported alcohol intoxication or a positive laboratory BAC (BAC greater than 0.01 g/dL). Specifically, this information was obtained from the DR_DRINK variable from the FARS vehicle data files. Of note, the FARS crash-level DRUNK_DR variable was miscoded in the database for the years 1999–2007. While every crash within the database with driver alcohol involvement was included in this study, alcohol data are often missing from the database, meaning that this analysis may undercount the actual number of alcohol-related fatalities.

While the entire study period ranged from 1995 to 2015, analyses of race and ethnicity were from the years 2000 to 2015, since the FARS database did not begin recording race until 1999, and the U.S. Census significantly modified how it recorded race and ethnicity starting in 2000. As a result, the year 2000 was selected as the starting point for race and ethnicity subanalyses. Importantly, because the FARS obtains race and ethnicity information from death certificates, data are only available for individuals who were fatally injured. Even in this group, race or ethnicity information was missing in 14 percent of those persons reported to have died. This led to reduced fatality rates in the study's analyses by race and ethnicity. Though the FARS had a small degree of missing data for other data elements, none of the absent data significantly affected analyses since the information was missing in well below 1 percent of persons fatally injured.

The FARS database is updated every year with several new and recoded variables, and this recoding did limit the urban and rural sub-analysis to a minor extent. While rural and urban designation was previously a dichotomous variable, in 2015, the FARS recoded its road classification data element to include a third interstate category. Since this led to reduced rural and urban crash rates, 2015 data were excluded and only the years 1995–2014 were examined. In addition, because the HCUP census uses a different criterion to distinguish rural and urban populations from the FARS, only adjusted fatality rates by VMT could be obtained for these urban and rural subanalyses.

REFERENCES

AHRQ (Agency for Healthcare Research and Quality). 2015. *Introduction to the Healthcare Cost and Utilization Project's (HCUP) Nationwide Emergency Department Sample (NEDS), 2013.* https://www.hcup-us.ahrq.gov/db/nation/neds/NEDS2013Introduction.pdf (accessed October 24, 2017).

Brady, J. E., S. P. Baker, C. Dimaggio, M. L. McCarthy, G. W. Rebok, and G. Li. 2009. Effectiveness of mandatory alcohol testing programs in reducing alcohol involvement in fatal motor carrier crashes. *American Journal of Epidemiology* 170(6):775–782.

Clark, D. E., K. L. Anderson, and D. R. Hahn. 2004. Evaluating an inclusive trauma system using linked population-based data. *Journal of Trauma-Injury, Infection, and Critical Care* 57(3):501–509.

FBI (Federal Bureau of Investigation). 2016. *FBI releases 2015 crime statistics from the national incident-based reporting system, encourages transition.* Washington, DC: FBI National Press Office. https://www.fbi.gov/news/pressrel/press-releases/fbi-releases-2015-crime-statistics-from-the-national-incident-based-reporting-system-encourages-transition (accessed March 7, 2018).

Loo, B. P., and K. Tsui. 2007. Factors affecting the likelihood of reporting road crashes resulting in medical treatment to the police. *Injury Prevention* 13(3):186–189.

Lopez, D. G., D. L. Rosman, G. A. Jelinek, G. J. Wilkes, and P. C. Sprivulis. 2000. Complementing police road-crash records with trauma registry data—An initial evaluation. *Accident Analysis & Prevention* 32(6):771–777.

Lujic, S., C. Finch, S. Boufous, A. Hayen, and W. Dunsmuir. 2008. How comparable are road traffic crash cases in hospital admissions data and police records? An examination of data linkage rates. *Australian and New Zealand Journal of Public Health* 32(1):28–33.

Miller, J. D., I. Cisin, and A. Harrel. 1986. *A new technique for surveying deviant behavior: Item-count estimates of marijuana, cocaine, and heroin.* Paper presented at the Annual Meeting of the American Association for Public Opinion Research, St. Petersburg, FL.

Schroeder, T., and K. Ault. 2001. *The NEISS sample (design and implementation) 1997 to present.* https://www.cpsc.gov/s3fs-public/pdfs/blk_media_2001d011-6b6.pdf (accessed October 24, 2017).

Sterne, J. A., I. R. White, J. B. Carlin, M. Spratt, P. Royston, M. G. Kenward, A. M. Wood, and J. R. Carpenter. 2009. Multiple imputation for missing data in epidemiological and clinical research: Potential and pitfalls. *BMJ* 338:B2393.

Subramanian, R. 2002. *Transitioning to multiple imputation—A new method to estimate missing blood alcohol concentration (BAC) values in FARS.* Washington, DC: National Center for Statistics and Analysis.

Subramanian, R., and D. Utter. 2003. *Multiple imputation of missing blood alcohol concentration (BAC) values in FARS.* Paper presented at the Federal Committee on Statistical Methodology Conference, Arlington, VA.

Warner, S. L. 1965. Randomized response: A survey technique for eliminating evasive answer bias. *Journal of the American Statistical Association* 60(309):63–69.

B

Content Analysis of Alcohol-Impaired Driving Stories in the News

Deborah A. Fisher, Ph.D.

INTRODUCTION

Throughout the 30-year period from 1980 to 2010, the United States made substantial gains in reducing alcohol-impaired driving fatalities, which fell from around 24,000 deaths annually in the early 1980s to just over 10,000 in 2010. Along with the number of fatalities, the rate of alcohol involvement in crash fatalities decreased from 60 percent in 1982 to 34 percent in 2010 (Alcoholalert.com, n.d.; NCSA, 2016). This progress came about through the efforts of grassroots community advocacy on alcohol and traffic safety, most notably with the advent of Mothers Against Drunk Driving and the legislative agendas supported at the state and federal levels, including raising the minimum legal drinking age and lowering the illegal per se blood alcohol concentration (BAC) limit for drivers.

Since 2010, however, fatalities and fatality rates associated with alcohol-impaired driving have remained stable. To provide guidance on how to resume progress on the issue, the Committee on Accelerating Progress to Reduce Alcohol-Impaired Driving Fatalities was established and tasked with identifying promising interventions for preventing impaired driving, barriers that exist and approaches to overcome them, and ways interventions may need to be changed or adapted to resume a downward trend.

One area for potentially refining or redirecting prevention approaches is the information environment around alcohol-impaired driving. The ways stories are told in the media (i.e., the slant, the frame, the lens used to view events and issues) have the potential to influence the ways people think about issues and, therefore, the solutions they believe will be effective and, thus, will support for alleviating problems. The framing of news stories around issues such as poverty, for example, has been shown to affect the way people think about them, with presentations that focus on general outcomes leading to attributions of responsibility to society at large, while those that focus on specific instances of low-income persons align with attributions of individual responsibility (Iyengar, 1990).

Evidence suggests that the way impaired driving is covered in the news can affect individuals' support for alcohol enforcement and may affect behavior. In a study that manipulated the presence or absence of alcohol as a causative factor in news stories about violent crime, motor vehicle crashes, and other unintended injuries, investigators found that participants who read news stories with alcohol mentions reported greater support for enforcement of alcohol-control laws compared to those who read news stories lacking alcohol mentions (Slater et al., 2012). Yanovitzky (2002) found in a longitudinal study using data from 1978 to 1995 that news coverage of alcohol-impaired driving significantly contributed to impaired-driving-related policy actions, which, in turn, were associated with a reduction in impaired driving among young and high-risk drivers.

The current content analysis of alcohol-impaired driving news stories was conducted to support the work of the committee by providing an assessment of the news environment around alcohol-impaired driving. Content analysis offers a rigorous methodology for qualitatively coding the content of media stories to gather insights into what topics are being presented to the public most often and how that information is being presented or framed (i.e., the context). The results help further our understanding of what messages viewers may be taking away from their interaction with media. Additionally, the results may suggest ways media messaging may need to be modified to support public health efforts.

METHODS

Sampling

As a first step in identifying the universe of news stories from which a sample could be drawn for coding purposes, four newspapers (*The Washington Post*, *The New York Times*, *USA Today*, and *The Wall Street Journal*) and three cable television news outlets (CNN, Fox News Network, and MSNBC) were selected as sources in an effort to obtain a balance of media outlets generally considered to represent the right, left, and center of the political spectrum. (Initially several other news outlets were targeted, including Politico, The Drudge Report, and Breitbart; however, the news stories of these outlets were not available as transcripts in LexisNexis and, therefore, they were dropped from the content analysis.)

After these sources were identified, a literature search was conducted in an attempt to gather as comprehensive a universe of stories as possible on alcohol-impaired driving spanning from 2010 through June 2017. The search strategy involved using a series of alcohol terms (e.g., *blood alcohol*) and driving terms (e.g., *drunk driving*) appearing in the headline, byline, or appearing at least four times in the story. The exact search strategy was as follows:

> **hlead** *(driving while impaired or driving while intoxicated or driving under the influence or crash or driving or driving fatalities or traffic accidents or traffic fatalities or traffic safety or automobile accidents or driving while intoxicated* **and** *blood alcohol or BAC or 0.05 or 0.05 blood alcohol content or alcohol impaired driver or drunk driving limit or drunk driving threshold or drink driving or drink! driving or drunk! driving or drunken driving or drunk driving or alcohol impaired driving or alcohol impaired fatalities or alcohol related deaths or alcohol related driving or alcohol intoxication or binge drinking or drinking behavior or drunken driving or alcohol involved driving)* **or** **atl4** (*driving while impaired or driving while intoxicated or driving under the influence or crash or driving or driving fatalities or traffic accidents or traffic fatalities or traffic safety or automobile accidents* **and** *blood alcohol or BAC or 0.05 or 0.05 blood alcohol content or alcohol impaired driver or drunk driving limit or drunk driving threshold or drink driving or drink! driving or drunk! driving or drunken driving or drunk driving or alcohol impaired driving or alcohol impaired fatalities or alcohol related deaths or alcohol related driving or alcohol intoxication or binge drinking or drinking behavior or drunken driving or alcohol involved driving).*

This search strategy cast a wide net to ensure that the vast majority of relevant stories were captured and initially led to the identification of 774 articles published across the seven news outlets. Upon further investigation, 156 stories were dropped because on cursory inspection, they did not focus on impaired driving, or full-text access via hyperlinks or transcripts in LexisNexis was not available. The stories eliminated from the sample at this point came from *The Wall Street Journal* and the three cable television news outlets. This resulted in a sample of 618 news stories for coding. The distribution of news stories across the seven sources is shown in Table B-1.

Coding Protocol

Guided by the work of Shanto Iyengar and other researchers who have conducted media content analyses focused on how issues such as tobacco are framed in the news media (Clegg Smith et al., 2002), a coding scheme was developed and reviewed by the committee members. The coding scheme contained five sections: story descriptors, story frame and

TABLE B-1 Number of News Stories by Media Outlet

Media Outlet	Alcohol-Impaired Driving Stories Identified
The New York Times	134
The Wall Street Journal	17
The Washington Post	234
USA Today	58
CNN	132
Fox	20
MSNBC	23
Total	618

focus, voices represented, values and themes, and story topics. A copy of the final version of the coding scheme is presented after the references section of this paper.

Story Descriptors

Fields completed to provide descriptive information for each story included title, source, date of publication, date of coding, word count, and type of article (e.g., news, editorial, opinion, other).

Story Frame and Focus

A story frame refers to the techniques used to tell a news story that are posited to influence viewers' attributions of responsibility for social problems and suggest the solutions needed to solve them. As described by Benjamin (2007), an *episodic* news frame focuses on individual case studies and discrete events; it is likened to taking a telephoto lens in that it gives a close-up picture. In contrast, a *thematic* frame focuses on trends over time, and highlights contexts and environment; it is likened to taking a wide-angle lens to the issue. Implications of news framing are that episodic frames tend to highlight solutions targeting the individual experiencing the problem; thematic frames, with their broader focus on the surrounding environment and public policies and institutions, highlight solutions aimed at fixing the underlying conditions that cause or contribute to the problem. Applied to alcohol-impaired driving news stories, those that focus on a specific incident of impaired driving (e.g., a crash, an arrest for driving under the influence of alcohol) represent the application of an episodic frame; those stories that focus on larger societal issues such as through historical and epidemiological pieces or calls for action by communities and officials to reduce the problem represent use of a thematic frame.

For each story about a specific incident of alcohol-impaired driving, several characteristics of the incident were coded, including the following:

- Type of incident: fatal crash, injury crash, property-damage-only crash, arrest without a crash, other;
- Time frame for reporting on the incident: less than 1 week, 1–4 weeks, more than 1 month later, unclear;
- Ramifications reported: physical injuries to victims and perpetrators, psychological impacts on victims and perpetrators, other impacts on victims and perpetrator (e.g., inability to work, financial), impacts on victims' families, various stages of the adjudication process, other;
- Whether the focus was on the victim versus the perpetrator;
- Whether the incident involved a celebrity or local person of prominence in the community; and
- What substances were reported as being involved in the incident.

For each story that included discussion of broader social or environmental issues, the technique(s) or approach(es) to presenting this wide-angle perspective, the focus, was coded. Coding categories for focus included historical/epidemiological, call for action, program/policy/legislation, alcohol/drinking culture, sales/marketing/promotion of alcohol, court challenges, and so forth. Stories that included discussion of an alcohol-impaired crash or arrest together with broader social issues related to alcohol-impaired driving were coded for both the specific incident (i.e., episodic frame) and the broader discussion (i.e., thematic frame).

Voices Represented

An extensive list of persons whose voices could be represented in stories by being directly quoted, cited, or referenced as sources of information for the story was developed. As with all variables, the list originally developed was expanded throughout the coding process. Voices included law enforcement and judicial officials, victims and their families, perpetrators and their families, attorneys (perpetrator's, victim's, and other/legal analyst), traffic safety advocates, government health and safety organizations, alcohol industry or trade association representatives, alcohol retailers, medical/health professionals, and others. Voices were coded for all stories.

Values or Themes

Values or themes represent the underlying message(s) embodied in the story. Examples of themes coded included victimization, injustice, punishment, individual problem/responsibility, collective problem/responsibility, liberty/personal freedom, and so forth. Values may be expressed directly by individuals represented in the story or implied by the type of information or way information is presented in the story. For example, one story reported on the advocacy efforts by the parents of one of two teenage passengers killed when their friend crashed the car they were all riding in after having been drinking at an underage party where the parent of the host joked with partygoers about the alcohol they were bringing into the home. The victim's parents were quoted calling for more severe penalties for the teen driver and the adult who knew about and permitted the teen drinking party in his home. In addition to the value/theme of punishment, this story was also coded based on the described actions of the adult social host for individual/problem responsibility as well as failure of family, the latter owing to the implied references to irresponsible parenting. Values were coded for all stories.

Story Topics

Story topics are the specific issues related to alcohol-impaired driving that were discussed explicitly in the story. In the coding scheme developed, these 41 topics fell into broad categories:

- Scope of the problem (e.g., societal toll, human toll);
- Responsibility for the problem (e.g., individual, enforcement of alcohol laws);
- Types of prevention or alcohol-impaired driving countermeasures discussed (e.g., prevention/general deterrence, intervention/specific deterrence, harm reduction);
- New tools or technology (e.g., for police, courts, retailers; for drinkers or drivers);
- Community mobilization;
- Impaired-driving system problems/failures (e.g., system overall, court system, alcohol retailers);
- Impaired-driving system successes (e.g., system overall, legislation/policy, alcohol industry); and
- Other topics that emerged during the coding process (e.g., politics/corruption, targeting social/moderate versus heavy/hardcore drinkers, underage drinking, two-tiered justice system).

Story topics were coded for all stories.

Coding Procedures

A single coder experienced in content analysis conducted the coding task during a 5-week period from July 23, 2017, through August 27, 2017. Once the coding process began and stories were read in their entirety, 31 additional stories of the 618 that were originally included in the sample were eliminated, mostly because they were too short and lacked sufficient information for coding (n = 17). This led to a criterion that stories had to be at least three paragraphs in length to provide enough information for coding. Other reasons for eliminating stories were incomplete transcripts or finding that a story did not actually involve impaired driving (e.g., an article on drowsy driving that had one mention of impaired driving as a comparison regarding degree of impairment; a story about how numerous red flags, one of which was impaired driving along with owing back taxes, multiple divorces, and so forth should have resulted in revocation of an individual's security clearance; a story on research from the Netherlands on effects of alcohol and cannabis on aggression).

Because of the project timeline, the full sample of 587 stories could not be coded. After flipping a coin to randomly start with the first or second story to begin the coding process, every fourth story was coded. If the fourth story was one of the 31 stories eliminated, the next story was coded. This yielded a final sample of 147 coded stories.

As each story was reviewed, in addition to checking the appropriate codes, extensive notes were entered on a hard copy of the coding form. All "other" responses were specified so that emerging issues could be tracked. This led to the addition of several new codes over the course of the task (e.g., pulling justice/judge out of the other category and making it a separate category in voices; adding effects on enforcement/prosecution and targeting social/moderate drinkers versus heavy/hardcore drinkers to values), which are represented in the coding scheme listed at the end of this paper. Given that most of these new codes had emerged about halfway through the coding process, after the full sample of 147 stories was coded, a second pass was made through the first half of the stories to supplement notes taken and see if material needed to be recoded.

Data from the coding forms, excluding handwritten notes, were entered into an electronic form in Survey Gizmo. Data were exported into an Excel file, which was used to develop counts for all data points.

Results

Overall Sample

Of the total sample of 147 coded stories, 139 (94.6 percent) were news focused, 4 (2.7 percent) were editorials, and 4 (2.7 percent) were opinion pieces. The number of stories in the sample by year of publication were 10 from 2010, 15 from 2011, 16 from 2012, 27 from 2013, 9 from 2014, 33 from 2015, 27 from 2016, and 10 from the first half of 2017.

Other descriptive information for the sample is presented in Table B-2. Seventy percent of the news stories coded came from the newspaper sources, mostly *The New York Times* and *The Washington Post*. Newspaper stories tended to be around 550–570 words in length, while cable television news stories were about double that in length. This differential in story length is attributable to the fact that when cable television news outlets cover a story on alcohol-impaired driving, it is often a story that receives national attention. Additionally, depending on the show on which it is televised, the story may be part of an hour-long news magazine show (e.g., *The Nancy Grace Show*, *Primetime Justice*, *The O'Reilly Factor*) in which stories may be discussed in one of three or four show segments or the entire show may be devoted to it.

Newspaper stories, on the other hand, are shorter, due in part to the diversity of types of stories covered in this platform. Newspapers like *The New York Times*, *The Washington Post*, and *The Wall Street Journal* tend to cover both local events in their respective communities and events of national interest. Thus, their coverage of alcohol-impaired driving events includes a combination of highly publicized national incidents as well as short stories of local arrests and crashes, many of which are covered within a day or two of the event's occurrence before much information is known. These variations in story length between cable television news outlets and newspaper sources may also reflect assumptions about the

TABLE B-2 Frequency Distribution of News Stories Across News Outlets for All Alcohol-Impaired Driving Stories, n = 147

News Source	Number of Stories	Percent of Sample	Average Word Count
The New York Times	30	20.4	571
The Washington Post	56	38.1	554
The Wall Street Journal	5	3.4	N/A*
USA Today	13	8.8	576
CNN	32	21.8	1,690
Fox News	5	3.4	1,115
MSNBC	6	4.1	509
Total	147	100.0	

* Transcripts of *The Wall Street Journal* articles did not provide a word count, and because they were locked, the content could not be copied into a Word file to determine story length.

differential attention spans of the public for material presented in a written versus visual format.

Episodic Versus Thematic Frames

Of the 147 alcohol-impaired driving news stories, 66 (44.9 percent) focused exclusively on discussing a specific incident of alcohol-impaired driving and, thus, are considered to have employed an episodic frame. The remaining 81 (55.1 percent) used a thematic frame, with a discussion of the broader societal issues either alone (e.g., a comparison of different versions of alcohol-impaired driving laws pending in a state's legislature, a traffic safety organization's recommendations that all states lower their illegal per se BAC limit from 0.08% to 0.05%) or in combination with an incident of alcohol-impaired driving (e.g., how a fiery school bus crash in a state was the impetus to a shift in norms and attitudes about alcohol-impaired driving and activism that resulted in stronger legislation, or renewed support for a stronger interlock law following the death of a police officer struck by an impaired driver while working on a holiday driving while impaired [DWI] task force).

Research question 1: Whose voices are represented most often and least often in alcohol-impaired driving news stories? Table B-3 presents the frequency distribution of voices that were represented across the 147 news stories. Most stories quoted or referenced information provided by multiple sources so the percentages do not total to 100 percent. The individuals and entities referenced most often in alcohol-impaired driving stories included law enforcement (27.2 percent; often via the public information officer or other official giving details from the police report), traffic safety advocates (21.1 percent), prosecutors (19.7 percent; typically discussing charges filed/to be filed or sentences sought), other attorney or legal analyst (18.4 percent; legal experts not directly involved in the prosecution or defense providing legal analysis and opinions on cases), and victim's family (15.6 percent; often in the aftermath of fatal crashes such as trial and sentencing of offenders or in stories that follow up on actions prompted by the crash such as new legislation), followed closely by perpetrators (15.0 percent) and the media (15.0 percent; investigative reporters on cable news shows). Those represented least often in alcohol-impaired driving stories were alcohol retailers (2.0 percent), perpetrator's family members (2.0 percent), victims (2.7 percent), medical and health professionals (3.4 percent), and callers into cable television shows (3.4 percent). The category "other" was represented in 40.8 percent of stories and consists of a diverse array of individuals and entities idiosyncratic to one or two stories, such as the director of public parks and a bicycle

TABLE B-3 Frequency of Voices Represented in Alcohol-Impaired Driving Stories, n = 147

Voice	Percent and Number of Stories	Voice	Percent and Number of Stories
Law enforcement	27.2 (40)	Government public health/safety organization	6.1 (9)
Traffic safety advocates	21.1 (31)	Researcher	5.4 (8)
Prosecutor	19.7 (29)	Alcohol industry or industry-funded lobby group	4.8 (7)
Other attorney/legal analyst	18.4 (27)	Medical/health professional	3.4 (5)
Victim's family	15.6 (23)	Callers into show	3.4 (5)
Perpetrator	15.0 (22)	Victim	2.7 (4)
Media	15.0 (22)	Perpetrator's family	2.0 (3)
Policy maker	14.3 (21)	Alcohol retailers	2.0 (3)
Perpetrator's attorney	14.3 (21)	Other	40.8 (60)
Judge/justice	6.1 (9)		

advocacy group representative quoted in a story about an injury crash in which a vehicle driven by a suspected impaired driver entered a biking path and struck a bicyclist, or an official with the National Conference of State Legislators in a story about calls for tougher state impaired driving legislation.

Research question 2: What values or themes are expressed most frequently in alcohol-impaired driving news stories? The frequency with which different values or themes were discussed in the sample of stories is presented in Table B-4. Because many stories were coded as having multiple themes, the percentages do not total 100 percent. The theme of individual problem/responsibility was the most frequently coded value/theme, occurring in half of the stories (50.3 percent). This is consistent with the fact that nearly half of the stories in the sample (44.9 percent) were incident-only stories that detailed an arrest or crash linked to alcohol consumption. In some cases, the perpetrator or others made a direct statement regarding the perpetrator's responsibility for the crash; however, in most cases, individual problem/responsibility was inferred by the fact that the story provided details of the incident (e.g., offender's

TABLE B-4 Frequency of Values/Themes Represented in Alcohol-Impaired Driving Stories, n = 147

Value/Theme	Percent and Number of Stories	Value/Theme	Percent and Number of Stories
Individual problem/ responsibility	50.3 (74)	Personal engagement/ activism	6.8 (10)
Victimization	28.6 (42)	Effects on enforcement/ prosecution	6.1 (9)
Punishment	27.9 (41)	Protective role of government	4.8 (7)
Injustice	16.3 (24)	Targeting social versus heavy/ hardcore drinkers	4.1 (6)
Getting serious/ tough	13.6 (20)	Avoiding holiday alcohol-impaired driving	4.1 (6)
Failure of family	13.6 (20)	Need for evidence-based prevention	3.4 (5)
Entitlement/ above the law	12.9 (19)	Economic interests	2.0 (3)
Collective problem/ responsibility	9.5 (14)	Experiential learning to prevent risky driving	2.0 (3)
Liberty/personal freedom	7.5 (11)	Influence of special interests beyond industry	1.4 (2)
Cultural change in norms	7.5 (11)	Recovery/personal transformation	1.4 (2)
Alcohol retailer/ industry problem or responsibility	6.8 (10)	Other	14.3 (21)

impairment, driving actions that led to the crash, charges filed/to be filed) with no information suggesting the event was attributable to causes beyond the perpetrator's decision to drink and drive and subsequent actions on the road.

Other values/themes expressed relatively frequently included other topics associated with crashes and linked to them immediately afterward, such as victimization (28.6 percent), or later at their legal resolution, such as punishment (27.9 percent) and injustice (16.3 percent). These values/

themes were followed by getting serious or tough on alcohol-impaired driving (13.6 percent) and failure of family (13.6 percent). The failure of family theme resulted, in large part, from the widespread media coverage of the Texas teen, dubbed the "affluenza" teen, who avoided prison for killing four and seriously injuring two persons in an alcohol-impaired driving crash he caused and instead was sentenced to rehabilitation and probation when his defense argued that his parents' coddling of him and failure to teach him responsibility or consequences for his actions led to his risky decision to drink and drive. Numerous stories about this crash appeared across media outlets in two spates—first in 2013 when the perpetrator's trial took place and again in 2015 after the perpetrator and his mother fled the United States for Mexico following the posting of a video on social media of an alleged probation violation.

Many values/themes incorporated throughout the coding process appeared with low frequencies (i.e., across six or seven stories), including the protective role of government (4.8 percent), targeting social versus heavy/hardcore drinkers (4.1 percent), avoiding holiday alcohol-impaired driving (4.1 percent), and five other values/themes were expressed even less frequently. Twenty-one stories (14.3 percent) were coded for "other" values/themes that occurred alone or in addition to more commonly expressed values/themes. Examples of these story-specific values/themes include the right to counsel of DWI offenders (in an opinion piece by a trial lawyer), positive-focused media messaging (in a news story on an alcohol-impaired driving campaign developed in one jurisdiction targeting young males), and possible public safety contributions of a ride-hailing service (in a story in which the company linked data on increases in its ridership to decreases in impaired driving).

Research question 3: What specific topics are included in alcohol-impaired driving news stories most and least often? Table B-5 displays the frequency of mentions of a wide array of topic categories and specific story topics across the sample of alcohol-impaired driving stories. The categories of topics represented most often in stories were prevention/intervention approaches to dealing with alcohol-impaired driving (63.9 percent; e.g., prevention/general deterrence, intervention/specific deterrence, sanctions, harm reduction), responsibility for the problem (61.2 percent), scope of the alcohol-impaired driving problem (53.1 percent), and the combination category of emergent issues (72.1 percent). The single-item category community, which consisted of grassroots advocacy efforts, and the category impaired-driving system successes were the categories that were least frequently mentioned, appearing in just 2.0 and 4.1 percent of news stories, respectively.

TABLE B-5 Frequency of Alcohol-Impaired Driving Issues and Specific Topics Represented in Alcohol-Impaired Driving Stories, n = 147

Impaired-Driving Issues and Topics	Percent and Number of Stories	Impaired-Driving Topics	Percent and Number of Stories
Scope of the Problem	53.1 (78)	*Alcohol-Impaired Driving System Successes*	4.1 (6)
Public health toll	23.1 (34)	Successes, unspecified	1.4 (2)
Human toll	37.4 (55)	Legislation/policy	1.4 (2)
Responsibility	61.2 (90)	Enforcement	1.4 (2)
Personal	52.4 (77)	Court system	0.7 (1)
Enforcement	0.7 (1)	Alcohol retailers	0.0 (0)
Court/probation system	0.7 (1)	Alcohol industry	0.7 (1)
Government/policy makers	6.8 (10)	Others	0.0 (0)
Alcohol retailers	2.7 (4)	*Emergent Issues*	72.1 (106)
Alcohol industry	3.4 (5)	Politics/corruption	4.1 (6)
Other	4.8 (7)	Entitlement/above the law	13.6 (20)
Prevention/Intervention	63.9 (94)	Two-tiered justice system	5.4 (8)
General deterrence	19.0 (28)	Irresponsible parenting	12.9 (19)
Specific deterrence	34.0 (50)	Targeting social versus heavy/hardcore drinkers	3.4 (5)
Sanctions	27.9 (41)	Change in lifestyle/direction	0.7 (1)
Harm reduction	8.8 (13)	Underage drinking	5.4 (8)
Other alcohol policies	6.8 (10)	Individual versus states' rights	4.8 (7)
Tools/Technology	7.5 (11)	Illegal immigration	2.7 (4)
Police, courts, retailers	0.7 (1)	Other	46.9 (69)
Drinkers/drivers	6.8 (10)		
Community	2.0 (3)		
Grassroots advocacy	2.0 (3)		
Alcohol-Impaired Driving System Failures/Problems	23.8 (35)		
Failure, unspecified	0.0 (0)		
Legislation/policy	8.8 (13)		
Enforcement	3.4 (5)		
Court system	10.2 (15)		
Alcohol retailers	1.4 (2)		
Alcohol industry	0.7 (1)		
Others	1.4 (2)		

NOTE: Because stories that address an impaired-driving issue or topic category may contain multiple mentions of the subsumed specific topics, the numbers and percentages for topic categories, which are unduplicated counts, and mentions of specific topics are not equal.

Among specific story topics, those with the most mentions were personal responsibility (52.4 percent), human toll (37.4 percent), specific deterrence strategies for reducing recidivism and protecting the public (34.0 percent), sanctions (27.9 percent), and public health toll (23.1 percent); the "other" category of story-specific topics was represented in 46.9 percent of stories. With few exceptions, the remaining specific topics related to alcohol-impaired driving appeared in less than 10 percent of stories. The topics alcohol-impaired driving system successes-alcohol retailer and alcohol-impaired driving system failure/problem-unspecified did not appear in any of the news stories in the sample. Numerous other topics were mentioned just once or twice across the 147 news stories.

Stories with Alcohol-Impaired Driving Incidents (n = 104)

Table B-6 presents the frequency with which news stories involving alcohol-impaired driving incidents involved different types of events (e.g., fatal crash, arrest without crash), substances used, and persons of public interest, including celebrities and local persons of prominence in the community (e.g., local politician, well-known businessperson). In terms of type of incident, more than half of the stories on impaired-driving events were about a fatal crash (56.7 percent) and just over a quarter of stories were about an arrest without a crash (26.9 percent); injury crashes and property-damage-only crashes each accounted for 6.7 percent of stories.

Regarding substance involvement, over 85 percent of stories suggested that alcohol was the sole substance used and the basis for intoxication. It should be noted that most stories of alcohol-impaired driving incidents did not directly specify alcohol involvement, but mentioned that a driver was "intoxicated" or "impaired" and/or that the driver was charged with DUI or DWI. In this overwhelming majority of cases, the assumption was that the substance involved was alcohol; if another drug was mentioned, then it was coded alone or together with alcohol, as described in the story. The combination of alcohol and prescription medications and alcohol and illicit drugs accounted for 3.8 and 2.9 percent of stories, respectively. In four cases (3.8 percent) the driver was reported to have tested positive for all three substances, and in one case (1.0 percent) the driver was speculated to have taken a prescription drug, GHB, alone.

Over the course of the coding process, it was noted that among some stories that appeared in the sample multiple times across sources and over time, reports of substance involvement for the same incident differed. In one crash that appeared in numerous stories in 2013 at the time of trial and again in 2015 after a potential probation violation, most stories referenced alcohol; only a few stories reported alcohol and cannabis

TABLE B-6 Frequency of Incident Types, Substances Involved, and Noted Persons in News Stories with Alcohol-Impaired Driving Incidents, n = 104

Type of Incident	Percent	Substance Involvement	Percent	Celebrity	Percent	Local Person of Prominence	Percent
Arrest	26.9	Alcohol only	86.5	Perpetrator	13.5	Perpetrator	15.4
Injury crash	6.7	Alcohol plus prescription drug	3.8	Victim	0.0	Victim	2.9
Fatal crash	56.7	Alcohol plus illicit drug	2.9	Passenger with perpetrator	0.0	Passenger with perpetrator	0.0
Property-damage crash	6.7	Alcohol plus drugs (unspecified)	1.9	Passenger with victim	0.0	Passenger with victim	0.0
Other	2.9	Prescription drugs only	1.0	Other	0.0	Other	0.0
		Alcohol plus prescription and illicit drugs	3.8				
Total	99.9	Total	99.9		13.5		18.3

or alcohol and Valium and a single story reported all three substances. Some of the discrepancies in substance involvement are likely attributable to the reporting of events within days of their occurrence before toxicology reports are available. In stories that run in one news cycle only, the information on other substances may become available after the story has ceased to be covered. Thus, the involvement of drugs may be underrepresented in news stories.

Celebrities were mentioned in 13.5 percent of stories with alcohol-impaired driving incidents, always as the perpetrator. For local persons of prominence in the community (i.e., those with name recognition and known widely in their community but not celebrities on a national or international scale), such individuals were represented in 15.4 percent of stories as perpetrators and 2.9 percent of stories as victims.

Research question 4: How extensively across time and consequences is the coverage of alcohol-impaired driving incidents in news stories? Information on the distribution of the news stories with alcohol-impaired driving incidents across different time frames and the frequency with which different consequences associated with alcohol-impaired driving events were reported is presented in Table B-7. Nearly two-thirds of stories (63.5 percent) were reported more than a month after their occurrence. This is associated with the fact that 38 of the 104 stories involving alcohol-impaired incidents also discussed broader societal issues, often dealing with advocacy or policy efforts undertaken in the aftermath of a crash. Just over one-quarter of the stories (26.0 percent) reported alcohol-impaired driving events that had occurred within a week.

Regarding consequences stemming from the alcohol-impaired driving incidents, those mentioned most frequently included pretrial processes (e.g., charges, jail, bond, indictment), which were covered in 44.2 percent of stories; victim's physical injuries, mentioned in 31.7 percent of stories; impacts on victim's family, found in 26.0 percent of stories; and sentencing of perpetrators, mentioned in 24.0 percent of stories. Again, the "other" category containing idiosyncratic or story-specific ramifications such as a swimmer's suspension from competition by USA Swimming and loss of corporate endorsements was coded in 55.8 percent of stories. The remaining consequences associated with impaired driving were each mentioned in less than 10 percent of news stories.

Research question 5: To what extent do news stories on alcohol-impaired driving incidents focus on victims compared to perpetrators? Stories on alcohol-impaired driving overwhelmingly focused on perpetrators (78.8 percent), owing in part to the fact that more than half of the stories involved fatal crashes. Although victims were mentioned, stories tended

TABLE B-7 Time Frame of Reporting and Extensiveness of Coverage Over Time of Alcohol-Impaired Driving Incidents, n = 104

Time Frame	Percent	Ramifications	Percent
Immediately after (within 6 days)	26.0	Victim's physical injuries	31.7
Short term (1–4 weeks)	5.8	Psychological effects on victims	5.8
Long term (more than 1 month later)	63.5	Other impacts on victims	8.7
Unclear	4.8	Impact on victim's family	26.0
		Perpetrator's physical injuries	5.8
		Psychological effects on perpetrators	9.6
		Other impacts on perpetrators	5.8
		Pretrial (bond, jail, charges)	44.2
		Trial	7.7
		Sentencing	24.0
		Other	55.8
Total	100.1		

to focus on the actions leading up to the incident and consequences for perpetrators in terms of charges, trial, and sentencing. Victims were the focus of stories in 11.5 percent of cases. In three cases (2.9 percent), stories about an alcohol-impaired driving incident focused equally on perpetrator and victim, and in seven cases (6.7 percent), the focus of the story was on another individual other than perpetrator or victim (e.g., a police officer standing trial for perjury for her testimony given in an earlier DWI case who was acquitted of charges; a father who allowed an underage drinking party in his home after which one of the partygoers caused a fatal crash; two teens facing charges for allowing a fellow underage drinking partygoer to drive home).

Stories with a Broader Social/Environmental Focus (n = 81)

Research question 6: What approach to discussing larger societal/ environmental issues do news stories taking a thematic frame to the issue of alcohol-impaired driving use? Table B-8 displays the occurrence of different approaches to discussing broader societal/environmental issues across the 81 thematically framed news stories on alcohol-impaired

TABLE B-8 Frequency of Approaches to Discussing Societal/Environmental Issues in Thematic News Stories on Alcohol-Impaired Driving, n = 81

Focus	Percent and Number of Thematic Stories
Program/policy/legislation	39.5 (32)
Historical/epidemiological	37.0 (30)
Call for action/more action	19.8 (16)
Alcohol/drinking culture	17.3 (14)
Links to other social issues	17.3 (14)
Politics/corruption	4.9 (4)
Two-tiered justice system	6.2 (5)
Illegal immigration	6.2 (5)
Court challenges	9.9 (8)
Sales/marketing/promotion of alcohol	3.7 (3)
Other	22.2 (18)

driving. Because thematic news stories often used multiple techniques to discuss social issues linked to alcohol-impaired driving, percentages do not sum to 100. Approaches or foci used to present a thematically framed story most often involved discussion of program/policy/legislation (39.5 percent), historical/epidemiological trends or information (37.0 percent), and calls for action/more action on the issue of alcohol-impaired driving (19.8 percent). In 17.3 percent of stories on alcohol-impaired driving there was discussion of broader societal issues by discussing alcohol/drinking culture or linking an incident to issues of politics/corruption, bias/preferential treatment by the judicial system, or illegal immigration. The most infrequently used approach to thematic framing was the discussion of sales/marketing/promotion of alcohol (3.7 percent).

Fifty-one unique stories presented a thematic frame through the discussion of a program, policy, and/or legislation; historical context or epidemiological trends; and/or calls to action. To investigate whether the use of these three approaches to thematic framing was associated with discussions about efforts to reduce the occurrence of alcohol-impaired driving through targeting individuals or the general population, the prevention/intervention approaches within specific topics were examined for these 51 stories. The prevention/intervention approaches included three that are focused on broad populations of all drivers or all drinkers. These include general deterrence strategies (e.g., per se BAC limits, information/educational campaigns relating to impaired driving), harm reduction efforts to separate drinking and driving (e.g., sober rides, use of designated drivers), and other alcohol policies (e.g., alcohol taxes, legislation on dram shop, responsible beverage service, furnishing alcohol to minors). The other two categories of prevention/intervention approaches to alcohol-impaired driving focus on individuals, specifically impaired-driving offenders, and include specific deterrence (i.e., strategies designed to reduce recidivism through means such as ignition interlocks, assessment/treatment, supervised probation) and punishment (e.g., fines, jail).

Across the 51 stories a fairly even distribution across the two foci of prevention and intervention strategies emerged, with 17 stories (33.3 percent) coded as focusing on an individually targeted policy related to specific deterrence or punishment only, 16 stories (31.4 percent) focused exclusively on a general population approach, and 12 stories (23.5 percent) that included a combination of general population and individually focused approaches to dealing with the problem of alcohol-impaired driving. Six stories (11.8 percent) were coded for using a broader social/environmental approach; however, the specific topics discussed were not related to prevention/intervention of impaired driving but issues such as illegal immigration, efforts to establish online criminal registries, and underage drinking education efforts.

Within each of the three framing techniques, there was considerable variability in the patterns of general population versus individual focus of prevention/intervention approaches. For the 32 stories within the program, policy, and legislation category, individually targeted strategies were discussed most often and were contained in 13 stories (40.6 percent), with 9 stories (28.1 percent) addressing strategies targeting the general population, and 7 stories (21.9 percent) focused on both prevention and intervention strategies. For the 16 stories in call to action, the most prevalent approach was a discussion of a combination of general population and individually focused approaches found in 8 stories (50.0 percent), with 4 stories (25.0 percent) discussing individually focused strategies and 2 stories (12.5 percent) discussing general population strategies exclusively. Finally, among the 30 stories employing a discussion of historical context or epidemiological trends, an even distribution was seen, with 10 stories (33.3 percent) focused on general population strategies, followed closely by 9 stories (30.0 percent) focused on individually targeted strategies and 9 stories (30.0 percent) on a combination of general population and individually focused approaches.

DISCUSSION

The current study was undertaken to determine how alcohol-impaired driving is framed in today's news environment. The sample of 147 news stories was split, with 45 percent using an episodic frame by focusing on a single incident of impaired driving and 55 percent using a thematic frame by placing the issue within a larger social context. Overall, news stories most frequently expressed values of individual problem/responsibility, victimization, and punishment. Within story topics covered, categories represented most often across all stories were prevention/intervention approaches, responsibility, and scope of the problem. Finally, for the entire sample, the voices most often represented in news stories included law enforcement, traffic safety advocates, prosecutors, and other attorneys/legal analysts. In terms of stories with alcohol-impaired driving events, stories overwhelmingly (almost 80 percent of the time) focused on perpetrators.

These findings suggest two trends in alcohol-impaired driving news stories over the past 7.5 years. First, the pattern of codes across these variables is consistent with the preponderance of fatal crashes among stories, which were nearly 57 percent of stories with alcohol-impaired driving incidents or 40 percent of the entire sample of stories. Such incidents evoke more sense of victimization and discussion of punishment than other types of impaired-driving incidents. Additionally, with a focus in stories on the actions of the perpetrator directly leading up to the incident, they communicate a message of personal responsibility for the arrest or crash, in which the individual is held responsible for drinking and driving. Second, the relatively high representation of the category, scope of the problem, and inclusion of traffic safety advocates as the voice with the second highest prevalence across stories reflect the influence of thematic-framed stories dealing with the issue of alcohol-impaired driving in terms of a community problem, with input from advocates who can speak to the statistics on the public health toll and the efforts aimed at reducing the problem.

Although thematic framing of stories places the problem of alcohol-impaired driving within a broader societal context, it does not ensure that approaches discussed for solving the problem necessarily target social and environmental factors. Among the stories using the most frequent techniques for thematic framing, a substantial proportion focused on individually targeted solutions (33 percent) or issues not directly associated with impaired driving (12 percent), often recounting the details of impaired driving events, highlighting individuals' bad decision making, and discussing the need for action or policy changes focused on efforts to punish offenders or control their drinking and driving. It should be noted that efforts to rehabilitate and control impaired driving offenders are advanced by traffic safety advocates and popular among policy makers because they not only target offenders but serve to support public health and safety by either keeping offenders off the road or ensuring that they do not drive with alcohol in their systems. Strategies such as ignition interlocks, electronic monitoring of offenders, and intensive supervision and probation allow offenders to remain with their families and keep their jobs while protecting the public and, therefore, are an important part of the arsenal of impaired driving countermeasures.

Focusing on individually targeted policy approaches to impaired driving, however, means that issues such as the culture of alcohol use, sales and promotion of alcohol, and the responsibility of persons and entities other than offenders often receive scant attention in news stories, even those with a thematic frame. Prevention efforts that target socio-cultural and policy contexts are critically important as they hold the promise of creating an environment in which heavy drinking and drinking and driving are not condoned or facilitated and, thus, help prevent the problem from occurring rather than dealing with offenders after an event has taken place. In the current analysis, slightly more than half of the stories in the entire sample used a thematic frame and, among those using the three most frequent thematic framing approaches, only 55 percent included a discussion of solutions targeting the broader social context of impaired driving and population-based approaches to the problem. To move forward in reducing impaired driving fatalities, efforts to engage news outlets in media advocacy on the issue should focus on encouraging news organizations to move away from stories of simple problem descriptions to those that contain more critical analysis of the social/environmental causal factors and discussion of broader-based solutions through primary prevention.

No other content analyses in the published literature were located that matched the focus of this one on alcohol-impaired driving in general or that used a similar sampling frame, with coding of both newspaper and cable television news stories. However, a comparison to another study of framing analysis of impaired driving stories is worth noting. In a study that examined motor vehicle crashes with injuries in U.S. newspapers between 1999 and 2002, researchers reported that among their sample of 473 stories, most reports in newspapers (97 percent) used an episodic frame. In summarizing their results, Rosales and Stallones (2008, p. 477) explained that "the majority of reports included information on the type of crash, but characteristics about people and vehicles were rarely reported." Thus, according to the authors, newspaper accounts are incomplete sources of information for influencing public attitudes and supporting public health agendas.

Because the current study examined stories involving crashes, arrest-only events, and alcohol-impaired driving without alcohol-impaired driving incidents, a lower percentage of stories were found to have an episodic frame (45 percent), a rate nearly one half of that found in the study by Rosales and Stallones (2008). This suggests that when assessing the news coverage of alcohol-impaired driving, the sampling methods used to select the platforms and the types of news stories to be included in the analysis may substantially affect the results. Stories confined to crashes are likely to recount details of the incident often in its immediate aftermath; stories on impaired driving without a crash event will more likely discuss causal factors beyond individuals and increase the prevalence of thematic framed stories.

The current study provides up-to-date information on alcohol-impaired driving in the news, yet has several limitations. First, the sample size of 147 stories is small. Unlike other content analyses undertaken as part of longer-term research projects, this content analysis had to be planned and executed within 6 to 8 weeks; thus, it was not possible to code a large sample.

Second, the short time frame also made it necessary to have the coding conducted by a single coder rather than a cadre of trained coders. Using multiple coders requires an extensive training and practice phase, ongoing reliability assessments throughout training and actual coding, retraining as needed, and a reconciliation process for the portion of the actual sample of stories that is double coded. Such a process was infeasible in this case, which resulted in a limited sample size and lack of reliability data. However, the fact that the sample was coded in a relatively short period of 5 weeks may have reduced the likelihood of changes in coding practices over time.

Third, because the purpose of the study was to look at the current and recent past years' news environment, stories had to be coded using archival means, primarily transcripts in LexisNexis. Although transcripts provide a full record of stories developed for dissemination in text format and presented in platforms such as newspapers, transcripts of stories broadcast on television are not as conducive to capturing information as comprehensively. For cable television programs, transcripts of stories can be incomplete for several reasons (e.g., video segments are not seen and the material transcribed is partial with persons in videos often identified simply as "unidentified male" or "unidentified female"). Additionally, because hosts and multiple guests often talk at the same time so that discussion is indecipherable by transcribers, information is missing as places in the transcript will simply designate "cross talk." Finally, because the coder cannot access the visual content, some material is harder to understand as context is lost. When information is not accessible in its originally developed format, there are inherent difficulties in coding stories across platforms.

Finally, because the current sample was drawn from a combination of a limited number of newspapers (mostly published on the East Coast) and several cable television news outlets, there may have been selection bias in terms of the types of stories covered in this content analysis. This may have influenced the results in several ways. First, to the extent that there are cultural differences across regions of the United States regarding impaired driving, the values/themes may have reflected those of East Coast and urban areas disproportionately. Second, news outlets that focus on a national audience (such as *USA Today* and the three cable television news outlets) cover only the most serious or egregious incidents and, thus, do not cover the number and breadth of impaired-driving crashes as news sources that focus on local events in the community or both local and national events (e.g., *The Washington Post* and *The New York Times*). The fact that this framing analysis adopted a broad focus on all types of impaired-driving stories not limited to crashes and the inclusion of several national news outlets together likely reduced the occurrence of incident-only (i.e., episodic) stories in this analysis.

In the future, content coding of news stories can be improved in several ways. First, with a longer planning phase, it will be possible to review stories and develop methods specifically tailored to the different story formats. Second, conducting content analyses of current news stories in which content can be recorded in real time in the format it is disseminated (e.g., recording television shows that can be watched by coders) would avoid problems of coding in formats different from that in which stories were originally developed. Third, digital media deserves more attention. Content analyses have already been conducted of posts to online news message boards covering alcohol-impaired driving enforcement, but young people are increasingly turning to nontraditional sources for their news, including online social networks such as Facebook and Twitter, and these are not as easy to access (Connor and Wesolowski, 2009). Use of these platforms and the rise in citizen journalism may have significant implications for what types of content on alcohol-impaired driving are covered as news and how.

REFERENCES

Alcoholalert.com. n.d. *2011 Drunk driving statistics*. http://www.alcoholalert.com/drunk-driving-statistics.html (accessed September 3, 2017).

Benjamin, D. 2007. *A FrameWorks Institute FrameByte: Episodic vs thematic stories*. https://www.frameworksinstitute.org/assets/files/framebytes/framebytethematic.pdf (accessed September 5, 2017).

Clegg Smith, K., M. Wakefield, C. Siebel, G. Szczypka, S. J. Slater, Y. Terry-McElrath, S. Emery, and F. J. Chaloupka. 2002. Coding the news: The development of a methodological framework for coding and analyzing newspaper coverage of tobacco issues. *ImpacTeen Research Paper Series*, No. 21, May.

Connor, S. M., and K. Wesolowoski. 2009. Posts to online news message boards and public discourse surrounding DUI enforcement. *Traffic Injury Prevention* 10:546–551.

Iyengar, S. 1990. Framing responsibility for political issues: The case of poverty. *Political Behavior* 12(1):19–40.

NCSA (National Center for Statistics and Analysis). 2016. *Traffic safety facts, 2015 data—Alcohol-impaired driving*. Washington, DC: National Highway Traffic Safety Administration.

Rosales, M., and L. Stallones. 2008. Coverage of motor vehicle crashes with injuries in U.S. newspapers, 1999–2002. *Journal of Safety Research* 39(5):477–482.

Slater, M. D., A. F. Hayes, C. E. Goodall, and D. R. Ewoldsen. 2012. Increasing support for alcohol-control enforcement through news coverage of alcohol's role in injuries and crime. *Journal of Studies on Alcohol and Drugs* 73:311–315.

Yanovitzky, I. 2002. Effect of news coverage on the prevalence of drunk-driving behavior: Evidence from a longitudinal study. *Journal of Studies on Alcohol* 63:342–351.

MEDIA CONTENT ANALYSIS: FRAMING OF ALCOHOL-IMPAIRED DRIVING NEWS STORIES

Article Title:	
Source:	
Date of pub:	
Date coded:	
Record No:	
Word count:	
Type of story (news, editorial, opinion, other):	

FRAME AND FOCUS (episodic versus thematic)

1. ***Alcohol-impaired driving incident*** featured [if N, skip to Broader Focus]
2. ***Incident type***

_________ Arrest without crash (i.e., based on driving behavior)
_________ Injury crash
_________ Fatal crash
_________ Property-damage-only crash
_________ Other
If Other, specify ___________________________

3. ***Time frame*** of reporting

_________ Immediately after incident (i.e., within 6 days)
_________ Short term (i.e., 1–4 weeks after incident)
_________ Long term (i.e., more than 1 month after incident)
_________ Unclear

4. ***Ramifications*** of incident covered [Code all that apply]

_________ Victim's physical injuries
_________ Psychological effects on victim
_________ Other impacts on victim—e.g., lost job/wages, disability
_________ Impact on victim's family
_________ Physical impact on perpetrator—e.g., injuries
_________ Psychological effects on perpetrator—e.g., guilt, remorse
_________ Other impacts on perpetrator—e.g., financial, job
_________ Pretrial—e.g., charges, bond, home confinement
_________ Trial

_________ Sentencing
_________ Other
If Other, specify _________________________

5. ***Perpetrator–Victim Focus***
[Code both Perpetrator and Victim only if 50-50 split in focus]

_________ Perpetrator
_________ Victim
_________ Other
If Other, specify _________________________

6. ***Celebrity***—involvement of national/international public figure (e.g., entertainer, athlete) [Code all that apply]

_________ Perpetrator
_________ Victim
_________ Passenger in vehicle with suspected impaired driver
_________ Passenger in vehicle with victim
_________ Other (e.g., party host)
If Other, specify _________________________

7. ***Local person of prominence/interest***—involvement of local person known in the community before incident such as high-profile businessperson, elected official [Code all that apply]

_________ Perpetrator
_________ Victim
_________ Passenger in vehicle with suspected impaired driver
_________ Passenger in vehicle with victim
_________ Other (e.g., party host)
If Other, specify _________________________

8. ***Substance involvement*** in incident [Code all that apply]

_________ Alcohol
_________ Rx drugs
_________ Illicit drugs
_________ Drugs, unspecified

9. ***Broader focus*** on societal/environmental issues [Code all that apply; If N, skip to Voices]

_________ Historical/epidemiological
_________ Call for action/more action on alcohol-impaired driving
_________ Program/policy/legislation

________ Alcohol/drinking culture
________ Sales/marketing/promotion of alcohol
________ Court challenges to laws, police practices

Links to other social issues

________ Politics/corruption
________ Two-tiered justice system
________ Illegal immigration
________ Other
If Other, specify ____________________

VOICES (all stories)

10. Whose voice is represented by providing information, being quoted or cited as source of info [Code all that apply]

________ Law enforcement
________ Prosecutor
________ Policy maker
________ Victim
________ Victim's family
________ Perpetrator
________ Perpetrator's family
________ Traffic safety advocates—e.g., MADD, IIHS, community alcohol-impaired driving task force/coalition
________ Government public health/safety org.—e.g., NHTSA, NTSB, CDC
________ Alcohol industry or industry-funded lobbying/advocacy groups
________ Alcohol retailers—e.g., owners/managers of local bars, clubs, or restaurants
________ Researcher
________ Medical/health professional
________ Perpetrator's attorney
________ Other attorney/legal analyst
________ Media
________ Callers into show
________ Other
If Other, specify ____________________

VALUES (all stories) [Record type of content included in categories]

11. *What are the* ***underlying values/themes*** *expressed in the story* [Code all that apply]

________ Victimization
________ Injustice
________ Punishment
________ Individual problem or responsibility
________ Collective problem or responsibility
________ Alcohol retailer/industry problem or responsibility
________ Failure of family
________ Entitlement/above the law
________ Liberty/personal freedom
________ Effects on alcohol-impaired driving enforcement/prosecution
________ Economic interests
________ Cultural change in norms/attitudes
________ Personal engagement/activism
________ Protective role of government
________ Influence of special interests beyond industry
________ Recovery/personal transformation
________ Targeting social versus heavy/hardcore drinkers
________ Need for evidence-based prevention
________ Experiential learning to prevent risky driving
________ Avoiding holiday alcohol-impaired driving
________ Getting serious/tough on alcohol-impaired driving
________ Other
If Other, specify ________________________

TOPICS (all stories)

12. *What* ***topics*** *are discussed in the story* [Code all that apply]

Scope of the Problem

________ Public health toll—effects on society in terms of deaths, injuries, costs
________ Human toll—impact on victims, survivors, offenders

Responsibility

________ Personal—responsibility of individual drinkers, parents of minors, other
________ Third party-enforcement (e.g., ABC, police)
________ Third party-court and/or probation system

_________ Third party-government/policy makers

_________ Third party-alcohol retailers

_________ Third party-alcohol industry

_________ Third party-other

Prevention/Intervention Approach

_________ Prevention/general deterrence—countermeasures directed at general driving population (e.g., per se BAC limits, public information/education, checkpoints)

_________ Intervention/specific deterrence—countermeasures directed at offenders to reduce recidivism and support public safety (e.g., license suspension/revocation, ignition interlocks, DWI courts/ISP, assessment/treatment services, court-mandated sobriety)

_________ Sanctions—countermeasures focused on punishment of offenders (e.g., fines, jail, home confinement)

_________ Harm reduction—efforts to separate drinking and driving (e.g., sober ride programs, designated driver, ridesharing [Uber, Lyft])

_________ Other alcohol policies (e.g., taxes, restrictions on use/density, dram shop, RBS, alcohol promotion)

Tools/Technology

_________ New tools/technology for police, courts/probation, retailers—geospatial mapping of crashes/calls for service, passive sensors, tools for checking IDs, etc.

_________ New tools/technology for drinkers/drivers—BAC estimators, breathalyzers in cars, driverless cars, etc.

Community

_________ Grassroots advocacy efforts—community-based efforts (e.g., alcohol-impaired driving coalition/task force, work of traffic safety advocates, other citizen-led efforts)

Alcohol-Impaired Driving System Failures/Problems

_________ Failures in alcohol-impaired driving system overall/unspecified

_________ Failures in/greater action needed on alcohol-impaired driving legislation/policy

_________ Failures in/greater action needed on enforcement of alcohol laws (e.g., sobriety checkpoints, compliance checks)

_________ Failures in/greater action needed from court system (e.g., sentencing offenders, monitoring offenders)

_________ Failures in/greater action needed from alcohol retailers (e.g., RBS training, improved ID checking, dram shop liability)

_________ Failures in/greater action needed from alcohol industry

Failures in/greater action needed from others (e.g., universities, fraternities)
__________ If Other, specify__________________________

Alcohol-Impaired Driving System Success

__________ Alcohol-impaired driving system overall/unspecified
__________ Successes on alcohol-impaired driving legislation/policy
__________ Successes on enforcement of alcohol laws
__________ Successes related to court system (i.e., judiciary, probation)
__________ Successes related to alcohol retailers (e.g., RBS training, improved ID checking)
__________ Successes related to alcohol industry
__________ Successes related to other entities (e.g., universities, fraternities)
If Other, specify __________________________

Emergent Issues

__________ Politics/corruption
__________ Entitlement/above the law
__________ Two-tiered justice system
__________ Irresponsible parenting/family dysfunction
__________ Targeting social versus heavy/hardcore drinkers
__________ Change in lifestyle/direction/purpose
__________ Underage drinking
__________ Individual vs. state's rights
__________ Illegal immigration
__________ Other issues (e.g., holiday drinking, gang violence)
If Other, specify __________________________

NOTES

C

The Role of the Alcohol Industry in Policy Interventions for Alcohol-Impaired Driving[1]

Thomas F. Babor, Ph.D., M.P.H., Katherine Robaina, M.P.H., and Jonathan Noel, Ph.D., M.P.H.

EXECUTIVE SUMMARY

Introduction

Through its corporate social responsibility (CSR) efforts, the alcoholic beverage industry has become increasingly active in the support, analysis, and promotion of drinking and driving countermeasures and policies, especially in relation to road traffic safety. The involvement of the alcohol industry in these initiatives has been questioned by some organizations and individuals in the public health community, as well as others involved in road traffic safety. In light of these concerns, the objectives of this paper are to (1) describe the structure and concentration of the alcohol industry in the United States and internationally; (2) review commercial and political activities of the alcohol industry that may influence alcohol-related harms, particularly in the area of drinking and driving; and (3) evaluate drinking and driving initiatives advanced by the alcohol industry from a public health perspective. In the final section, we consider the implications of the findings for public health professionals, road traffic safety advocates, the alcohol industry, nongovernmental organizations (NGOs), researchers, and other interested individuals.

[1] This is an abridged version of the paper. A full version including all tables and figures can be found in the public access file for the Committee on Accelerating Progress to Reduce Alcohol-Impaired Driving Fatalities. Available by request from the National Academies of Sciences, Engineering, and Medicine's Public Access Records Office (PARO@nas.edu).

Methods

The information presented in this paper was compiled using two methods: (1) a narrative review of the relevant literature and (2) a content analysis of industry activities related to drinking and driving. The source materials for the narrative review consisted of industry documents, organizational websites, annual reports, industry trade journals, and an extensive search of the world scientific literature including articles, reviews, editorials, commentaries, newspaper articles, books, book chapters, and unpublished documents. The analysis of industry activities was based on a systematic evaluation of 97 "industry actions" that were conducted by alcohol producers and related organizations in support of the World Health Organization's (WHO's) 2010 Global Strategy to Reduce the Harmful Use of Alcohol.

Findings

Global Concentration

- The global concentration of the alcohol industry into a small number of transnational alcohol corporations has increased the industry's capacity to act individually and in concert in order to influence alcohol policy at the national, regional, and local levels.
- Market expansion by transnational producers of alcoholic beverages is likely to result in increased alcohol availability, which in turn can impact alcohol consumption and the prevalence of alcohol-related health consequences, including traffic injuries and fatalities.

Commercial Activities

- Evidence suggests that some of the alcohol industry's commercial activities have the potential to not only increase the frequency and amount of alcohol consumption, but also the likelihood of alcohol-impaired driving.
- The alcohol industry's marketing and product design activities contribute to the ongoing recruitment of young people, women, and other vulnerable populations, and may increase alcohol consumption through the promotion of more frequent drinking occasions. Evidence suggests that the relationship between the alcohol industry and the energy drink industry is mutually beneficial, despite the significant risks associated with alcohol mixed with energy drinks, such as increased alcohol consumption and related harms.

- Through industry trade associations and self-regulatory alcohol marketing codes, U.S. alcohol producers have pledged not to promote alcohol-impaired driving and to avoid associating driving with alcoholic beverages in their marketing activities. Associating alcoholic beverages with race car driving is likely in violation of these pledges as well as the industry's own self-regulatory advertising codes because the brand is being identified with a sport that displays vehicles driving in a manner that would be deemed unsafe and illegal if it occurred on a public road.

Corporate Political Activities

Corporate political activities are conducted in many parts of the alcohol industry to create a favorable regulatory environment. The main political strategies are

- Using information and other means to gain access to political decision makers;
- Indirect targeting of political decision makers through constituent support;
- Promoting alternative policies or voluntary measures (policy substitution);
- Providing financial incentives to influence government policy makers; and
- Employing legal preemption, litigation, or circumvention.

Each strategy includes a variety of tactics, and many of these tactics are carried out under the umbrella of corporate social responsibility.

In most cases, it is difficult to establish a direct link to alcohol policies that either reduce or increase alcohol-impaired driving and alcohol-related traffic injuries, but there is considerable circumstantial evidence that some of these activities are detrimental to public health and traffic safety, and that many others serve to dilute the public health response.

In many instances, the industry has built partnerships or is involved in collaborations with government agencies and civil society organizations with the aim of developing alcohol-impaired driving countermeasures. There is little evidence that they achieve their intended aims, and in some cases they have been criticized because of industry domination of the committee process and failure to consider effective policies.

Content Analysis of Industry Actions

A content analysis of 97 industry actions conducted in support of the WHO's Global Strategy to Reduce the Harmful Use of Alcohol provides strong evidence that the alcohol industry does not fund or support public health policies that have been shown to prevent alcohol-impaired driving and reduce alcohol-related harm. Nearly all (97.9 percent)[2] of the alcohol industry's U.S. drinking and driving initiatives were rated as either ineffective or of unknown effectiveness.

Conclusions

Three general conclusions are derived from the evidence presented in this paper. First, some of the industry's promotional activities, combined with product innovations, have the potential to increase not only the frequency and amount of alcohol consumption but also the likelihood of impaired driving. Second, some of the alcohol industry's corporate political activities are used to oppose effective alcohol policies whereas others are used to improve the public image of the producers as good corporate citizens. Third, based on current scientific research, neither of these activities is likely to reduce the incidence of alcohol-impaired driving because most of the policies and programs favored by the alcohol industry are ineffective. The findings reinforce recent concerns expressed by NGOs, the scientific community, and international health agencies in relation to the alcohol industry's road traffic safety initiatives.

Recommendations

We close with a set of recommendations regarding the role of the alcohol industry in the development of policy aimed at reducing alcohol-impaired driving and its negative consequences.

- The alcohol industry has the capacity and the responsibility to minimize the harm caused by its products at all stages of the production chain, especially in terms of product design and marketing.
- In setting and implementing their public health policies with respect to alcohol control, federal and state agencies as well as civil society organizations need to protect the integrity of these policies from commercial and other vested interests.
- In the absence of clear evidence that the industry is fulfilling its responsibilities, civil society organizations and professional groups should not enter into partnerships with the commercial alcohol industry, its community outreach public relations organizations,

[2] This information was updated after the prepublication release.

and other groups substantially funded by the commercial alcohol industry.

- Research on drinking and driving should be funded only by sources that are independent of commercial and other vested interests.

INTRODUCTION

A United Nations General Assembly resolution (#64/2551) proclaimed 2011–2020 the Decade of Action for Road Safety. According to WHO, nearly 1.2 million people die in road crashes annually throughout the world. Because alcohol-impaired driving is one of the main factors contributing to crashes, the alcohol industry has expressed concern about the abuse of its products and has focused on the need to prevent drinking and driving as a reflection of their corporate social responsibility (Hawkins et al., 2012). For example, at a press conference in October 2012, representatives of 11 of the world's largest alcohol producers and two trade associations issued a list of "Commitments," one of which was to prevent driving under the influence of alcohol (Producers' Commitments, 2015). At the same time, a website listing more than 3,500 "Industry Actions"[3] was released to demonstrate the alcohol industry's ability to address harmful drinking in support of WHO's Global Strategy to Reduce the Harmful Use of Alcohol (WHO, 2010). Among these activities, nearly 100 (n = 97) were classified as drinking and driving initiatives in the United States, and many others (n = 169) were promoted by U.S.-based producers in other countries (Esser et al., 2016).

The involvement of the alcohol industry in the promotion of these initiatives has been questioned by some in the public health community, as well as others involved in road traffic safety. More than 500 individuals and 27 organizations from 14 countries endorsed a "Statement of Concern" that was addressed to the director general of WHO (Babor et al., 2013). The statement questioned the alcohol industry's unilateral assumption of public health responsibilities in the implementation of the WHO Global Strategy, arguing that the producers' proposed actions were unlikely to reduce harmful alcohol use.

Objectives

In light of growing concerns about the inherent conflict of interest and lack of expertise in the promotion of public health measures by the

[3] The website that hosted the database was shut down in April 2016. A snapshot of the website can be seen at https://web.archive.org/web/20121015022208/http://initiatives.global-actions.org (accessed November 22, 2017).

alcohol industry, the objective of this paper is to document and critically evaluate the strategies used by the alcohol industry to influence public health policy related to road traffic safety, and to consider the implications of the findings for public health professionals, road traffic safety advocates, the alcohol industry, NGOs, researchers, and other individuals and organizations.

This paper is divided into five sections. The introduction provides an overview of the alcoholic beverage industry and explains the rationale for addressing alcohol consumption, promotion, and policy in relation to road traffic safety. The second section describes alcohol industry marketing practices and commercial strategies, including CSR activities designed to improve brand image. The third part reviews corporate political activities undertaken by the alcohol industry in relation to drinking and driving. The fourth section presents the results of a content analysis of industry activities conducted during the past decade in relation to drinking and driving. The final part draws conclusions and makes recommendations that may have implications for various stakeholders and constituencies involved in public health and traffic safety.

Methods

This paper was compiled using two methods: a narrative review of the relevant literature and a mixed method analysis of industry activities related to drinking and driving. The results of the literature review are summarized in the second and third sections of this paper. The source materials consisted of industry documents, organizational websites, annual reports, industry trade journals, publicly available presentations, and business meeting reports and transcripts. Additional information was obtained from an extensive search of the world scientific literature including articles, reviews, editorials, commentaries, newspaper articles, books, book chapters, and unpublished documents. Google and other search engines were used to obtain grey literature (e.g., unpublished documents and reports relevant to health issues) as well as industry documents. As described in a later section, the second method consisted of a quantitative and qualitative analysis of recent industry activities in the United States focused on drinking and driving.

The Alcohol Industry

The term *alcohol industry* refers to the producers of beer, wine, and distilled spirits and their networks of distributors and retailers. Trade associations and social aspects/public relations organizations, which are funded to promote industry interests, are also included in this definition.

TABLE C-1 Largest U.S. Beer, Wine, and Distilled Spirits Companies in 2015

Company	Market Share by Volume (%)
Beer	
Anheuser-Busch InBev NV	44.3
SABMiller	28.1
Constellation Brands Inc.	7.0
Heineken NV	4.8
Boston Beer Company	2.2
Wine	
E&J Gallo Winery	24.6
Constellation Brands Inc.	15.9
The Wine Group	15.5
Trinchero Family Estates	5.1
St. Michelle Wine Estates	2.9
Distilled Spirits	
Diageo PLC	16.7
Beam Suntory Inc.	10.1
Bacardi & Company Limited	9.0
Sazerac Company, Inc.	8.7
Pernod Ricard SA	6.9

SOURCES: Mintel Group, 2016a,b,c.

In the past decade, transnational corporations have concentrated the market in the malt beverage sector by purchasing local companies and regional breweries (see Table C-1). For example, Anheuser-Busch (AB) InBev, the world's largest brewer, recently acquired SABMiller to create the largest overall alcohol producer in the world. The distilled spirits industry has also become more concentrated with Constellation Brands and Diageo emerging as two of the largest transnational owners of distilled beverage brands, although the U.S. market share for Constellation Brands remains relatively small (less than 5 percent). Consolidation has occurred in the wine industry as well, with three wine producers controlling more than 50 percent of the market share. However, the wine industry remains relatively decentralized in the United States, and large corporations, such as Mondavi, Gallo, and Kendall-Jackson, have focused on international, rather than U.S., investments.

In a broader sense, the alcohol industry also includes proprietors of local hospitality outlets and entertainment industries such as restaurants, clubs, hotels, tourism, and sports. Another group, although not under the direct control of alcohol producers and trade associations, consists of advertising, marketing, research, and other organizations that are substantially dependent on alcohol industry funding for their activities.

TABLE C-2 Major Segments of the U.S. Alcoholic Beverage Industry: Large Producers, Trade Associations, and Social Aspects/Public Relations Organizations

	Beer	Distilled Spirits	Wine
Largest producers (parent company)	Anheuser-Busch InBev	Diageo	E&J Gallo Winery
	Molson Coors	Pernod Ricard	Kendall-Jackson
	Heineken	Bacardi	
	Blue Ribbon	Brown-Forman	
	Boston Beer Company		
	Constellation Brands, Inc.		
	Yuengling		
Trade associations	Beer Institute	Distilled Spirits Council (DISCUS)	Wine Institute
	Brewers Association		California Association of Winegrape Growers
Social aspects/public relations organizations	Foundation for Advancing Alcohol Responsibility (FAAR) (formerly Century Council)		
	International Association for Responsible Drinking (IARD) (formerly ICAP)		

Table C-2 describes the structure of the U.S. alcoholic beverage industry in terms of major producers, trade associations, and social aspects/public relations organizations.

Other segments of the alcohol industry include local producers and on- and off-premises vendors. There are several types of local producers: craft brewers and those making premium alcoholic drinks including wine, whiskey, and rum. This paper primarily focuses on large national and transnational alcohol producers because they are more involved in lobbying, policy initiatives, marketing, and product development that may affect alcohol consumption and alcohol control policy related to road traffic safety. The results of this analysis may not apply to other segments of the industry, as noted in the Conclusion.

On-premises vendors refers to establishments that sell alcoholic beverages for consumption at the establishment (e.g., bars, nightclubs, restaurants). Off-premises vendors refers to establishments that sell alcoholic beverages that are consumed elsewhere (e.g., package stores, grocery stores).

U.S. states differ in the number and density of on- and off-premises alcohol retailers, and in many states, small retailers account for the majority of alcohol sales. But this is changing rapidly with the growth of large retail outlets and supermarkets, which has increased the number of off-premises locations where alcohol is sold. As suggested below, policies that affect the number and density of retail outlets are likely to affect the prevalence of drinking and driving.

Impact Assessment and Implications for Public Health

The global concentration of the alcohol industry into a small number of large transnational alcohol corporations has increased the industry's capacity to act individually and in concert in order to influence alcohol policy at the national, regional, and local levels (Jernigan, 2009; Jernigan and Babor, 2015). The alcohol industry plays an important role in the development of new products (e.g., caffeinated alcohol "energy drinks" and alcopops) and the promotion of these products through sophisticated marketing techniques. These promotional activities, combined with market expansion by the transnational producers, result in increased alcohol availability and sales, which in turn can affect alcohol consumption levels and the prevalence of alcohol-related problems. Although there is some evidence (Babor, 2014; Babor et al., 2015; Ferreira-Borges et al., 2016) that these activities are leading to increased alcohol consumption in low- to middle-income countries, consumption in high-income countries such as the United States is stable or declining. The following section describes how the alcohol industry uses marketing practices and other commercial tactics in ways that could contribute to the harmful use of alcohol.

MARKETING PRACTICES AND COMMERCIAL STRATEGIES

A significant amount of alcohol industry revenue is spent on the marketing and promotion of alcoholic beverages. According to *Advertising Age* (AdAge, 2016), the top 100 global advertisers in 2016 include 7 alcohol companies operating in the United States. The alcohol industry's marketing activities play an important role in defining the environment in which harmful drinking patterns are learned and practiced (Babor et al., 2015; Robaina and Babor, 2017).

From the perspective of road traffic safety, at least three strategies are noteworthy: (1) the targeting of young adults; (2) product innovations that facilitate heavy drinking; and (3) sponsorship of sporting and auto racing events.

Promotion of Alcohol to Selected Target Groups

Young adults, women, and racial and ethnic minorities (e.g., Hispanics) are mentioned in numerous industry documents as a key growth sector and a demographic category of strategic importance (e.g., AB InBev, 2016a; SABMiller, 2016). Representing over half the population and 85 percent of purchasing power (Omazic, 2014; Silverstein et al., 2009), women are seen by many of the major alcohol producers as a consumer group where sales are likely to increase (O'Reilly, 2014). For example, multiple instances were found of alcoholic beverages being advertised in concert with breast cancer awareness messages (Mart and Giesbrecht, 2015). Additionally, marketing programs like "Make it a Margarita Moment" for AB InBev's Lime-a-Rita products have been specifically designed for women (Anheuser-Busch, 2017). Making beer more appealing to women is mentioned in SABMiller's (2016) annual report as one of the key elements of their growth strategy. The company's marketing chief, Nick Fell (Joseph, 2014), was quoted as saying: "It's time to change the image of beer as just a drink for guys watching sport."

Young populations have become the focus of efforts to build brand recognition, strengthen brand loyalty, and initiate regular alcohol consumption. One mechanism is through digital marketing, which has become increasingly common in part because it is relatively inexpensive and online campaigns can be closely tailored to specific target audiences. There are neither voluntary nor statutory regulations restricting when or where alcohol advertising should be published, and procedures that are designed to prevent minors from entering company websites can be easily circumvented. For this reason, nearly all producers and brands in the United States have some type of online presence, with many using multiple social media channels (e.g., Facebook, Twitter, YouTube, Instagram, Foursquare) (Lobstein et al., 2017). Websites and social media platforms are often designed to encourage personal interactions with a brand in various ways, including interactive games, the sharing of messages, images, and videos, and links to other websites.

Product Innovations

Alcoholic beverage sales can be increased in key demographic groups through product innovation and product design. For example, high-strength premixes and spirit-based, ready-to-drink (RTD) products are aimed at price-conscious younger consumers, specifically students, as are alcoholic energy drinks. Sweet RTD alcohol products appeal to women and young people, particularly underage drinkers, who are not always aware of the beverage's alcohol content (CHOICE, 2008; Copeland et al., 2007; Euromonitor International, 2017).

One area where product innovations have been implicated in drinking and driving in a more direct way is alcoholic energy drinks. Premixed alcoholic energy drinks entered the U.S. market in the early 2000s after the successful introduction of the nonalcoholic energy drink Red Bull in 1997. Among these early entrants were Sparks (Miller Brewing) in 2002, Tilt (AB) in 2005, and FourLoko (Phusion Projects) in 2005. In 2008, the Center for Science in the Public Interest (CSPI) sued AB InBev and Miller Brewing, alleging that caffeine and other stimulant additives were not officially approved for use in alcoholic beverages (Cronin and Stone, 2008). The CSPI suit, as well as pressure from more than a dozen U.S. attorneys general, led to several products being either removed from the market or reformulated to reduce or eliminate the product's stimulants prior to the suit reaching trial. In 2010, premixed alcoholic energy drinks were functionally banned after the Food and Drug Administration (FDA) labeled caffeine as an "unsafe food additive" for alcoholic malt beverages (FDA, 2010), although other premixed drinks (e.g., p.i.n.k. vodka) are still on the market.

Despite the ban on premixed alcoholic energy drinks, official relationships between some alcohol producers and some segments of the energy drink industry have continued. For example, in 2007, AB InBev signed a distribution deal with Monster Energy, the second most popular energy drink in the United States, to manage and coordinate the distribution of Monster Energy products to on-premises alcohol retailers, such as bars, nightclubs, and restaurants.[4] The distribution deal still appears to be active following AB's merger with SABMiller.[5] In 2017, AB InBev agreed to purchase the energy drink maker Hiball for an undisclosed amount (Snider, 2017).

Sponsorships

Strategies designed to integrate alcohol consumption into particular lifestyles, as well as cultural and ethnic experiences, have been documented in promotions that associate alcohol products with sports, cultural events, and music. While some countries (e.g., Costa Rica, France, and Guatemala) have banned sponsorship in sports and youth events, this is not the case in the United States. Sports and popular music events that appeal to young people are widely sponsored by alcohol brands.

---

[4] Canadean. 2016. *History, Monster Beverage Company*. Progressive Media Group. Available by request from the National Academies of Sciences, Engineering, and Medicine's Public Access Records Office (PARO@nas.edu).

[5] Hoover's, Inc. 2017. *Hoover's Company Records—In-depth records*. Anheuser-Busch Companies, LLC. Available by request from the National Academies of Sciences, Engineering, and Medicine's Public Access Records Office (PARO@nas.edu).

Reuters Knowledge Direct. 2017. *Anheuser-Busch Companies, LLC*. Thomson Financial. Available by request from the National Academies of Sciences, Engineering, and Medicine's Public Access Records Office (PARO@nas.edu).

TABLE C-3 Alcohol Brand Sponsorships in U.S. Motorsports in 2017

Motorsport Series	ARCA	Formula Drift	IndyCar	IHRA
Does an alcohol brand sponsor the series?	N	N	Y	N
If yes, what brands?			Coors Light	
Does an alcohol brand sponsor one or more races in the series?	N	N	N	N
If yes, what brands?				
Does an alcohol brand sponsor one or more drivers/teams in the series?	Y	N	Y	N
If yes, what brands?	Captain Ron Craft Beer		Fuzzy's Ultra Premium Vodka; Domaine Tour Saint-Michel; Jim Beam	
Number of drivers/teams	66		94	
% driver/team brand sponsorship	1.5%		3.2%	

NOTES: ARCA = Automobile Racing Club of America; IHRA = International Hot Rod Association; IMSA = International Motor Sports Association; NASA = National Auto Sport Association; NASCAR = National Association for Stock Car Racing; NHRA = National Hot Rod Association; SCCA = Sports Car Club of America; USAC = United States Auto Club; USHRA = United States Hot Rod Association.
* ? = Information unknown.

Sponsorships provide a direct way for the alcohol industry to promote their products and to create a positive, emotional relationship between the brand and consumers.

All major U.S. professional sports leagues, including auto racing, are sponsored by at least one alcohol brand and sporting events attract substantial audiences, particularly young adults and middle-aged men, who are the heaviest consumers of alcoholic beverages. By sponsoring leagues, events, and/or teams, the alcohol industry is able to incorporate the brand

IMSA	NASA	NASCAR	NHRA	Rally America	SCCA	USAC	USHRA
Y	N	Y	N	N	N	N	N
Tequila Patrón		Coors Light					
N	?*	N	N	Y	N	?*	N
				Budweiser; Coors Light			
Y	?*	Y	Y	N	?*	?*	Y
Tequila Patrón (two teams); Adobe Road Winery		Twisted Tea (two teams); Wagner Family of Wine; Caymus Vineyards; Busch Beer; Miller Lite; Dale's Pale Ale	Tequila Patrón				Norman Vineyards (two teams)
101		111	87				79
3.0%		5.4%	1.1%				2.5%

SOURCES: Information retrieved from ARCA, 2017; Formula Drift, 2017; IHRA, 2017; IMSA, 2017; IndyCar, 2017; Monster Jam, 2016; NASA, 2017; NASCAR, 2017; NHRA, 2017; Rally America, 2017; SCCA, 2017; USCA, 2015.

into the name of the event through verbal pronouncements in sports commentaries, as well as signage on clothing, sporting arenas, and products sold to fans (Amis and Cornwell, 2005). Table C-3 describes the range of corporate sponsorships in auto racing leagues in the United States.

According to a report on the extent of alcohol advertising during the 2014 Formula One (F1) Monaco Grand Prix, alcohol sponsorship of F1 provides a platform for an extremely high exposure of alcohol advertising to audiences (Eurocare, 2015). During the broadcast of the 2014 Monaco

F1 race, the worldwide audience of 500 million people was exposed to an alcohol brand every 5 seconds on average.

In the United States, professional motorsports were the fourth most popular sport in 2014, surpassed by only the National Football League, Major League Baseball, and college football (Schwartz and McGarry, 2014). Motorsports were more popular than both the National Hockey League and the National Basketball League. This level of popularity allows motorsport sponsors to capture significant brand exposure. For example, there is approximately $100 million worth of advertising exposure during races held on the Sunday of Memorial Day weekend (Katzmark, 2015), and any alcohol brand sponsorships of motorsports would be able to capitalize on such exposure.

Through industry trade associations and self-regulatory alcohol marketing codes, U.S. alcohol producers have pledged not to promote alcohol-impaired driving and to avoid having driving associated with alcoholic beverages. Associating alcoholic beverages with race car driving is likely in violation of these pledges as well as the industry's own self-regulatory advertising codes because the brand is being associated with a sport that displays vehicles driving in a manner that would be deemed unsafe and illegal if it occurred on a public road. For examples of alcohol brand sponsorships in U.S. motorsports, see (1) the 2017 NASCAR race car sponsored by Twisted Tea (see Figure C-1); (2) the 2005 IndyCar race car[6] sponsored by Jim Beam; (3) the 2015 IMSA race car[7] sponsored by Tequila Patrón; and (4) the 2017 NASCAR race car[8] sponsored by Miller Lite. This suggests a need for better enforcement of the codes by the industry and other regulatory bodies.

In an effort to evaluate compliance with these guidelines by U.S. alcohol brands, we estimated the prevalence of alcohol sponsorships among professional U.S. motorsports series in 2017 as a proxy for associating alcoholic beverages with potentially unsafe driving. Unlike other U.S. professional sports, there are multiple types of sponsorships in motorsports. A brand can sponsor the entire professional series, a race, or an individual racing team and driver. To estimate the prevalence of alcohol brand sponsors at the series, race, and team/driver level, U.S. motorsports series were identified through a series of Google searches. Initial keywords included "(U.S. OR United States) AND motorsports." A

---

[6] For the associated image, see https://www.motorsport.com/indycar/photo/main-gallery/michael-andretti-s-distinctive-helmet-with-the-new-jim-beam-vonage-colors-on-his-dallara-2 (accessed December 12, 2017).

[7] For the associated image, see http://autoweek.com/gallery/sports-cars/photo-galler-tequila-patron-tests-ligier-j2-p2-prototype-race-cars-france (accessed December 12, 2017).

[8] For the associated image, see http://nascar.nbcsports.com/2017/11/03/discount-tire-miller-lite-to-sponsor-brad-keselowskis-cup-car-in-2018 (accessed December 12, 2017).

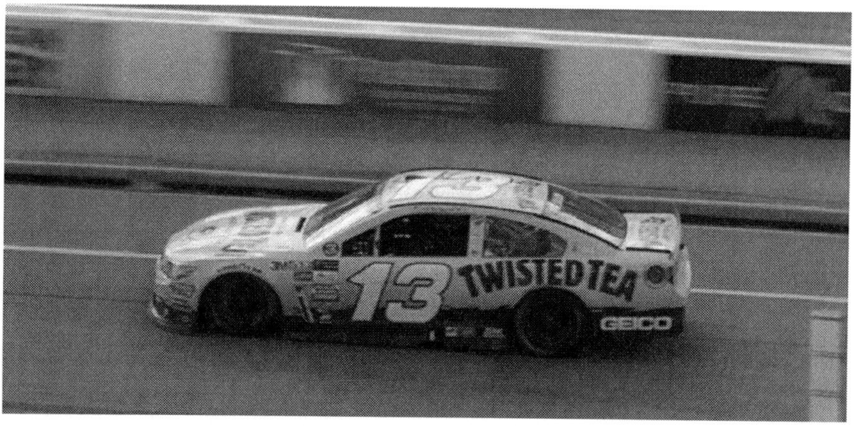

FIGURE C-1 Example of alcohol brand sponsorships in U.S. motorsports—NASCAR race car sponsored by Twisted Tea.
NOTE: Photograph by Joseph Tregembo, licensed under CC BY-SA 4.0.
SOURCE: Wikimedia Commons, 2017.

snowball approach was then used to identify additional keywords to expand the search. Additionally, general sport and motorsport news sites that appeared in the search results were reviewed to identify additional motorsport series that did not appear in the Google search results. All searches were conducted in May and June 2017. A U.S. motorsport series was defined as a professional racing league whose headquarters were in the United States and that held the majority of its races in the United States. Once a motorsport series was identified, official series, race, and team/driver sponsors were identified based on the information available through the primary series website, race websites, and/or team/driver websites.

As shown in Table C-3, 12 U.S. professional motorsport series were identified. Three (25 percent) were sponsored by alcohol brands (Coors Light [IndyCar and NASCAR] and Tequila Patrón [IMSA]). Based on the information available, races from only one series (Rally America) were sponsored by alcohol brands (Budweiser and Coors Light). However, at least one team or driver from six series (50 percent) was sponsored by an alcohol brand. Although the prevalence of alcohol brand sponsorship at the team/driver level is very low in any particular series, the effect of such sponsorships may be large because an entire race car is decorated in the name, colors, and logos of that brand, and such branding can be made available to the audience throughout a race (see Figure C-1).

Impact Assessment

The strategies reviewed here suggest that the alcohol industry's marketing and product design activities contribute to the ongoing recruitment of young people, women, and other vulnerable populations, and such activities may increase consumption through the promotion of more frequent drinking. The industry's online presence is likely to reach a large number of young people (Winpenny et al., 2014) and encourage drinking (Litt and Stock, 2011; McCreanor et al., 2012; Moewaka Barnes et al., 2016). The use of alcohol-related social media is associated with alcohol consumption, engagement in risky behaviors, and intention to consume alcohol (Litt and Stock, 2011; McCreanor et al., 2012; Moewaka Barnes et al., 2016; Winpenny et al., 2014), although heavy drinking and engagement with alcohol marketing on social media may both be affected by a common confounder, such as positive alcohol expectancies or sensation-seeking tendencies.

Despite industry claims that marketing is only used for capturing market share (see, e.g., Lambright, 1985), research demonstrates that exposure to alcohol marketing is associated with earlier initiation of drinking among young people, increased alcohol consumption among current young drinkers, and increased alcohol-related problems (Anderson et al., 2009; Austin et al., 2006; Jernigan et al., 2017; Smith and Foxcroft, 2009). Moreover, there is ample evidence that young drivers are disproportionately involved in alcohol-impaired motor vehicle crashes. Of all drivers involved in fatal crashes who had blood alcohol concentration (BAC) levels of 0.08 g/dL or higher in 2014, 47 percent were 16–24 years of age (NHTSA, 2015). To the extent that alcohol companies may be targeting young drinkers (Bond et al., 2009, 2010; Hastings, 2009), alcohol industry marketing activities may increase the prevalence of heavy drinking and alcohol-related negative consequences, including traffic crashes. This hypothesis is supported by an econometric analysis conducted by Saffer (1994), which found that alcohol broadcast advertising has a significant and positive effect on motor vehicle fatalities in the United States.

Policies that limit exposure to advertising and other marketing can affect sales, consumption levels, and profits (AB InBev, 2016b). According to the econometric analysis conducted by Saffer (1997), a ban on alcohol broadcast advertising could reduce the number of traffic fatalities by 2,000 to 3,000 per year. A more recent analysis concluded that a complete ban on alcohol advertising would prevent 7,610 alcohol-related deaths and save 156,413 years of potential life lost (Hollingworth et al., 2006).

Regarding alcohol and energy drinks, evidence suggests that alcohol mixed with energy drinks may facilitate drinking and related harms via their effects on intoxication. Systematic reviews have concluded that adolescents and young adults who consume alcohol mixed with energy drinks are more likely to consume more alcohol, drive after binge drinking, ride in a car with an intoxicated driver, and be arrested for driving under the influence (McKetin et al., 2015; Striley and Khan, 2014). A separate review of randomized controlled studies found that while energy drinks may counteract some minor cognitive effects of alcohol consumption, such effects disappear when drinkers engage in complex tasks such as driving (Lalanne et al., 2017).

These previously accepted scientific findings into the harmful effects of alcohol mixed with energy drinks have in some cases been contradicted by industry-sponsored research. Red Bull GmbH funded a survey of 6,002 Dutch university students that concluded that alcohol mixed with energy drink consumption was associated with significantly decreased alcohol consumption, binge drinking, and instances of driving while impaired (de Haan et al., 2012). These findings are indicative of a larger pattern. Without exception, all industry-funded studies included in a systematic review of studies on alcohol mixed with energy drinks determined that drinking alcohol mixed with energy drinks either decreased or did not significantly increase the risk of alcohol-related harms (McKetin et al., 2015). The authors who reviewed these studies concluded that there is difficulty in comparing studies according to funding source because industry-funded studies used substantially different methods and outcomes.

The findings suggest that the relationship between the alcohol industry and the energy drink industry may be mutually beneficial, despite the significant harms caused by alcohol mixed with energy drinks, and distribution deals may allow such products to be more easily and more closely associated with each other. Moreover, the funding of research on alcoholic products by the energy drink industry may equip these producers with evidence designed to create doubt about the emerging scientific consensus. In their review, McKetin et al. (2015) concluded that the influence of industry involvement in this area of research needs to be monitored because of conflicts of interest.

Industry sponsorship of festivals and other public events may contribute to the social acceptance of alcohol and influence the frequency and volume of drinking by increasing public acceptance of a wide variety of drinking occasions (Amis and Cornwell, 2005; Brown, 2016). They also expose children and adolescents to alcohol marketing messages. The findings suggest that the alcohol industry should refrain from sponsoring events where children are likely to be present. In particular, alcohol sponsorship of auto racing events is a marketing strategy that seeks to incorporate alcohol brands and products into the national culture and into the enjoyment of leisure activities (Klein, 2000).

A recent systematic review on the relationship between alcohol sports sponsorship and alcohol consumption found an association between alcohol industry sponsorship of sports and risky drinking among school children and adult athletes (Brown, 2016). Sports sponsorship is also associated with heavier drinking by individual players, teams, and clubs (O'Brien and Kypri, 2008). This is particularly true for university sports sponsored by the alcohol industry. Among university sports in the United Kingdom, those receiving alcohol industry sponsorship were four times more likely to report hazardous drinking than nonsponsored athletes (O'Brien et al., 2014). Although collegiate sports in the United States do not have official alcohol sponsors yet, the National Collegiate Athletic Association (NCAA) has recently sanctioned the sale of beer and wine at NCAA events (Dodd, 2016).

In summary, the evidence suggests that some of the alcohol industry's commercial activities have the potential to increase not only the frequency and amount of alcohol consumption, but also the likelihood of alcohol-impaired driving.

CORPORATE POLITICAL ACTIVITIES

In addition to commercial activities designed to promote alcoholic beverages, some segments of the alcohol industry may act indirectly to create a favorable regulatory environment. These corporate political activities are conducted in many areas of business (Getz, 1997; Hillman and Hitt, 1999; Savell et al., 2014, 2016; Schuler, 1996; Schuler et al., 2002). As described in Table C-4, the main political strategies are (1) using information and other means to gain access to political decision makers; (2) indirectly targeting political decision makers through constituent support; (3) promoting alternative policies or voluntary measures (policy substitution); (4) providing financial incentives to influence government policy makers; and (5) employing legal preemption, litigation, or circumvention. As described below, each strategy includes a variety of tactics, and many of these tactics are carried out under the umbrella of corporate social responsibility.

Access and Information

Gaining access to those who decide public policy may be the alcohol industry's single most important political goal (Hillman and Hitt, 1999; Keim and Zeithaml, 1986; Schuler et al., 2002). The industry attempts to shape policy makers' perceptions of the scientific evidence through the funding and dissemination of information and research (Jiang and Ling, 2013; McCambridge and Hartwell, 2015). Industry activities used to gain and maintain access to political decision makers and to influence the evidence base include donations and campaign contributions, placement of

TABLE C-4 Corporate Political Strategies Used by the Alcohol Industry

Strategy	Tactics
Access or information	• Campaign contributions • Direct and indirect lobbying (meetings and correspondence with policy makers) • Shaping the evidence base (e.g., funding and dissemination of research, use of paid consultants, position papers, technical reports) • Partnerships/collaboration (e.g., working industry competitors, civil society groups, and academia to provide technical support and advice)
Constituency building	• Forming alliances with trade associations and other industry sectors • Forming alliances with or mobilizing civil society organizations, consumers, employees, and/or the public • Creation of social aspects/public relations organizations • Corporate-image advertising[a] • Advocacy advertising[b] (press releases, publicity campaigns)
Policy substitution	• Developing and promoting self-regulation • Developing and promoting alternative regulatory policy, often under the umbrella of "modernization" of state regulatory regimes • Developing and promoting voluntary activities
Financial	• Contributions to political parties • Hiring or offering future employment to people with political, regulatory, governmental, or academic connections • Other financial enticement (travel, honoraria)
Legal actions	• Preemption • Litigation (or threat of litigation)

[a] Corporate-image advertising seeks to build a favorable image and keep the company's name in the public eye.

[b] Advocacy advertising is defined as an advertisement or public communication that attempts to influence public opinion on a specific issue.

SOURCES: Adapted from Hillman and Hitt (1999) and Savell et al. (2014).

key personnel in positions of authority, partnerships with civil society and governmental organizations, political lobbying, and alcohol advertising (Moodie et al., 2013).

Donations and Campaign Contributions

Through its business presence, the alcohol industry maintains strong connections to the federal government, state governments, and local communities. In addition, the industry uses political action committees to support candidates in ways that may allow them to influence the political process. For example, alcohol producers and other industry organizations contributed a total of $23,424,228 to the campaigns of both Republicans and Democrats in 2016, according to the Federal Election Commission. This includes $3,939,367 of unregulated "soft money." The industry's top two campaign contributors were the National Beer Wholesalers Association and AB InBev. Other top contributors include Total Wine & More, Kendall-Jackson, and Silver Eagle Distributors (Center for Responsive Politics, 2017).

Industry Lobbying

Lobbying has been identified as a key strategy used by the alcohol industry, particularly to oppose tax increases (Bakke and Endal, 2010; Bond et al., 2010; Collin et al., 2014; Hope, 2006; McCambridge et al., 2013), even though tax increases can significantly reduce harmful alcohol consumption and the prevalence of alcohol-impaired driving (Wagenaar et al., 2010; Xu and Chaloupka, 2011). The alcohol industry spent approximately $27 million on lobbying in 2016, the highest yearly amount on record. Of the 296 lobbyists hired by the industry in 2016, 220 (74.3 percent) were "revolving door" lobbyists who previously worked for the federal government. The top three alcohol industry lobbying organizations in 2016 were the Distilled Spirits Council of the United States, AB InBev, and the Beer Institute.

While the industry tends to lobby Congress primarily on taxes and regulations, other issues listed on 2016 disclosure forms obtained from https://lobbyingdisclosure.house.gov (accessed August 13, 2017) using the Lobbying Disclosure Filing Search include

- Impaired driving and underage drinking prevention issues;
- Centers for Disease Control and Prevention—alcohol research and alcohol programs;
- S. 728/H.R. 1717—Sober Truth on Preventing Underage Drinking Reauthorization Act and H.R. 6 and H.R. 34—21st Century Cures

Act—to provide for programs and activities with respect to the prevention of underage drinking;
- Surgeon General's Report on Substance Use, Addiction, and Health;
- Nominations to the National Highway Traffic Safety Administration (NHTSA) and Federal Communications Commission; and
- Distracted driving and NHTSA issues.

From the information provided, it is difficult to determine whether the industry's positions are consistent with evidence-based public health practice, but some industry literature, such as press releases, internal documents, and testimony, suggest that they generally oppose tax increases, while supporting policies and programs that have either been shown to be ineffective (e.g., classroom education, social norms approaches) or have not been sufficiently evaluated (e.g., safe ride programs) (AB InBev, 2016a; Bakke and Endal, 2010; Bond et al., 2009; House of Commons Health Committee, 2010; McCambridge et al., 2013).

One example of industry-sponsored activities that oppose effective drinking and driving policies is a campaign against Utah's attempt to lower the BAC limit set by state law. In 2017, Utah became the first U.S. state to lower the BAC limit to 0.05%, a policy that was recommended by the National Transportation Safety Board in 2013 (NTSB, 2013). According to a 2014 tax form, the American Beverage Institute (ABI), which has been sponsored by numerous alcohol producers (ABI, 2013), "continued in aggressive opposition to a recommendation by the National Transportation Safety Board to lower the drunk-driving arrest threshold to a 0.05% BAC level" (ABI, 2015). To this end, ABI published a series of ads in Utah and neighboring states mocking the law and implying the law significantly threatens Utah's tourist industry. ABI has also likened the law to "driving while older" (Weber, 2017), identified lawmakers that would be considered "older" drivers (Weber, 2017), organized a national petition against the law (ABI, 2017a), and wrote several op-eds against the law (ABI, 2017b). Beyond the new BAC law, ABI has "opposed state and federal legislation that would mandate the use of ignition interlock devices or alcohol detection devices for all drunk-driving offenders" in favor of focusing only on repeat and high BAC offenders, according to the 2014 tax form (ABI, 2015).

Partnerships and Collaboration

In many instances, the alcohol industry has built partnerships or is involved in collaborations with government agencies and civil society organizations. These partnerships are generally established to recommend or develop alcohol-impaired driving countermeasures. However, there is little evidence that they achieve their intended goals, and in some cases they have been criticized because of industry domination of the committee process and failure to consider effective policies. For example, in 2013, the Wisconsin Bureau of Transportation Safety created the Operating While Impaired (OWI)/Impaired Driving Task Force to help shape Wisconsin's Impaired Driving Plan. One year later, four members of the task force resigned, citing the role played by the Tavern League of Wisconsin (the only nongovernmental partner), which advanced ineffective policies such as educational programs and opposed evidence-based interventions (Brown et al., 2014; Marley and Ferguson, 2014). These individuals also documented numerous instances of alcohol industry influence on department of transportation staff members, including exclusive use of industry data that misrepresented underage drinking. The resigning members concluded that their "continued participation on the OWI Task Force simply lends credibility to a hollow process." Other instances of failed industry–government partnerships have been reported in the United Kingdom (Brown, 2015; Gornall, 2014; Knai et al. 2015; Panjwani and Caraher, 2014) in relation to many of the same transnational alcohol producers listed in Table C-2.

Activities to Shape the Evidence Base

The support of research to generate scientific evidence and to demonstrate corporate social responsibility is another strategy used by the industry. In 2015, the International Center for Alcohol Policies (ICAP), the largest alcohol industry social aspects organization, merged with the Global Alcohol Producers Group (GAPG), a major lobbying organization established "to support a constructive policy dialogue with the World Health Organization, member state governments, and the public health community to reduce harmful drinking" (Associated Press, 2008). The merger resulted in the creation of the International Alliance for Responsible Drinking (IARD), which, like its predecessor ICAP, is funded by a consortium of the world's leading alcohol producers (IARD, 2017a).

According to one analysis, most of ICAP's activities were focused on countering the influence of WHO and the public health community (Jernigan, 2012), which have promoted both population-wide and targeted measures (e.g., evidence-based drinking and driving laws) to reduce alcohol-related harms. ICAP publications, conferences, monographs, policy implementation guides, and toolkits, often developed through collaborations between industry-paid academics and industry representatives, emphasized education for heavy drinkers (among the least effective measures to reduce alcohol-related harms) and treatment (among the most costly), while they attempted to reframe the debate from reducing population levels of consumption to the more limited goal of changing individual patterns of drinking. Since the ICAP/GAPG merger, IARD has continued to claim its activities are intended to support the WHO Global Strategy, but without official authorization or collaboration with WHO (Chan, 2013; IARD, 2017b).

Beyond its corporate social responsibility activities, some segments of the alcohol industry (e.g., Diageo) have been highly critical of academics who have been involved in alcohol policy research. A Diageo presentation, for example, labeled public health academics "alcophobes" who have threatened industry accomplishments, citing declines in the prevalence of drinking and driving.[9] Several academics, scientific journals, and research organizations, including the Centers for Disease Control and Prevention, and the Center for Alcohol Marketing and Youth, were accused of being "serial alcophobes" for their research on alcohol marketing and the health benefits of higher alcohol taxes.

Funding of Research

A major research organization funded in part by the alcohol industry is the Traffic Injury Research Foundation (TIRF), a registered charity in Canada, and TIRF, USA, which received 501(c)(3) status in 2014 "in order to meet the needs of its U.S. funders, stakeholders, and partners."[10] TIRF conducts studies of drinking and driving interventions, education measures, and issues related to road traffic safety, such as ignition interlock devices and apprehension of high-risk offenders. TIRF makes it a priority to share its research findings with the media, advocacy organizations, and members of the general public and provides testimony to governments in many states to inform decisions about road safety legislation. TIRF has received support from AB InBev, and it currently lists Beer Canada and the Beer Institute as financial supporters.

Another source of research funding was channeled through an independent organization called the Alcoholic Beverage Medical Research Foundation (ABMRF), which, from 1982 to 2016, supported 570 grantees from around the world.[11] Most of these grants were provided to novice researchers, initially to investigate the positive effects of moderate drink-

---

[9] Smith, G. 2012. Impact of globalization upon the U.S. alcohol environment. *Responsible Retailing Forum* April 11. Available by request from the National Academies of Sciences, Engineering, and Medicine's Public Access Records Office (PARO@nas.edu).

[10] For more information, see http://tirf.us (accessed December 20, 2017).

[11] ABMRF. 2015. *Research reference guide: 1982–present*. Available by request from the National Academies of Sciences, Engineering, and Medicine's Public Access Records Office (PARO@nas.edu).

ing, and later on a broader range of topics including alcohol-impaired driving. Only 25 grants were awarded on drinking and driving, whereas 171 grants were funded for research on cell biology and 219 grants focused on specific organ systems.[12] While investigators funded by ABMRF were free from direct industry influence, the ABMRF Scientific Advisory Board prioritized research grants with little public health impact.

Constituency Building

The industry collaborates with several allied groups that profit from the sale of alcohol, such as convenience stores, restaurants, bars, hotels, and advertising agencies. The alcohol industry also creates front groups or third-party organizations to lobby on its behalf and forms alliances with NGOs and other civil society organizations. According to Savell et al. (2014, 2016), this generally occurs when the industry is facing a significant regulatory threat.

Forming Alliances with Trade Associations and Other Sectors

Trade associations represent alcohol industry interests to the media, the public, and the government. Within the United States, trade associations are well developed, bringing together industry members to advance common interests. The largest alcohol industry trade associations in the United States are the Beer Institute, the Distilled Spirits Council of the United States, and the Wine Institute. Alcohol producers have also supported other trade associations, and the largest alcohol producers (e.g., AB InBev) often hold affiliate memberships in alcohol retailer and wholesaler associations. Some segments of the alcohol industry have also established alliances with business associations (especially regarding taxes), the tobacco industry, and groups that sell their products to the alcohol industry. The relationship between the alcohol industry and the American Beverage Institute is one specific example of such an alliance.

Policy Substitution

As suggested by the foregoing examples, the alcohol industry often exerts its influence through its investment in alliances and related CSR activities, which sometimes involves partnerships with members of civil society and government. In a review of corporate political activities, Hillman et al. (2004) noted that by sponsoring community projects, a company's or an industry's social activities become new ways to achieve

[12] Ibid.

strategic aims. CSR activities allow the industry to gain access to the public domain and policy makers while improving their reputation and responding to public demands for socially responsible behavior. Alcohol industry prevention and CSR activities include responsible drinking campaigns and educational programs, which emphasize voluntary (rather than legislative) solutions to alcohol-related problems. These activities are designed to improve the public image of the producers as good corporate citizens who are attempting to ensure that their product is used responsibly. As noted in the next section, there is little evidence that the policies and programs favored by the industry are effective.

In 2015, AB InBev pledged to invest more than $1 billion in projects in the United States and other countries that would reduce the harmful effects of alcohol (AB InBev, 2017). Called "Smart Drinking Goals," one of the three areas targeted by this initiative is alcohol-impaired driving, and behavior change is to occur primarily through social norms programs, which a Cochrane Review (Foxcroft et al., 2015) concluded were ineffective at changing alcohol consumption.

Conflicts of interest may develop when a highly profitable business enters the public health arena. In a discussion in the *Bulletin of the World Health Organization*, it was argued that industry–civil society partnerships "lend legitimacy and provide a platform for the distilled spirits industry to lobby against proposals to reduce the availability of alcohol, increase the price of alcohol through raising excise taxes, and place restrictions on the marketing of alcohol, despite the global evidence that these measures are the most cost-effective way to decrease alcohol-related harm" (Matzopoulos et al., 2012, p. 67).

These concerns are supported by the business literature that argues that a company's credibility is the most important characteristic of lobbying (Hillman, 2003; Hillman et al., 2004). A company's reputation or credibility is associated with a company's ability to affect public policy decisions (Boddewyn and Brewer 1994; Hillman, 2003; Hillman et al., 2004). According to Boddewyn and Brewer (1994), industry–government partnering conveys a derivative "seal of approval" of what international firms are doing. Perhaps most importantly, industry partnerships divert resources and attention away from evidence-based interventions (Brown, 2015). Speaking at a global conference on health promotion, WHO Director General Margaret Chan (2013) said it was "dangerous" when industry gets "involved in policy making."

Impact Assessment

The wide variety of political activities described in this section has been used by the alcohol industry to influence the policy environment related to drinking and driving. Many of these activities are promoted as corporate social responsibility, but they also have the potential to serve the strategic aims of commercial interests, one of which is to sell more alcohol. In most cases, it is difficult to establish a direct link to alcohol policies that either reduce or increase alcohol-impaired driving and alcohol-related traffic injuries, but there is considerable circumstantial evidence that some of these activities are detrimental to public health and traffic safety and that many others serve to dilute the public health response. Furthermore, efforts to increase overall alcohol consumption will inevitably lead to negative alcohol-related consequences including increased alcohol-impaired driving.

For example, political donations to finance electoral campaigns for presidential, congressional, state, and local elections are often bipartisan and may be effective at promoting the industry's agenda. Donations and campaign contributions may create financial dependencies and influence over an organization or individual (Adams, 2016; Bion, 2009; Dana and Loewenstein, 2003). Conflicts of interest can further influence behavior by imposing a "sense of indebtedness," and thereby the obligation to reciprocate (Adams, 2016; Katz et al., 2003).

Regarding the support of scientific research, the alcohol industry may influence available scientific data by commissioning studies that set the research agenda. For example, in a public opinion poll conducted by TIRF and funded by AB InBev, approximately 5,000 U.S. drivers were asked about the suitability of designated driver programs and safe rides (Meister et al., 2015; Powell et al., 2016), which are likely ineffective policies (Ditter et al., 2005). Although media campaigns, local programs, and ridesharing companies may increase the use of designated drivers and/or safe ride services, it is less clear whether these programs lead to a reduction in alcohol-impaired driving and alcohol-related crashes (Brazil and Kirk, 2016; Nielson and Watson, 2009).

Potentially effective policies, such as alcohol tax increases, availability restrictions, and BAC limits, have not been investigated by means of industry-funded studies. According to some observers (Pantani et al., 2012; Wolburg, 2005), the industry finances academic researchers to disseminate messages regarding "responsible drinking" and "alcohol and health" to use scientific arguments to influence public policy and establish a positive public image.

Even when the industry supports evidence-based policies, such as the use of ignition interlock devices, these policies often have limited practical applicability because they focus on individuals who have already committed a drinking and driving offense ("hard-core drink drivers") and cannot prevent first-time offenders.

Although research across a wide range of health and environmental areas (Bero et al., 2007; DeAngelis, 2007; Jørgensen et al., 2008; Kassirer, 2005; Krimsky, 2003; Lesser et al., 2007; Yank et al., 2007) suggests that conflicts of interests are associated with biased research findings that favor commercial interests, there is no evidence from the traffic safety field. Nevertheless, the alcohol industry and its surrogate organizations have been suspected of distorting the science base on a more general level to promote alcohol policies that favor industry economic interests rather than public health (Babor, 2009; Babor and Miller, 2014; Babor and Xuan, 2004; Miller et al., 2017).

There is little research on the potential effect of alcohol industry lobbying, but a news article written by a lobbyist for the Nevada wine and spirits distributors suggests that some alcohol industry lobbyists provide access for their clients and help to arrange campaign contributions on or about the time that legislation is being considered (Williams, 2017).

In the following section we analyze a database collected by the world's largest alcohol producers to demonstrate their collective commitment to good corporate citizenship. As many of these initiatives concern drinking and driving, they provide a way to evaluate the extent to which corporate social responsibility is consistent with evidence-based public health practices concerning road traffic safety. These initiatives also provide a way to evaluate the extent to which policy substitution is evident in the alcohol industry's attempts at corporate social responsibility over an extended period of time.

CONTENT ANALYSIS OF INDUSTRY ACTIVITIES CONDUCTED IN RELATION TO ALCOHOL-IMPAIRED DRIVING

In 2012, a consortium of transnational alcohol corporations and other industry segments released a set of more than 3,500 "industry actions," which they claimed were being conducted in support of the WHO's Global Strategy to Reduce the Harmful Use of Alcohol (WHO Global Strategy). A full list of the actions was posted on the industry actions website (initiatives.global-actions.org), but the website was removed without explanation in 2016. According to the website, 97 industry-sponsored activities had been initiated in the United States in the area of drinking and driving. To the extent that this information represents the alcohol industry's own inventory of activities that were conducted or were considered ongoing at the time of the release of the WHO Global Strategy in 2010, it is likely to be a relatively complete accounting of what various industry segments consider to be their main initiatives in this area. Although the database was created in 2012, many of the initiatives were listed as "ongoing" and the only major new initiative that was identified was the Smart Drinking Goals program, which was discussed previously.

We analyzed the 97 drinking and driving industry actions to determine what proportion of them

- Conform to the drinking and driving target area as described in the WHO Global Strategy;
- Can be considered as evidence-based activities likely to have a positive impact on drinking behavior or alcohol-impaired driving;
- Have the potential to promote a brand or product (i.e., marketing potential); and
- Have the potential to affect policy or create harm.

Methods

We conducted a content analysis and rated each of the 97 actions on scales developed to evaluate marketing potential, potential to influence policy, and estimated population reach (see Pantani et al., 2017, and Esser et al., 2016, for a more complete description of the methods). Each initiative posted on the industry website consisted of a short description of the program (approximately 100–150 words) as well as information about the program's year of initiation, the sponsoring company or organization, the WHO Global Strategy area it was intended to address (e.g., alcohol-impaired driving), and whether it was the subject of an evaluation.

Trained raters coded each initiative according to 65 activity types that have been evaluated for evidence of effectiveness in the literature. Actions that did not fall into any of the 65 activity types were coded as 1 of 12 "other" subcodes. Actions coded under these "other" subcodes include online BAC calculators and designated driver posters in bars (coded as "Miscellaneous").

We also conducted a literature review to identify interventions, strategies, and programs that have been evaluated scientifically for their effect on alcohol-impaired driving and alcohol-related traffic injuries. These ratings were based on procedures developed by Babor et al. (2010) and Nelson et al. (2013) to evaluate the strength of evidence, the extent of research, and the population reach of 29 policy options that have been the subject of research on alcohol-impaired driving.

In addition, each industry action was rated in terms of the type of CSR activity it represented: risk management, as defined by Lantos (2001); strategic; or altruistic philanthropy. Ratings were also made depending on unintended consequences (i.e., potential for harm) and whether the program or initiative had a process or outcome evaluation.

Findings

AB InBev was the leading sponsor of the industry actions (33.0 percent), followed by SABMiller (24.7 percent). Our analysis also found that 37.1 percent of the 97 actions classified by the industry as addressing the WHO Global Strategy target area of "drink-driving" were only tangentially related to alcohol-impaired driving and therefore did not fit into this or any of the other 10 areas for policy options and interventions described in the WHO Global Strategy.

Table C-5 shows the percentage of industry actions classified according to type of activity, estimated effectiveness, strength of evidence, and population reach. The table includes only the 97 activities conducted by the alcohol industry in the United States.

Nearly all (97.9 percent) of the alcohol industry's U.S. drinking and driving initiatives were rated as either ineffective or of unknown effectiveness. The remaining 2.1 percent consisted of support for more severe punishment of impaired drivers, which has mixed evidence of effectiveness because effects decay over time and depend on enforcement (Babor et al., 2010).

Nearly 15 percent (14.4%) involved a designated driver or responsible drinking message being added to packaging or marketing materials. Approximately 7 percent of actions were coded as "unrelated," such as a contest for journalists. Only three actions met minimum criteria for promoting designated drivers as described in the literature.

Whereas some activities (e.g., research, miscellaneous, unrelated) did not have sufficient empirical support to even evaluate the strength of the evidence, others (e.g., designated driver programs, safe rides, information campaigns, social norms programs, support of severe punishment for alcohol-impaired drivers) had considerable evidence indicating that they were *ineffective*. In total, 56.2 percent of the actions supported by the industry had evidence of ineffectiveness, and most of the others had either not been evaluated or were unrelated to alcohol-impaired driving.

We also rated the population reach of each action. Population reach refers to the number of individuals likely to be affected by a program initiative. The majority of actions (53.6 percent) were limited to a small number of people, such as patrons within one community or workplace employee programs; 33.0 percent were considered to have no population reach. These included activities like the funding of social aspects organizations and an award presented to AB InBev. Only 13.4 percent had moderate population reach, and none of the actions were found to have large or national reach.

Common industry actions were the distribution of flyers or brochures about designated drivers or responsible drinking, which often doubled as marketing for the alcohol brands. More than 45 percent (45.5 percent)

TABLE C-5 Percentage of Industry Actions Classified According to Type of Activity, Estimated Effectiveness, Strength of Evidence, and Population Reach of 97 Activities Conducted by the Alcohol Industry in the United States in Support of the WHO Global Strategy to Reduce the Harmful Use of Alcohol

Activity	%	Effectiveness[a]	Strength of Evidence[b]	Population Reach[c]
Severity of punishment	2.1	0/+	+++	++
Designated driver programs	3.1	0	+++	0
Social marketing	1.0	0	++	0
Social norms programs	1.0	0	+++	0
Safe ride programs	19.6	0	++	+
Other	73.2	?	?	?
Miscellaneous[d] (e.g., online BAC)	28.9	?	?	?
Activity secondary to alcohol marketing	14.4	?	?	?
Public information/ conferences	14.4	?	?	?
Activities unrelated to alcohol-impaired driving (e.g., journalism award)	7.2	?	?	?
Research on alcohol-impaired driving	5.2	?	?	0
Training for staff other than responsible beverage service	2.1	?	?	?
Alcohol policy development	1.0	?	?	?

[a] – net negative effect; 0 no effect; + minimal positive effect; ++ positive effect but secondary efforts required; +++ independent positive effect; 0/+ mixed evidence; ? insufficient evidence.

[b] 0 no evidence; + only one to three studies; ++ more than three studies but no systematic reviews or meta-analysis published; +++ one or more systematic reviews or meta-analysis published on the topic.

[c] 0 no population effect; + effect only on a small, well-defined group of individuals; ++ community or citywide effect; +++ effect likely felt on a state or national level; ? unknown.

[d] Includes campaigns that do not meet minimum criteria to be coded as mass media or social marketing.

were considered to have the potential to promote a brand or product, for example, by means of brand advertising associated with the activity. Raters also found that 20.6 percent of the actions had the potential to affect national or local policy (e.g., Diageo's support for a congressional Stop-DUI caucus event that brought together members of Congress and the industry-funded Century Council, and Heineken's sponsorship of the 2006 Congressional Black Caucus Foundation Legislative Conference).

Ratings of corporate social responsibility consisted of classifying each action into one of the three previously mentioned CSR categories. Most (83.5 percent) of the actions were found to meet the definition of corporate social responsibility as a risk-management strategy (i.e., to prevent legal liability, as defined by Lantos, 2001). The remaining 16.5 percent were classified as strategic (i.e., promoting the industry's commercial objectives). None were considered to be altruistic philanthropy.

Regarding the ratings of unintended consequences, 13.4 percent were found to have the potential for harm. These include safe ride programs that were considered to have the potential to encourage or sanction heavy drinking.

Almost all of the activities lacked a systematic evaluation capable of determining program effectiveness. The industry website reported that 8.2 percent had some type of evaluation component. Raters also coded the type of evaluation based on the industry's description and found that only 5.2 percent met the minimum criteria to be classified as a process evaluation, with only a few reporting what appeared to be an outcome evaluation.

Impact Assessment

The appropriateness of the industry's more than 3,500 global "Industry Actions to Reduce Harmful Drinking," of which the 97 drinking and driving initiatives analyzed here were a part, were questioned in a public statement of concern (Babor et al., 2013) addressed to the director general of WHO by an international group of 17 alcohol policy experts. The statement claimed that the global alcohol producers had misinterpreted their roles with respect to the implementation of the WHO Global Strategy, and therefore should not be conducting public health activities on behalf of WHO other than to allow effective, evidence-based alcohol control measures to be adopted by WHO member states.

According to a similar content analysis of industry actions in Latin America and the Caribbean region (Pantani et al., 2017), only 4 percent of the initiatives could be considered as evidence-based activities capable of affecting drinking behavior or alcohol-related problems, and 55 percent of the actions were considered to have the potential to promote a brand or product, for example, by means of brand advertising associated with the activity. This analysis also showed that actions considered to have marketing potential were more likely to have a large population reach than those that did not. As this analysis covered many of the same transnational producers operating in the United States, it suggests the alcohol industry's CSR activities are potentially conducted in part for marketing purposes. In another analysis of the 266 drinking and driving initiatives conducted worldwide, which included the 97 U.S. initiatives described above, most actions were conducted by industry-funded social aspects/public relations organizations, and only 0.2 percent met the minimum definition of evidence based (Esser et al., 2016).

The findings provide strong evidence that the industry does not fund or support public health policies that have been shown to affect alcohol-impaired driving and reduce alcohol-related harm. Although the industry has supported the development of ignition interlock devices in the United States and Canada for repeat and high BAC offenders, the population impact of this technology has been limited because of its expense and limited population reach (Elder et al., 2011).

Many of the industry actions included responsible drinking campaigns or messages. Since the 1990s, researchers have analyzed the use of such messages and have concluded that instead of encouraging moderate consumption, the messages create a favorable image of the alcohol brand without influencing excessive drinking (Barry and Goodson, 2010; DeJong et al., 1992; Pantani et al., 2012; Smith et al., 2006; Wolburg, 2005). Therefore, responsible drinking campaigns can potentially be considered another form of alcohol marketing and may even encourage alcohol consumption. Furthermore, the industry has not produced any evidence of their effectiveness, other than to note that message recipients like them.

Consistent with the political activities described in the previous section, segments of the alcohol industry have actively resisted efforts to promote effective, evidence-based drinking and driving policies, such as lower legal permissible blood alcohol concentrations and increased alcohol taxes. Instead, industry-sponsored designated driver or safe ride campaigns are widely promoted, despite the lack of evidence regarding their effectiveness. Research suggests that users of safe rides have significantly higher BAC levels and are more likely to be heavy drinkers compared to nonusers (Caudill et al., 2000), and BAC levels are significantly greater when using free safe rides compared to other occasions when drinking outside the home (Harding et al., 2001). Research shows that designated drivers often do not abstain from alcohol, but rather drink less (Barry, 2013; Rivara et al., 2007). Such voluntary efforts have been interpreted by some as attempts to avoid stricter regulations (Knai et al., 2015; McCambridge et al., 2013; Savell et al., 2016), and to draw attention away from the alcohol industry's role in opposing effective policies by giving the appearance of extensive collaboration with governments and NGOs.

CONCLUSIONS

This paper has attempted to critically evaluate the strategies and tactics used by the alcohol industry that have implications for road traffic safety. We have provided a general assessment of several major industry segments and a wide range of activities, but it is important to note that the alcohol industry is not monolithic. Some segments of the industry have at times supported laws to reduce underage drinking and have promoted efforts to enforce drinking and driving laws and to punish alcohol-impaired drivers. Other segments, perhaps the large majority of retailers, distributors, and producers, do not engage in political or commercial activities that are likely to affect alcohol-impaired driving. This analysis has focused primarily on the transnational producers, large trade associations, and multistate retailers, so generalizations of the entire industry may be limited. Furthermore, our qualitative analysis of commercial and political activities is limited to information that can be accessed through news reports, industry websites, and the reports of NGOs and watchdog groups. To the extent that this information tends to be anecdotal and circumstantial, it may not be representative of the entire industry. Nevertheless, the industry's own inventory of local, state, and national initiatives provides an indication of the scope and effect of their drinking and driving programs. Most of them were considered to have low population reach, primarily because they were local in nature, and even when their media campaigns reached a larger audience, they simultaneously were considered to have a marketing function.

Taking into account these caveats and limitations, we conclude that activities of the large producers, both in their commercial initiatives (e.g., advertising, product design) and their political activities (e.g., opposition to effective drinking and driving laws and regulations), have been documented in a number of areas that conflict with a public health approach to the management of alcohol-related problems. Three general conclusions are consistent with the evidence presented in this paper. First, some of the industry's promotional activities, combined with product innovations, may increase the frequency and amount of alcohol consumption, as well as the likelihood of alcohol-impaired driving. Second, the alcohol industry's corporate political activities may interfere with effective alcohol policies and improve the public image of the producers as good corporate citizens, rather than reduce the incidence of alcohol-impaired driving. Third, the evidence suggests that the policies and programs favored by the alcohol industry are ineffective.

Commercial Activities

The strategies reviewed here suggest that some of the alcohol industry's marketing and product design activities contribute to the ongoing recruitment of young people, women, and other potentially vulnerable populations, and may increase consumption through the promotion of more frequent drinking occasions. By recruiting new drinkers from the majority population of abstainers and by implementing measures designed to increase the frequency of drinking, there is likely to be an increase in the prevalence of heavy drinking and alcohol-related problems, including motor vehicle crashes. This is illustrated by our analysis of the relationship between the alcohol industry and the energy drink industry, and the use of marketing in association with professional motorsports leagues. Industry sponsorship of festivals and other youth-oriented public events may contribute to the social acceptance of alcohol and influence the frequency and volume of drinking by increasing public acceptance of a wide variety of drinking occasions.

Corporate Political Activities

Activities such as lobbying, image advertising, and strategic alliances may be used to influence industry-favorable policies in relation to alcohol-impaired driving countermeasures. The findings suggest that multiple tactics are often practiced simultaneously to achieve favorable policy outcomes. Many of the industry's CSR activities were found to be public relations exercises and largely attempts to promote ineffective policies. In its CSR activities, the industry has supported the need to address impaired driving and has actively collaborated with a wide array of civil society and governmental groups seeking to prevent it. At the same time, the industry's corporate political activities have blocked effective measures (e.g., restrictions on outlets and hours of sale; server liability laws; alcohol tax increases) that might reduce overall alcohol consumption.

The findings of this paper suggest that the economic interests of the large transnational producers, combined with their extensive campaign contributions to political parties and politicians, create the conditions for a strong industry influence in the policy-making process around road traffic safety. Some of this influence may be exercised through a set of key agenda items that promote the industry's interests, such as low alcohol taxes, minimum regulation of alcohol availability, and industry self-regulation of alcohol marketing, all of which contribute to alcohol consumption and alcohol-related problems. At the same time, the industry's increasing investments in CSR activities have coalesced around a few themes, such as designated driver programs and increased enforcement of existing laws regardless of their effectiveness.

Promotion of Ineffective Programs and Policies

As indicated in our review of the evidence (Table C-5 and additional appendix tables[13]), the most effective policies to promote road traffic safety and to combat drinking and driving are not only direct interventions such as sobriety checkpoints, but also indirect alcohol control policies in public health that are typically aimed at decreasing per capita consumption to minimize alcohol problems. There is an impressive amount of evidence (Babor et al., 2010) that universal measures to raise the price of alcohol (Elder et al., 2010) and control its availability (Campbell et al., 2009) are among the most effective policy options to reduce alcohol-impaired driving. This evidence is reinforced by the results of a Delphi panel composed of 10 U.S. alcohol policy experts. The experts rated alcohol control policies in terms of their impact on binge drinking and alcohol-impaired driving (Nelson et al., 2013). The highest ratings of efficacy were given to policies limiting price, increasing alcohol taxes, and regulating alcohol availability.

The industry has opposed these approaches and instead champions voluntary action alongside targeted interventions that focus on a minority of heavy drinkers (Babor and Robaina, 2013; Babor et al., 2015; Jernigan, 2012; Knai et al., 2015; Pantani et al., 2017). Of the 29 strategies and interventions that have been evaluated in terms of their effectiveness in preventing or reducing alcohol-impaired driving, few if any are promoted by the industry. On the contrary, we found that the industry's initiatives were largely considered to be either ineffective by current scientific standards or have not been evaluated.

There is concern among some road safety experts that the alcohol industry's activities may compromise the development of public health policy and the work of public health experts (Brown, 2015; Esser et al., 2016). Whereas some would argue that any efforts by the alcohol industry to improve traffic safety should be welcomed, alcohol producers have a major conflict of interest in the policies they promote and oppose.

Recommendations

We close with a set of recommendations regarding the role of the alcohol industry in the development of policy aimed at reducing alcohol-impaired driving and its negative consequences. We also consider the role of federal and state agencies as well as the road traffic safety community.

---

[13] Available by request from the National Academies of Sciences, Engineering, and Medicine's Public Access Records Office (PARO@nas.edu).

Alcohol Producers and Other Industry Segments

The alcohol industry has the ability and the responsibility to minimize the harm caused by its products at all stages of the production chain, especially in terms of product design and marketing. This responsibility cannot be regarded solely as a national issue. Transnational corporations should adhere to minimal ethical standards for responsible product design and marketing practices regardless of the country where their products are sold. Global alcohol producers, their trade associations, and community outreach and public relations organizations have an ethical responsibility to do the following:

- Reduce the alcohol content of existing products when warranted to reduce the risk of injury while intoxicated and the toxic effects of chronic drinking.
- Refrain from all marketing that is likely to encourage underage consumption or unsafe driving, including motorsport sponsorship activities.
- Refrain from traffic safety educational activities that purport to protect the public health but do not do so.
- Support research bearing on the public health consequences of alcohol use through independent organizations, rather than through direct funding that raises concerns about agenda setting and research bias.

Role of Federal and State Agencies

Federal and state agencies engaged in public health and traffic safety need to protect the integrity of these policies from commercial and other vested interests, and should be informed by the following considerations:

- Government-sponsored activities for developing and implementing public health and traffic safety measures should be conducted by professionals free of conflicts of interest who have appropriate expertise in these areas. Participation of developers, producers, distributors, marketers, and sellers of alcoholic beverages should be advisory.
- In the absence of clear evidence that the industry is fulfilling its ethical responsibilities, civil society organizations and professional groups should be extremely cautious about entering into partnerships with the commercial alcohol industry, its community outreach and public relations organizations, and other groups substantially funded by the commercial alcohol industry.

Road Traffic Safety Community, Including Research Scientists, NGOs, and Other Public Interest Organizations

Financial support from the alcohol industry and its third-party organizations has the potential to affect professional judgment and may strengthen the influence of private interests in the policy-making process. All participating parties should keep in mind that the evolution of ethical thresholds and standards in recent decades has generally been toward more stringent standards, such as in the case of tobacco. This has led organizations such as Mothers Against Drunk Driving (MADD) Canada to refuse funding from alcohol industry sources (Solomon et al., 2004). The following actions are warranted by the road traffic safety community:

- Do not accept direct funding from industry sources for prevention, research, education, and information dissemination activities.
- Encourage industry support for evidence-based policies.
- Promote rigorous adherence to conflict-of-interest principles.
- Make all information relating to funding and/or partnership work transparent and available for public scrutiny.
- Support funding for research, prevention, and public health surveillance activities through hypothecated tax revenues that are proportionate to the societal costs of alcohol problems.

REFERENCES

AB (Anheuser-Busch) InBev. 2016a. *Anheuser-Busch annual report*. http://annualreport.ab-inbev.com/index.html (accessed November 17, 2017).

AB InBev. 2016b. *Form 20-F*. http://www.ab-inbev.com/content/dam/universaltemplate/ab-inbev/investors/reports-and-filings/sec-filings/SEC_filings_20-F_0909.pdf (accessed November 17, 2017).

AB InBev. 2017. *Global smart drinking goals*. http://www.ab-inbev.com/better-world/a-healthier-world/global-smart-drinking-goals.html (accessed November 24, 2017).

ABI (American Beverage Institute). 2013. *Join us*. http://big.assets.huffingtonpost.com/abi_2013_promo.pdf (accessed November 17, 2017).

ABI. 2015. *Form 990. Return of Organization Exempt from Income Tax 2014*. https://projects.propublica.org/nonprofits/organizations/521730954 (accessed November 27, 2017).

ABI. 2017a. *American Beverage Institute garners 10,000 signatures opposing Utah's .05 law*. https://abionline.org/press_release/american-beverage-institute-garners-10000-signatures-opposing-utahs-05-law (accessed November 17, 2017).

ABI. 2017b. *Op-eds & letters*. https://abionline.org/newsroom (accessed November 17, 2017).

AdAge. 2016. *World's largest advertisers 2016*. http://adage.com/datacenter/globalmarketers2016 (accessed November 17, 2017).

Adams, P. 2016. *Moral jeopardy*. Cambridge, UK: Cambridge University Press.

Amis, J., and T. B. Cornwell. 2005. *Global sports sponsorship*. Oxford, UK: Oxford University Press.

Anderson, P., A. de Bruijn, K. Angus, R. Gordon, and G. Hastings. 2009. Impact of alcohol advertising and media exposure on adolescent alcohol use: A systematic review of longitudinal studies. *Alcohol and Alcoholism* 44(3):229–243.

Anheuser-Busch. 2017. *Lime-A-Rita announces brand makeover created by women, for women.* http://www.anheuser-busch.com/newsroom/2017/03/lime-a-rita-announces-brand-makeover-created-by-women--for-women.html (accessed November 17, 2017).

ARCA (Automobile Racing Club of America). 2017. *Main page.* https://www.arcaracing.com (accessed November 27, 2017).

Associated Press. 2008. Correction: Alcohol group lobbying story. Associated Press Newswires. 20 Feb. https://global.factiva.com/ha/default.aspx#./!?&_suid=1511382472516041972327029832135 (accessed November 22, 2017, from Factiva.com).

Austin, E. W., M. J. Chen, and J. W. Grube. 2006. How does alcohol advertising influence underage drinking? The role of desirability, identification, and skepticism. *Journal of Adolescent Health* 38(4):376–384.

Babor, T. F. 2009. Alcohol research and the alcoholic beverage industry: Issues, concerns and conflicts of interest. *Addiction* 104(Suppl 1):34–47.

Babor, T. F. 2014. The gathering storm: Alcohol abuse among the Chinese in Asia, and the public health response. *Malaysian Journal of Chinese Studies* 3(1):1–20.

Babor, T. F., and P. G. Miller. 2014. McCarthyism, conflict of interest and Addiction's new transparency declaration procedures. *Addiction* 109(8):341–344.

Babor, T. F., and K. Robaina. 2013. Public health, academic medicine, and the alcohol industry's corporate social responsibility activities. *American Journal of Public Health* 103(2):206–214.

Babor, T. F., and Z. Xuan. 2004. Alcohol policy research and the grey literature. *Nordic Studies on Alcohol and Drugs* 21(English Suppl):125–137.

Babor, T., R. Caetano, S. Casswell, G. Edwards, N. Giesbrecht, K. Graham, J. Grube, L. Hill, H. Holder, R. Homel, M. Livingston, E. Osterberg, J. Rehm, R. Room, and I. Rossow. 2010. *Alcohol: No ordinary commodity—Research and public policy.* 2nd ed. Oxford, UK: Oxford University Press.

Babor, T., K. Brown, D. Jernigan, N. Tumwesigye, G. Hastings, R. Laranjeira, I. Obot, S. Carlsson, E. Gillian, W. Hao, M. Daube, K. Robaina, P. Miller, P. Anderson, A. Veryga, S. Casswell, and S. Chun. 2013. *Statement of concern—The international public health community responds to the global alcohol producers' attempts to implement the WHO strategy on the harmful use of alcohol.* http://www.iogt.org/wp-content/uploads/2013/02/WHO-statement-of-concern-final-8-Feb-2013.pdf (accessed November 17, 2017).

Babor, T. F., K. Robaina, and D. Jernigan. 2015. The influence of industry actions on the availability of alcoholic beverages in the African region. *Addiction* 110(4):561–571.

Bakke, Ø., and D. Endal. 2010. Vested interests in addiction research and policy alcohol policies out of context: Drinks industry supplanting government role in alcohol policies in sub-Saharan Africa. *Addiction* 105(1):22–28.

Barry, A. E. 2013. Breath alcohol concentrations of designated drivers. *Journal of Studies on Alcohol and Drugs* 74(4):509–513.

Barry, A. E., and P. Goodson. 2010. Use (and misuse) of the responsible drinking message in public health and alcohol advertising: A review. *Health Education and Behavior* 37(2): 288–303.

Bero, L., F. Oostvogel, P. Bacchetti, and K. Lee. 2007. Factors associated with findings of published trials of drug-use comparisons: Why some statins appear more efficacious than others. *PLoS Medicine* 4(6):184.

Bion, J. 2009. Financial and intellectual conflicts of interest: Confusion and clarity. *Current Opinion in Critical Care* 15:583–590.

Boddewyn, J., and T. Brewer. 1994. International-business political behavior: New theoretical directions. *Academy of Management Review* 19(1):119–143.

Bond, L., M. Daube, and T. Chikritzhs. 2009. Access to confidential alcohol industry documents: From "Big Tobacco" to "Big Booze." *American Medical Journal* 1(3):1–26.

Bond, L., M. Daube, and T. Chikritzhs. 2010. Selling addictions: Similarities in approaches between Big Tobacco and Big Booze. *American Medical Journal* 3(6):325–332.

Brazil, N., and D. S. Kirk. 2016. Uber and metropolitan traffic fatalities in the United States. *American Journal of Epidemiology* 184(3):192–198.

Brown, K. 2015. The public health responsibility deal: Why alcohol industry partnerships are bad for health. *Addiction* 110(8):1227–1228.

Brown, K. 2016. Association between alcohol sports sponsorship and consumption: A systematic review. *Alcohol and Alcoholism* 51(6):747–755.

Brown, R., M. Busalacchi, S. Hargarten, and J. Sherman. 2014. *Letter to Secretary Mark Gottlieb, P.E., Wisconsin Department of Transportation*. http://media.jrn.com/documents/FINAL+ltr+to+Sec+DOT+OWI.pdf (accessed November 20, 2017).

Campbell, C. A., R. A. Hahn, R. Elder, R. Brewer, S. Chattopadhyay, J. Fielding, T. S. Naimi, T. Toomey, B. Lawrence, J. C. Middleton, and Task Force on Community Preventive Services. 2009. The effectiveness of limiting alcohol outlet density as a means of reducing excessive alcohol consumption and alcohol-related harms. *American Journal of Preventive Medicine* 37(6):556–569.

Caudill, B. D., W. M. Harding, and B. A. Moore. 2000. At-risk drinkers use safe ride services to avoid drinking and driving. *Journal of Substance Abuse* 11(2):149–159.

Center for Responsive Politics. 2017. *Beer, wine, and liquor*. http://www.opensecrets.org/industries/indus.php?ind=N02 (accessed November 20, 2017).

Chan, M. 2013. Re: Doctors and the alcohol industry: An unhealthy mix? *BMJ* 346:f2647.

CHOICE. 2008. *Alcopops*. https://www.choice.com.au/food-and%20drink/drinks/alcohol/articles/alcopops (accessed July 3, 2017).

Collin, J., E. Johnson, H. Officer, and S. Hill. 2014. Government support for alcohol industry: Promoting exports, jeopardizing global health? *BMJ* 348:g3648.

Copeland, J., R. J. Stevenson, P. Gates, and P. Dillon, P. 2007. Young Australians and alcohol: The acceptability of ready-to-drink (RTD) alcoholic beverages among 12–30-year-olds. *Addiction* 102(11):1740–1746.

Cronin, J., and A. Stone. 2008. *CSPI to sue Anheuser-Busch, Miller over alcoholic energy drinks*. https://cspinet.org/news/cspi-sue-anheuser-busch-miller-over-alcoholic-energy-drinks-20080228 (accessed November 20, 2017).

Dana, J., and G. Loewenstein. 2003. A social science perspective on gifts to physicians from industry. *JAMA 290*(2):252–255.

de Haan, L., H. A. de Haan, J. van der Palen, B. Olivier, and J. C. Verster. 2012. Effects of consuming alcohol mixed with energy drinks versus consuming alcohol only on overall alcohol consumption and negative alcohol-related consequences. *International Journal of General Medicine* 5:953–960.

DeAngelis, C. 2007. Comment on "Conflict of interest in medical research: Facts and friction" in meeting proceedings, *Call to Action: Managing Financial Relationships Between Academia and Industry in Biomedical Research*, pp. 15–16. http://www.faseb.org/portals/2/PDFs/opa/July17CalltoActionSummary.pdf (accessed November 20, 2017).

DeJong, W., C. Atkin, and L. Wallack. 1992. A critical analysis of "moderation" advertising sponsored by the beer industry: Are "responsible drinking" commercials done responsibly? *Milbank Quarterly* 661–678.

Ditter, S., R. Elder, R. Shults, D. Sleet, R. Compton, J. Nichols, and Task Force on Community Preventive Services. 2005. Effectiveness of designated driver programs for reducing alcohol-impaired driving: A systematic review. *American Journal of Preventive Medicine* 28(5 Suppl):280–287.

Dodd, D. 2016. *Alcohol: Coming soon to a college football stadium near you*. https://www.cbssports.com/college-football/news/alcohol-coming-soon-to-your-college-football-stadium-if-its-not-there-already (accessed November 20, 2017).

Elder, R. W., B. Lawrence, A. Ferguson, T. S. Naimi, R. D. Brewer, S. K. Chattopadhyay, T. L. Toomey, J. E. Fielding, and Task Force on Community Preventive Services. 2010. The effectiveness of tax policy interventions for reducing excessive alcohol consumption and related harms. *American Journal of Preventive Medicine* 38(2):217–229.

Elder, R. W., R. Voas, D. Beirness, R. A. Shults, D. A. Sleet, J. L. Nichols, R. Compton, and Task Force on Community Preventive Services. 2011. Effectiveness of ignition interlocks for preventing alcohol-impaired driving and alcohol-related crashes: A Community Guide systematic review. *American Journal of Preventive Medicine* 40(3):362–376.

Esser, M. B., J. Bao, D. H. Jernigan, and A. A. Hyder. 2016. Evaluation of the evidence base for the alcohol industry's actions to reduce drink driving globally. *American Journal of Public Health* 106(4):707–713.

Eurocare. 2015. *Alcohol advertising and sponsorship in Formula One: A dangerous cocktail*. http://www.ias.org.uk/uploads/pdf/Marketing/Alcohol_Advertising_And_Sponsorship_In_Formula_One__A_Dangerous_Cocktail_May_2015.pdf (accessed November 22, 2017).

Euromonitor International. 2017. *Alcoholic drinks dashboard*. http://www.portal.euromonitor.com/portal/dashboard/Statistics (accessed May 30, 2017).

FDA (U.S. Food and Drug Administration). 2010. *Update on caffeinated alcoholic beverages*. https://www.fda.gov/NewsEvents/PublicHealthFocus/ucm234900.htm (accessed November 20, 2017).

Ferreira-Borges, C., J. Rehm, S. Dias, T. Babor, and C. Parry. 2016. The impact of alcohol consumption on African people in 2012: An analysis of burden of disease. *Tropical Medicine & International Health* 21(1):52–60.

Formula Drift. 2017. *Home page*. Formula Drift Holdings LLC. http://www.formulad.com (accessed November 27, 2017).

Foxcroft, D. R., M. Moreira, N. M. L. Almeida Santimano, and L. A. Smith. 2015. Social norms information for alcohol misuse in university and college students. *Cochrane Database of Systematic Reviews* 12.

Getz, K. 1997. Research in corporate political activity: Integration and assessment. *Business and Society* 36:32–77.

Gornall, J. 2014. Under the influence. *BMJ* 348:f7646.

Harding, W. M., B. D. Caudill, B. A. Moore, and K. C. Frissell. 2001. Do drivers drink more when they use a safe ride? *Journal of Substance Abuse* 13(3):283–290.

Hastings, G. 2009. "They'll drink bucket loads of the stuff": An analysis of internal alcohol industry advertising documents. *Alcohol and Education Research Council*. http://oro.open.ac.uk/22913/1/AERC_FinalReport_0060.pdf (accessed November 20, 2017).

Hawkins, B., C. Holden, and J. McCambridge. 2012. Alcohol industry influence on UK alcohol policy: A new research agenda for public health. *Critical Public Health* 22(3):297–305.

Hillman, A. J. 2003. Determinants of political strategies in US multinationals. *Business & Society* 42(4):455–484.

Hillman, A., and M. Hitt. 1999. Corporate political strategy formulation: A model of approach, participation, and strategy decisions. *The Academy of Management Review* 24(4):825–842.

Hillman, A. J., G. D. Keim, and D. Schuler. 2004. Corporate polictical activity: A review and research agenda. *Journal of Management* 30(6):837–857.

Hollingworth, W., B. Ebel, C. McCarty, M. Garrison, D. Christakis, and F. Rivara. 2006. Prevention of deaths from harmful drinking in the United States: The potential effects of tax increases and advertising bans on young drinkers. *Journal of Studies of Alcohol* 67(2):300–308.

Hope, A. 2006. The influence of the alcohol industry on alcohol policy in Ireland. *Nordic Studies on Alcohol and Drugs* 23:467–481.

House of Commons Health Committee. 2010. *Alcohol: First report of session 2009–2010*. http://www.publications.parliament.uk/pa/cm200910/cmselect/cmhealth/151/15102.htm (accessed November 20, 2017).

IARD (International Alliance for Responsible Drinking). 2017a. *Members*. http://www.iard.org/about/members (accessed November 22, 2017).

IARD. 2017b. *About IARD*. http://www.iard.org/about (accessed November 22, 2017).

IHRA (International Hot Rod Association). 2017. *Home page*. http://www.ihra.com (accessed November 27, 2017).

IMSA (International Motor Sports Association). 2017. *Home page*. International Motor Sports Association, Inc. https://www.imsa.com (accessed November 27, 2017).

IndyCar. 2017. *Home page*. http://www.indycar.com (accessed November 27, 2017).

Jernigan, D. H. 2009. The global alcohol industry: An overview. *Addiction* 104(Suppl 1):6–12.

Jernigan, D. H. 2012. Global alcohol producers, science, and policy: The case of the International Center for Alcohol Policies. *American Journal of Public Health* 102(1):80–89.

Jernigan, D. H., and T. F. Babor. 2015. The concentration of the global alcohol industry and its penetration in the African region. *Addiction* 110(4):551–560.

Jernigan, D., J. Noel, J. Landon, N. Thornton, and T. Lobstein. 2017. Alcohol marketing and youth alcohol consumption: A systematic review of longitudinal studies published since 2008. *Addiction* 112(Suppl 1):7–20.

Jiang, N., and P. Ling. 2013. Vested interests in addiction research and policy. Alliance between tobacco and alcohol industries to shape public policy. *Addiction* 108:852–864.

Jørgensen, A. W., K. L. Maric, B. Tendal, A. Faurschou, and P. C. Gøtzsche. 2008. Industry-supported meta-analyses compared with meta-analyses with non-profit or no support: Differences in methodological quality and conclusions. *BMC Medical Research Methodology* 8:60.

Joseph, M. 2014. *SABMiller: "No one wants to buy pink beer, including women."* https://www.marketingweek.com/2014/10/07/sabmiller-no-one-wants-to-buy-a-pink-beer-including-women (accessed November 20, 2017).

Kassirer, J. P. 2005. *On the take: How medicine's complicity with big business can endanger your health*. Oxford, UK: Oxford University Press.

Katz, D., A. L Caplan, and J. F. Merz. 2003. All gifts large and small. *American Journal of Bioethics* 3(3):39–46.

Katzmark, G. 2015. *Motorsports' $100 Million Day in the U.S.* Nielsen Sports. http://nielsensports.com/motorsports-100-million-day-in-the-u-s (accessed November 27, 2017).

Keim, G. D., and C. P. Zeithaml. 1986. Corporate political strategy and legislative decision making: A review and contingency approach. *The Academy of Management Review* 11(4):828–843.

Klein, N. 2000. *No space, no choice, no jobs, no logo*. London: HarperCollins.

Knai, C., M. Petticrew, A. Durand, E. Eastmure, and N. Mays. 2015. Are the Public Health Responsibility Deal alcohol pledges likely to improve public health? An evidence synthesis. *Addiction* 110:1232–1246.

Krimsky, S. 2003. *Science in the private interest: Has the lure of profits corrupted biomedical research?* Lanham, MD: Rowman & Littlefield.

Lalanne, L., P. E. Lutz, and F. Paille. 2017. Acute impact of caffeinated alcoholic beverages on cognition: A systematic review. *Progress in Neuropsychopharmacology and Biological Psychiatry* 76:188–194.

Lambright, S. 1985. Testimony submitted by Stephen K. Lambright Vice President and Group Executive Anheuser-Busch Companies, Inc. to the U.S. House Of Representatives Subcommittee on Telecommunications, Consumer Protection and Finance May 21, 1985; testimony by Miller Brewing Company to the U.S. House Of Representatives Subcommittee on Telecommunications, Consumer Protection and Finance May 21, 1985; and beer and wine advertising: Impact of electronic media. Hearing before the Subcommittee on Telecommunications, Consumer Protection, and Finance of the Committee on Energy and Commerce of the House of Representatives. 99th Congress. 21 May, 1985. http://files.eric.ed.gov/fulltext/ED263489.pdf (accessed November 27, 2017).

Lantos, G. P. 2001. The boundaries of strategic corporate social responsibility. *Journal of Consumer Marketing* 18(7):595–632.

Lesser, L. I., C. B. Ebbeling, M. Goozner, D. Wypoj, and D. S. Ludwig. 2007. Relationship between funding source and conclusion among nutrition-related scientific articles. *PLoS Medicine* 4(1):e5.

Litt, D. M., and M. L. Stock. 2011. Adolescent alcohol-related risk cognitions: The role of social norms and social networking sites. *Psychology of Addictive Behaviors* 25(4):708–713.

Lobstein, T., J. Landon, N. Thornton, and D. Jernigan. 2017. The commercial use of digital media to market alcohol products: A narrative review. *Addiction* 112(Suppl 1):21–27.

Marley, P., and D. Ferguson. 2014. *Four Wisconsin OWI task force members quit*. http://archive.jsonline.com/news/statepolitics/four-wisconsin-owi-task-force-members-quit-b99285141z1-262006681.html (accessed November 20, 2017).

Mart, S., and N. Giesbrecht. 2015. Red flags on pinkwashed drinks: Contradictions and dangers in marketing alcohol to prevent cancer. *Addiction* 110(10):1541–1548.

Matzopoulos, R., C. Parry, J. M. Corrigall, S. Goldstein, and L. London. 2012. Global Fund collusion with liquor giant is a clear conflict of interest. *Bulletin of the World Health Organization* 90:67–69.

McCambridge, J., and G. Hartwell. 2015. Has industry funding biased studies of the protective effects of alcohol on cardiovascular disease? A preliminary investigation of prospective cohort studies. *Drug and Alcohol Review* 34:58–66.

McCambridge, J., B. Hawkins, and C. Holden. 2013. Industry use of evidence to influence alcohol policy: A case study of submissions to the 2008 Scottish Government Consultation. *PLoS Medicine* 10(4):e1001431.

McCreanor, T., A. Lyons, C. Griffin, I. Goodwin, H. Moewaka Barnes, and F. Hutton. 2012. Youth drinking cultures, social networking and alcohol marketing: Implications for public health. *Critical Public Health* 23(1):110–120.

McKetin, R., A. Coen, and S. Kaye. 2015. A comprehensive review of the effects of mixing caffeinated energy drinks with alcohol. *Drug and Alcohol Dependence* 151:15–30.

Meister, S. R., W. G. M. Vanlaar, T. C. Powell, and R. D. Robertson. 2015. *Alcohol-impaired driving in the United States*. http://tirf.ca/wp-content/uploads/2017/02/RSM-TIRF-USA-Alternatives-to-Alcohol-Impaired-Driving2016-8.pdf (accessed November 20, 2017).

Miller, P., F. Martino, S. Gross, A. Curtis, R. Mayshak, N. Droste, and K. Kypri. 2017. Funder interference in addiction research: An international survey of authors. *Addiction Behaviors* 72:101–105.

Mintel Group. 2016a. *US-Beer: Company retail market share by volume (%)*. Information Resources, Inc., Mintel. http://marketsizes.mintel.com.ezproxy.lib.uconn.edu/snapshots/USA/4/shares/single (accessed November 27, 2017).

Mintel Group. 2016b. *US-Wine and Sparking Wines: Company retail market share by volume (%)*. Information Resources, Inc., Mintel. http://marketsizes.mintel.com.ezproxy.lib.uconn.edu/snapshots/XNA/947/shares/market (accessed November 27, 2017).

Mintel Group. 2016c. *US-Spirits: Company retail market share by volume (%)*. Information Resources, Inc., Mintel. http://marketsizes.mintel.com.ezproxy.lib.uconn.edu/snapshots/USA/116/shares/single (accessed November 27, 2017).

Moewaka Barnes, H., T. McCreanor, I. Goodwin, A. Lyons, C. Griffin, and F. Hutton. 2016. Alcohol and social media: Drinking and drunkenness while online. *Critical Public Health* 26(1):62–76.

Monster Jam. 2016. *Home page*. Feld Motor Sports, Inc. https://www.monsterjam.com (accessed November 27, 2017).

Moodie, R., D. Stuckler, C. Monteiro, N. Sheron, B. Neal, T. Thamarangsi, P. Lincoln, S. Casswell, and Lancet NCD Action Group. 2013. Profits and pandemics: Prevention of harmful effects of tobacco, alcohol, and ultra-processed food and drink industries. *The Lancet 381*(9867):670–679.

NASA (National Auto Sport Association). 2017. *Home page*. https://www.nasaproracing.com (accessed November 27, 2017).

NASCAR (National Association for Stock Car Auto Racing). 2017. *Home page*. NASCAR Digital Media, LLC. https://www.nascar.com (accessed November 27, 2017).

Nelson, T. F., Z. Xuan, T. Babor, R. D. Brewer, F. J. Chaloupka, P. Gruenewald, H. Holder, M. Klitzner, J. Mosher, R. L. Ramirez, R. Reynolds, T. L. Toomey, V. Churchill, and T. S. Naimi. 2013. Efficacy and strength-of-evidence of U.S. alcohol control policies. *American Journal of Preventive Medicine* 45(1):19–28.

NHRA (National Hot Rod Association). 2017. *Home page*. https://www.nhra.com/nhra (accessed November 27, 2017).

NHTSA (National Highway Traffic Safety Administration). 2015. *Alcohol-Impaired Driving. 2014 Data*. https://crashstats.nhtsa.dot.gov/Api/Public/ViewPublication/812231 (accessed November 22, 2017).

Nielson, A. L., and B. Watson. 2009. The effectiveness of designated driver programs. *Journal of the Australasian College of Road Safety* 20(2):32–37.

NTSB (National Transportation Safety Board). 2013. *Safety report: Reaching zero: Actions to eliminate alcohol-impaired driving*. https://www.ntsb.gov/safety/safety-studies/Documents/SR1301.pdf (accessed November 20, 2017).

O'Brien, K., and K. Kypri. 2008. Alcohol industry sponsorship and hazardous drinking among sportspeople. *Addiction* 103(12):1961–1966.

O'Brien, K. S., J. Ferris, I. Greenlees, S. Jowett, D. Rhind, P. A. Cook, and K. Kypri. 2014. Alcohol industry sponsorship and hazardous drinking in UK university students who play sport. *Addiction* 109(10):1647–1654.

Omazic, T. 2014. *What women want*. https://www.qsrmagazine.com/consumer-trends/what-women-want (accessed November 20, 2017).

O'Reilly, L. 2014. *Brewers desperately want women to drink more beer—and they've learned that pink beer isn't the answer*. http://www.businessinsider.com/brewers-marketing-female-friendly-beer-2014-10. (accessed November 20, 2017).

Panjwani, C., and M. Caraher. 2014. The Public Health Responsibility Deal: Brokering a deal for public health, but on whose terms? *Health Policy* 114(2):163–173.

Pantani, D., R. Sparks, Z. Sanchez, and I. Pinsky. 2012. "Responsible drinking" programs and the alcohol industry in Brazil: Killing two birds with one stone? *Social Science* 75:1387–1391.

Pantani, D., R. Peltzer, M. Cremonte, K. Robaina, T. Babor, and I. Pinsky. 2017. The marketing potential of corporate social responsibility activities: The case of the alcohol industry in Latin America and the Caribbean. *Addiction* 112:74–80.

Powell, T., M. Hing, W. Vanlaar, and R. Robertson. 2016. *Alcohol-impaired driving in the United States. Results from the 2016 TIRF USA Road Safety Monitor*. http://us.tirf.ca/wp-content/uploads/2016/12/RSM-TIRF-USA-Alcohol-Impaired-Driving-in-the-United-States-10.pdf (accessed November 20, 2017).

Producers' Commitments. 2015. *About the commitments*. http://www.producerscommitments.org/about (accessed November 22, 2017).

Rally America. 2017. *Home page*. Rally America, Inc. http://www.rally-america.com (accessed November 27, 2017).

Rivara, F. P., A. Relyea-Chew, J. Wang, S. Riley, D. Boisvert, and T. Gomez. 2007. Drinking behaviors in young adults: The potential role of designated driver and safe ride home programs. *Injury Prevention* 13(3):168–172.

Robaina, K., and T. F. Babor. 2017. Alcohol industry marketing strategies in Latin America and the Caribbean: The way forward for policy research. *Addiction* 112(1):122–124.

SABMiller, plc. 2016. *SABMiller annual report, 2016*. http://www.ab-inbev.com/content/dam/universaltemplate/ab-inbev/investors/sabmiller/reports/annual-reports/annual-report-2016.pdf (accessed November 20, 2017).

Saffer, H. 1994. *Alcohol advertising and motor vehicle fatalities*. National Bureau of Economic Research Working Paper 4708. Cambridge, MA: National Bureau of Economic Research.

Saffer, H. 1997. Alcohol advertising and motor vehicle fatalities. *Review of Economics and Statistics* 89(3):431–442.

Savell, E., A. B. Gilmore, and G. Fooks. 2014. How does the tobacco industry attempt to influence marketing regulations? A systematic review. *PLoS ONE* 9(2):e87389.

Savell, E., G. Fooks, and A. B. Gilmore. 2016. How does the alcohol industry attempt to influence marketing regulations? A systematic review. *Addiction* 111:18–32.

SCCA (Sports Car Club of America). 2017. *Home page*. https://www.scca.com (accessed November 27, 2017).

Schuler, D. 1996. Corporate political strategy and foreign competition: The case of the steel industry. *Academy of Management Journal* 39(3):720–737.

Schuler, D., K. Rehbein, and R. Cramer. 2002. Pursuing strategic advantage through political means: A multivariate approach. *Academy of Management Journal* 45(4):659–672.

Schwartz, N., and T. McGarry. 2014. *The NFL is the most popular sport in America for the 30th year running. USA Today*. http://ftw.usatoday.com/2014/01/nfl-most-popular-sport-poll (accessed November 27, 2017).

Silverstein, M. J., K. Sayre, and J. Butman. 2009. *Women want more: How to capture your share of the world's largest, fastest-growing market*. New York: HarperBusiness.

Smith, L. A., and D. R. Foxcroft. 2009. The effect of alcohol advertising, marketing and portrayal on drinking behaviour in young people: Systematic review of prospective cohort studies. *BMC Public Health* 9:51.

Smith, S. W., C. K. Atkin, and J. Roznowski. 2006. Are "drink responsibly" alcohol campaigns strategically ambiguous? *Health Communication* 20(1):1–11.

Snider, M. 2017. *Anheuser-Busch buys drink maker Hiball Energy*. https://www.usatoday.com/story/money/business/2017/07/20/anheuser-busch-buys-drink-maker-hiball-energy/495803001 (accessed November 20, 2017).

Solomon, R., E. Chamberlain, and A. Murie. 2004. *The alcohol industry: Friend or foe in the fight against impaired driving: A MADD perspective*. http://www.icadtsinternational.com/files/documents/2004_118.pdf (accessed November 20, 2017).

Striley, C. W., and S. R. Khan. 2014. Review of the energy drink literature from 2013: Findings continue to support most risk from mixing with alcohol. *Current Opinion in Psychiatry* 27(4):263–268.

USCA (Ultimate Street Car Association). 2015. *Home page*. http://driveusca.com (accessed November 27, 2017).

Wagenaar, A., A. Tobler, and K. Komro. 2010. Effects of alcohol tax and price policies on morbidity and mortality: A systematic review. *American Journal of Public Health* 100(11):2270–2278.

Weber, S. 2017. *American Beverage Institute compares Utah's .05 DUI law to "Driving While Older."* http://kutv.com/news/local/american-beverage-institute-compares-utahs-05-dui-law-to-driving-while-older (accessed November 20, 2017).

WHO (World Health Organization). 2010. *Global strategy to reduce the harmful use of alcohol.* http://www.who.int/substance_abuse/msbalcstragegy.pdf (accessed November 20, 2017).

Wikimedia Commons. 2017. File: Ty Dillon in the Firekeepers 400.jpg. https://commons.wikimedia.org/w/index.php?title=File:Ty_Dillon_in_the_Firekeepers_400.jpg&oldid=266459113 (accessed December 19, 2017).

Williams, J. 2017. *I was a lobbyist for more than 6 years. I quit. My conscience couldn't take it anymore. "The hypocrisy from both sides is staggering."* https://www.vox.com/first-person/2017/6/29/15886936/political-lobbying-lobbyist-big-money-politics (accessed November 20, 2017).

Winpenny, E. M., T. M. Marteau, and E. Nolte. 2014. Exposure of children and adolescents to alcohol marketing on social media websites. *Alcohol and Alcoholism* 49(2):154–159.

Wolburg, J. 2005. How responsible are "responsible" drinking campaigns for preventing alcohol misuse. *Journal of Consumer Marketing* 22:176–177.

Xu, X., and F. Chaloupka. 2011. The effects of prices on alcohol use and its consequences. *Alcohol Research and Health* 34(2):236–245.

Yank, V., D. Rennie, and L. A. Bero. 2007. Financial ties and concordance between results and conclusions in meta-analyses: Retrospective cohort study. *BMJ* 335:1202–1205.

D

Reducing Alcohol-Impaired Driving: Lessons from a Global Review[1]

Adnan A. Hyder, M.D., Ph.D., M.P.H., Lead Consultant;
Andres Vecino, M.D., M.Ec., Ph.D., Co-Author for Part 1
(Thanks to Nukhba Zia, Ph.D., Research Assistant, for help with Part 2)

INTRODUCTION

Road injuries accounted for more than 67 million disability-adjusted life years in 2015, representing a 4.6 percent increase since 1990 (GBD, 2016). Each year, more than 1.3 million people are killed on roadways and another 50 million are injured. Recognizing this serious global public health problem, the World Health Organization (WHO) declared 2011–2020 as the Decade of Action on Road Safety (WHO, 2013).

Drink-driving[2] is a major cause of global road traffic fatalities. The United Nations General Assembly has expressed its concern that only 7 percent of the world's population is covered by adequate laws that address all road safety behavioral risk factors including driving under the influence of alcohol. According to WHO's 2015 Global Status Report on Road Safety, only 34 countries have drink-driving laws in line with best practices, and only 46 countries rated their enforcement of drink-driving laws as "good." Accordingly, it is critical to support stronger legislation

[1] This is an abridged version of the paper. A full version including all tables and figures can be found in the public access file for the Committee on Accelerating Progress to Reduce Alcohol-Impaired Driving Fatalities. Available by request from the National Academies of Sciences, Engineering, and Medicine's Public Access Records Office (PARO@nas.edu)

[2] *Drink-driving* is a colloquial term commonly used in countries outside of the United States to refer to driving or operating a motor vehicle while impaired or while one's blood alcohol concentration is above the permissible limit set by law. This term will be used in lieu of "alcohol-impaired driving" for the purpose of this background paper.

and stricter enforcement to curb drunk driving and mitigate its harmful effect on public health (WHO, 2015).

Approximately 17 percent of all global deaths that are caused by road traffic injuries have been attributed to alcohol consumption (Shield et al., 2012). A strong body of global evidence confirms that alcohol consumption is a risk factor for road traffic injuries and deaths (Aguilera et al., 2015; Bachani et al., 2013; Gururaj, 2004; Peden et al., 2004; WHO, 2013). For that reason, WHO included the prevention of drink-driving as one of the five leading areas to focus on to reduce road injuries and deaths during the Decade of Action on Road Safety (WHO, 2013).

GOALS AND OBJECTIVES

At the direction of the Committee on Accelerating Progress to Reduce Alcohol-Impaired Driving Fatalities (the committee), this commissioned paper was requested to offer insights into the international landscape of drink-driving interventions. The commissioned paper was asked to conduct a purposive review of international drink-driving interventions with a focus on driving policies and countermeasures that target individuals and system changes, and identify how they have been carried out abroad (part 1). The paper was asked to make conclusions on which interventions have worked and why, and in general discuss the potential applicability of those interventions in the United States. In addition, it was requested to focus on countries that are economically and culturally analogous to the United States (part 1). The commission was also asked to conduct a smaller (part 2) scoping review to provide recommendations regarding data collection and application to support the reduction of drink-driving. The paper was also asked to focus the data review and discussion points to highlight new or unique data and tools that the United States could learn from and international data variables that have not been done in the United States, that should be considered, and innovative ways of linking data (part 2). Therefore, this paper responds to the charge from the committee and includes both lessons on interventions (see part 1) and data systems (see part 2).

APPROACH

As requested, this paper provides a purposive review of available knowledge and experiences from global road safety in the prevention and control of alcohol-related harm that may be important for the United States. This last element was critical to the screening of all materials and experiences, and guided the work culminating in this paper. It is to be noted that a general review of alcohol-related interventions and programs would be more extensive and wide ranging and would include relevance to low- and middle-income countries, which was not the focus of this paper.

Overall, this paper is based on the experience of the authors, interviews with a selected number of global experts, a review of the peer-reviewed literature (since 2000), and a careful screening of key international publications from organizations such as WHO. This paper has been informed by previous discussions in meetings (such as the partner meetings of the United Nations Road Safety Collaboration) and workshops (such as those in the Bloomberg Initiative for Global Road Safety).

The review is presented below in two parts. Part 1 proposes selected intervention domains against drink-driving that may have important lessons for the United States. This is a selection of those interventions considered effective, implemented by other countries (or states), and worthy of consideration in the United States. A deeper discussion of those interventions is described using a systematic approach so the background, details, outcomes, and challenges associated (as reported) are captured for consideration by the committee. References are provided in the event the committee wants more nuanced details.

Part 2 is a review of data around drink-driving and is based on analysis of the best systems currently existing in other high-income countries. Specifically, the section analyzed recommendations from global agencies and a select group of Organisation for Economic Co-operation and Development (OECD) countries, and compares with the Fatality Analysis Reporting System (FARS) data in the United States. Recommendations around both variables and indicators are provided.

The paper ends with a brief conclusion and encourages active discussion on the issues raised here by the National Academies of Sciences, Engineering, and Medicine (the National Academies) committee.

PART 1—INTERVENTIONS AND PROGRAMS

This section proposes a set of domains for interventions against drink-driving for consideration by the National Academies committee. Each proposal is followed by a summary of the evidence, a detailed case study with references, description of some key challenges, and a brief conclusion. Tables 1–4 support the section,[3] and the references provide other materials for the committee to obtain more information.

[3] Available by request from the National Academies of Sciences, Engineering, and Medicine's Public Access Records Office (PARO@nas.edu).

Proposal 1: Enforcement Interventions

The Evidence on Its Effectiveness

During the review of global experiences, enforcement interventions were found among the most effective strategies to reduce mortality, morbidity, and crashes on the road. The evidence found reveals that enforcement interventions, specifically general deterrence strategies, and the performance of random breath-testing stops, have demonstrated improvements in drink-driving outcomes in high-income countries. The characteristics of some key analysis around these interventions can be found in Table 1.[4]

In the case of *deterrence strategies*, we found that the evidence on effectiveness is heterogeneous; such heterogeneity is likely to be due to differences in the intensity of enforcement and media coverage accompanying such campaigns. Important examples of such varying effectiveness have been observed in Serbia (specifically on enforcement for pedestrians to prevent mortality) (Zivkovic et al., 2016) and Canada (increased enforcement on drivers reducing alcohol-related crashes and casualties) (Mercer, 1985; Vingilis and Salutin, 1980).

The specific case of France is relevant because despite the penalties being increased by 52 percent, drink-driving behavior increased threefold. It has been argued that the legislation change was not properly enforced, leading to increasing drink-driving and highlighting the importance of enforcement accompanying legislation change (Constant et al., 2009).

Random breath-testing (RBT) stops are very effective in reducing serious crashes, with an effectiveness on mortality of up to 35 percent. The key for sustainability of RBT interventions seems to reside in the characteristics of *randomness* of the stops, the high level of enforcement, and the deployment of mass media campaigns during the RBT intervention (with the purpose of increasing the perception of enforcement and creating the risk of apprehension) (Henstridge et al., 1997; Mercer, 1985; Vingilis and Salutin, 1980).

One example of the relevance of the latter has been revealed in the specific case of Canada, where two campaigns (called blitz) with equal enforcement characteristics were deployed and compared based on the level of media coverage that accompanied the blitz. The study found that the blitz with no mass media coverage campaign failed in reducing drink-driving behaviors when compared to the baseline (Mercer, 1985). Similar findings were found in Australia where RBT interventions (deployed

[4] Ibid.

in Tasmania) were found to be less effective, likely owing to the lack of an accompanying mass media campaign (Henstridge et al., 1997), and in the United Kingdom in the 1970s in a study that showed that media combined with random breath testing reduced crashes but the impact faded without renewed media activity (Ross et al., 1970). These findings emphasize the key role of mass media campaigns to effectively deter drink-driving behavior.

Case Study 1: Learning from Random Breath-Testing Activities in Australia

Background Victoria was the first Australian state where RBT campaigns were introduced in 1976 amid public controversy (Henstridge et al., 1997; WHO, 2007). Since then, RBT interventions have been implemented in other states after learning about the successes in Victoria. Most RBT campaigns have usually been implemented in combination with mass media coverage to both increase the perception of enforcement and facilitate the creation of social norms rejecting drink-driving behavior.

One example in Australia highlighting the relevance of concurrent mass media campaigns has been described in Tasmania, where despite some limitations, the general understanding is that the interventions were not as successful as in other states because of the lack of media campaigns associated with the enforcement activities (Henstridge et al., 1997).

Intervention and its characteristics RBT interventions in Australia, and specifically in Victoria, are not implemented as an isolated primary enforcement intervention. Importantly, RBT campaigns are a more general policing approach known in Australia as "problem-oriented policing." This approach requires police to redirect the focus of enforcement interventions toward prevention. More broadly, this approach allows the police to emphasize solving the problems of safety issues instead of relying on its traditional role of detection and arrest.

Problem-oriented policing is a strategy that requires close collaboration between police departments and state authorities to plan a strategic approach, coordinate safety interventions, and importantly share data on trends on crashes and risk factors. The use of data is extremely important in this approach because it provides police with a surveillance tool to target locations and driver profiles that are found to be at higher risk of drinking and driving.

As part of this policing approach, RBT campaigns make up a key element, and the effectiveness of RBT interventions relies on three main features. First, RBT campaigns are by nature a *primary enforcement* strategy. Therefore, drivers are pulled over to be tested for drink-driving with no need for another offense to have been committed. This is different from "selective stops," when the stop and tests are carried out when another offense has been committed. Random stops are around 50 percent more effective than selective stops in reducing mortality, which reflects the importance of the primary enforcement component in policing drink-driving (Elder et al., 2002; Shults et al., 2001).

The second aspect that has been key to the success of RBT is its *actual randomness*. This implies that all drivers truly face the same probability of being pulled over and tested. To create a truly random RBT system, the Victoria State Police relies on a computer-generated random assignment of patrols to perform the RBT stops in specific locations and times. The uncertainty around times and locations of the RBT stops effectively increases the perception of risk of detection, improving the effectiveness of the preventive enforcement approach (Henstridge et al., 1997).

The third key aspect for the success of RBT campaigns is their *intensity*. Experts indicate that the Victoria State Police sets the aim of testing each driver twice per year. However, measures on the optimal intensity of enforcement are not available and need to be the focus of future research (Henstridge et al., 1997).

In Australia, the guidelines around RBT vary across states. For example, in some states alcohol tests are conducted on all drivers stopped, whereas in others this is not necessarily the case. Also, in some states, vehicles are pulled over only for the test to be conducted without a license check (the stop might take less than 30 seconds).

Importantly, a meta-analysis found that the country with the largest crash reduction was Australia, precisely for the use of the blitz type of checkpoints including buses and large media coverage (Erke et al., 2009). One study found that the most effective types of checkpoints are those covering both minor and major roads simultaneously; those that cover at least 20 hours per 100 square kilometers per week; and the level of enforcement is cost-effective when it aims at 1.5 breath tests per year per licensed driver (benefit-cost ratio equal to 2.05) (Cameron, 2013).

Challenges The main challenges faced by Australia around the implementation of RBT are related to resources (Henstridge et al., 1997). The high targets in terms of intensity and randomness requires investment of scarce police resources and the involvement of general duty officers to perform drink-driving checks. The involvement of these police officers increases the coverage of the enforcement activities but at the same time leads to the implementation of low-profile "mobile testing" stations manned by these general duty officers. These mobile stations have low visibility and lack the traditional visible blitz equipment (cones, lights, heavy presence of police and a bus where the tests are taken commonly called the "booze bus") and other highly visible signs. The low visibility of the intervention, however, is thought to lead to an overall less effective intervention (Henstridge et al., 1997).

Another challenge is that despite the sharing of data by state authorities with the police, police officers did not necessarily keep records on the key features of enforcement activities. These features have been cited as potential factors determining the variability of the effectiveness of RBT across Australian states. However, since such data were not systematically collected, there is some uncertainty as to which aspects of enforcement make it more or less effective. Finally, public opinion was initially unfavorable toward the implementation of RBT stops, but currently it is a widely accepted strategy.

Conclusion

Overall, RBT campaigns demonstrated an "immediate, substantial, and fairly permanent impact" on drink-driving outcomes including mortality and crashes (Henstridge et al., 1997). Therefore, it is worth serious consideration for the United States. However, it needs to be emphasized that there is an understanding in Australia that the successful implementation of the RBT campaigns is not isolated from other institutional changes that led the Australian police to establish closer collaborations with the state authorities and to change its focus to a preventive emphasis rather than a punitive one (Sweedler and Stewart, 2009).

Proposal 2: Reduction in Blood Alcohol Concentration (BAC) Levels

The Evidence on Effectiveness

A policy option that was detected during our review and was consistently mentioned in expert interviews as a potential strategy to reduce drink-driving in the United States was a reduction of the current legal blood alcohol concentration (BAC) level. All of the experts spoken with for this paper believe that the 0.08% BAC per se laws currently in place in most states in the United States are too high. Such views are confirmed in clinical and experimental research that demonstrates that a level of BAC of 0.05% (Kennedy et al., 1993; Tagawa et al., 2000) or even lower (Breitmeier et al., 2007) is enough to impair a driver. In fact, the literature shows clear evidence on the effectiveness of reducing BAC to 0.05% and the characteristics of such evidence is summarized in Table 2.[5]

[5] Available by request from the National Academies of Sciences, Engineering, and Medicine's Public Access Records Office (PARO@nas.edu).

During our review, we found consistent evidence on the effectiveness of reducing BAC levels on drink-driving outcomes. An important example is Australia, in which the reduction of BAC levels from 0.08% to 0.05% led to a reduction of fatal and nonfatal serious injuries of 8 and 7 percent, respectively, in New South Wales, and 18 and 14 percent, respectively, in Queensland (Henstridge et al., 1997). Another example of successful reduction of BAC is Austria, which reduced the BAC levels from 0.08% to 0.05% in 1998, and this was associated with an initial decrease in injuries of about 10 percent (Bartl and Esberger, 2000).

In the Netherlands, the alcohol limit of 0.05% was imposed in 1974, leading to a 10 percent reduction in the prevalence of drivers with positive alcohol levels both over and below the limit (Noordzij, 1994). Such reduction was followed by a 10-year period of stability in the prevalence figures, followed by a further drop over time. Even though the long-term reduction in the prevalence of drink-driving cannot be attributable to the establishment of the 0.05% legal limit alone, it is understood that the downward trend started with this intervention.

In Norway, the reduction of BAC limit from 0.08% to 0.05% did not show statistically significant reductions in nighttime and weekend single-vehicle crashes and deaths (Assum, 2010). It is possible that the lack of effect in this study was caused by measurement issues or the lack of a control group. Reductions lower than 0.05% have also shown positive results (Table 2)[6] such as in Japan (Desapriya et al., 2007) and Brazil (Andreuccetti et al., 2011). Japan showed a marked decrease in alcohol-related crashes after the reduction of BAC limit from 0.05% to 0.03%; Brazil also had marked reductions in mortality after the BAC limit set by law changed from 0.06% to 0.02%. Studies on changes in BAC limit have limitations as some of them were carried out several decades ago when road safety studies did not often report statistical test results; however, the changes observed in these earlier studies present point estimates of relevant magnitude in large populations.

Case Study 2: Lessons from Europe and National Legislation on BAC

Background In Europe, the BAC limits are defined by national legislation in each country. In 1984, the European Parliament recommended to the European Commission (one of the institutions belonging to the legislative arm of the then European Communities) that it should submit a proposal to establish a single 0.08% limit for all European countries. This was based on the high cross-border traffic in Europe and the fact that one-third of road traffic deaths had drink-driving as a contributory factor (European

[6] Ibid.

Commission, 1989a). In 1988 the European Commission proposed a directive to reduce the BAC limits for all countries, but established a different lower limit of 0.05%, considering preliminary evidence of its effectiveness (European Commission, 1989a). This was very progressive and made Europe lead the change in this space for the world.

Legislative change and its characteristics The legislative change in 1988 was aimed at reducing drink-driving. At the time, the Section for Transport and Communications of the European Commission challenged the proposal, arguing that the new 0.05% limit "would seem unjustified in the absence of conclusive evidence that it will enhance road safety." Furthermore, the committee requested the commission to do the following:

> compile detailed statistics on the link between high blood alcohol concentrations and the number of accidents. The link between blood alcohol levels and the number of fatal accidents should also be carefully assessed, as should the effects of medicines and drugs on road safety. If necessary, the maximum permissible limit should be amended after an appropriate transitional period has elapsed. Research findings should be widely publicized, as should the maximum permissible limit, so that drivers can sensibly decide when and how to consume alcohol so as not to exceed the legal limit. (European Commission, 1989b)

The main issues around the proposal (according to the committee) were the lack of conclusive evidence supporting the proposal, and the potential effect on public opinion, as they requested a transitional period and that research findings should be publicized to generate support (European Commission, 1989b).

Despite this the European Commission's proposal did not pass the committee. However, 8 out of the 15 member countries in 2003 adopted national legislation to reduce BAC levels between 1988 (when the reduction in BAC levels was first proposed) and 2003 (Albalate, 2008). Even though the adoption of reduced levels in these European countries cannot be solely attributed to the failed proposal, it is understood that this was the first step in a series of institutional changes that led to the reduction of national BAC limits.

In 1997 the European Commission released a 4-year program for "Promoting Road Safety in the European Union: The Programme for 1997–2001." The European Commission brought back the 1988 proposal and this time included evidence obtained by the same commission in which they estimated reductions in 5 to 40 percent in mortality if a comprehensive intervention (legislation + enforcement + telematics + education) reduced drivers with alcohol levels above 0.05% (European Commission, 1997). This second attempt is thought to have led to changes in legislation for BAC in five countries in 2 years, including Germany, which had opposed the reduction of BAC limits through common European legislation 10 years before (Albalate, 2008).

In 2001, the European Commission brought back the proposal to change BAC limits in all member countries to 0.05% and added a further reduction of BAC for inexperienced and commercial drivers as well as motorcyclists to 0.02% (European Commission, 2001). For example, Italy reduced the BAC levels to 0.05% in that year as a consequence of the recommendation.

The evidence assessing these changes has shown that the continuous efforts of the European Commission throughout these years, as well as the peer effects generated across country members of the European Union (EU), led to the reduction of BAC levels in Europe (Albalate, 2008). The assessment of the reduction of the BAC levels in Europe was associated with a reduction in mortality of 5.7 percent among males and 11.5 percent among younger road users, especially in urban areas (Albalate, 2008). This trend has continued since the end of the program in 2001.

In 2006 Cyprus joined the 0.05% limit, while Luxemburg reduced its limit to 0.05% in 2007. All but two member states have changed their BAC limits to at least 0.05%, four countries have a zero BAC limit, and half of EU states have implemented 0.02% limits for inexperienced/commercial drivers (Anderson et al., 2012; EU Directorate General for Health and Consumers, 2009).

In addition, it has been shown that awareness about drink-driving among citizens of countries with BAC levels of 0.05% is higher than in the countries in which the limit remains 0.08% (Babor, 2010; EU Directorate General for Health and Consumers, 2009). This adds a social and public perception value for this approach.

Challenges Three main challenges have been reported in the reduction of BAC levels in European countries. The first challenge was the passage of the European law itself, which was not passed as European legislation. The issue appeared to have been that the original proposal was not presented with enough evidence at the time and the fact that the law included neither a transitional period, nor a comprehensive approach including mass media interventions (European Commission, 1989a). Also, other sources have reported heavy lobbying efforts from the alcohol industry to prevent reducing BAC limits, particularly in countries where the BAC limit remains to be 0.08%, specifically Ireland (Hope, 2006) and the United Kingdom (Hawkins et al., 2012). (This is a point we discuss later in the paper.)

The second issue has been the low levels of national enforcement accompanying these legislative changes. Enforcement levels in Europe are relatively low implying that even though road traffic injuries have been reduced all over Europe as a consequence of the changes in BAC limits, there is a potential to further decrease such deaths if more intensive enforcement, including random breath-testing strategies, would be implemented (Anderson, 2008).

Finally, this experience (like other reviews on BAC laws) found the importance of mass media campaigns accompanying the interventions as critical to maximize effectiveness. BAC laws require media campaigns accompanying the legislation change (Killoran et al., 2010).

Conclusion

Overall, BAC legislation is critical for a national or state-level effort and has been demonstrated to have a substantial effect on drink-driving outcomes. Therefore, such laws and their revisions are worth serious consideration for states in the United States.

Proposal 3: Social Interventions on Alcohol

The Evidence on Effectiveness

Social interventions on alcohol have been shown to have heterogeneous effects on drink-driving outcomes. In Table 3,[7] we present evidence of different interventions and their effects. These social interventions have varied designs, are applied in diverse settings, and are not always easy to evaluate in a comprehensive way. However, it is relevant to take them into account because the evidence shows that they are necessary complements of other interventions (as stated in this paper), such as reduction of BAC levels or the deployment of random breath-testing checkpoints.

The results of our review reveal that mass media campaigns have a small but significant effect in reducing alcohol-related crashes of around 13 percent (Elder et al., 2004). School-based programs have shown reductions in the prevalence of drunk drivers and riding with drunk drivers (and associated behaviors), which reflect the effect of knowledge and a "social norm effect," especially on younger people (Elder et al., 2005).

Designated driver programs have shown a much smaller effect, and the evidence available is not very strong (Ditter et al., 2005). In fact, our interviews revealed that these interventions were not favored by our experts. The reasons stated were that these programs tend to be pushed by the alcohol industry as feasible interventions, but the evidence supporting

[7] Available by request from the National Academies of Sciences, Engineering, and Medicine's Public Access Records Office (PARO@nas.edu).

them is weak and that the effects are small. Furthermore, from a policy standpoint it is not sensible to rely solely on individual-level choices (with no need for accountability) rather than interventions that implement a structural or institutional restriction to drink-driving behavior.

During expert interviews, social interventions often considered "ideal" were those outside the specific scope of drink-driving and those that target alcohol consumption more broadly. Even though no direct evaluations are available for the effect of the STAD (Stockholm Prevents Alcohol and Drug Problems) program on road safety, and the focus has been on process outcomes (refusal rates to pseudo-intoxicated patrons) and on alcohol-related violence outcomes, our experts consider that to tackle drink-driving in the United States, alcohol policy needs to be considered more broadly than only targeting individuals drinking while driving. For example, comprehensive interventions need to be made at the point of distribution since in the United States, about half of individuals who get alcohol and then drink and drive get it from licensed stores (Gruenewald et al., 1996). Therefore, the STAD intervention, such as in Stockholm, is worth considering for state and county authorities in the United States.

Case Study 3: A Program for Bartenders in Sweden

Background In the last decade of the 20th century, Stockholm created the STAD program as a comprehensive approach to reduce the consequences of alcohol consumption, primarily to reduce alcohol-related violence (Norström and Trolldal, 2013).

Intervention and its characteristics The STAD program was implemented in northern Stockholm in 1996 with the aim of reducing episodic heavy (binge) drinking. The STAD intervention was implemented through three different strategies: community mobilization, training for bartenders in responsible beverage service, and strict enforcement (Norström and Trolldal, 2013). The training strategy for bartenders became compulsory for all licensed premises that stayed open until 1 a.m. or later, and was aimed at (1) preventing sales of alcohol to minors; (2) preventing sales of alcohol to intoxicated customers; (3) improving the ability of staff to recognize high-risk situations and intervene appropriately; and (4) helping staff from licensed establishments to develop their own alcohol service guidelines (Wallin et al., 2005). The 2-day training program, which issues a certification, focuses on six main subjects:

1. The effects of alcohol,
2. Alcohol legislation,

3. The extent of alcohol-related violence and how this can be prevented,
4. Service refusal issues and skills,
5. Drug issues, and
6. Conflict management skills (Wallin et al., 2005).

The enforcement component of the program includes fines for the establishment, and fines and even prison for the server if he or she provides alcohol to an intoxicated individual (Wallin et al., 2005).

Five years after starting the intervention, the program had trained 1,318 restaurant employees (Wallin et al., 2005) and initial monitoring using pseudo-intoxicated patrons revealed that the serving refusal rate increased from 5 to 70 percent. These results have been disputed since control areas also increased refusal rates in similar magnitude, but this is thought to be attributable to contamination effects of the intervention, which was widely publicized in the media (Rehnman et al., 2005). Further evaluations of this intervention concluded that the intervention reduced violent crimes between 21 and 32 percent (Norström and Trolldal, 2013; Wallin et al., 2003), which proved the effectiveness of the intervention in reducing problematic alcohol consumption. Therefore, it is not difficult to infer that an effect on drink-driving is likely; furthermore, a study considering only the direct costs of the intervention found it to be cost-effective in terms of cost per quality-adjusted life years gained (Mansdotter et al., 2007). The success of the STAD interventions has led the European Commission to expand the program and tailor it to seven European countries (Ames et al., 2016).

Challenges One obvious challenge is the ability to measure the effect of this, and other social interventions, as the target population and measurement strategies are difficult to define. Also, context matters in this type of intervention, and a successful strategy in one setting will not always be replicable in another.

It is important to note that there are no reports of any types of "resistance" to this intervention, and actually other areas (the "control" areas) freely adopted the intervention, making it difficult to measure its effect. This in turn provides a strength to this approach.

Conclusion

Even though the evidence for this intervention is programmatic, such types of interventions combine legal aspects, with strict enforcement, and training in high-risk establishments. Therefore, we suggest that this be considered for potential implementation in the United States.

Proposal 4: Alcohol Ignition Interlock Devices

The Evidence on Effectiveness

Expert interviews highlighted the role of alcohol ignition interlock programs in Australia as exemplary for their role in reducing recidivism and contributing to rehabilitation of drink-driving offenders. For that reason, this type of intervention is considered here and the evidence summarized in Table 4.[8]

Studies in the United States demonstrated a reduction of 15 percent in mortality of alcohol-involved road traffic fatalities among states that implemented ignition devices (Kaufman and Wiebe, 2016); this is attributable to its effect on recidivism among repeat offenders. A Cochrane review on the effectiveness of interlock devices showed a consistent average reduction in recidivism of 64 percent (Willis et al., 2004). One caveat is that this reduction was only during the time in which the devices were installed, so sustainability of the measure needs to be further assessed. A study in Canada also showed a (lower) reduction in recidivism of around 6 percent (Voas et al., 1999); this was attributed to the selection effect of the devices since they are not consistently applied to all offenders.

Case Study 4: Alcohol Ignition Interlock Devices in Australia

Background Several states in Australia demonstrated interest in implementing alcohol ignition interlock devices for convicted drink drivers. With this aim, road authorities from all jurisdictions were consulted to create national standards in 1995. The purpose of these standards was to make sure the devices and the implementation were technically, economically, administratively, and logistically harmonized across Australian states. Such guidelines implied the following:

- The devices would be legally recognized and enforced across all states;
- At the discretion of courts they must be restricted to participants in interlock programs who must be repeat offenders or high BAC offenders and they can appeal;
- The devices should be installed for at least 3 years with a minimum service period of 1–3 months;
- Some minimum period of license cancellation and conditional license categories need to be set with its use;

[8] Available by request from the National Academies of Sciences, Engineering, and Medicine's Public Access Records Office (PARO@nas.edu).

- Costs must be contained for both the state and the user; and
- The program needs to be evaluated (Christie et al., 1995).

As a result, some states in Australia had to delay implementation to address the conditions stated above. For example, alcohol ignition interlocks were actually not introduced until 2001, first in Queensland, with the specific aim of reducing repeated drink-driving behavior. This case study summarizes lessons to help inform implementation of this strategy in the United States in order to reduce repeated drink-driving behaviors (Schonfeld and Sheehan, 2004).

Intervention and its characteristics The implementation of alcohol ignition interlocks by the justice system in Australian states was significantly delayed since the establishment of the national guidelines in 1995 until its final implementation in Queensland in 2001. Multiple reasons have been suggested for this delay, and these comprise lessons for other countries attempting similar interventions. First, some doubts about the effectiveness and compliance of the devices were raised and more evidence on this was required before moving on with the actual implementation of the devices. Second, the costs of the devices for the offenders were too high, which was against specified national standards. Third, there was a marked unwillingness to modify the license suspension provisions and to complement such suspension sentences with the use of the devices as part of the penalty. Together, these had to be addressed before the program was implemented at scale in the country.

Postimplementation analysis has revealed that certain characteristics differentiate a set of different models of interlock programs, all of them with pros and cons (Bailey et al., 2013; Fitzharris et al., 2015; Klipp, 2013; Schonfeld and Sheehan, 2004). For example:

- Some states established compulsory interlock device programs; this increases the coverage of the program but tends to more heavily affect lower-income individuals.
- There are differences across states on the use of the device data to measure compliance, and to use those data to identify individuals with alcohol dependence who may need specific (or further) treatment for their condition.
- There has been variable use of interlock device data for monitoring improvement and increasing awareness about drink-driving behavior.
- Given the issue that losing a license can generate among convicted drivers, including problems in their recovery programs and the risk of driving unlicensed, there is a general tendency

to understand the period of "suspended license" as a protective rather than a punitive measure. Therefore, the program in most states encourages the early adoption of interlock devices to allow the offender to drive as soon as he or she has finished the rehabilitation program. This makes the interlock device a protective and punitive measure that is taken against the driver for even longer than the length of an alternative suspended license period, but allows them to recover and get back to normal life as soon as possible.

- Interlock device programs are pragmatically used for both offenders who were, and were not, licensed at the time of the offense, recognizing the high risk for the latter to attempt to drive unlicensed again as a protective measure.

Evidence on the economics of alcohol ignition interlocks found that the cost-benefit ratio of these devices ranges between 1 and 3.4 depending on the assumptions of the model—this is for all devices with effectiveness in terms of "noncircumvention rates" (the rate at which the device can be tampered) higher than 50 percent (Lahausse and Fildes, 2009).

Challenges The main issues reported are costs associated with the ignition device. Nearly 70 percent of offenders were deemed unable to use the device during the first year of the program in Queensland because of high costs (Terer and Brown, 2014). This was despite the argument that since the larger society will benefit from ignition locks, it ought to be the society that should pay for it.

Another significant issue was the difficulty for states to adopt the proposed standard legislation (Schonfeld and Sheehan, 2004). This was deemed key when the national standards were established in Australia since drivers should not face different legal frameworks while driving across the country. This was also deemed to be important for consistency in the legislation regarding administrative or judicial sentences and because administrative sentences cannot provide discretionary powers for specific conditions that might make the adoption of the program exceptionally difficult. A final issue is the sustainability of the effect of the device, which appears to disappear when the device is uninstalled. It is for this reason that rehabilitation programs must be combined with ignition interlock programs (Terer and Brown, 2014).

Conclusion

Alcohol interlock devices are effective and offer a safe way to recovery for repeat offenders, allowing them to return to their usual lives sooner.

Particularly important are the high costs of the devices, which are usually faced by the offender. It is important to take this into consideration in terms of the overall social benefits of having those offenders driving with interlock devices in the United States.

Proposal 5: Alcohol Is the New Tobacco

Introduction

One of the reasons for the lack of effective drink-driving policies in many countries is the alcohol industry's opposition to meaningful regulations, including effective drunk-driving policies, alcohol taxation, and restrictions on the sale of alcohol. Instead, the alcohol industry has been promoting weak interventions to control drink-driving; a 2016 study showed that less than 1 percent of the industry's actions to reduce drink-driving aligned with evidence-based recommendations (Esser et al., 2016). Under the umbrella of corporate social responsibility, the industry has not only continued to market its products but has also increased its involvement in policy making and scientific research (Babor and Robaina, 2013) while continuing their lobbying efforts to prevent legislation that saves lives (Hawkins et al., 2012; Hope, 2006).

The globalization of the alcohol industry and growth of multinational beverage alcohol corporations is a potential barrier to the implementation and enforcement of effective drink-driving policies (Caetano and Laranjeira, 2006; Casswell, 2011a,b; Jernigan, 2009; WHO, 2014). Furthermore, alcohol industry-sponsored alcohol programs are rarely evaluated around the world (Mosher, 2012), and when they are evaluated, have shown little or no effect (Ditter et al., 2005).

These concerns have been raised and are becoming more acute globally. For example, the International Network on Brief Interventions for Alcohol & Other Drugs (INEBRIA) released a strong position statement dissuading their members from engaging with the alcohol industry altogether and highlighting that any form of industry involvement in evidence-based interventions should be of concern (INEBRIA, 2015).

Case Study 5: Understanding the Alcohol Industry

This case study will demonstrate examples to show the ease with which the alcohol industry is able to gain access to high levels of the United Nations (UN) and national policy processes, and obtain valuable brand association. Alcohol companies and their funded organizations such as the International Center for Alcohol Policies (ICAP) and the International Alliance for Responsible Drinking have a history of promoting ineffective drink-driving strategies such as education and awareness, and undermining effective approaches such as lower BAC limits. It is important for the United States to recognize, understand, and then develop a strategy to address this potential challenge. The examples listed below provide a glimpse into the types of issues raised by the previous and current working activities of the alcohol industry.

Example: Coalition formation In 2015, the alcohol industry sponsored road safety events involving the International Telecommunications Union (ITC), the United Nations Economic Commission for Europe (UNECE), and the UN Headquarters. The ITC and UNECE symposium on the Future Networked Car was held in Geneva on March 5–6, 2014, and gave prominent and equal branding to the world's largest beverage company AB InBev alongside UN logos. On November 13, 2014, the UN played a major role in the launch of a private-sector road safety initiative led by AB InBev called Together for Safer Roads. The event was held in the UN, broadcast on UN Web TV, and involved the participation of Mrs. Amina Mohammed, Special Advisor on Post 2015 Development Planning. On March 23, 2015, the UNECE, UNECA, and the newly formed alcohol industry-sponsored International Alliance for Responsible Drinking launched an e-book titled *Preventing Drink-Driving in Africa*[9] on the UN premises in Geneva, Switzerland.

Given that the ITC and the UNECE have a direct involvement in setting both global and European regulatory standards and, therefore, there is room for conflicts of interest, it is disturbing to see an alcohol company with obvious commercial interests obtaining such privileged access possibly in exchange for an undisclosed sponsorship fee. Because WHO has led responsibility for road safety within the UN system, it is important to note that it was reportedly not asked for their advice before approval was given for the events stated above and were not officially present at the event.

Example: Platforms for marketing In mid-2016, the beverage giant Heineken struck an agreement with Formula One (F1), which allowed the company to become one of the main sponsors of F1 races, rendering Heineken a global platform for aggressive alcohol marketing. Already, F1 was predominantly sponsored by the alcohol industry; a 2015 report showed that audiences of F1 are exposed to alcohol brands every 5 seconds. In fact, the UN Special Ambassador for Road Safety was involved

[9] See http://www.unece.org/trans/roadsafe/ece-eca-icap_ebook.html (accessed January 2, 2018).

in the ceremonies related to this event. This is alarming as it sends mixed messages about alcohol and driving.

Example: Obscuring independent research The alcohol industry's ICAP, for example, funded six countries (China, Colombia, Mexico, Nigeria, Russia, and Vietnam) to conduct reviews of available data on drink-driving outcomes and policies (Stewart et al., 2012). Between 2000 and 2006, the Worldwide Brewing Alliance showed that 23 grants were given to university-based alcohol researchers in 13 countries. Such partnerships may interfere with the public health agenda, as the alcohol industry's involvement in drink-driving initiatives may serve to promote corporate interests (Jernigan, 2009). Concerns about scientific publications funded by the alcohol industry have been expressed, including their potential to jeopardize the integrity of science and reliable health information, their potential to obscure the evidence on the effectiveness of alcohol policies, and at times their promotion of findings that favor the alcohol industry and undercut those of public health (Babor, 2009; Caetano, 2008).

The public and policy makers may not be aware of the alcohol industry's involvement in this line of research, especially without statements of funding sources, leaving them vulnerable to uncritically accept studies as research from public health professionals (Babor, 2009). Many drink-driving studies published in scientific journals (Johnson, 2012; Li et al., 2012; Ngoc et al., 2012; Stewart et al., 2012) fail to include a statement disclosing that they are funded by the alcohol industry or even an acknowledgment to support from the alcohol industry.

Stenius and Babor (2010) have argued for the need to sever financial ties with the alcohol industry in order to uphold the integrity of scientific research and prevent potential conflicts of interest. As stated by the Director-General of WHO, "In the view of WHO, the alcohol industry has no role in the formulation of alcohol policies, which must be protected from distortion by commercial or vested interests" (Chan, 2013). Countries may face pressure, as the alcohol industry typically emphasizes the importance of partnerships between themselves and public health professionals (Babor, 2009; Caetano, 2008; Jernigan, 2012). Furthermore, several studies have found that the alcohol industry goals (including ICAP initiatives) are at odds with those of public health (Babor, 2009; Hawkins and McCambridge, 2014; Jernigan, 2012; McCambridge et al., 2013, 2014; Miller et al., 2011).

Conclusion

Given this context and the ongoing debate about alcohol industry funding, this paper makes the case to the alcohol and road safety communities in the United States, as well as policy researchers, to take these issues seriously. It is important to generate the data needed to take action against stakeholder marketing and other alcohol industry-sponsored activities that undermine effective, evidence-based, alcohol control policies and encroach on the integrity of scientific research. It is critical for the health and scientific community to hold the alcohol industry to high standards for the promotion and protection of public health, especially that of vulnerable and younger communities. It is also imperative that public health scientists work to prevent any efforts that seek to undermine evidence-based best practices and that policy makers keep a critical view of industry-sponsored studies, as has been the case with studies sponsored by pharmaceutical and nutritional companies in recent years.

Recommendations for Programs

The proposals above, including the case studies, provide both evidence and stories of how intervention programs have been implemented in other high-income countries. They provide guidance on what lessons global experiences provide to inform the recommendations of the National Academies committee, which are being formulated separately. This paper suggests serious consideration of the following:

- Enhance enforcement, including random breath testing and creation of an environment where effective and data-based policing becomes the norm.
- Enhance national (and state) legislation around BAC to become consistent with other high-income countries for all drivers (≤0.05%) and focusing on high-risk groups (~0.02%).
- Implement specific, evidence-based social interventions that target high-risk situations and include not only awareness creation but legal and individual consequences.
- Promote alcohol ignition interlocks for repeat offenders together with rehabilitation programs.
- Control the unrestricted marketing and engagement of the alcohol industry through a unified multifaceted approach across sectors, and maybe this can begin by interdepartmental dialogues at the national level.

These remain strategic recommendations for the National Academies committee to compare with its own analysis of the U.S. situation and consider where global lessons enhance its own advice. These are not meant to stand alone in the absence of focused U.S.-based analysis of the current climate of alcohol-based interventions and their effect. Of course, if picked up by the committee and the National Highway Traffic Safety Administration (NHTSA), then more detailed work will need to be done in each area, to understand the specifics of how such a change or introduction of new programs can be done within the U.S. (or state) context.

Finally, it is important to caution against the use of facile comparisons between countries—each context is specific and the relevant complexities need to be understood. To the extent that despite these realities lessons can be transferred, cross-national learning can be a useful strategy for global road safety.

PART 2—DATA PROPOSALS

This section provides suggestions for the United States on data variables and indicators that are either recommended by international organizations or used by other countries for drink-driving. The section provides details on the approach used, descriptions of data systems in selected countries, and recommendations for consideration by the committee.

Drink-Driving Data and Variables

Introduction

The main objective of this section of the paper is to understand the architecture of drink-driving data in the United States and compare it with other high-income countries that have well-established data systems. Furthermore, innovative ways in which databases in selected high-income countries link drink-driving data with other data, such as hospital data and insurance data, are also explored. This section provides a review of drink-driving databases in selected high-income countries and compares them to the United States to provide recommendations that can improve such data and data collection processes.

Methods

Our approach is based on the following:

- Assessing drink-driving data in selected high-income countries by understanding the type of variables collected, frequency of data collection, reporting, and dissemination;
- Comparing U.S. data with those of selected countries to identify variables that are in the databases of the selected high-income countries and not in the U.S. database;

- Understanding innovative ways of linking different data; and
- Providing recommendations for improvement in the U.S. drink-driving database.

The information in this section was primarily collected by searching websites of road traffic crash and injury databases, their manuals (when available), reports related to the databases, peer-reviewed literature, and suggestions from global road safety experts (see Annex 1).[10] This is further described below.

Recommended Drink-Driving Variables

Drink-driving evidence is crucial to the understanding of development, implementation, and evaluation of drink-driving laws. Efforts have been made by WHO to guide countries toward establishing standardized data systems. In this regard, two manuals—*Drinking and Driving: A Road Safety Manual for Decision-Makers and Practitioners* (2007) and *Data Systems: A Road Safety Manual for Decision-Makers and Practitioners* (2010)—list variables that should be part of any drink-driving database (WHO, 2007, 2010). Table 5 lists the WHO-recommended variables and compares them to the U.S. fatality database, FARS.[11]

The recommended road traffic injury variables are categorized into person, crash, road, vehicle characteristics, and cost. *Person* characteristics include age, sex, road user type, seating position, safety equipment, and so on. *Crash* characteristics include date and time of crash, weather, location, type, effect of crash, and lighting conditions. *Road* characteristics include road type, surface, obstacles, and speed limit (WHO, 2007, 2010). Variables specific to drink-driving include suspected use of alcohol, status of alcohol test, type of testing conducted, and test results. The suspected use of alcohol is reported by police and is a binary (yes/no) variable. The responses for alcohol test status include test not given, test refused, test given, and unknown if tested. Test type includes blood, breath, urine, other, or unknown; test results report value, pending value, or results unknown (WHO, 2007, 2010).

Drink-driving needs involvement of multiple stakeholders, which means that data from other organizations, such as insurance and hospital data, are also needed for a holistic understanding (WHO, 2007). Reporting of data through standardized indicators provides a common language for data presentation. It is useful for understanding time trends, thus

[10] Available by request from the National Academies of Sciences, Engineering, and Medicine's Public Access Records Office (PARO@nas.edu).

[11] Ibid.

enabling stakeholders to assess and evaluate the effectiveness of interventions. Table 6 compares recommended drink-driving-related indicators with the FARS.[12]

The Fatality Analysis Reporting System (FARS)

The FARS is a data system established in the United States in 1975 by NHTSA to collect data on fatal road traffic crashes that resulted in the death of a road user within 30 days of the crash event. The data are collected from the 50 U.S. states, the District of Columbia, and Puerto Rico. It includes more than 150 variables that relate to person, vehicle, crash, and road characteristics from various data sources including police reports, emergency medical services reports, hospital records, state driver and vehicle registration records, death certificates, coroner reports, and state highway department data (FARS, 2014). The FARS data can be used based on the requirements of researchers through a data query system that allows selections of variables based on research objectives and questions[13] (FARS, 2014). Specific variables in the FARS related to drink-driving include police-reported alcohol involvement, method of alcohol determination by police, alcohol test status, test type, and test results.

However, NHTSA has found that there are significant data missing for BAC (FARS, 2014). This vacancy is handled using multiple imputation methods (FARS, 2017; Jewett et al., 2015). NHTSA, with support from the National Center for Statistics and Analysis, publishes reports that provide national and state-level statistics related to road traffic crashes and fatalities, including drink-driving data (FARS, 2014).

Data Linkage

Linking drink-driving and road traffic crash and injury data is important for understanding the full spectrum of issues associated with drink-driving. Several data sources including police data and hospital data can be linked for this purpose (Amorima et al., 2014; Derriks and Mak, 2007). However, there are challenges associated with linking various databases.

The International Traffic Safety Data and Analysis Group reports that one of the main reasons for lack of data linkage is protection of individual-level data as no personal identifiers are part of such databases. The majority OECD countries deidentify the data to protect individual identity, which has resulted in development of mechanisms that can link databases based on other variables such as date, time, location of crash, age, and sex

---

[12] Ibid.

[13] See https://www-fars.nhtsa.dot.gov/Main/index.aspx (accessed January 10, 2018).

(Derriks and Mak, 2007). Exploring innovative mechanisms employed by other high-income countries is crucial to holistically addressing risk factors of drink-driving.

Selection Criteria

For this section of the paper, our approach was to present case studies from countries that have databases that collect drink-driving data. Two main criteria for selection of countries for case studies were high-income countries with similar levels of economic development to the United States, the presence of data systems (or databases) related to road traffic injuries that also collect alcohol-related data, and the demonstrated use of such data for interventions or programs against drink-driving.

Based on the above selection criteria, drink-driving-related information for 35 OECD countries was collected from the 2015 *Global Road Safety Status* report. This included data related to BAC limits for general population and young drivers, self-reported enforcement of drink-driving law, estimated fatality rates caused by road traffic crashes, reported number of road traffic deaths, and percentage of road traffic deaths caused by alcohol. In addition, information related to data sources for drink-driving percentages was also recorded (WHO, 2015).

The 2017 report *OECD Health Statistics* for injuries in road traffic crashes was also reviewed for additional databases for road traffic crashes and injuries (OECD, 2017). All the 35 OECD countries were found to have road traffic databases that collected data related to drink-driving. However, for this section of the paper, a sample of the 35 OECD countries were selected as case studies: Australia, France, New Zealand, Sweden, and Switzerland. These countries were selected because each has a comprehensive road traffic database with drink-driving variables. These databases have been shown to generate data that has led to the development and implementation of law enforcement and social media campaigns to address the issue of drink-driving in these countries.

Assessment of Selected Countries

To understand the differences between the FARS and databases from selected high-income countries, a set of five questions was selected to analyze these databases:

1. What type of data system is available in the country to collect data on drink-driving?
2. What agencies or organizations are collecting the data?
3. Who collects the data (i.e., police or hospital)?

4. What is the frequency of data dissemination?
5. If available, how is the database linked with other databases?

Table 5 compares the FARS with a recommended list of variables and databases from selected high-income countries.[14] Described below are a series of case studies of data systems based on the above criteria.

Case Study A: Australia

Australia has a population of 24 million with a gross national income per capita of US$54,420 (World Bank, 2017). In 2015, the estimated rate of road traffic fatalities was 7.5 per 100,000 population and the estimated number of road traffic deaths was 1,823 (GBD, 2016). The BAC limit for the general population is 0.049 g/dl, and it is 0.00 for young drivers. The percentage of road traffic deaths involving alcohol is reported to be 28 to 30 percent (OECD, 2016; WHO, 2015). Australia has two main crash datasets that collect data on road traffic fatalities: the Australian Road Deaths Database and the National Crash Database.

Australian Road Deaths Database

The Australian Road Deaths database provides basic information (demographics and crashes) related to road traffic fatalities. The database has been hosted by the Bureau of Infrastructure, Transport and Regional Economics (BITRE) since 1989. The data are collected by police on a monthly basis, reporting both fatalities and crashes, and are linked through a unique ID (BITRE, 2014). BITRE also collects data on economic development, infrastructure, and regional developmental issues including social capital, household wealth, and industry structure. In addition to road data, it also collects data on aviation, maritime, and rail transport incidents (BITRE, 2017a). A steering committee helps improve data collection systems for timely and efficient dissemination of information to stakeholders for planning and implementation of interventions focusing on infrastructure and transportation (BITRE, 2017b).

National Crash Database

This is a national database on fatal and injurious crashes, and it is updated annually (BITRE, 2017c). Crash data in Australia are collected from eight states by police and transport authorities. Uniformity

[14] Available by request from the National Academies of Sciences, Engineering, and Medicine's Public Access Records Office (PARO@nas.edu).

in methods of crash data collection has resulted in development of this national crash database, which is maintained by the Department of Infrastructure and Regional Development. It gives fatality counts related to deaths from drink-driving, the number of drivers and motorcycle riders killed with a BAC above the limit set by law, and the number of deaths from crashes involving a driver or motorcycle rider with a BAC above the limit set by law (BITRE, 2017c).

Developing a national data system for serious injuries is a priority in Australia. The effort is directed to have a data system that links road crash data and hospital data. Currently, there is great variation in the data collected for serious road traffic injuries and hence a lack of a national database for serious injuries (OECD, 2016). However, there is a database that provides data related to nonfatal road traffic crashes, including variables related to drink-driving.

Australian Institute of Health and Welfare (AIHW)

AIHW collects data on many health-related issues including expenditure data, hospital data, alcohol, and disability (AIHW, 2017a). It reports injuries from road traffic as the "number of people injured in road traffic crashes per million population." The data also report on "hospitalized injury that results from road traffic crashes" (OECD, 2017). In addition, the agency collects alcohol-related data from the National Drug Strategy Household Survey, which is conducted every 3 years with the latest one conducted in 2016 (AIHW, 2017b). The data are reported as the percentage of disease burden attributable to alcohol and alcohol-related hospitalizations including road traffic injuries that resulted from the use of alcohol (AIHW, 2017b). AIHW collects data on multiple aspects of health and social issues including maternal child health, youth health, ageing, disability, welfare, burden of disease, noncommunicable diseases, and injuries; it therefore offers an opportunity for linking different databases (AIHW, 2017a).

In Australia, data linkage is possible because AIHW is based within a national agency and has access to national and state-level databases. The example of AIHW is relevant in this case as it collects data on several different aspects of health. It is an accredited data integrating authority in Australia and has access to non-AIHW databases such as the National Hospitals Morbidity Database. It has a dedicated group that helps investigators and researchers by putting together linked data. AIHW facilitates data linkage by developing a customized database on requests from researchers and policy makers. Furthermore, the data linkage requires approval from the AIHW Ethics Committee (AIHW, 2017c,d; BITRE, 2017b).[15]

The data from the Australian Road Deaths Database are disseminated through monthly bulletins on fatal road traffic crashes and quarterly reports on fatal road crashes involving heavy vehicles; however, these do not report data specific to drink-driving. The monthly bulletin on fatal road traffic crashes is available around the 14th of each month and contains information on counts, provides trends of fatalities since the beginning of the year and over the past 5 years for the reporting month, and the percentage change in trend. The monthly bulletin also reports count of fatalities by road user type, age group, gender, crash type, day, and time of day. Annual death rates per 100,000 population for each jurisdiction over the past 5 years for the reporting month are also given (BITRE, 2017d). The quarterly reports on fatal road crashes involving heavy vehicles include count on deaths by jurisdiction, crash type, and road user type over the past year. It also reports the percentage change over the past 1 year and 3 years.

Data from the above data sources are compiled for two annual reports: one related to fatal crashes and the other to fatal crashes involving heavy vehicles. The annual report on road traffic crashes reports the number and standardized rates of fatal crashes, injuries, and fatalities for the previous 10 years. These data are reported based on jurisdiction, road user type, age group, gender, crash type, day and time of day, and hospitalized injuries. The annual report includes a section on historical series covering data on fatalities, crashes, and rates for the past 30 years and exposure series with data in population, age group, and registered vehicles for the past 30 years. The data from this database have been used to follow progress on targets identified in Australia's National Road Safety Strategy 2011–2020. The targets are assessed with their baseline that was reported in 2008–2010. A specific target related to drink-driving is "Number of deaths from crashes involving a driver or motorcycle rider with a BAC above the legal limit." It was reported to be 205 at baseline and 134 in 2015, showing a 37.4 percent reduction in drink-driving-related fatalities (BITRE, 2017c,d).

The annual report for heavy vehicle crashes includes data on counts and rates of fatal road crashes involving heavy vehicles, as well as fatalities and injuries requiring hospitalization. The percentage change in these parameters is reported for the last calendar year as well as for the past few years. This report also has historical series and exposure data, such as the annual report on all road traffic crashes. It reports the BAC status of drivers involved in heavy vehicle crashes that resulted in deaths (BITRE,

[15] A list of approved research projects is available at https://www.aihw.gov.au/our-services/data-linkage (accessed January 10, 2018).

2017d). In addition to national reports, these data are also reported in the *Annual International Road Safety Comparisons Report* published for OECD nations, allowing for comparisons to be made with other OECD nations (BITRE, 2017d).

The innovation related to data use from these databases is that the process addresses the needs of various stakeholders in multiple jurisdictions at national and international levels including the public, government officials, policy makers, several ministries, and even international road safety organizations. Public availability of these data and reports allows stakeholders to understand gaps in road safety. Specifically, these reports have been used to assess time series trends in road traffic fatalities in Australia and provide evidence related to implementation of laws and their effect on reduction in fatalities. Furthermore, the use of these data to report on progress of the National Road Safety Strategy is an effective way for the country and each jurisdiction to assess improvements in road safety interventions and policies, and to plan for future road safety strategy.

Efforts of the steering committee for timely dissemination of these results to stakeholders are crucial to the effective use of these data. The data are used for developing information sheets for sharing with the public and to raise awareness among the masses. The database is also available for research and publication related to various aspects of road safety, including vulnerable users and assessments of road safety measures in improving outcomes (BITRE, 2017d).

Case Study B: New Zealand

New Zealand has a population of 4 million with a gross national income per capita of US$39,070 (World Bank, 2017). The estimated rate of road traffic fatalities was 8.3 per 100,000 population, and the estimated number of deaths was 378 in 2015 (GBD, 2016). The BAC limit for the general population is ≤0.05 g/dl and 0.00 for young drivers. The estimate for percentage of road traffic deaths involving alcohol is reported to be 31 percent (WHO, 2015). It is reported that for every 100 people who die on roads in New Zealand because of their drink-driving, about 47 of their passengers and 24 road users who were sober also die in the *same* traffic crash (Ministry of Transport, 2016a).

The Ministry of Transport in New Zealand reports road traffic injuries per 100,000 people using injury and crash data from several resources, including police crash reports, hospitalization data, and the Accident Compensation Corporation (ACC) new claims data from the Motor Vehicle Authority. Road traffic crash data are collected by the police on all fatal crashes. Information collected includes crash location, drivers, vehicles, road, number of injured, and deaths in the crash. Detailed description of the crash site and a diagram are also included as part of crash reports. Once the data are collected, they are submitted to the New Zealand Transport Agency for coding and data entry into the Crash Analysis System (CAS) (New Zealand Transport Agency, 2017). Data from the CAS are accessible through a secure login system. The process of data collection and data availability takes time; therefore, police develop an initial report that is made available within 24 hours of the crash.

Data related to person characteristics, crash event, and road conditions are collected for each crash along with road user behavior. It also includes data on the number of infringements and offences collected on a monthly basis. For fatal drink-driving crashes, the type of vehicle is also recorded. Specific to drink-driving, the number of deaths in alcohol crashes, proportion of total road traffic deaths, number of drivers tested, and number found to be over the legal alcohol limit is reported using this data (Ministry of Transport, 2016b; OECD, 2016).

In addition to crash data, linking of data is done to calculate social costs of crashes and injuries. The social cost data differ from the ACC, which collects data related to the claims cost incurred by ACC (Ministry of Transport, 2017a). These data have been reported since 2006 and are updated annually after accounting for inflation. The cost is reported for fatal and nonfatal road injuries and includes the total cost of road crashes to the nation (loss of life and life quality, loss of productivity, medical, legal, and vehicle damage costs) and average social cost per injury and per crash (Ministry of Transport, 2017a). It is important to note that the social cost data are based on crash and injury estimates and are calculated by using injury and crash conversion factors (ratio of estimated to reported numbers of injuries or crashes). This gives an estimate of the total number of road traffic incidents and accounts for nonreporting crashes and injuries (Ministry of Transport, 2006; OECD, 2017).

The data are reported on a monthly basis and are available on the website. The monthly overview of crash statistics reports deaths and injuries by age, sex, road user type, outcome of crashes, road user behavior, and social cost-related factors that contribute to crashes. It also gives time trends related to road traffic deaths since 1990. The monthly report also includes the numbers and percentage of drivers killed because of excess alcohol; this has been available since 2005. Drink-driving data for earlier years are not reported because the data are not comparable owing to changes in the crash reporting processes (Ministry of Transport, 2017b). There is also an annual statistical statement, the *Motor Vehicle Crashes in New Zealand Report*, which collects data from the CAS and reports annual statistics on injuries, crashes, and deaths for different road user types and ethnicities. It also gives historical trends since 1950, and includes data on population and vehicles. This annual statement also gives international comparisons by road user type and age; this is reported as percentage and rates per 100,000 people. These annual data are available in the form of Excel sheets that are freely available from the website (Ministry of Transport, 2017b).

The ministry also publishes *Crash Fact Sheets* on an annual basis using the data from the CAS. It highlights key findings of drink-driving data from the previous year and reports drink-driving-related crashes based on road type, age group, gender, license status, day and time of crash, and other risk factors like use of seat belts. Time series data on fatal crashes, deaths, and injuries have been reported since 1990, and time series based on age groups and gender have been reported since 1995. The *Crash Fact Sheets* also summarize the history of legislation related to drink-driving in New Zealand (Ministry of Transport, 2017b; RoadSafetyBC, 2016). In addition, ad hoc reporting is also done; for example in 2012, the Ministry of Transport published a special report, *High-Risk Drivers Statistics*, which reported statistics from data available to the ministry. It reported on two drink-driving-related high-risk behaviors: drivers with a BAC of at least 50 percent over the adult legal limit and repeat alcohol offenders, specifically drivers in alcohol-related crashes who have at least one prior alcohol conviction in the previous 5 years (Ministry of Transport, 2012).

Road safety is a high-priority area identified by the government of New Zealand. These data are used for planning safe road and transport systems and for assessing programs that are planned and implemented to achieve goals based on New Zealand's road safety strategy 2010–2020 (Ministry of Transport, 2017c). In this regard, the data have been used by stakeholders involved in planning and legislation related to road safety. In addition, the data are used for developing targeted campaigns for the public. They also serve to track road safety trends since 2010 and have helped to address gaps and identify opportunities that can drive work at the national level to make roads safer in New Zealand.

Specific drink-driving-related goals that have been achieved since 2010 include implementation of an alcohol interlock program, implementation of zero BAC levels for drivers under 20 years of age, and lowered BAC limit to 0.05% for those above 20 years of age. In addition, efforts to increase community responsibility for reducing drink-driving were also implemented. These efforts resulted in a reduction in road crashes caused by drink-driving (National Road Safety Committee, 2016). Currently, collaborative efforts between the Ministry of Transport and the police are under way to enforce, educate, and use social media to reduce drink-driving.

Like Australia, in New Zealand multiple stakeholders work in collaboration and have taken a data-driven approach to address the issue of drink-driving. This approach is innovative in the context of New Zealand because it considers road safety a systems-level issue and is addressing it using a systems approach that accounts for infrastructure, roads users, and road behaviors, and uses a multiprong method to address these components of road systems to make them safer (National Road Safety Committee, 2016).

Case Study C: Sweden

The population of Sweden is 9 million with a gross national income per capita of US$54,630 (World Bank, 2017). In 2016, the estimated rate of road traffic fatalities was 4.6 per 100,000 people, and the estimated number of fatalities was 447, respectively (GBD, 2016; OECD, 2016; WHO, 2015). The BAC limit for the general population and young drivers is 0.02 g/dl. The estimate for the percentage of road traffic deaths involving alcohol is reported to be 19 to 24 percent (OECD, 2016; WHO, 2015).

The database related to road traffic injuries in Sweden is called the *Swedish Traffic Accident Data Acquisition* (STRADA). This national-level database was established in 2003 and collects data from the police and hospitals. Police reporting is mandatory and no additional funding is given to the police, while hospital reporting is voluntary and each participating hospital receives fixed funding each year to cover costs related to meetings, training, and materials (Howard and Linder, 2014). The police data provide details related to the crash (date, location weather, road conditions, type of crash), traffic elements (road user type, injury severity), and person (age). In terms of drink-driving data, only information related to the driver being under the influence of alcohol is collected. No further information on drink-driving is reported by the police (Howard and Linder, 2014). More than 60 out of 80 Swedish hospitals share data with STRADA (Howard and Linder, 2014). Together, these two sources of data facilitate the understanding of circumstances of road traffic crashes and their severity in the country (Howard and Linder, 2014; OECD, 2016).

Although the STRADA data system is a comprehensive source of data on serious crashes, it does not include data on individuals, crashes that were less severe, injured persons not seen in an emergency department (ED), or crashes not reported to the police. In cases where the police have information related to a minor crash or individual with minor injury, data are sent to STRADA (OECD, 2016; Transport Styrelsen, 2015). In addition, the STRADA is linked with national-level registries that collect data related to driver's licenses and vehicles registered in the country (Howard and Linder, 2014). The STRADA data are available for use by the Swedish Transport Agency in the form of a Microsoft Access database and

Web-based system. The agency also provides 1 day of training to those interested in using the data (Howard and Linder, 2014).

Even though STRADA collects data from the police and hospitals, these two sources of data are not always linked. Only 40 percent of police data are linked with hospital data, and 30 percent of the hospital data are found to be linked to police data. The data are linked based on predefined matching criteria that develop an algorithm with the STRADA. The criteria for matching include a patient identification number, crash timing within 24 hours, and crash location within a 1,000-meter radius (person, time, and place matching). The linked data are then given a unique crash number. This unique identification number is stored in the database along with a quality estimate which is a value between 0 and 100 and is based on differences in time and location (Howard and Linder, 2014). Several reasons have been identified for the lack of 100 percent matching; police may not have registered crash and person information related to vulnerable road users (cyclists, pedestrians) or the information needed for matching is not available or it is incorrect. Hospital data may not match because individuals involved in the crash may not have gone to a hospital that is part of the STRADA system (Howard and Linder, 2014). Duplicate cases are checked through monthly quality checks performed by the Swedish Transport Agency and by collecting hospital data from the first hospital where the crash victim was seen. No data from hospitals to where the patient are later transferred are collected (Howard and Linder, 2014).

Data are disseminated through monthly and annual reports (Howard and Linder, 2014; Transport Styrelsen, 2015, 2016, 2017). Sweden has implemented Vision Zero to address the issue of road safety in the country and targets zero road traffic-related deaths by the year 2050. The innovation for the use of data in Sweden is to make road systems safe for its users so that there is no crash, injury, or fatality where the road system is a contributing factor; thus the focus is more on engineering rather than enforcement of laws.

The data from the STRADA are used for understanding changes in road traffic crashes and fatalities because of road interventions. The data have been used for making improvements in the existing system through collaborations with stakeholders (engineers, transport agencies, and ministries) as well as government. The data identify areas of improvement and facilitate development and implementation of new road safety interventions in the country. These data were also presented at the Vision Zero conference held in Sweden annually for the past 9 years. One of the major steps taken in this regard was the relaunch of Vision Zero by the Swedish government in 2016 with the key focus on stakeholder engagement to achieve the zero target (Swedish Transport Administration, 2017a,b).

The hospital component of the data is used for different research projects. These include analysis of vulnerable road users, such as pedestrians and bicycle users; accuracy of data in terms of response rate; and classification of injury. Some work is more regional while the rest is at the national level (Howard and Linder, 2014). The data are also used for assessing interventions implemented for achieving Vision Zero in Sweden, such as interlock systems (Transport Styrelsen, 2015).

Case Study D: France

The population of France is 66 million with a gross national income per capita of US$38,950 (World Bank, 2017). In 2016, the estimated rate of road traffic fatalities was 7.9 per 100,000 people, and the estimated number of road traffic deaths was 5,179 (GBD, 2016; WHO, 2015). The BAC limit is ≤0.05 g/dl for both the general population and young drivers. The percentage of road traffic deaths involving alcohol is reported to be 19 to 29 percent (OECD, 2016; WHO, 2015).

In France, road traffic crashes that result in an injury are recorded by the police. Variables collected include information related to vehicle occupants and classification of injury severity into four categories: noninjured, slightly injured (outpatients or inpatients with less than a 6-day hospital stay), seriously injured (those requiring a longer hospital stay), or killed (individuals who die within 6 days of the crash) (Amoros et al., 2008). These data are then collected centrally, which has led to the development of a national road traffic crash database. The data management is done by the French Road Safety Observatory (ONISR, Observatoire National Interministériel de la Sécurité Routière) within the Ministry of Interior (Ministry of Road Safety, 2015a, 2017).

Data from the national database are accurate for fatal and serious crashes; however, crashes resulting in minor injuries are underreported owing to variation across the country in reporting such events (OECD, 2016). The database has data related to person, road, vehicle, and crash characteristics. Drink-driving-related data include variables related to BAC levels; the ONISR reports data on fatal crashes that involve at least one driver with a known BAC level (Ministry of Road Safety, 2015a).

ONISR also assesses road user behavior using three data sources that include observations of road user behavior; these observations are conducted by ONISR. In addition, it also collects data on offenses and permits that are gathered by law enforcement agencies. Data on convictions associated with road traffic offenses are collected from the Ministry of Justice (Ministry of Road Safety, 2015b). There is a lack of information related to how these data sources can be linked to provide a complete picture related to road safety risk factors.

There are no county-level data in France except for Rhone County, where police data are compared with the Rhone trauma registry that collects medical care data from health facilities. The facilities include primary care clinics, EDs, and rehabilitation units. The data from police and health care facilities are linked based on date and time of crash, crash location, year, month, and gender of crash victims (Amoros et al., 2008).

ONISR has multiple stakeholders, including enforcement agencies and road safety departments. These data are shared with them on a regular basis to help with the enforcement of road safety and drink-driving laws in the country (Ministry of Road Safety, 2015a, 2017). These data are disseminated via monthly reports that provide the number of injuries, casualties, and hospitalizations. It reports trends from the current year and the previous year and helps identify areas of road safety that need immediate action (Ministry of Road Safety, 2017). The annual report gives fatality trends since 2010. It also gives comparisons of crashes, fatalities, injured people, and hospitalization from the current year and previous year and presents the percentage change in these data. Data also include road type, day of the week, road user type, age group, and sex. It also gives a comparative analysis of data on vulnerable road users in France and the rest of Europe. Specific to drink-driving, data on percentage of crashes caused by the use of alcohol are reported for the overall population and for different age groups (Ministry of Road Safety, 2017).

In the year 2014, ONISR reported local performance indicators for France and its counties. These indicators were developed based on main road safety issues in France and included drivers driving under the influence of alcohol (Ministry of Road Safety, 2016). Data from ONISR are also made available for the *IRTAD Annual Report* to provide a comparison with OECD nations by providing annual trends in road safety based on road user type, age group, sex, and road safety risk factors including drink-driving (Ministry of Road Safety, 2017).

Case Study E: Switzerland

Switzerland has a population of 8 million with a gross national income per capita of US$81,240 (World Bank, 2017). In 2015, the estimated rate of road traffic fatalities was 4.7 per 100,000 people, and the reported road traffic deaths were 390 in 2015 (GBD, 2016). The BAC limit for the general population is ≤0.05 g/dl and ≤0.01 g/dl for young drivers. The percentage of road traffic deaths involving alcohol is reported to be 14 to 16 percent (OECD, 2016; WHO, 2015).

The Federal Roads Office (FEDRO) in Switzerland is responsible for the collection of road traffic crash data in the country. These data are collected by police. It is hosted by the Federal Department of the Environment, Transport, Energy and Communications (DETEC) (FEDRO, 2017).

Like other high-income countries, Switzerland also collects data on person, crash, vehicle, and road characteristics. The data have been available since 2002. They are accessible via Excel spreadsheets available free of cost at the FEDRO website (FEDRO, 2017).

The crash data reported by police are compared with insurance claim data related to road traffic crashes. This comparison is done to make an accurate estimation of road traffic injuries. It also accounts for underreporting based on road user type and age group. Recently, efforts were made to link police and hospital data, and data are reported by age group and road user type (FEDRO, 2016; OECD, 2016). A pilot program was conducted that showed promising results and led to the implementation of data linkage procedures in the national database (OECD, 2016).

The data are disseminated via monthly and annual reports and shared with national and international organization partners to plan interventions and assess their effect (FEDRO, 2016). FEDRO uses these data to plan changes in infrastructure and then assesses the changes to see their effect on reduction in road traffic crashes (FEDRO, 2016). Table 7 compares databases from the above countries.[16]

Recommendations for Data Systems

Based on the analysis above on a sample of high-income countries similar to the United States, key points include the following:

- All data systems collect basic data related to road traffic crashes, fatalities, and injuries and present them based on road user type, sex, age groups, day, time of day, and in some cases road type. Most of these data are available in the form of time series to assess trends in road traffic mortality and injuries.
- In all of these countries there is a national-level data system that collects detailed data on road traffic crashes. These data are collected by police and managed at a central level for coding and cleaning. The cleaned data are available in most cases to the public (except for New Zealand, where special training is needed to use the data).
- Data from these countries are reported on a monthly and annual basis and used by local and national governments to inform decision making about road safety measures that are identified within national road safety strategies in these countries (e.g., New Zealand and Sweden).

[16] Available by request from the National Academies of Sciences, Engineering, and Medicine's Public Access Records Office (PARO@nas.edu).

- Data are also available for use by researchers and international road safety agencies to generate evidence that is available for policy makers to develop and implement road safety policies within countries based on gaps identified in the data.
- Data systems in New Zealand and Switzerland are linked with other data systems, such as insurance data; in Australia fatal and nonfatal data are linked by AIHW because it has access to several sources of health-related data.

Some considerations in applying findings from the above case studies to the FARS are as follows:

- The FARS has a comprehensive set of variables on fatal crashes including person, vehicle, road, and crash characteristics. There are a few variables, such as passenger position, injury position (arm, head), activity of road user at the time of crash (reversing), and purpose of journey, that are not in the FARS and could be included for better understanding of risk factors associated with drink-driving in the United States. However, it is important to note that the FARS collects all WHO-recommended variables for drink-driving.
- While the FARS collects data on fatal injuries from the participating states, there is a need to establish a similar system that collects nonfatal data at a central level. This requires engagement with various stakeholders, including hospitals, emergency services, police, and state authorities.
- There is no combined database for fatal and nonfatal injuries at the national level in the United States. Several states in the United States have databases that combine fatal and nonfatal data on road traffic crashes and injuries; however, the true burden of road injuries and crashes attributed to alcohol requires analysis of both fatal and nonfatal databases *at the national level*. Such a system at the national level will help in cost estimations and planning, implementation, and evaluation of interventions geared toward reducing road traffic crashes and injuries caused by drink-driving (Amorima et al., 2014; Derriks and Mak, 2007).

Finally, this paper recommends further study and analysis of U.S.-based data to explore the quality of data collected and associated analytic limitations around alcohol-related data in the FARS and relevant state databases. More work is needed in this area to help efforts to curb drink-driving.

REFERENCES

Aguilera, S. L., P. Sripad, J. C. Lunnen, S. T. Moyses, A. Chandran, and S. J. Moyses. 2015. Alcohol consumption among drivers in Curitiba, Brazil. *Traffic Injury Prevention* 16:219–224.

AIHW (Australian Institute of Health and Welfare). 2017a. *AIHW: A–Z topics.* https://www.aihw.gov.au/reports-statistics/a-z-topics (accessed October 31, 2017).

AIHW. 2017b. *National drug strategy household survey 2016: Detailed findings.* Drug Statistics series no. 31. Cat. no. PHE 214. Canberra: AIHW.

AIHW. 2017c. *AIHW: Our data collections.* https://www.aihw.gov.au/about-our-data/our-data-collections (accessed October 31, 2017).

AIHW. 2017d. *AIHW: Data linkage.* https://www.aihw.gov.au/our-services/data-linkage (accessed October 31, 2017).

Albalate, D. 2008. Lowering blood alcohol content levels to save lives: The European experience. *Journal of Policy Analysis and Management* 27(1):20–39.

Ames, C. L., Y. Lu, and R. Weaver. 2016. Evaluating the effectiveness of "no refusal" blood draw search warrant programs to reduce alcohol-related traffic crashes in central Texas. *Papers in Applied Geography* 2(1):113–120.

Amorima, M., S. Ferreiraa, and A. Coutoa. 2014. A conceptual algorithm to link police and hospital records based on occurrence of values. *Transportation Research Procedia* 3:224–233.

Amoros, E., J. L. Martin, S. Lafont, and B. Laumon. 2008. Actual incidences of road casualties, and their injury severity, modelled from police and hospital data, France. *European Journal of Public Health* 18(4):360–365.

Anderson, P. 2008. *Reducing drinking and driving in Europe.* London: Institute of Alcohol Studies.

Anderson, P., L. Moeller, and G. Galea. 2012. *Alcohol in the European Union: Consumption, harm and policy approaches.* Copenhagen, Denmark: World Health Organization Regional Office for Europe.

Andreuccetti, G., H. B. Carvalho, C. J. Cherpitel, Y. Ye, J. C. Ponce, T. Kahn, and V. Leyton. 2011. Reducing the legal blood alcohol concentration limit for driving in developing countries: A time for change? Results and implications derived from a time-series analysis (2001–10) conducted in Brazil. *Addiction* 106(12):2124–2131.

Assum, T. 2010. Reduction of the blood alcohol concentration limit in Norway—Effects on knowledge, behavior and accidents. *Accident Analysis & Prevention* 42(6):1523–1530.

Babor, T. F. 2009. Alcohol research and the alcoholic beverage industry: Issues, concerns and conflicts of interest. *Addiction* 104(Suppl 1):34–47.

Babor, T. F. 2010. *Alcohol: No ordinary commodity: Research and public policy,* 2nd ed. New York: Oxford University Press.

Babor, T. F., and K. Robaina. 2013. Public health, academic medicine, and the alcohol industry's corporate social responsibility activities. *American Journal of Public Health* 103(2):206–214.

Bachani, A. M., N. S. Jessani, V. C. Pham, L. N. Quang, P. N. Nguyen, J. Passmore, and A. A. Hyder. 2013. Drinking & driving in Viet Nam: Prevalence, knowledge, attitudes, and practices in two provinces. *Injury* 44(Suppl 4):S38–S44.

Bailey, T., V. Lindsay, and J. Royals. 2013. Best practice in alcohol ignition interlock schemes. *Australasian College of Road Safety "A Safe System: The Road Safety Discussion,"* Adelaide, Australia, 6–8 November.

Bartl, G., and R. Esberger. 2000. *Effects of lowering the legal BAC limit in Austria.* Vienna: Austrian Road Safety Board.

BITRE (Bureau of Infrastructure, Transport and Regional Economics). 2014. *Australian road deaths database*. https://bitre.gov.au/statistics/safety/fatal_road_crash_database.aspx (accessed October 31, 2017).

BITRE. 2017a. *Regional databases*. https://bitre.gov.au/databases/regional.aspx (accessed October 31, 2017).

BITRE. 2017b. *National infrastructure data collection and dissemination plan*. https://bitre.gov.au/data_dissemination/index.aspx (accessed October 31, 2017).

BITRE. 2017c. *Road trauma Australia 2016 statistical summary*. https://bitre.gov.au/publications/ongoing/files/Road_Trauma_Australia_2016_Web.pdf (accessed October 31, 2017).

BITRE. 2017d. *Safety statistics—road safety statistics*. https://bitre.gov.au/statistics/safety (accessed October 31, 2017).

Breitmeier, D., I. Seeland-Schulze, H. Hecker, and U. Schneider. 2007. The influence of blood alcohol concentrations of around 0.03% on neuropsychological functions—a double-blind, placebo-controlled investigation. *Addiction Biology* 12(2):183–189.

Caetano, R. 2008. About smoke and mirrors: The alcohol industry and the promotion of science. *Addiction* 103:175–178.

Caetano, R., and R. Laranjeira. 2006. A "perfect storm" in developing countries: Economic growth and the alcohol industry. *Addiction* 101(2):149–152.

Cameron, M. 2013. *Best practice in random breath testing and cost-effective intensity levels*. 20th International Conference on Alcohol, Drugs and Traffic Safety (T2013), Brisbane, Queensland, Australia.

Casswell, S. 2011a. Alcohol harm—the urgent need for a global response. *Addiction* 106(7):1205–1207.

Casswell, S. 2011b. Alcohol marketing research agenda—let us look at how the industry maintains its hegemony. *Addiction* 106(3):476–477.

Chan, M. 2013. Re: Doctors and the alcohol industry: An unhealthy mix? *BMJ* 346:f2647.

Christie, R., D. Carseldine, and S. Brown. 1995. *National guidelines for alcohol ignition interlock programs for drink driving offenders*. Sydney, Australia: Austroroads.

Constant, A., L. R. Salmi, S. Lafont, M. Chiron, and E. Lagarde. 2009. Road casualties and changes in risky driving behavior in France between 2001 and 2004 among participants in the gazel cohort. *American Journal of Public Health* 99(7):1247–1253.

Derriks, H. M., and P. M. Mak. 2007. *IRTAD special report—underreporting of road traffic casualties*. The Netherlands: OECD and International Transport Forum.

Desapriya, E., S. Shimizu, I. Pike, S. Subzwari, and G. Scime. 2007. Impact of lowering the legal blood alcohol concentration limit to 0.03 on male, female and teenage drivers involved alcohol-related crashes in Japan. *International Journal of Injury Control and Safety Promotion* 14(3):181–187.

Ditter, S. M., R. W. Elder, R. A. Shults, D. A. Sleet, R. Compton, J. L. Nichols, and Community Preventive Services Task Force. 2005. Effectiveness of designated driver programs for reducing alcohol-impaired driving: A systematic review. *American Journal of Preventive Medicine* 28(5 Suppl):280–287.

Elder, R. W., R. A. Shults, D. A. Sleet, J. L. Nichols, S. Zaza, and R. S. Thompson. 2002. Effectiveness of sobriety checkpoints for reducing alcohol-involved crashes. *Traffic Injury Prevention* 3(4):266–274.

Elder, R. W., R. A. Shults, D. A. Sleet, J. L. Nichols, R. S. Thompson, W. Rajab, and Community Preventive Services Task Force. 2004. Effectiveness of mass media campaigns for reducing drinking and driving and alcohol-involved crashes: A systematic review. *American Journal of Preventive Medicine* 27(1):57–65.

Elder, R. W., J. L. Nichols, R. A. Shults, D. A. Sleet, L. C. Barrios, R. Compton, and Community Preventive Services Task Force. 2005. Effectiveness of school-based programs for reducing drinking and driving and riding with drinking drivers: A systematic review. *American Journal of Preventive Medicine* 28(5 Suppl):288–304.

Erke, A., C. Goldenbeld, and T. Vaa. 2009. *Good practice in the selected key areas of speeding, drink driving and seat belt wearing; results from meta-analysis.* Police Enforcement Policy and Programmes on European Roads. Contract No. 019744.

Esser, M. B., J. Bao, D. H. Jernigan, and A. A. Hyder. 2016. Evaluation of the evidence base for the alcohol industry's actions to reduce drink driving globally. *American Journal of Public Health* 106(4):707–713.

EU (European Union) Directorate General for Health and Consumers. 2009. *First progress report on the implementation of the EU alcohol strategy.* Brussels, Belgium: European Union Directorate General for Health and Consumers.

European Commission. 1989a. Proposal for a council directive relating to the maximum permitted blood alcohol concentration for vehicle drivers. *Official Journal of the European Communities* 32:9.

European Commission. 1989b. Opinion on the proposal for a council directive relating to the maximum permitted blood alcohol concentration for vehicle drivers. *Official Journal of the European Communities* 32:54–55.

European Commission. 1997. *Promoting road safety in the EU: The Programme for 1997–2001.* http://webcache.googleusercontent.com/search?q=cache:ZXSkku-AdDcJ:aei.pitt.edu/4729/1/4729.pdf+&cd=1&hl=en&ct=clnk&gl=us (accessed December 12, 2017).

European Commission. 2001. Recommendation of 17 January 2001 on the maximum permitted blood alcohol content (BAC) for drivers of motorised vehicles. *Official Journal of the European Communities* 44.

FARS (Fatal Analysis Reporting System). 2014. *Fatality Analysis Reporting System.* https://crashstats.nhtsa.dot.gov/Api/Public/ViewPublication/811992 (accessed October 31, 2017).

FARS. 2017. *FARS alcohol data.* https://www-fars.nhtsa.dot.gov/QueryTool/Common/alcohol_warning.html (accessed October 31, 2017).

FEDRO (Federal Roads Office). 2016. *Developments, facts and figures: Roads and traffic.* https://www.astra.admin.ch/astra/en/home/documentation/facts-and-figures/archive.html (accessed October 31, 2017).

FEDRO. 2017. *About FEDRO.* https://www.astra.admin.ch/astra/en/home.html (accessed October 31, 2017).

Fitzharris, M., S. Liu, S. Peiris, A. Devlin, K. Young, M. Lenne, D. Bowman, and J. Gatof. 2015. Options to extend coverage of alcohol interlock programs. *Austroads,* September 30.

GBD (Global Burden of Disease). 2016. *Global burden of disease study.* https://vizhub.healthdata.org/gbd-compare (accessed October 31, 2017).

Gruenewald, P. J., P. R. Mitchell, and A. J. Treno. 1996. Drinking and driving: Drinking patterns and drinking problems. *Addiction* 91(11):1637–1649.

Gururaj, G. 2004. Alcohol and road traffic injuries in south Asia: Challenges for prevention. *Journal of the College of Physicians and Surgeons Pakistan* 14(12):713–718.

Hawkins, B., and J. McCambridge. 2014. Industry actors, think tanks, and alcohol policy in the United Kingdom. *American Journal of Public Health* 104(8):1363–1369.

Hawkins, B., C. Holden, and J. McCambridge. 2012. Alcohol industry influence on UK alcohol policy: A new research agenda for public health. *Critical Public Health* 22(3):297–305.

Henstridge, J., R. Homel, and P. Mackay. 1997. *The long-term effects of random breath testing in four Australian states: A time series analysis.* Canberra: Department of Transport and Regional Development, Federal Office of Road Safety.

Hope, A. 2006. The influence of the alcohol industry on alcohol policy in Ireland. *Nordic Studies on Alcohol and Drugs* 23(6):467–481.

Howard, C., and A. Linder. 2014. *Review of Swedish experiences concerning analysis of people injured in traffic accidents.* Brussels, Belgium: Belgian Road Safety Institute.

INEBRIA (International Network on Brief Interventions for Alcohol & Other Drugs). 2015. *INEBRIA position statement on the alcohol industry.* http://inebria.net/wp-content/uploads/2016/02/position_statement_on_the_alcohol_industry.pdf (accessed January 10, 2018).

Jernigan, D. H. 2009. The global alcohol industry: An overview. *Addiction* 104(Suppl 1):6–12.

Jernigan, D. H. 2012. Global alcohol producers, science, and policy: The case of the International Center for Alcohol Policies. *American Journal of Public Health* 102(1):80–89.

Jewett, A., R. A. Shults, T. Banerjee, and G. Bergen. 2015. Alcohol–impaired driving among adults—United States, 2012. *Morbidity and Mortality Weekly* 64(30):814–817.

Johnson, M. 2012. Assessing a country's drink driving situation: An overview of the method used in 6 low- and middle-income countries. *Traffic Injury Prevention* 13(2):96–100.

Kaufman, E. J., and D. J. Wiebe. 2016. Impact of state ignition interlock laws on alcohol-involved crash deaths in the United States. *American Journal of Public Health* 106(5):865–871.

Kennedy, R. S., J. J. Turnage, R. L. Wilkes, and W. P. Dunlap. 1993. Effects of graded dosages of alcohol on nine computerized repeated-measures tests. *Ergonomics* 36(10):1195–1222.

Killoran, A., U. Canning, N. Doyle, and L. Sheppard. 2010. *Review of effectiveness of laws limiting blood alcohol concentration levels to reduce alcohol-related road injuries and deaths.* London: National Institute for Health and Clinical Excellence.

Klipp, S. 2013. *Towards a national alcohol interlock field trial in Germany. Achievements and challenges.* Bundesanstalt für Straßenwesen (BASt). https://kuldoc.com/download/towards-a-national-alcohol-interlock-field-trial-in-germany-achievements-and-challenges-_5948bd121723dd36bf5a1655_pdf (accessed December 19, 2017).

Lahausse, J. A., and B. N. Fildes. 2009. Cost-benefit analysis of an alcohol ignition interlock for installation in all newly registered vehicles. *Traffic Injury Prevention* 10(6):528–537.

Li, Y., D. Xie, G. Nie, and J. Zhang. 2012. The drink driving situation in China. *Traffic Injury Prevention* 13(2):101–108.

Mansdotter, A. M., M. K. Rydberg, E. Wallin, L. A. Lindholm, and S. Andreasson. 2007. A cost-effectiveness analysis of alcohol prevention targeting licensed premises. *European Journal of Public Health* 17(6):618–623.

McCambridge, J., B. Hawkins, and C. Holden. 2013. Industry use of evidence to influence alcohol policy: A case study of submissions to the 2008 Scottish government consultation. *PLoS Medicine* 10(4):e1001431.

McCambridge, J., K. Kypri, P. Miller, B. Hawkins, and G. Hastings. 2014. Be aware of Drinkaware. *Addiction* 109(4):519–524.

Mercer, G. W. 1985. The relationships among driving while impaired charges, police drinking-driving roadcheck activity, media coverage and alcohol-related casualty traffic accidents. *Accident Analysis & Prevention* 17(6):467–474.

Miller, P. G., F. de Groot, S. McKenzie, and N. Droste. 2011. Vested interests in addiction research and policy. Alcohol industry use of social aspect public relations organizations against preventative health measures. *Addiction* 106(9):1560–1567.

Ministry of Road Safety. 2015a. *Statistical series.* http://www.securite-routiere.gouv.fr/la-securite-routiere/l-observatoire-national-interministeriel-de-la-securite-routiere/series-statistiques (accessed October 31, 2017).

Ministry of Road Safety. 2015b. *User behaviors.* http://www.securite-routiere.gouv.fr/la-securite-routiere/l-observatoire-national-interministeriel-de-la-securite-routiere/comportements-des-usagers (accessed October 31, 2017).

Ministry of Road Safety. 2016. *Local performance indicators 2014.* http://www.securite-routiere.gouv.fr/la-securite-routiere/l-observatoire-national-interministeriel-de-la-securite-routiere/english-version/local-performance-indicators (accessed October 31, 2017).

Ministry of Road Safety. 2017. *Road accidents.* http://www.securite-routiere.gouv.fr/la-securite-routiere/l-observatoire-national-interministeriel-de-la-securite-routiere/english-version (accessed October 31, 2017).

Ministry of Transport. 2006. *The social cost of road crashes and injuries: June 2006 update.* Wellington: New Zealand Ministry of Transport.

Ministry of Transport. 2012. *High-risk drivers in fatal and serious crashes: 2006–2010.* http://www.transport.govt.nz/assets/Import/Documents/High-risk-drivers-in-fatal-and-serious-crashes-2006-2010.pdf (accessed October 31, 2017).

Ministry of Transport. 2016a. *Motor vehicle crashes in New Zealand 2015.* http://www.transport.govt.nz/research/roadcrashstatistics/motorvehiclecrashesinnewzealand/motor-vehicle-crashes-in-new-zealand-2015 (accessed October 31, 2017).

Ministry of Transport. 2016b. *Alcohol and drugs.* http://www.transport.govt.nz/research/crashfacts/alcohol-and-drugs (accessed October 31, 2017).

Ministry of Transport. 2017a. *The social cost of road crashes and injuries.* http://www.transport.govt.nz/research/roadcrashstatistics/thesocialcostofroadcrashesandinjuries (accessed October 31, 2017).

Ministry of Transport. 2017b. *Road crash statistics.* 2017. http://www.transport.govt.nz/research/roadcrashstatistics (accessed October 31, 2017).

Ministry of Transport. 2017c. *Our work.* http://www.transport.govt.nz/ourwork (accessed October 31, 2017).

Mosher, J. F. 2012. Joe Camel in a bottle: Diageo, the Smirnoff brand, and the transformation of the youth alcohol market. *American Journal of Public Health* 102(1):56–63.

National Road Safety Committee. 2016. *Safer journeys: Action plan 2016–2020.* http://www.saferjourneys.govt.nz/assets/Safer-journeys-files/Safer-Journey-Action-Plan-2016-2020.pdf (accessed October 31, 2017).

New Zealand Transport Agency. 2017. *Crash Analysis System (CAS).* https://www.nzta.govt.nz/safety/safety-resources/crash-analysis-system (accessed October 31, 2017).

Ngoc, L. B., N. T. Thieng, and N. L. Huong. 2012. The drink driving situation in Vietnam. *Traffic Injury Prevention* 13(2):109–114.

Noordzij, P. C. 1994. *Decline in drinking and driving in the Netherlands.* Paper presented at Transportation Research Circular, The Hague, The Netherlands.

Norström, T., and B. Trolldal. 2013. Was the STAD programme really that successful? *Nordic Studies of Alcohol and Drugs* 30(3):171–178.

OECD (Organisation for Economic Co-operation and Development). 2016. *Road safety annual report 2016.* Paris, France: OECD/International Transport Forum.

OECD. 2017. *Injuries in road traffic accidents—OECD health statistics. Definitions, sources and methods.* Paris, France: Organisation for Economic Co-operation and Development.

Peden, M., R. Scurfield, D. Sleet, D. Mohan, A. A. Hyder, E. Jarawan, and C. Mathers. 2004. *World report on road traffic injury prevention.* Geneva, Switzerland: World Health Organization.

Rehnman, C., J. Larsson, and S. Andreasson. 2005. The beer campaign in Stockholm—attempting to restrict the availability of alcohol to young people. *Alcohol* 37(2):65–71.

RoadSafetyBC. 2016. *Immediate roadside prohibition fact sheet.* Victoria, British Columbia: Ministry of Public Safety and Solicitor General.

Ross, H. L., D. T. Campbell, and G. V. Glass. 1970. Determining the social effects of a legal reform: The British "Breathalyser" crackdown of 1967. *American Behavioral Scientist* 13(4):493–509.

Schonfeld, C., and M. Sheehan. 2004. *Critical overview of alcohol ignition interlock programs in Australia.* Carseldine, Australia: Centre for Accident Research and Road Safety-Queensland.

Shield, K. D., G. Gmel, J. Patra, and J. Rehm. 2012. Global burden of injuries attributable to alcohol consumption in 2004: A novel way of calculating the burden of injuries attributable to alcohol consumption. *Population Health Metrics* 10(1):9.

Shults, R. A., R. W. Elder, D. A. Sleet, J. L. Nichols, M. O. Alao, V. G. Carande-Kulis, S. Zaza, D. M. Sosin, R. S. Thompson, and Community Preventive Services Task Force. 2001. Reviews of evidence regarding interventions to reduce alcohol-impaired driving. *American Journal of Preventive Medicine* 21(4 Suppl):66–88.

Stenius, K., and T. F. Babor. 2010. The alcohol industry and public interest science. *Addiction* 105(2):191–198.

Stewart, K., D. Silcock, and F. Wegman. 2012. Reducing drink driving in low- and middle-income countries: Challenges and opportunities. *Traffic Injury Prevention* 13(2):93–95.

Swedish Transport Administration. 2017a. *The number of fatalities on Swedish roads is not decreasing.* https://www.trafikverket.se/en/visionzero/vision-zero-conference-2017/news/2017/2017-05/the-number-of-fatalities-on-swedish-roads-is-not-decreasing (accessed October 31, 2017).

Swedish Transport Administration. 2017b. *Vision zero and ways to work.* https://www.trafikverket.se/en/startpage/operations/Operations-road/vision-zero-academy/Vision-Zero-and-ways-to-work (accessed October 31, 2017).

Sweedler, B. M., and K. Stewart. 2009. Worldwide trends in alcohol and drug impaired driving. In *Drugs, driving and traffic safety*, edited by J. C. Verster, S. R. Pandi-Perumal, J. G. Ramaekers, and J. J. de Gier. Basel, Switzerland: Birkhäuser Basel. Pp. 23–41.

Tagawa, M., M. Kano, N. Okamura, M. Itoh, E. Sakurai, T. Watanabe, and K. Yanai. 2000. Relationship between effects of alcohol on psychomotor performances and blood alcohol concentrations. *Japanese Journal of Pharmacology* 83(3):253–260.

Terer, K., and R. Brown. 2014. Effective drink driving prevention and enforcement strategies: Approaches to improving practice. *Trends & Issues in Crime and Criminal Justice.* Canberra: Australian Institute of Criminology 472.

Transport Styrelsen. 2015. *Swedish traffic accident data acquisition (STRADA).* http://www.transportstyrelsen.se/sv/vagtrafik/statistik-och-strada/STRADA-informations system-for-olyckor-skador (accessed October 31, 2017).

Transport Styrelsen. 2016. *Alkola lock after steering wheel.* http://www.transportstyrelsen.se/sv/Publikationer/Vag (accessed October 31, 2017).

Transport Styrelsen. 2017. *Accident statistics.* http://www.transportstyrelsen.se/sv/vagtrafik/statistik-och-strada/Vag/Olycksstatistik (accessed October 31, 2017).

Vingilis, E., and L. Salutin. 1980. A prevention programme for drinking driving. *Accident Analysis & Prevention* 12(4):267–274.

Voas, R. B., P. R. Marques, A. S. Tippetts, and D. J. Beirness. 1999. The Alberta interlock program: The evaluation of a province-wide program on DUI recidivism. *Addiction* 94(12):1849–1859.

Wallin, E., T. Norstrom, and S. Andreasson. 2003. Alcohol prevention targeting licensed premises: A study of effects on violence. *Journal of Studies of Alcohol* 64(2):270–277.

Wallin, E., J. Gripenberg, and S. Andreasson. 2005. Overserving at licensed premises in Stockholm: Effects of a community action program. *Journal of Studies of Alcohol* 66(6):806–814.

WHO (World Health Organization). 2007. *Drinking and driving: A road safety manual for decision-makers and practitioners.* Geneva, Switzerland: World Health Organization and Global Road Safety Partnership.

WHO. 2010. *Data systems: A road safety manual for decision-makers and practitioners.* Geneva, Switzerland: World Health Organization.

WHO. 2013. *Global plan for the decade of action for road safety 2011-2020.* Geneva, Switzerland: World Health Organization.

WHO. 2014. *Global status report on alcohol and health.* Geneva, Switzerland: World Health Organization.

WHO. 2015. *Global status report on road safety.* Geneva, Switzerland: World Health Organization.

Willis, C., S. Lybrand, and N. Bellamy. 2004. Alcohol ignition interlock programmes for reducing drink driving recidivism. *Cochrane Database Systematic Review* (4):CD004168.

World Bank. 2017. *World Bank open data 2016.* https://data.worldbank.org (accessed October 31, 2017).

Zivkovic, V., V. Lukic, and S. Nikolic. 2016. The influence of alcohol on pedestrians: A different approach to the effectiveness of the new traffic safety law. *Traffic Injury Prevention* 17(3):233–237.

E

Committee Meeting Agendas

MEETING 1

Thursday, February 16, 2017
National Academy of Sciences Building
2101 Constitution Avenue, NW
Washington, DC 20418

10:00–10:10 **Welcome and Opening Remarks**
Steven M. Teutsch
Committee Chair

10:10–11:00 **Presentation of the Statement of Task, Background, and Discussion**
Jeff Michael
Associate Administrator for Research and Program Development
National Highway Traffic Safety Administration

11:00–11:30 **Overview and History of Interventions for Alcohol-Impaired Driving and Discussion**
Diane Wigle
Chief, Impaired Driving Division
National Highway Traffic Safety Administration

11:30–12:30 **Lunch**

12:30–2:00 **Laws, Policies, Enforcement, and Discussion**
Ralph Hingson
Director, Division of Epidemiology and Prevention Research
National Institute on Alcohol Abuse and Alcoholism
National Institutes of Health

Thomas Woodward
Lt. (Retired) Maryland State Police

Rebecca Ramirez
Executive Director
National Liquor Law Enforcement Association

2:00–2:40 **Interventions and Policies in Canada and Discussion**
Doug Beirness
Canadian Centre on Substance Abuse
Chair, Committee on Alcohol, Other Drugs, and Transportation, Transportation Research Board

3:00 **Adjourn**

MEETING 2

Wednesday, March 22, 2017
Keck Center of the National Academies
500 Fifth Street, NW
Washington, DC 20001

9:45–10:00 **Welcome and Opening Remarks**
Steven M. Teutsch
Committee Chair

10:00–11:00 **PANEL 1**

Policies and Systems Change and Discussion
Steve Schmidt
Senior Vice President of Public Policy and Communications
National Alcohol Beverage Control Association

Frank Harris
State Legislative Director
Mothers Against Drunk Driving

Anne Teigen
Program Principal
National Conference of State Legislatures
(*participating remotely*)

11:00–12:00 **PANEL 2**

The Alcohol Environment and Behaviors and Discussion

M. J. Paschall
Senior Research Scientist
Pacific Institute for Research and Evaluation

Thomas Greenfield
Scientific Director
Alcohol Research Group (*participating remotely*)

Debra Furr-Holden
C. S. Mott Endowed Professor of Public Health
Michigan State University

12:00–1:00 **Lunch**

1:00–2:00 **PANEL 3**

Stakeholder Activities and Discussion

Jacqueline Gillan
President
Advocates for Highway and Auto Safety

J. T. Griffin
Chief Government Affairs Officer
Mothers Against Drunk Driving

Jessica Cicchino
Vice President, Research
Insurance Institute for Highway Safety

Russ Martin
Director of Government Relations
Governors Highway Safety Association

2:00–3:00 **PANEL 4**

Surveillance Systems, Approaches, and Strategies and Discussion

Tara Kelley-Baker
Principal Research Scientist
NORC at The University of Chicago

Robert Voas
Senior Research Scientist
Pacific Institute for Research and Evaluation

James C. Fell
Principal Research Scientist
NORC at The University of Chicago

3:00–3:45 **PANEL 5**

Social Movements and Discussion

Craig Reinarman
Professor Emeritus, Professor of Sociology and Legal Studies Emeritus
University of California, Santa Cruz

Francesca Polletta
Professor of Sociology
University of California, Irvine (*participating remotely*)

3:45–4:10 **Public Comment**

4:10 **Adjourn**

MEETING 3

Tuesday, May 9, 2017
Keck Center of the National Academies
500 Fifth Street, NW
Washington, DC 20001

8:15–8:25	**Welcome and Opening Remarks** Steven M. Teutsch Committee Chair
8:25–9:15	**Automobile and Insurance Industry Perspectives and Discussion** Jessica Cicchino Vice President, Research Insurance Institute for Highway Safety Brooke Stringer Financial Policy and Legislative Advisor National Association of Insurance Commissioners Robert Strassburger Vice President, Vehicle Safety and Harmonization Alliance of Automobile Manufacturers
9:15–10:15	**Technology and Innovative Strategies and Discussion** Keith Nothacker CEO, BACtrack Nadia Anderson Manager, Public Policy, Road and Traffic Safety Uber Steve Taylor General Manager, Washington, DC Region Lyft
10:15–10:30	**Break**
10:30–11:00	**Alcohol Policy and Discussion** Phil Cook ITT/Terry Sanford Professor of Public Policy Studies Duke University

11:00–11:50 **Highway Safety and Law Enforcement and Discussion**

Jim McDonnell
Program Director for Engineering
American Association of State Highway and Transportation Officials

Sheriff Clint Shrum
Grundy County Sheriff's Office

11:50–12:20 **Lunch**

12:20–1:10 **Alcohol-Impaired Driving in Tribal Communities and Discussion**

Nancy Bill
Injury Prevention Program Manager
Indian Health Service

Lawrence Robertson
Director, Indian Highway Safety Program
Bureau of Indian Affairs

1:10–2:00 **Perceptions of Alcohol Impairment, Warning Labels, Cognitive Processing when Impaired and Discussion**

Bill Kerr
Senior Scientist, Center Director
Alcohol Research Group (*presenting remotely*)

Nick Van Dyke
Department of Psychology
University of Kentucky

2:00–2:15 **Public Comment**

3:00 **Adjourn**

F

Committee Biosketches

Steven M. Teutsch, M.D., M.P.H. (*Chair*), is an independent consultant, Adjunct Professor at the Fielding School of Public Health, University of California, Los Angeles; Senior Fellow, Public Health Institute; and Senior Fellow, Leonard D. Schaeffer Center for Health Policy and Economics, University of Southern California. Until 2014 he was the Chief Science Officer, Los Angeles County Public Health, where he continued his work on evidence-based public health and policy. He had been in the Outcomes Research and Management program at Merck since October 1997 where he was responsible for scientific leadership in developing evidence-based clinical management programs, conducting outcomes research studies, and improving outcomes measurement to enhance quality of care. Prior to joining Merck he was Director of the Division of Prevention Research and Analytic Methods (DPRAM) at the Centers for Disease Control and Prevention (CDC) where he was responsible for assessing the effectiveness, safety, and the cost-effectiveness of disease and injury prevention strategies. DPRAM developed comparable methodology for studies of the effectiveness and economic impact of prevention programs, provided training in these methods, developed CDC's capacity for conducting necessary studies, and provided technical assistance for conducting economic and decision analysis. DPRAM also evaluated the impact of interventions in urban areas, developed the *Guide to Community Preventive Services*, and provided support for CDC's analytic methods. He has served as a member of that Task Force and the U.S. Preventive Services Task Force, which develops the *Guide to Clinical Preventive Services*, as well as on the

American Health Information Community's Personalized Health Care Workgroup and the Evaluation of Genomic Applications in Practice and Prevention Workgroup. He chaired the Secretary's Advisory Committee on Genetics, Health, and Society and has served on and has chaired Institute of Medicine panels, Medicare's Evidence Development and Coverage Advisory Committee, and several subcommittees of the Secretary's Advisory Committee on Healthy People 2020 and 2030.

Dr. Teutsch joined CDC in 1977, where he was assigned to the Parasitic Diseases Division and worked extensively on toxoplasmosis. He was then assigned to the Kidney Donor and subsequently the Kidney Disease Program. He developed the framework for CDC's diabetes control program. He joined the Epidemiology Program Office and became Director of the Division of Surveillance and Epidemiology where he was responsible for coordinating CDC's disease monitoring activities. He became Chief of the Prevention Effectiveness Activity in 1992.

Dr. Teutsch was born in Salt Lake City, Utah. He received his undergraduate degree in biochemical sciences at Harvard University in 1970, an M.P.H. in epidemiology from the University of North Carolina School of Public Health in 1973, and his M.D. from Duke University School of Medicine in 1974. He completed his residency training in internal medicine at The Pennsylvania State University, Hershey. He was certified by the American Board of Internal Medicine in 1977, the American Board of Preventive Medicine in 1995, and is a Fellow of the American College of Physicians and American College of Preventive Medicine. Dr. Teutsch has published more than 200 articles and eight books in a broad range of fields in epidemiology, including parasitic diseases, diabetes, technology assessment, health services research, and surveillance.

Julie A. Baldwin, Ph.D., earned her doctorate in behavioral sciences and health education in 1991 from the Johns Hopkins University School of Hygiene and Public Health. From 1994 to 2004, she served as a tenured faculty member at Northern Arizona University, with a joint appointment in the Mel and Enid Zuckerman Arizona College of Public Health. She joined the faculty at the University of South Florida College of Public Health in the Department of Community and Family Health in 2005. She returned to Northern Arizona University's Department of Health Sciences in August 2015, where she now directs the Center for Health Equity Research.

Dr. Baldwin's research has focused on both infectious and chronic disease prevention. Cross-cutting themes that have characterized her work include using community-based participatory research approaches, working with underserved and/or marginalized populations, and addressing health disparities by developing and implementing culturally competent public health interventions. As an enrolled member of the Cherokee Nation of Oklahoma, she has made a life-long commitment to serving diverse communities and to advocating for health promotion programs for children, adolescents, and families.

Linda C. Degutis, Dr.P.H., MSN, is the Executive Director of Defense Health Horizons, sponsored by the Henry M. Jackson Foundation and based at the Uniformed Services University of the Health Sciences, which envisions and develops promising ideas to assist the Assistant Secretary of Defense (Health Affairs), the service surgeons general, and the Defense Health Agency achieve the goals outlined in the Military Health System Quadruple Aim. In addition to holding an appointment as adjunct professor at Rollins School of Public Health, Emory University, she serves as the Chief Science Officer (pro bono) for the Avielle Foundation, which focuses its efforts on the relationships between brain health, compassion, and violence. Her research has focused on substance abuse prevention; screening, brief intervention, and referral to treatment (SBIRT); alcohol policy; alcohol-impaired driving; and injury and violence prevention.

Previously, Dr. Degutis was Director of the National Center for Injury Prevention and Control at CDC. She came to Atlanta from Yale University, where she was on the faculty of the Department of Emergency Medicine and the Department of Environmental Health at the School of Public Health, where she was Director of the Research Division in Emergency Medicine, and Director of the Yale Center for Public Health Preparedness. She served as a Robert Wood Johnson Foundation Health Policy Fellow in the office of the late Senator Paul Wellstone (D-MN). She has held multiple leadership roles in state and national organizations and currently serves on the boards of the Pacific Institute for Research and Evaluation, the Society for the Advancement of Violence and Injury Research, and the advisory board of the College of Sciences and Health at DePaul University. She is a Past President of the American Public Health Association and a member of the National Academy of Medicine.

Mucio Kit Delgado, M.D., M.S., is an assistant professor of emergency medicine and epidemiology in the Perelman School of Medicine at the University of Pennsylvania. He is committed to discovering innovative approaches to improve the outcomes of acutely ill and injured patients and mitigating the impulsive behaviors that lead to injuries in the first place. Dr. Delgado has two complementary lines of research. First, he analyzes large existing datasets and uses decision analytic modeling to guide policy-aimed care for injuries and substance use disorders. Second, he has recently developed a novel research program leveraging smartphones, connected devices, and insights from behavioral economics for injury prevention. He is currently testing smartphone-based "nudge" interventions to reduce cellphone use and drinking and driving. His research is currently funded by the Federal Highway Administration, the National Institutes of Health, and the Agency for Healthcare Research and Quality. He has joint faculty appointments in the Center for Health Incentives and Behavioral Economics, the Penn Injury Science Center, and the Center for Injury Research and Prevention at the Children's Hospital of Philadelphia.

David H. Jernigan, Ph.D., is an associate professor in the Department of Health, Behavior, and Society at the Johns Hopkins Bloomberg School of Public Health. Dr. Jernigan has 30 years of experience researching and implementing effective alcohol policies. He was a founding member of the National Alliance to Prevent Impaired Driving in the 1990s, formed in response to Surgeon General C. Everett Koop's 1989 recommendations on preventing impaired driving. He was principal author of the World Health Organization's (WHO's) first *Global Status Report on Alcohol and Health* and for subsequent reports has taken the lead on the reporting and analysis of policy responses being under taken by WHO member states. As such, he has a broad familiarity with policy approaches regarding alcohol use and related problems being undertaken in other countries as well as the research base that informs those interventions. His work has encompassed development, dissemination, implementation, and evaluation of public health approaches to excessive alcohol use and related problems, and he has authored more than 100 peer-reviewed articles and numerous book chapters and reports on those topics. He is also well versed in community-based prevention, and has provided training and technical assistance to thousands of individuals and coalitions across the United States and around the world in methods for implementing effective prevention strategies. He is a recipient of the Award of Excellence from the National Association of State Alcohol and Drug Abuse Directors and the Addiction Book Prize for his co-authorship of *Alcohol in Developing Societies: A Public Health Approach*. He is also an expert in media advocacy and serves or has served as an expert advisor to numerous organizations and campaigns, including the Substance Abuse and Mental Health Services Administration Underage Alcohol Use Prevention Media Campaign, the World Bank, the World Health Organization (including the Director General's Alcohol Policy Strategy Advisory Committee), the United Kingdom Center for Tobacco and Alcohol Studies, and the Cancer Research UK/Bupa Foundation Cancer Prevention Initiative.

Katherine Keyes, Ph.D., M.P.H., is an associate professor of epidemiology at the Columbia University Mailman School of Public Health. Dr. Keyes' research focuses on life-course epidemiology with particular attention to psychiatric disorders, including examination of fetal origins of child and adult health, long-term outcomes of adverse childhood environments, and cross-generational cohort effects of substance use, mental health, and chronic disease. She is particularly interested in the development of epidemiological theory to measure and elucidate the drivers of population health. Dr. Keyes is an expert in methodological issues in age-period-cohort effect estimation, and her empirical work in age-period-cohort effect has examined a range of outcomes including obesity, perinatal outcomes, substance use disorders, and psychological distress. She is the author of more than 170 peer-reviewed publications as well as two textbooks published by Oxford University Press with co-author Sandro Galea: *Epidemiology Matters: A New Introduction to Methodological Foundation* published in 2014 and *Population Health Science* published in 2016.

Ricardo Martinez, M.D., FACEP, is the Chief Medical Officer of Adeptus Health. Prior to that he served as the Chief Medical Officer of North Highland Worldwide Consulting, a global consulting company. A recognized health care innovator, he provides thought leadership, strategic advisory, program design, and frontline implementation activities across North Highland's four main health care transformations—digital, clinical, financial, and organizational. He has served in senior roles in academics, federal government, and business including faculty at both Emory and Stanford University Schools of Medicine; as President of Division East and Executive Vice President of Medical Affairs for the Schumacher Group, an emergency medicine practice management company serving more than 170 hospitals in 22 states with more than 3,000 providers and 3 million patients; and as the Administrator of the National Highway Traffic Safety Administration from 1994 to 1999 in Washington, DC. He also developed and served as the Executive Director of the Medical Leadership Academy, emphasizing patient-centered teamwork, data-driven quality care, systems thinking, continuous learning, and dynamic leadership. He was elected to the National Academy of Medicine in 2004.

Timothy S. Naimi, M.D., is a clinician-investigator at Boston Medical Center and an associate professor in the Boston University Schools of Medicine and Public Health. Prior to coming to Boston Medical Center, he served as a Senior Medical Epidemiologist on the Excessive Alcohol Use Prevention Team in the National Center for Chronic Disease Prevention and Health Promotion at CDC. His areas of expertise include alcohol epidemiology and alcohol policy. He has authored and co-authored many papers on binge drinking, alcohol-impaired driving, and the relationship between the two, and is currently working on a National Institutes of Health (NIH)-funded grant to assess the relationship between state alcohol control policies (e.g., alcohol taxes) and alcohol-related mortality, including motor vehicle crash fatalities. Dr. Naimi completed a combined internal medicine–pediatrics residency program at Massachusetts General Hospital in Boston and served as a Preventive Medicine Resident and Epidemic Intelligence Service Officer at CDC. He is board certified in internal medicine, pediatrics, and preventive medicine.

Jeff Niederdeppe, Ph.D., is an associate professor in the Department of Communication at Cornell University. His research examines the mechanisms and effects of mass media campaigns, strategic health messages, and news coverage in shaping health behavior, health disparities, and social policy. He has worked on several projects which seek to advance theorizing about the conditions under which various forms of strategic messages (including narratives, counterframing, refutation, and graphic imagery) can undermine or enhance public and policy-maker support for health policies and other collective, multisector solutions to social problems. Dr. Niederdeppe has also focused recent attention on understanding how variations in graphic warning labels on cigarette packages influence smoking-related cognitions and emotions among youth and adults from socioeconomically disadvantaged backgrounds, and testing the influence of alcohol control public service announcements in shaping drinking behavior and rates of alcohol-related fatal vehicle accidents. He has published more than 110 peer-reviewed articles in journals that include the *Journal of Communication, Health Communication, Social Science and Medicine, American Journal of Public Health, Milbank Quarterly,* and *New England Journal of Medicine*. His work has been funded in recent years by the National Institutes of Health, U.S. Department of Agriculture, Environmental Protection Agency, and Robert Wood Johnson Foundation.

Dr. Niederdeppe was awarded the Lewis Donohew Outstanding Scholar in Health Communication Award from the Kentucky Conference on Health Communication in 2014 and the Early Career Award from the Public Health Education and Health Promotion Section within the American Public Health Association in 2016. He is an Associate Editor for *Communication Methods & Measures* and serves on the editorial boards for eight other communication and public health journals.

Charles P. O'Brien, M.D., Ph.D., received his M.D. and Ph.D. degrees from Tulane University and received residency training in psychiatry, neurology, and medicine at Harvard, the University of London, Tulane, and the University of Pennsylvania (Penn). He is board certified in psychiatry, neurology, and addiction psychiatry. One of the most prominent addiction researchers in the world, Dr. O'Brien has made many important discoveries and contributions over the past 30 years that have become the standard of care in addiction treatment throughout the world. He pioneered the use of naltrexone as a treatment for alcoholism, ushering in a new era of alcoholism treatment. Dr. O'Brien also conducted research on genetic variations in alcoholism and discovered genes that determine the extent of pleasure one feels when drinking alcohol. Aside from developing medications to treat alcohol, opioid, and cocaine dependence, his work has also increased the understanding of the clinical aspects of addiction and the neurobiology of relapse. Among his numerous honors, Dr. O'Brien was elected to the National Academy of Medicine in 1991 and received the Nathan B. Eddy award for research from the College on Problems of Drug Dependence in 2003. He has advised the federal government on drug policy for decades and was President of the American College of Neuropsychopharmacology and President of the Association for Research in Nervous and Mental Disease. Dr. O'Brien is the Vice-Chair of Psychiatry at Penn and the founding director of the prestigious Center for Studies of Addiction.

Jody L. Sindelar, Ph.D., is a professor of public health and a health economist in the Department of Health Policy and Management at the Yale School of Public Health. Dr. Sindelar is also a research associate at the National Bureau of Economic Research, Research Fellow at IZA (the Institute of Labor Economics), and a member of the Associated Faculty at the Institution for Social and Policy Studies at Yale. She has been President-Elect, President, Past President, and a founding member of the American Society of Health Economists. She serves on several editorial, advisory, and review boards nationally and internationally.

Dr. Sindelar is an expert on the economics of substance abuse, including alcohol misuse, illicit drug misuse, and smoking. Within these areas her focus is on social costs and policy issues, particularly policy-related issues in economics, addiction, and health. She has published in health economics, addiction, policy, and medical journals. She has served on numerous editorial, review, advisory, and other boards and committees; has presented her research at seminars and conferences both nationally and internationally; and has been a visiting faculty member nationally and internationally.

Currently, she heads a project on economics and health issues related to regulation of tobacco products (NIH, Food and Drug Administration). Recently, she headed a multiyear project funded by the Centers for Medicare & Medicaid Services via the Connecticut Department of Social Services and the National Institute on Drug Abuse (NIDA). She has also been the Principal Investigator and a collaborator on numerous past research projects funded by the Agency for Healthcare Research and Quality, Robert Wood Johnson Foundation, National Institute on Aging,

National Institute on Alcohol Abuse and Alcoholism, National Institute of Mental Health, Yale Center for Clinical Investigation, U.S. Department of Veterans Affairs, and NIDA, among others.

Joanne E. Thomka, J.D., is a Program Counsel at the National Association of Attorneys General (NAAG). NAAG staff work to help attorneys general respond effectively—individually and collectively—to emerging state and federal issues. Mrs. Thomka is staff liaison to the attorney general community for traffic safety, substance abuse, and elder issues.

Prior to coming to NAAG, Mrs. Thomka served as the director of the National Traffic Law Center (NTLC) of the National District Attorneys Association (NDAA) in Alexandria, Virginia. The NTLC provides technical assistance, legal research, and training support to prosecutors, law enforcement, and other traffic safety professionals across the country. Prior to NDAA, she was a Senior Assistant District Attorney for the Onondaga County District Attorney's Office in Syracuse, New York. She was Bureau Chief of the DWI Unit. The DWI bureau is responsible for the prosecution of all alcohol-related crimes and all vehicular fatalities. Mrs. Thomka was previously a member of both the Special Victims and Violent Felony Bureaus within the Onondaga County District Attorney's Office.

Mrs. Thomka is a graduate of Salem State College (now Salem State University) and Vermont Law School. She was President of the Onondaga County Bar Association in 2003. Mrs. Thomka continues to be an instructor to assistant attorneys general, prosecutors, law enforcement officers, and other traffic safety personnel on all issues pertaining to impaired driving, other highway safety issues, trial advocacy, and various other areas of criminal law and procedure. She is one of the authors of the New York Prosecutors Training Institute's *Vehicular Homicide Manual for Prosecutors* and the National Traffic Law Center and National Highway Traffic Safety Administration's (NHTSA's) manuals: *DWI Prosecutor's Notebook*; *The Criminal Justice System: A Guide for Law Enforcement Officers and Expert Witnesses in Impaired Driving Cases*; *Cross Examination for Prosecutors*; and the *Traffic Safety Resource Prosecutor's Manual*. In addition, she is a co-author of a manual developed with the Century Council: *Hardcore Drunk Driver Prosecutorial Guide*.

Mrs. Thomka is a member of several committees that pertain to traffic safety: the Transportation Research Board's Traffic Law Enforcement Committee, the National Sheriffs' Association's Traffic Safety Committee, the Highway Safety Coalition, and the Traffic Injury Research Foundation's DWI Working Group. She is also the recipient of the 2013 J. Stannard Baker Award, presented by the National Sheriffs' Association and NHTSA in Recognition for Outstanding Achievement in Highway Safety and a 2016 Public Service Award from NHTSA for protecting communities and enhancing traffic safety through legal information and training to the nation's criminal justice community.

Douglas Wiebe, Ph.D., is an associate professor of epidemiology in the Perelman School of Medicine at the University of Pennsylvania and an expert in injury epidemiology and research on the impact of places and policies on health and injury outcomes. Having completed his Ph.D. in social ecology at the University of California, Irvine, and postdoctoral studies in injury epidemiology at the University of California, Los Angeles, Dr. Wiebe brings a unique multidisciplinary and place-based perspective to bear in his research on injury prevention science. His 2016 national study, published in the *American Journal of Public Health,* is one example that found that alcohol-impaired driving fatalities declined significantly in states upon passing universal ignition interlock legislation. It is likely that the study influenced the universal ignition interlock law that was passed in Pennsylvania just weeks after this work was published. Dr. Wiebe has contributed significantly to the science of injury prevention for the past 15 years. His research has been federally funded continually over that time with grants from the National Institutes of Health, the National Institute of Justice, and the Agency for Healthcare Research and Quality. He serves on study sections for the Center for Scientific Review, the National Science Foundation, and the Social Sciences and Humanities Research Council of Canada. He is a past president of the Society for Advancement of Violence and Injury Research and is the incoming director of the Penn Injury Science Center, 1 of 10 injury control research centers in the United States funded by CDC.